Rare Tumors and Tumor-like Conditions in Urological Pathology

Antonio Lopez-Beltran
Carmen L. Menendez
Rodolfo Montironi
Liang Cheng

Rare Tumors and Tumor-like Conditions in Urological Pathology

Springer

Antonio Lopez-Beltran, MD, PhD
Department of Surgery and Pathology
University of Cordoba Faculty
of Medicine
Cordoba
Spain

Carmen L. Menendez, MD
Pathology Department
Hospital de Cabueñes
Gijón
Spain

Rodolfo Montironi, MD
Department of Biomedical
Sciences and Public Health
Polytechnic University of the Marche
Region (Ancona)
Torrette
Italy

Liang Cheng, MD
Department of Pathology
Indiana University School of Medicine
Indianapolis, Indiana
USA

ISBN 978-3-319-10252-8 ISBN 978-3-319-10253-5 (eBook)
DOI 10.1007/978-3-319-10253-5
Springer Cham Heidelberg New York Dordrecht London

Library of Congress Control Number: 2014953767

Printed on acid-free paper

Springer is part of Springer Science+Business Media (www.springer.com)

Contents

1 Renal Tumors and Tumor-Like Conditions 1
1.1 Basic Anatomy and Histology 2
1.2 Overview 2
1.3 Familial Renal Cancer 4
1.3.1 Von Hippel-Lindau (VHL) Clear Cell Renal Cell Carcinoma (RCC) 4
1.3.2 Hereditary Papillary RCC 4
1.3.3 Hereditary Leiomyomatosis RCC. 4
1.3.4 Birt-Hogg-Dube Syndrome. 5
1.4 Renal Cell Carcinoma 6
1.4.1 Clear Cell RCC. 6
1.4.2 Multilocular Cystic Clear Cell Renal Cell Neoplasm of Low Malignant Potential. 6
1.4.3 Papillary RCC. 9
1.4.4 Chromophobe RCC 11
1.4.5 Hybrid Oncocytic Chromophobe Tumor (HOCT). . . 12
1.4.6 Collecting Duct Carcinoma 14
1.4.7 Renal Medullary Carcinoma. 16
1.4.8 Mucinous, Tubular and Spindle Cell Carcinoma . . . 16
1.4.9 Renal Cell Carcinoma After Neuroblastoma 20
1.4.10 RCC with Sarcomatoid or Rhabdoid Differentiation. 20
1.4.11 Renal Cell Carcinoma, Unclassified. 21
1.5 Proposed New and Emerging Epithelial Renal Tumors. 22
1.5.1 Tubulocystic Renal Cell Carcinoma. 22
1.5.2 Acquired Cystic Disease-Associated RCC. 22
1.5.3 Clear Cell Papillary (Tubulo-Papillary) RCC. 23
1.5.4 MiT Family Translocation RCC. 25
1.5.5 Thyroid-Like Follicular Renal Cell Carcinoma 27
1.5.6 Succinic Dehydrogenase B Deficiency Associated Renal Cell Carcinoma 27
1.5.7 ALK-Translocation Renal Cell Carcinoma 28
1.5.8 Renal Cell Carcinoma with Smooth Muscle Stroma 28

1.5.9 Tuberous Sclerosis-Associated Renal Cell Carcinoma . . . 29
1.6 Benign Tumors . . . 30
1.6.1 Papillary Adenoma . . . 30
1.6.2 Metanephric Tumors . . . 30
1.6.3 Renal Oncocytoma . . . 30
1.7 Percutaneous Biopsy of Renal Tumours . . . 33
1.8 Cystic Nephroma and Mixed Epithelial and Stromal Tumors . . . 34
1.9 Soft Tissue Tumors . . . 37
1.9.1 Medullary Fibroma . . . 37
1.9.2 Juxtaglomerular Cell Tumor . . . 38
1.9.3 Glomus Tumor . . . 39
1.9.4 Angiomyolipoma . . . 39
1.9.5 Epithelioid Angiomyolipoma . . . 40
1.9.6 Leiomyoma . . . 41
1.9.7 Lipoma . . . 41
1.9.8 Hemangioma . . . 42
1.9.9 Lymphangioma . . . 42
1.9.10 Schwannoma . . . 43
1.9.11 Solitary Fibrous Tumor . . . 43
1.9.12 Leiomyosarcoma . . . 43
1.9.13 Angiosarcoma . . . 44
1.9.14 Liposarcoma . . . 44
1.9.15 Rhabdomyosarcoma . . . 45
1.9.16 Malignant Fibrous Histiocytoma . . . 45
1.9.17 Hemangiopericytoma . . . 45
1.9.18 Hemangioblastoma . . . 46
1.9.19 Osteosarcoma . . . 46
1.9.20 Other Soft Tissue Tumors . . . 47
1.10 Wilms' Tumor and Other Renal Neoplasms in Children . . . 48
1.10.1 Nephrogenic Rests and Nephroblastomatosis . . . 48
1.10.2 Nephroblastoma (Wilms' Tumor) . . . 48
1.10.3 Cystic Partially Differentiated Nephroblastoma . . . 49
1.10.4 Congenital Mesoblastic Nephroma (CMN) . . . 50
1.10.5 Clear Cell Sarcoma of Kidney . . . 52
1.10.6 Rhabdoid Tumor of Kidney . . . 52
1.10.7 Neuroblastoma . . . 52
1.10.8 Primitive Neuroectodermal Tumor (PNET) . . . 52
1.10.9 Desmoplastic Small Round Cell Tumor . . . 52
1.10.10 Synovial Sarcoma . . . 53
1.10.11 Ossifying Renal Tumor of Infancy . . . 54
1.11 Other Rare Tumors and Tumor-Like Conditions . . . 54
1.11.1 Neuroendocrine Tumors . . . 54
1.11.2 Hematopoietic and Lymphoid Tumors . . . 54
1.11.3 Germ Cell Tumors . . . 54
1.11.4 Other Rare Epithelial Tumors and Renal Cell Carcinoma in Children . . . 55
1.11.5 Tumor-Like Conditions . . . 55

1.12 Secondary Tumors 56
Suggested Reading 56

2 Tumors and Tumor-Like Conditions of Urinary Bladder, Renal Pelvis, Ureter and Urethra 63
2.1 Introduction 63
2.1.1 Basic Anatomy and Histology 63
2.2 Urinary Bladder 68
2.2.1 Urothelial Carcinoma 68
2.2.2 Flat Intraepithelial Lesions 68
2.2.3 Urothelial Carcinoma 84
2.2.4 Benign Urothelial Neoplasms 122
2.2.5 Glandular Neoplasms 128
2.2.6 Squamous Cell Neoplasms 135
2.2.7 Neuroendocrine Tumors 139
2.2.8 Soft Tissue Tumors 148
2.2.9 Malignant Melanoma 166
2.2.10 Germ Cell Tumors 167
2.2.11 Hematologic Malignancies 167
2.2.12 Tumor-Like Conditions 168
2.2.13 Metastatic Tumors and Secondary Extension 176
2.2.14 Metastatic Urothelial Carcinoma 176
2.3 The Renal Pelvis and Ureter 177
2.4 The Urethra 181
Suggested Reading 187

3 The Prostate and Seminal Vesicles 195
3.1 Basic Anatomy and Histology 196
3.1.1 The Prostate 196
3.1.2 The Seminal Vesicles and Ejaculatory Ducts 201
3.2 Adenocarcinoma of the Prostate 202
3.2.1 Preneoplastic Lesions and Conditions 202
3.3 Diagnostic Criteria for Prostate Adenocarcinoma 214
3.3.1 Histologic Features of Prostate Cancer 215
3.4 Rare Histologic Subtypes of Prostatic Carcinoma 224
3.4.1 Pseudohyperplastic Adenocarcinoma 224
3.4.2 Foamy Gland Adenocarcinoma 225
3.4.3 Atrophic Adenocarcinoma 226
3.4.4 Adenocarcinoma with Glomeruloid Features 228
3.4.5 Mucinous and Signet Ring Cell Adenocarcinoma 228
3.4.6 Oncocytic Adenocarcinoma 229
3.4.7 Lymphoepithelioma-Like Carcinoma of the Prostate 230
3.4.8 Prostatic Ductal Adenocarcinoma 232
3.4.9 Intraductal Carcinoma 237
3.4.10 Small Cell Carcinoma 239
3.4.11 Sarcomatoid Carcinoma (Carcinosarcoma) 241
3.4.12 PIN-Like Carcinoma 243
3.4.13 Pleomorphic Giant Cell Carcinoma 244

3.5 Gleason Grading of Prostate Cancer 247
3.5.1 Gleason Patterns. 248
3.5.2 Reporting Gleason Scores in Prostate Needle Biopsies 250
3.5.3 Reporting Gleason Scores in Radical Prostatectomies 251
3.5.4 Grading Variants and Variations of Adenocarcinoma of the Prostate 252
3.5.5 Correlation Between Needle Biopsy and RP Gleason Scores 252
3.5.6 Pathology of the Prostate After Treatment. 254
3.6 Pathologic Prognosis of Prostate Cancer 261
3.6.1 Prostate Biopsy 261
3.6.2 Prognostic Factors After Radical Prostatectomy ... 266
3.7 Basic Molecular Pathology of Prostate Cancer 271
3.8 Rare Forms of Prostatic Tumours 274
3.9 Tumors and Tumor-Like Conditions of the Prostate Stroma 288
3.10 Miscellaneous Primary Tumours of the Prostate 298
3.11 Secondary Tumours Involving the Prostate 298
3.12 Seminal Vesicles 302
Suggested Reading 306

4 Testis and Paratesticular Structures 311
4.1 Basic Anatomy and Histology 312
4.2 Classification of Tumors and Tumor-Like Conditions. 313
4.2.1 Germ Cell Tumors 314
4.2.2 Intratubular Germ Cell Neoplasia, Unclassified (IGCNU) 315
4.2.3 Germ Cell Tumors of One Histologic Type. 316
4.2.4 Seminoma 316
4.2.5 Spermatocytic Seminoma 320
4.3 Non-seminomatous Germ Cell Tumors (NSGCTs). 322
4.3.1 Embryonal Carcinoma 322
4.4 Yolk Sac Tumor 326
4.4.1 Pathology 326
4.4.2 Immunohistochemistry 327
4.4.3 Genetics 330
4.5 Polyembryoma 331
4.6 Choriocarcinoma and Other Types of Throphoblastic Neoplasia 331
4.6.1 Pathology 331
4.6.2 Morphologic Variants. 332
4.6.3 Immunohistochemistry 333
4.6.4 Genetics 334
4.7 Teratoma 334
4.7.1 Pathology 334
4.7.2 Variants 334
4.7.3 Genetics 335

4.8 Burned Out GCTs 335
4.9 Tumors of More than One Histologic Type (Mixed Forms) 335
4.9.1 Pathology 336
4.9.2 Prognostic Factors 337
4.10 Tumors of Sex Cord/Gonadal Stroma 338
4.11 Benign and Malignant Leydig Cell Tumors 339
4.11.1 Pathology of Benign Tumors 339
4.11.2 Pathology of Malignant Tumors 339
4.11.3 Genetics 342
4.12 Benign and Malignant Sertoli Cell Tumors 342
4.12.1 Pathology of Benign Tumors 342
4.12.2 Pathology of Malignant Tumors 346
4.12.3 Genetics 346
4.13 Large Cell Calcifying Sertoli Cell Tumor (LCCST) 346
4.13.1 Pathology 346
4.14 Granulosa Cell Tumor of Adult Type 347
4.15 Granulosa Cell Tumor of Juvenile Type 347
4.16 Thecoma–Fibroma Type Tumors 347
4.17 Mixed or Incompletely Differentiated (Undifferentiated) Gonadal Stromal Tumors 348
4.18 Mixed Germ Cell/Sex Cord Stromal Tumor 348
4.18.1 Gonadoblastoma 348
4.18.2 Germ Cell Sex Cord/Gonadal Stromal Tumor, Unclassified 350
4.19 Other Tumors of the Testis 350
4.19.1 Carcinoid 350
4.19.2 Nephroblastoma 350
4.19.3 Lymphoma and Plasmacytoma 350
4.19.4 Leukemia 351
4.20 Other Rare Tumors 352
4.21 Testicular Metastases 353
4.22 Tumors of the Paratesticular Region 355
4.23 Tumors of Ovarian (Müllerian) Epithelial Types 355
4.24 Tumors of Collecting Ducts and Rete Testis 355
4.24.1 Adenoma 355
4.24.2 Adenocarcinoma of Rete Testis 355
4.25 Epithelial Tumors of the Epididymis 356
4.25.1 Papillary Cystadenoma of the Epididymis 356
4.25.2 Adenocarcinoma of the Epididymis 357
4.25.3 Adenomatoid Tumor 358
4.26 Mesothelioma of the Tunica Vaginalis Testis 358
4.26.1 Pathology 359
4.27 Melanotic Neuroectodermal Tumor of Infancy 360
4.28 Desmoplastic Small Round Cell Tumor 360
4.29 Soft Tissue Tumors of the Spermatic Cord 361
4.30 Tumor-Like Conditions 362
4.30.1 Intratesticular Hemorrhage 362
4.30.2 Segmental Testicular Infarction 362

4.30.3 Organized Testicular Hematocele 362
4.30.4 Inflammatory Lesions 362
4.31 Meconium Periorchitis. 363
4.32 Sperm Granuloma 364
4.33 Sclerosing Lipogranuloma. 364
4.34 Cysts. 364
4.34.1 Epidermoid Cyst 364
4.34.2 Tubular Ectasia of the Rete Testis 364
4.34.3 Epididymal Cysts and Spermatoceles 364
4.34.4 Spermatic Cord Cysts 365
4.35 Ectopic Tissues 365
4.35.1 Ectopic Adrenocortical Tissue. 365
4.35.2 Splenic-Gonadal Fusion. 365
4.35.3 Lipomatosis Testis 365
4.36 Testicular Appendages. 366
4.37 Other Tumor-Like Lesions. 366
4.37.1 Fibrous Pseudotumor. 366
4.37.2 Amyloidosis. 366
4.37.3 Polyorchidism 366
4.37.4 Sertoli Cell Hyperplasia. 366
4.37.5 Leydig Cell Hyperplasia 366
4.37.6 Hyperplasia of the Rete Testis 366
4.37.7 Cribriform Hyperplasia and Atypical Nuclei in the Epididymis. 367
4.37.8 Reactive Mesothelial Hyperplasia 367
4.37.9 Vasitis/Epididymitis Nodosa 367
4.37.10 Proliferative Funiculitis 367
4.37.11 Embryonic Remnants. 367
Suggested Reading 367

5 Penis and Scrotum. 373
5.1 Basic Anatomy and Histology 374
5.1.1 Penis. 374
5.1.2 Scrotum 374
5.2 Carcinoma of the Penis 374
5.2.1 Overview 374
5.2.2 Preneoplastic and Other Intraepithelial Lesions . 376
5.2.3 Squamous Cell Carcinoma, Usual Type 387
5.2.4 Variants of Squamous Cell Carcinoma 393
5.2.5 Other Carcinomas 409
5.3 Benign Tumors and Tumor-Like Conditions. 411
5.3.1 Benign Tumors of Epithelial Origin 411
5.3.2 Benign Human Papillomavirus-Associated Lesions. 411
5.3.3 Myointimoma. 413
5.3.4 Other Benign Tumors. 416
5.4 Malignant Soft Tissue Tumors. 416
5.4.1 Kaposi Sarcoma 417
5.4.2 Leiomyosarcoma 418

5.4.3 Epithelioid Sarcoma 419
5.4.4 Other Soft Tissue Sarcomas. 419
5.5 Other Rare Tumors. 420
5.5.1 Primary Malignant Melanoma of the Penis. 420
5.5.2 Clear Cell Sarcoma (Malignant Melanoma of Soft Parts) 420
5.5.3 Lymphoma. 420
5.6 Secondary Tumors 421
5.7 Carcinoma of the Scrotum 422
5.7.1 Overview 422
5.7.2 Preneoplastic Lesions 423
5.7.3 Squamous Cell Carcinoma 423
5.8 Other Carcinomas 423
5.8.1 Basal Cell Carcinoma 423
5.8.2 Merkel Cell Carcinoma 423
5.8.3 Extramammary Paget Disease. 423
5.9 Benign Tumors and Tumor-Like Conditions. 427
5.9.1 Scrotal Calcinosis 427
5.9.2 Sclerosing Lipogranuloma of the Scrotum 429
5.9.3 Angiokeratoma 429
5.9.4 Fat Necrosis. 430
5.9.5 Verruciform Xanthoma 430
5.9.6 Spindle Cell Nodule (Inflammatory Myofibroblastic Tumor). 432
5.9.7 Epidermal Cyst 432
5.9.8 Other Benign Lesions 432
5.10 Soft Tissue Tumors 433
5.11 Other Rare Tumors. 433
5.12 Secondary Tumors 433
Suggested Reading 435

Renal Tumors and Tumor-Like Conditions

1

Contents

1.1 **Basic Anatomy and Histology** 2

1.2 **Overview** 2

1.3 **Familial Renal Cancer** 4
1.3.1 Von Hippel-Lindau (VHL) Clear Cell Renal Cell Carcinoma (RCC) 4
1.3.2 Hereditary Papillary RCC 4
1.3.3 Hereditary Leiomyomatosis RCC 4
1.3.4 Birt-Hogg-Dube Syndrome 5

1.4 **Renal Cell Carcinoma** 6
1.4.1 Clear Cell RCC 6
1.4.2 Multilocular Cystic Clear Cell Renal Cell Neoplasm of Low Malignant Potential 6
1.4.3 Papillary RCC 9
1.4.4 Chromophobe RCC 11
1.4.5 Hybrid Oncocytic Chromophobe Tumor (HOCT) 12
1.4.6 Collecting Duct Carcinoma 14
1.4.7 Renal Medullary Carcinoma 16
1.4.8 Mucinous, Tubular and Spindle Cell Carcinoma 16
1.4.9 Renal Cell Carcinoma After Neuroblastoma 20
1.4.10 RCC with Sarcomatoid or Rhabdoid Differentiation 20
1.4.11 Renal Cell Carcinoma, Unclassified 21

1.5 **Proposed New and Emerging Epithelial Renal Tumors** 22
1.5.1 Tubulocystic Renal Cell Carcinoma 22
1.5.2 Acquired Cystic Disease-Associated RCC 22
1.5.3 Clear Cell Papillary (Tubulo-Papillary) RCC 23
1.5.4 MiT Family Translocation RCC 25
1.5.5 Thyroid-Like Follicular Renal Cell Carcinoma 27
1.5.6 Succinic Dehydrogenase B Deficiency Associated Renal Cell Carcinoma 27
1.5.7 ALK-Translocation Renal Cell Carcinoma 28
1.5.8 Renal Cell Carcinoma with Smooth Muscle Stroma 28
1.5.9 Tuberous Sclerosis-Associated Renal Cell Carcinoma 29

1.6 **Benign Tumors** 30
1.6.1 Papillary Adenoma 30
1.6.2 Metanephric Tumors 30
1.6.3 Renal Oncocytoma 30

1.7 **Percutaneous Biopsy of Renal Tumours** 33

1.8 **Cystic Nephroma and Mixed Epithelial and Stromal Tumors** 34

1.9 **Soft Tissue Tumors** 37
1.9.1 Medullary Fibroma 37
1.9.2 Juxtaglomerular Cell Tumor 38
1.9.3 Glomus Tumor 39
1.9.4 Angiomyolipoma 39
1.9.5 Epithelioid Angiomyolipoma 40
1.9.6 Leiomyoma 41
1.9.7 Lipoma 41
1.9.8 Hemangioma 42
1.9.9 Lymphangioma 42
1.9.10 Schwannoma 43
1.9.11 Solitary Fibrous Tumor 43
1.9.12 Leiomyosarcoma 43
1.9.13 Angiosarcoma 44
1.9.14 Liposarcoma 44
1.9.15 Rhabdomyosarcoma 45
1.9.16 Malignant Fibrous Histiocytoma 45
1.9.17 Hemangiopericytoma 45
1.9.18 Hemangioblastoma 46
1.9.19 Osteosarcoma 46
1.9.20 Other Soft Tissue Tumors 47

A. Lopez-Beltran et al., *Rare Tumors and Tumor-like Conditions in Urological Pathology*,
DOI 10.1007/978-3-319-10253-5_1,

1.10 **Wilms' Tumor and Other Renal Neoplasms in Children** 48
1.10.1 Nephrogenic Rests and Nephroblastomatosis 48
1.10.2 Nephroblastoma (Wilms' Tumor) 48
1.10.3 Cystic Partially Differentiated Nephroblastoma..................... 49
1.10.4 Congenital Mesoblastic Nephroma (CMN) 50
1.10.5 Clear Cell Sarcoma of Kidney.......... 52
1.10.6 Rhabdoid Tumor of Kidney............ 52
1.10.7 Neuroblastoma...................... 52
1.10.8 Primitive Neuroectodermal Tumor (PNET)....................... 52
1.10.9 Desmoplastic Small Round Cell Tumor......................... 52
1.10.10 Synovial Sarcoma 53
1.10.11 Ossifying Renal Tumor of Infancy...... 54
1.11 **Other Rare Tumors and Tumor-Like Conditions** 54
1.11.1 Neuroendocrine Tumors.............. 54
1.11.2 Hematopoietic and Lymphoid Tumors............................ 54
1.11.3 Germ Cell Tumors 54
1.11.4 Other Rare Epithelial Tumors and Renal Cell Carcinoma in Children 55
1.11.5 Tumor-Like Conditions 55
1.12 **Secondary Tumors**................. 56
Suggested Reading.......................... 56

1.1 Basic Anatomy and Histology

- The kidneys are paired retroperitoneal organs that normally extend from 12th thoracic vertebra to the 3rd lumbar vertebra. The average adult kidney is 11–12 cm long. It weighs 125–170 g in men and 115–155 g in women.
- The three defined regions, upper polo, middle zone and lower pole usually reflect regions drained by three lobar veins.
- The normal adult kidney has a minimum of 10–14 lobes, each composed of medullary pyramid surrounded by a cap of cortex.
- The renal parenchyma consists of the cortex and the medulla. The cortex is the nephron-containing parenchyma. The renal medulla is divided into outer medulla and the inner medulla or papilla. The papilla protrudes into a minor calyx. Its tip has 20–70 openings of the papillary collecting ducts (Bellini ducts).
- The cortex contains glomeruli, proximal and distal convoluted tubules, connecting tubules, and the initial portion of the collecting ducts, as well as interlobular vessels, arterioles, capillaries, and lymphatics. The interstitial space is scant; it contains the peritubular capillary plexus and inconspicuous numbers of interstitial fibroblasts and reticulum cells.

1.2 Overview

- The current classification of renal cell tumors was proposed in 2004 by the World Health Organization (WHO) and has been recently updated by the International Society of Urological Pathologists (Table 1.1). It describes categories and entities based on pathological and genetic analyses. A number of emerging or provisional categories are also incorporated (Table 1.2)
- Rare new entities and morphologic variants of common categories have recently been described and represent important diagnostic challenges in daily practice.

Table 1.1 International Society of Urological Pathologists (ISUP) Vancouver modification of WHO (2004) Histologic Classification of Renal Tumors

Renal cell tumors
Papillary adenoma
Oncocytoma
Clear cell renal cell carcinoma
Multilocular cystic clear cell renal cell neoplasm of low malignant potential
Papillary renal cell carcinoma
Chromophobe renal cell carcinoma
Hybrid oncocytic chromophobe tumor
Carcinoma of the collecting ducts of Bellini
Renal medullary carcinoma
MiT family translocation renal cell carcinoma
Xp11 translocation renal cell carcinoma
t(6;11) renal cell carcinoma
Carcinoma associated with neuroblastoma
Mucinous tubular and spindle cell carcinoma
Tubulocystic renal cell carcinoma
Acquired cystic disease associated renal cell carcinoma
Clear cell (tubulo) papillary renal cell carcinoma
Hereditary leiomyomatosis renal cell carcinoma syndrome-associated renal cell carcinoma
Renal cell carcinoma, unclassified
Metanephric tumors
Metanephric adenoma
Metanephric adenofibroma
Metanephric stromal tumor
Nephroblastic tumors
Nephrogenic rests
Nephroblastoma
Cystic partially differentiated nephroblastoma
Mesenchymal tumors occurring mainly in children
Clear cell sarcoma
Rhabdoid tumor
Congenital mesoblastic nephroma
Ossifying renal tumor of infants
Mesenchymal tumors occurring mainly in adults
Leiomyosarcoma (including renal vein)
Angiosarcoma
Rhabdomyosarcoma
Malignant fibrous histiocytoma
Hemangiopericytoma
Osteosarcoma
Synovial sarcoma
Angiomyolipoma
Epithelioid angiomyolipoma
Leiomyoma

Table 1.1 (continued)

Hemangioma
Lymphangioma
Juxtaglomerular cell tumor
Renomedullary interstitial cell tumor
Schwannoma
Solitary fibrous tumor
Mixed mesenchymal and epithelial tumors
Cystic nephroma/mixed epithelial stromal tumor
Neuroendocrine tumors
Carcinoid (low-grade neuroendocrine tumor)
Neuroendocrine carcinoma (high-grade neuroendocrine tumor)
Primitive neuroectodermal tumor
Neuroblastoma
Pheochromocytoma
Hematopoietic and lymphoid tumors
Lymphoma
Leukemia
Plasmacytoma
Germ cell tumors
Teratoma
Choriocarcinoma
Metastatic tumors
Other tumors

Table 1.2 Proposed New Renal Epithelial Tumors and emerging Tumor Entities

New epithelial tumors
Tubulocystic renal cell carcinoma
Acquired cystic disease associated renal cell carcinoma
Clear cell (tubulo) papillary renal cell carcinoma
MiT family translocation renal cell carcinoma including t(6;11) renal cell carcinoma
Hereditary leiomyomatosis renal cell carcinoma syndrome associated renal cell carcinoma
Emerging tumor entities
Thyroid-like follicular renal cell carcinoma
Succinic dehydrogenase B deficiency associated renal cell carcinoma
ALK-translocation renal cell carcinoma
Other
Renal cell carcinoma with smooth muscle stroma
Tuberous Sclerosis-associated Renal Cell Carcinoma

1.3 Familial Renal Cancer

- Hereditary renal cancers show a tendency to be multiple and bilateral, may have a family history, and present at an earlier age. Known inherited syndromes that predispose to renal tumors are listed in Table 1.3.

1.3.1 Von Hippel-Lindau (VHL) Clear Cell Renal Cell Carcinoma (RCC)

- Like its sporadic counterpart, VHL clear cell RCC harbors defective VHL tumor suppressor genes. Genetic alteration in the VHL gene in the tumor can include deletion, nonsense or frame-shift mutations, mis-sense mutations or methylation.

1.3.2 Hereditary Papillary RCC

- Hereditary papillary RCC are typically bilateral, multifocal type 1 papillary RCC. Genetic alterations involve a proto-oncogene, c-MET, located at 7q31.1. Similar to what is found in sporadic papillary renal cell carcinoma, trisomy 7 and 17 are identified.

1.3.3 Hereditary Leiomyomatosis RCC

- Hereditary leiomyomatosis associated-RCC patients develop cutaneous and uterine leiomyomas and one third of patients develop RCC. It was considered as a variant of type 2 papillary RCC. The pathologic findings in this disease are caused by germline mutations in the fumarate hydratase gene located at 1q42.
- Architectural patterns are papillary, tubulopapillary, tubular, solid or mixed. The morphologic hallmark of the hereditary leiomyomatosis-RCC, is the presence of large nucleus with a very prominent eosinophilic nucleolus, surrounded by a clear halo. These tumors are associated with poor prognosis.
- It is now recognized a unique morphotype of RCC. The renal tumors have a papillary, alveolar, solid or tubular architecture with the characteristic features being a large nucleus and a prominent nucleolus, with a clear peripheral halo These tumors behave aggressively and have a poor prognosis when compared to other hereditary forms of RCC, or clear cell and papillary RCC (Fig. 1.1).

Table 1.3 Familial renal tumors

Syndrome	Gene	Tumor
Von Hippel-Lindau (VHL)	VHL (3p25)	Clear cell
Tuberous Sclerosis	TSC1, TSC2	Angiomyolipoma, clear cell, other
Familial renal carcinoma	Gene not identified	Clear cell
Constitutional chromosome 3 translocation	Responsible gene not found[a]	Clear cell
Hereditary PRCC	c-MET	Papillary type 1
Birt-Hogg-Dube (BHD)	BHD	Chromophobe[b]
Familial oncocytoma	Loss of multiple chromosomes	Oncocytoma
Hereditary leiomyomatosis RCC	FH	Papillary type 2

[a]VHL gene mutated in some families
[b]Renal oncocytomas, hybrid oncocytic and clear cell carcinomas may occur

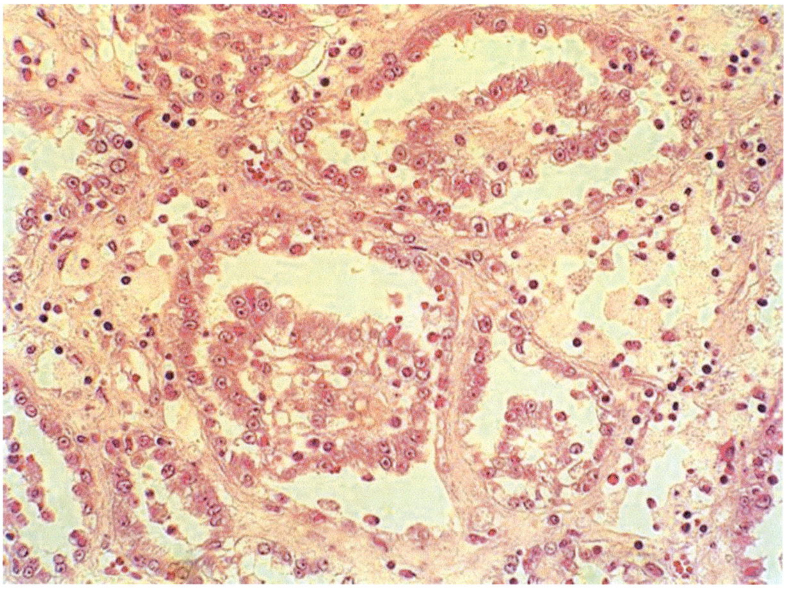

Fig. 1.1 Hereditary leiomyomatosis associated renal cell carcinoma

- HLRCC leiomyomas frequently have increased cellularity, multinucleated cells, and atypia. All cases show tumor nuclei with large orangeophilic nucleoli surrounded by a perinucleolar halo similar to the changes found in HLRCC. Occasional mitoses may be seen; however, the tumors did not fulfill the criteria for malignancy.

1.3.4 Birt-Hogg-Dube Syndrome

- Birt-Hogg-Dubé is an autosomal dominant cancer syndrome characterized by benign skin and renal tumors, and spontaneous pneumothorax. The disease related gene has been mapped to chromosome 17p11.2.
- Birt-Hogg-Dubé is characterized by a spectrum of mutations, and clinical heterogeneity among and within families. Renal epithelial tumors with hybrid features are seen in this syndrome (Figs. 1.2 and 1.3).

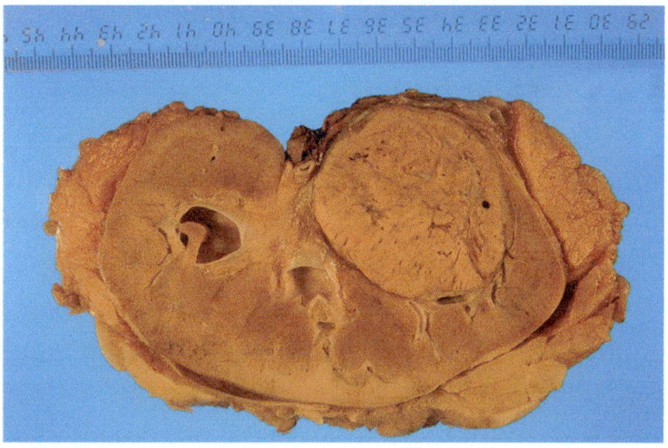

Fig. 1.2 Gross features in RCC associated with Birt-Hogg-Dubé syndrome

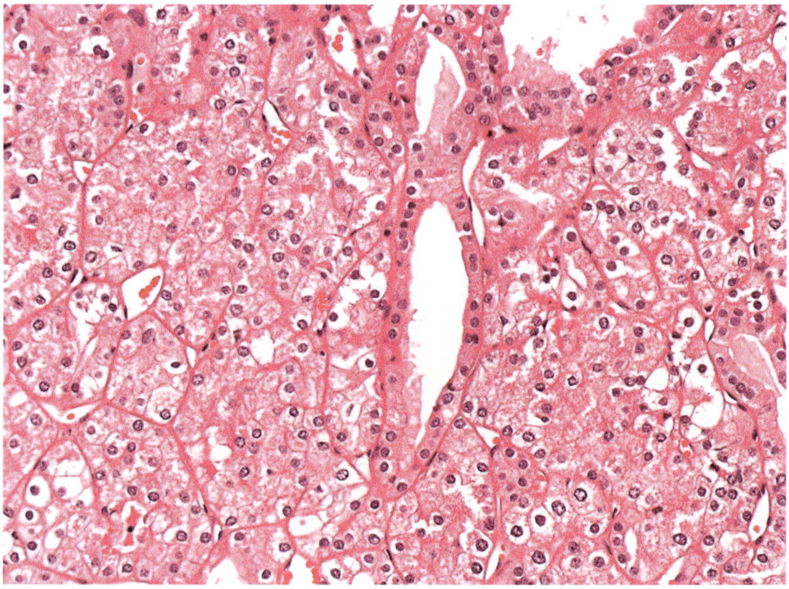

Fig. 1.3 Hybrid RCC with oncocytic and clear cells associated with Birt-Hogg-Dubé syndrome

1.4 Renal Cell Carcinoma

1.4.1 Clear Cell RCC

- Most clear cell RCC are variably sized solitary cortical neoplasms, rarely bilateral (<5 %) or multicentric (4 %), typically golden yellow. Necrosis, cystic degeneration, hemorrhage, calcification, ossification, and extension into the renal vein may occur. Clear cell tumors of any size are considered malignant.
- Microvascular invasion and microscopic tumor coagulative necrosis may be relevant predictors in low stage RCC (Table 1.4). Clear cell RCC has a worse prognosis when compared with chromophobe or papillary subtypes, and may progress into a sarcomatoid carcinoma which is an ominous prognostic sign (Figs. 1.4 and 1.5).
- The international Society of Urological Pathologists (ISUP) suggested that clear cell RCC grading should be based upon nucleolar features and not Fuhrman grading (Table 1.5). Sporadic clear cell RCC displays frequent chromosome 3p losses.
- Clear cell RCC may have acidophilic cytoplasm, hemangioblastoma-like, angioleiomyoma-like stroma or pseudo-papillary architecture but retains the characteristic 3p loss.

1.4.2 Multilocular Cystic Clear Cell Renal Cell Neoplasm of Low Malignant Potential

- The ISUP modification of the current 2004 WHO classification of kidney tumors recognizes multilocular cystic clear cell renal cell neoplasm of low malignant potential (MCNLMP) as a variant of clear cell RCC with a good prognosis.
- This is a tumor entirely composed of cysts of variable size separated from the kidney by a fibrous capsule. The cyst are lined by a single layer of clear to pale cells but occasionally shows a few small papillae. The septa are composed of fibrous tissue that may have epithelial cells with clear cytoplasm that resemble those lining the cysts (Figs. 1.6, 1.7 and 1.8).
- Cases with expansive nodules are excluded. VHL gene mutations in MCNLMP supports its classification as a type of clear cell RCC.
- No progression of MCNLMP has been reported.

Table 1.4 TNM classification of renal cell carcinoma (2010)

PrimaryTumor (T)	
TX	Primary tumor cannot be assessed
T0	No evidence of primary tumor
T1	Tumor ≤7 cm in greatest dimension, limited to the kidney
T1a	Tumor ≤4 cm in greatest dimension, limited to the kidney
T1b	Tumor >4 cm but ≤7 cm in greatest dimension, limited to the kidney
T2	Tumor >7 cm in greatest dimension, limited to the kidney
T2a	Tumor >7 cm but ≤10 cm in greatest dimension, limited to the kidney
T2b	Tumor >10 cm, limited to the kidney
T3	Tumor extends into major veins or perinephric tissues but not into the ipsilateral adrenal gland and not beyond the Gerota fascia
T3a	Tumor grossly extends into the renal vein or its segmental (muscle-containing) branches, or tumor invades perirenal and/or renal sinus fat but not beyond the Gerota fascia
T3b	Tumor grossly extends into the vena cava below the diaphragm
T3c	Tumor grossly extends into the vena cava above the diaphragm or invades the wall of the vena cava
T4	Tumor invades beyond the Gerota fascia (including contiguous extension into the ipsilateral adrenal gland)
Regional lymph nodes (N)	
NX	Regional lymph nodes cannot be assessed
N0	No regional lymph node metastasis
N1	Metastasis in regional lymph node(s)
Distant metastasis (M)	
M0	No distant metastasis
M1	Distant metastasis

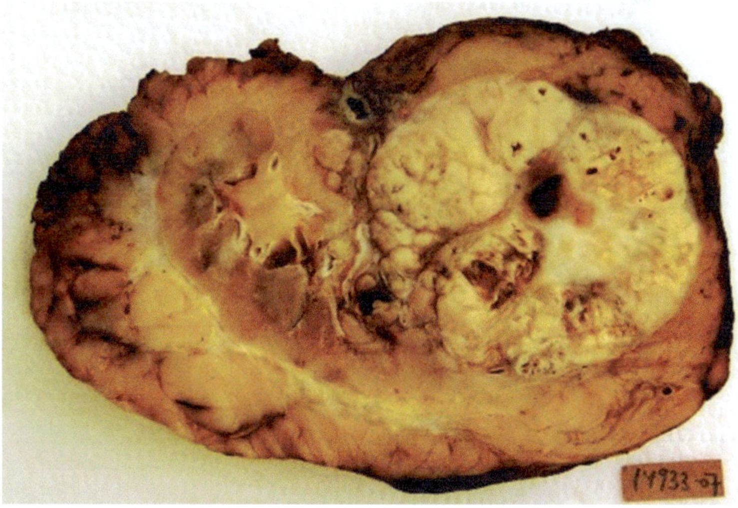

Fig. 1.4 Gross features of clear cell renal cell carcinoma

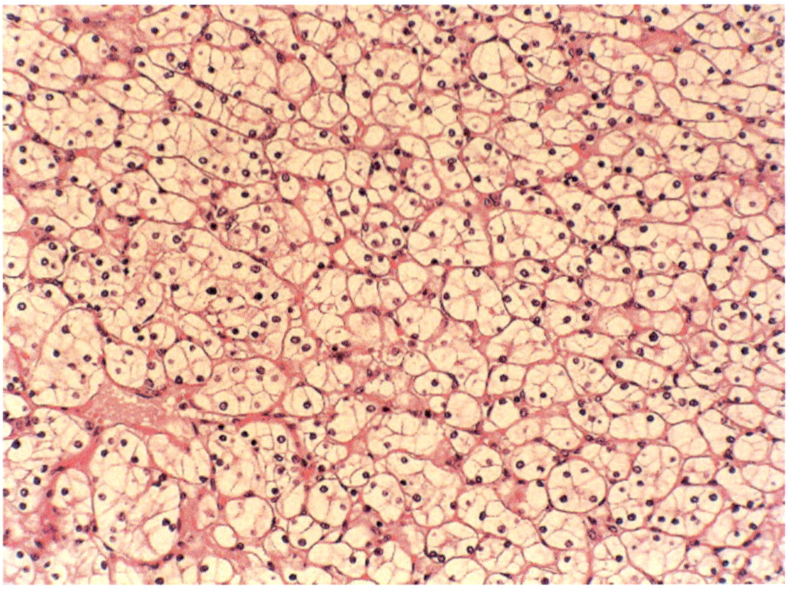

Fig. 1.5 Microscopic features of clear cell renal cell carcinoma

Table 1.5 International Society of Urological Pathology Nucleolar Grading System

Grade	Tumor description
1	Inconspicuous or absent nucleoli at 400× magnification
2	Nucleoli distinctly visible at 400× but inconspicuous or invisible at 100× magnification
3	Nucleoli distinctly visible at 100× magnification
4	Rhabdoid or sarcomatoid differentiation, or containing tumor giant cells or showing extreme nuclear pleomorphism with clumping of chromatin

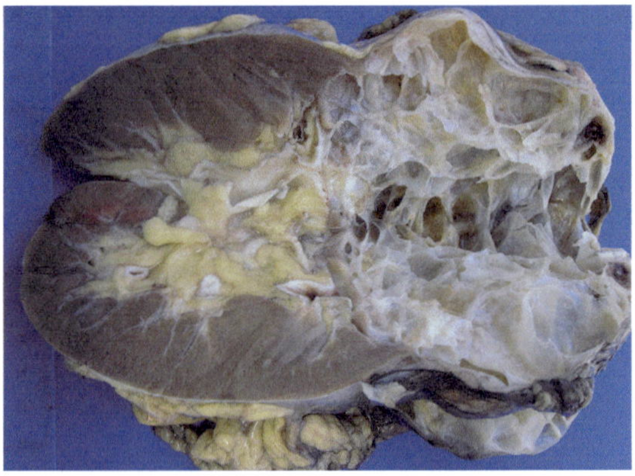

Fig. 1.6 Multilocular cystic renal cell neoplasia of low malignant potential (gross features)

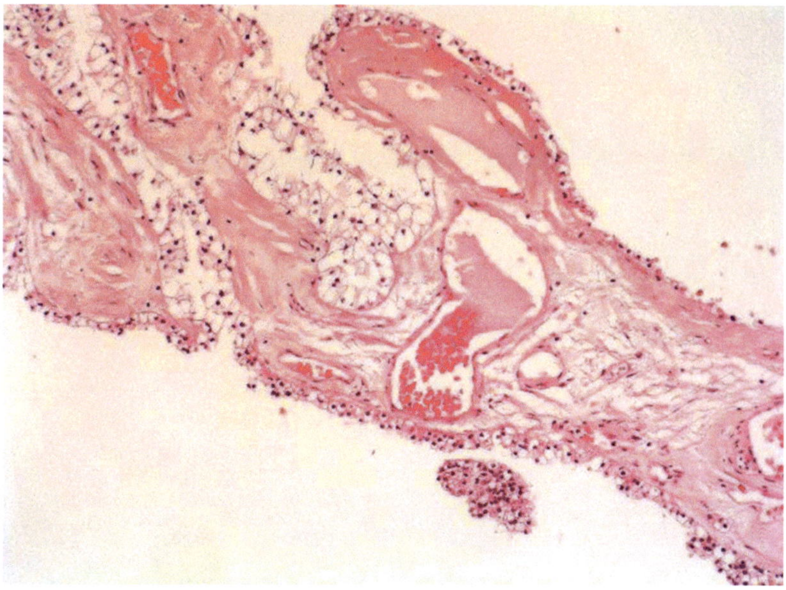

Fig. 1.7 Multilocular cystic renal cell neoplasia of low malignant potential (histologic features)

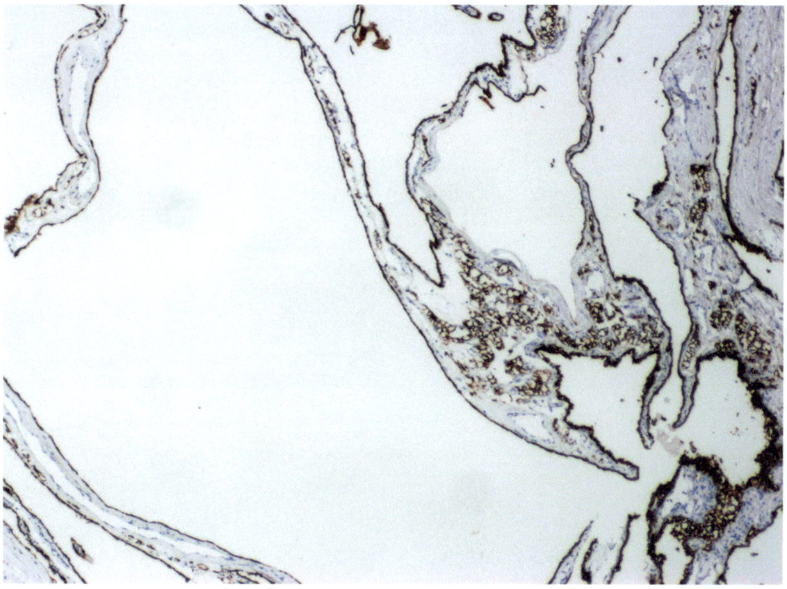

Fig. 1.8 Multilocular cystic renal cell neoplasia of low malignant potential. Expression of CAIX in the neoplastic cells

1.4.3 Papillary RCC

- Papillary RCC has a less aggressive clinical course than clear cell RCC. Papillary RCC has variable proportions of papillae and may be bilateral or multifocal with hemorrhage, necrosis or cystic degeneration. The papillae contain a fibrovascular core with aggregates of foamy macrophages, calcified concretions and frequent hemosiderin granules.
- Cellular type 1 and type 2 tumors have papillae covered by small cells with scanty cytoplasm arranged in a single layer in type1, and tumor cells of higher nuclear grade, eosinophilic cytoplasm and pseudostratified nuclei in type 2. Type 1 tumors have longer survival (Figs. 1.9, 1.10 and 1.11).
- Trisomy or tetrasomy 7, trisomy 17 and loss of chromosome Y are the cytogenetic signature. Stage, tumor proliferation and sarcomatoid change being correlated with outcome. It has been suggested that papillary RCC grading should be based upon nucleolar features and not Fuhrman grading.

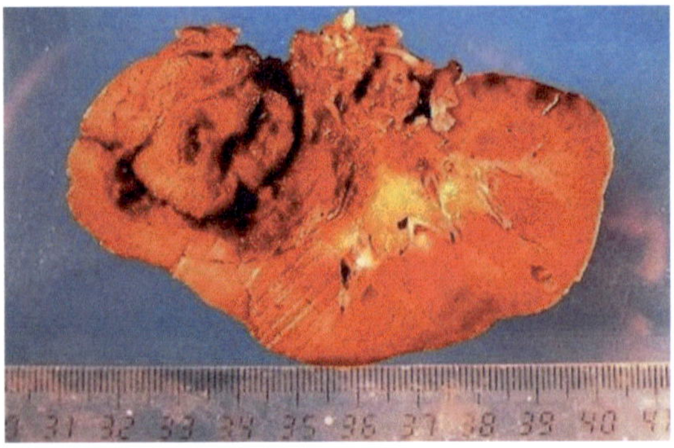

Fig. 1.9 Gross features of papillary renal cell carcinoma

- Age and sex distribution of papillary RCC is similar to clear cell RCC. Recent molecular genetic studies provide evidences for the independent origin of multifocal papillary tumors in patients with papillary RCC. An oncoytic variant of papillary RCC has been reported. One patient died of metastases on follow-up (Figs. 1.12 and 1.13).

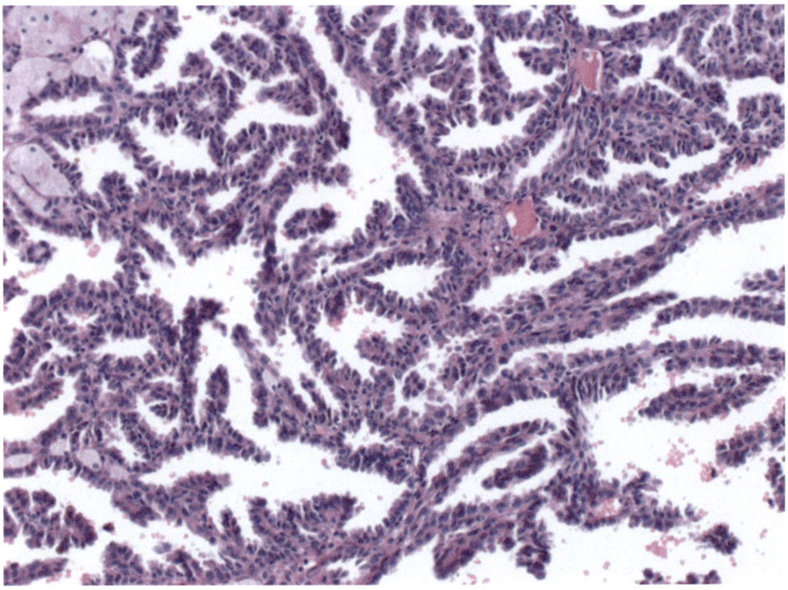

Fig. 1.10 Microscopic features of papillary carcinoma type 1

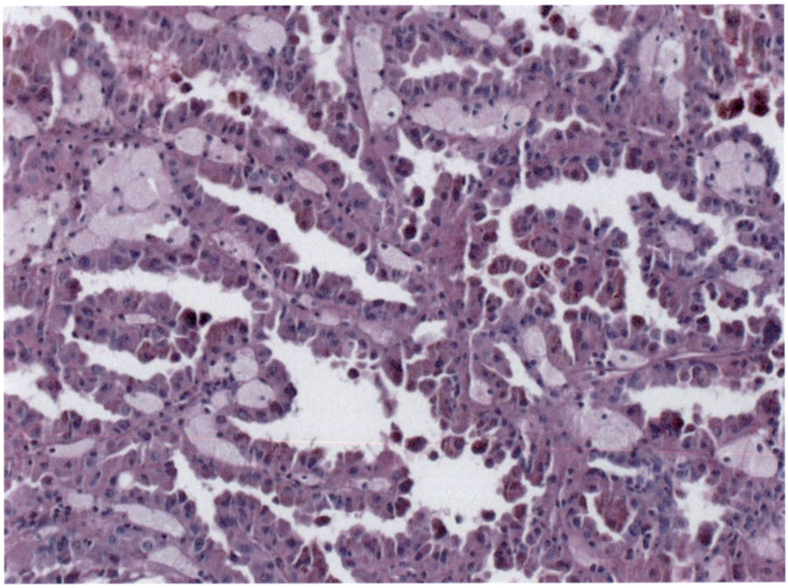

Fig. 1.11 Microscopic features of papillary carcinoma type 2

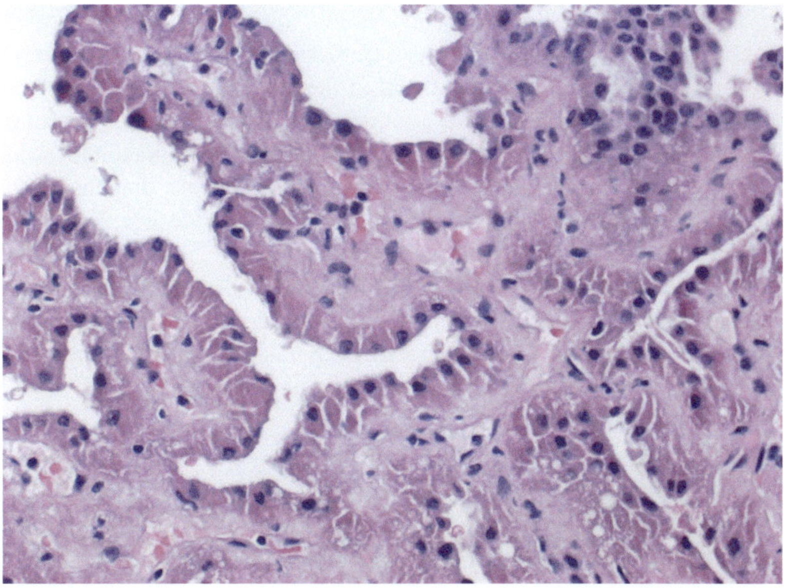

Fig. 1.12 Microscopic features of the oncocytic type of papillary carcinoma

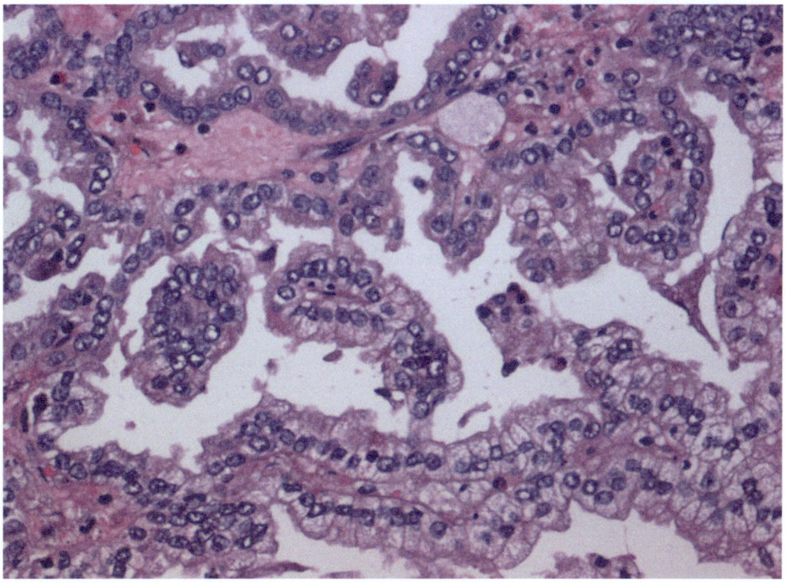

Fig. 1.13 Papillary carcinoma with focal clear cell change

1.4.4 Chromophobe RCC

- Less aggressive than other RCC, the chromophobe type is characterised by huge pale cells with reticulated cytoplasm and prominent cell membrane. It accounts for 5 % of renal epithelial tumors.
- Chromophobe RCC is solid and appears orange turning grey or sandy after fixation. The eosinophilic variant needs to be differentiated from oncocytoma. Sarcomatoid transformation is associated to aggressive disease. Diffuse cytoplasmic Hale's iron colloid stain is characteristic (Figs. 1.14, 1.15 and 1.16).

- The relationship between oncocytoma and chromophobe RCC is still unclear. Both seems to derive from the intercalated cell of the collecting duct, both have rearrangement of mitochondrial DNA, increased mitochondria in oncocytoma and numerous mitochondria-derived microvesicles in chromophobe RCC, and both are frequently observed in oncocytosis with or without Birt-Hogg-Dubé syndrome.
- There are reports of hybrid tumor composed of oncocytic and chromophobe elements. Therefore, oncocytoma might be the benign counterpart of chromophobe RCC. Loss of several chromosomes characterises chromophobe RCC. Recognising occassional occurrence of metastases and 10 % mortality is of clinical relevance.
- At diagnosis most patients are in the sixth decade, stage T1 or T2 (86 %) and similar gender incidence. Fuhrman grading is not appropriated to grade chromophome RCC with an international consensus on that chromophobe RCC should not be graded at present.

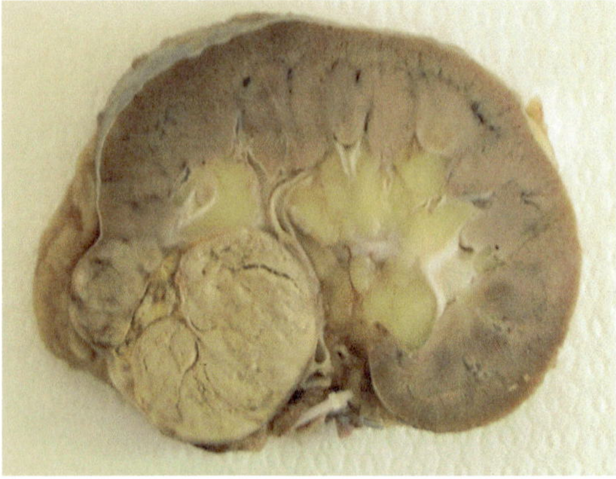

Fig. 1.14 Gross features of chromophobe renal cell carcinoma

1.4.5 Hybrid Oncocytic Chromophobe Tumor (HOCT)

- Described as tumors having a mixture of cells with the morphologic features of those seen in chromophobe RCC and renal oncocytoma (Figs. 1.17 and 1.18).
- HOCTs occur in three clinical situations: (i) being sporadic, (ii) in association with renal oncocytosis/oncocytomatosis, and (iii) in patients with the Birt-Hogg-Dubé syndrome (BHD). It seems that tumors from all three groups share similar morphologic features but that they have a differing molecular genetic background.

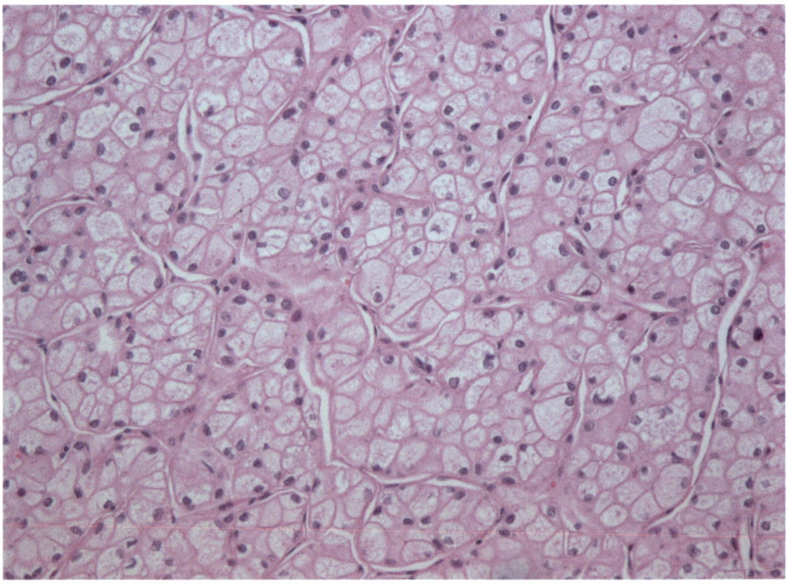

Fig. 1.15 Microscopic features of classic-type chromophobe renal cell carcinoma

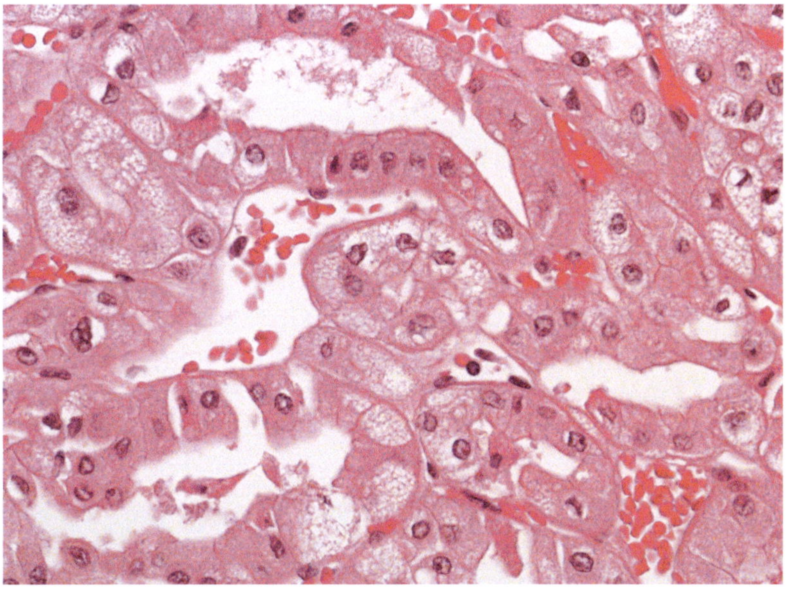

Fig. 1.16 Microscopic features of eosinophilic chromophobe renal cell carcinoma

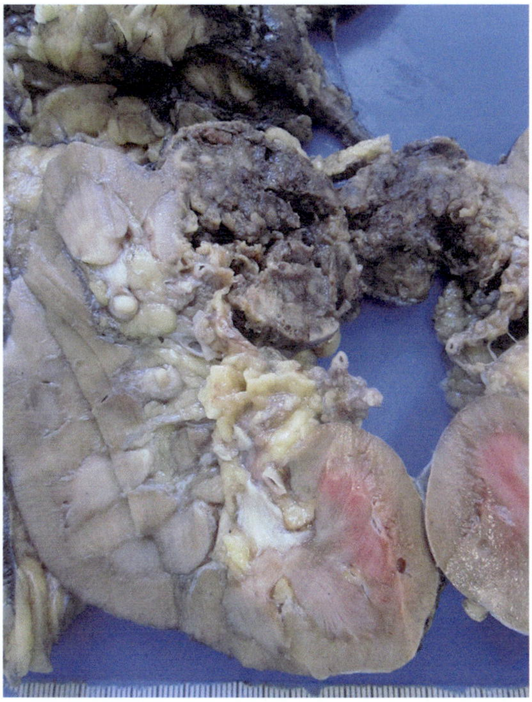

Fig. 1.17 Gross features of a case of hybrid chromophobe-oncocytoma tumor

- Sporadic HOCTs are composed of neoplastic cells predominantly arranged in a solid-alveolar pattern, with nuclei showing mild nuclear pleomorphism and abundant granular eosinophilic to oncocytic cytoplasm. Neoplastic cells have a perinuclear halo and are occasional binucleate. No raisinoid nuclei of the type seen in classic chromophobe RCC are present. Usually tumor cells resemble cells of oncocytoma with perinuclear cytoplasmic clearing, and, occasional, small tubules may be present.
- HOCTs in oncocytosis/oncocytomatosis are almost identical to those tumors that occur sporadically, being composed of sheets of cells separated by a delicate vasculature. The cells are round to polygonal with finely granular cytoplasm, and the nuclei are slightly pleomorphic and irregular with visible nucleoli. No typical raisinoid nuclei are seen, and mitotic figures are rare.
- HOCTs associated with BHD typically show three morphologic patterns: (i) an admixture of areas typical of oncocytoma and chromophobe RCC; (ii) scattered chromophobe cells in the background of a typical oncocytoma; and (iii) large eosinophilic cells with intracytoplasmic vacuoles. In these tumors, the nuclei are often more pleomorphic than other forms of HOCT and occasionally have a "raisinoid" morphology.

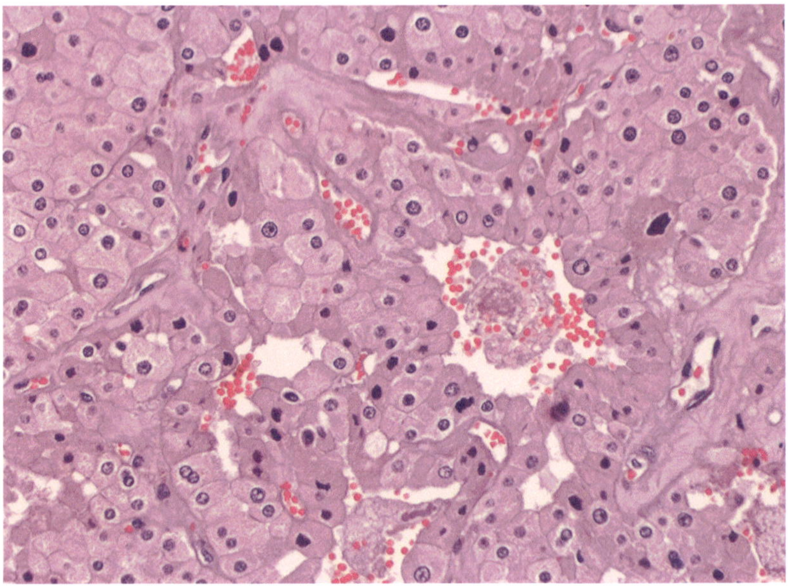

Fig. 1.18 Microscopic features of a case of hybrid chromophobe-oncocytoma tumor

- The majority of the tumors express parvalbumin, antimitochondrial antigen, CK7, and CD117 by immunohistochemistry. Monosomy of chromosome 20 is the most frequent genetic alteration, a finding highly unusual for both oncocytoma and chromophobe RCC.
- HOCTs usually occur in adult patients, with no sex predilection; some are associated with long term hemodialysis. Can be unilateral and solitary or being bilateral and multiple lesions. Necrosis is not frequently, but central fibrotic strands/scars may be occasionally present. Tumors are usually well circumscribed and nonencapsulated with homogenous tan to brown cut surface.
- HOCT, regardless of clinical association, seems to behave indolently and no evidence of aggressive behavior has been documented.

1.4.6 Collecting Duct Carcinoma

- Collecting duct carcinoma (CDC), also known as Bellini's tumor, accounts for <1 % of renal malignancies and derives from the "principal cells" of the collecting duct; ranges 2.5–12 cm, is centraly located and shows a firm grey-white appearance.
- Mean patient age is 55 years with male predominance. When small, origin within a medullary pyramid may be seen at gross examination. At diagnosis, most tumors are in advanced stage with metastasis and morphologic criteria for diagnosis are the presence of an infiltrative tubular or tubulopapillary pattern, associated with desmoplastic stromal reaction, necrosis and cells displaying high Fuhrman grade (Figs. 1.19, 1.20 and 1.21).
- CDC is positive for low and high molecular weight keratins, CD117 and vimentin, EMA, p63, CK7, Pax 2, Pax 8, but molecular alterations of CDC are poorly understood (Table 1.3). The main differential diagnoses of CDC include type 2 PRCC, renal pelvic adenocarcinoma or urothelial carcinoma with glandular differentiation. Immunohistochemistry is a valuable adjunct in this setting (Table 1.6).
- One recent experience identified complete loss of expression of INI1 in 15 % and focal/weak expression of INI1 in up to 30 % of CDC, with no difference in survival by INI1 status.

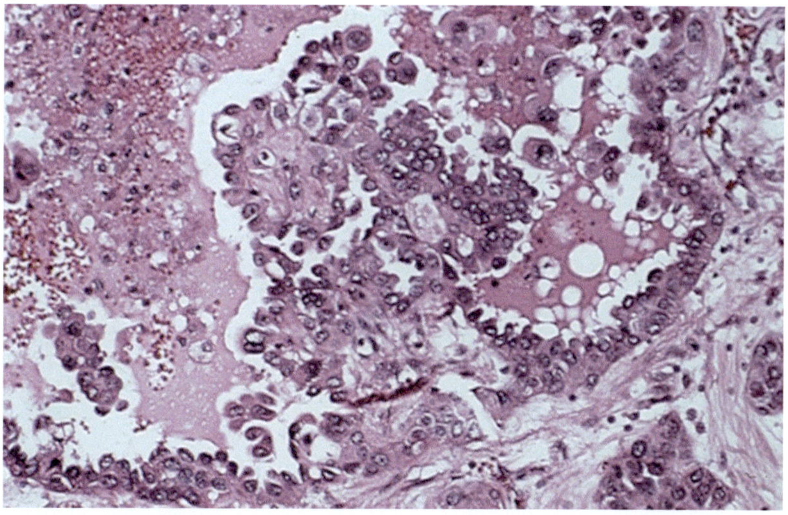

Fig. 1.19 Microscopic features of collecting duct carcinoma with papillary features

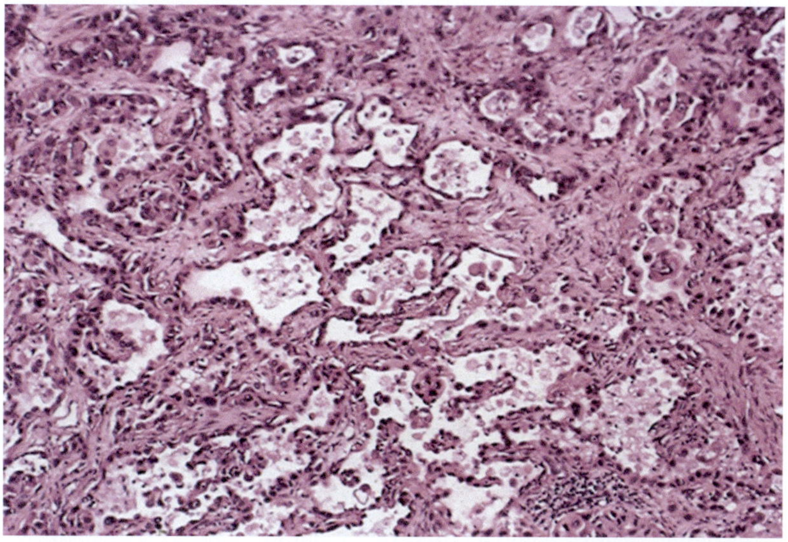

Fig. 1.20 Microscopic features of collecting duct carcinoma with anastomosing glandular channels

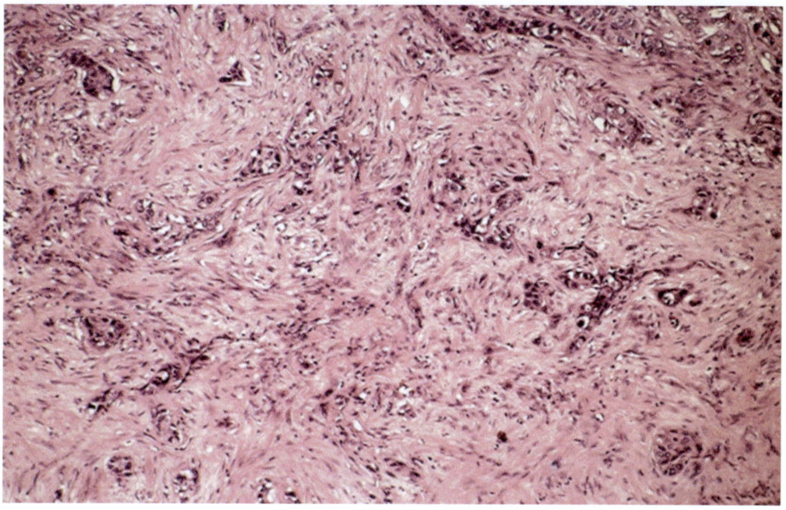

Fig. 1.21 Microscopic features of collecting duct carcinoma with desmoplastic stroma

Table 1.6 Main histotypes of renal cell tumors seen in adults with associated genetic alterations

Malignant renal cell tumors	**Main genetic alterations**
Clear cell renal cell carcinoma	−3p, +5q22, −6q, −8p, −9p, −14q
Multilocular cystic renal cell neoplasm of low malignant potential	VHL gene mutation
Papillary renal cell carcinoma	+3q, +7, +8, +12, +16, +17, +20, −Y
Chromophobe renal cell carcinoma	−1, −2, −6, −10, −17, −21, hypodiploidy
Carcinoma of the collecting ducts of Bellini	−1q, −6p, −8p, −13q, −21q, −3p (rare)
Tubulocystic carcinoma	Variable trisomy of chromosome 17
Renal medullary carcinoma	Rare loss of chromosome 22
MiT family translocation RCC (Renal carcinoma associated with Xp11.2 translocations/TFE3 gene fusions)	t(X;1)(p11.2;q21), t(X;17)(p11.2;q25), t(X;1)(p11.2;p34), t(X;17)(p11.2;q23), others
Renal cell carcinoma in long term survivors after neuroblastoma	Allelic imbalance at 20q13
Mucinous tubular and spindle cell carcinoma	−1, −4, −6, −8, −13, −14, +7, +11, +16, +17
Renal cell carcinoma unclassified	Variable, unknown
Acquired cystic disease-related RCC	Variable gains chromosomes 7 and 17, no VHL gene deletions, rare gains 1,2,6, 10
Clear cell papillary RCC	Lacked the gains of chromosome 7, no loss of Y chromosome, lack 3p deletions
Benign renal cell tumors	
Papillary adenoma	Similar to papillary RCC but less extensive
Oncocytoma	Chromosomes 1 and/or 14 loss and frequent alterations of mitochondrial DNA, 11q13 translocation, no chromosome 3p loss
Metanephric tumors: adenoma, adenofibroma, stromal metanephric	Normal karyotypes, 2p deletion, others
Mixed stromal and epithelial tumors	
Cystic nephroma/mixed epithelial and stromal tumor	Nonrandom X chromosome
	Inactivation, others

1.4.7 Renal Medullary Carcinoma

- It is a rapidly growing rare tumor of the renal medulla regarded as an aggressive variant of collecting duct carcinoma that was initially considered of renal pelvis origin. Some may have solid, spindled or rhabdoid phenotype (Figs. 1.22 and 1.23).
- Immunohistochemistry analysis shows that the neoplastic cells are positive for CEA (7/8), AE1/3 (8/8), CAM5.2 (7/7), CK7 (5/5), CK20 (4/6), and vimentin (6/6)
- Essentially all cases of RMC show loss of nuclear expression of the transcriptional regulator INI1/SMARCB1, reflecting prevalent mutation of the gene.
- With few exceptions this tumor is seen in young male blacks with sickle cell trait (mean age 22 years), presenting with hematuria, flank pain, weight loss and palpable mass.
- Metastatic disease may be the initial clinical evidence and the reported prognosis is poor.

1.4.8 Mucinous, Tubular and Spindle Cell Carcinoma

- Low-grade carcinoma composed of tightly packed tubules separated by pale mucinous stroma and a spindle cell component. It seems to derive from the distal nephron (Figs. 1.24, 1.25, 1.26, 1.27 and 1.28).
- This tumor has a combination of losses involving chromosomes 1, 4, 6, 8, 13 and 14 and gains of chromosome 7, 11, 16 and 17. Immunohistochemical analysis found a significant overlap with papillary RCC, and some authors believe this is a variant of papillary RCC with spindle cell differentiation.

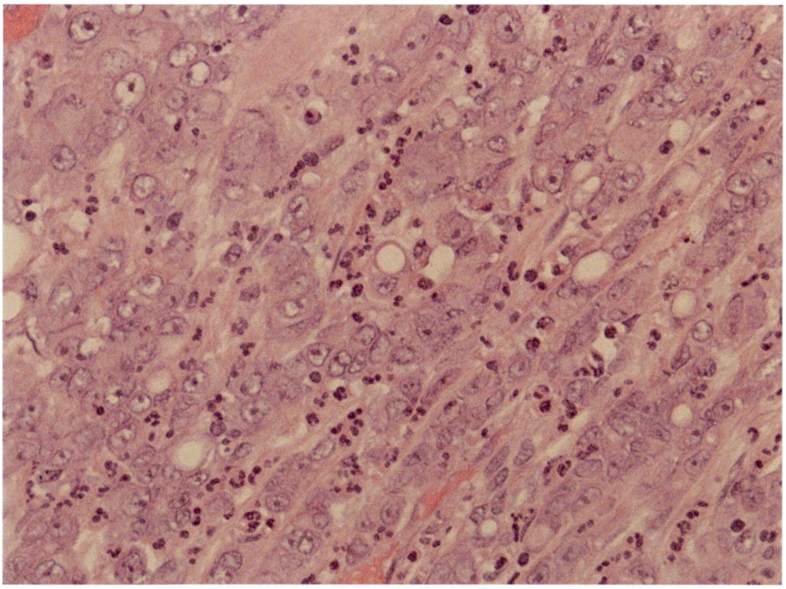

Fig. 1.22 Microscopic appearance of medullary carcinoma with associated inflammation

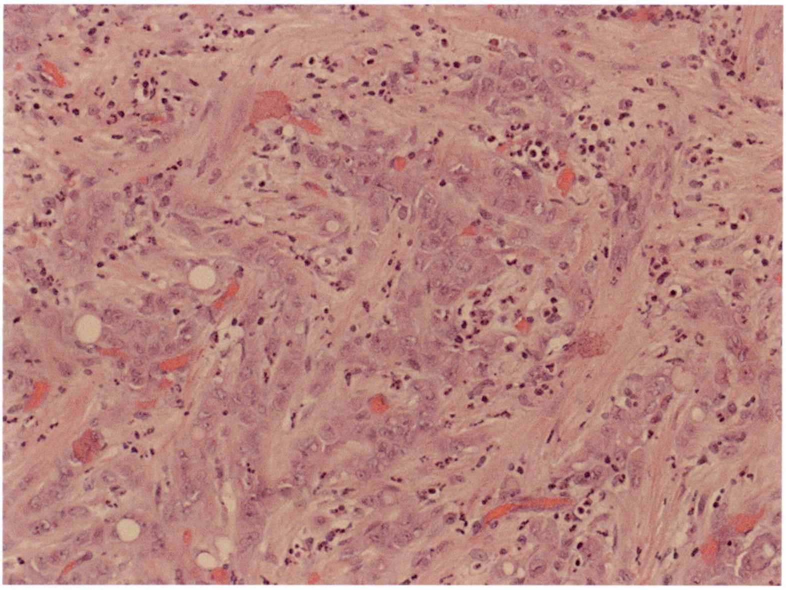

Fig. 1.23 Microscopic appearance of medullary carcinoma with desmoplasia

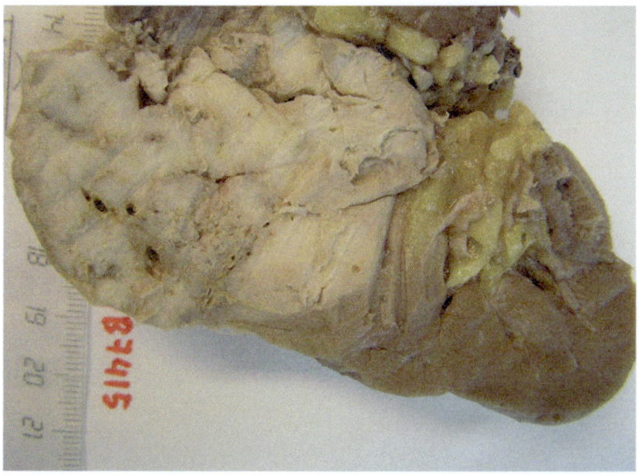

Fig. 1.24 Gross features of mucinous, spindle and tubular tumor

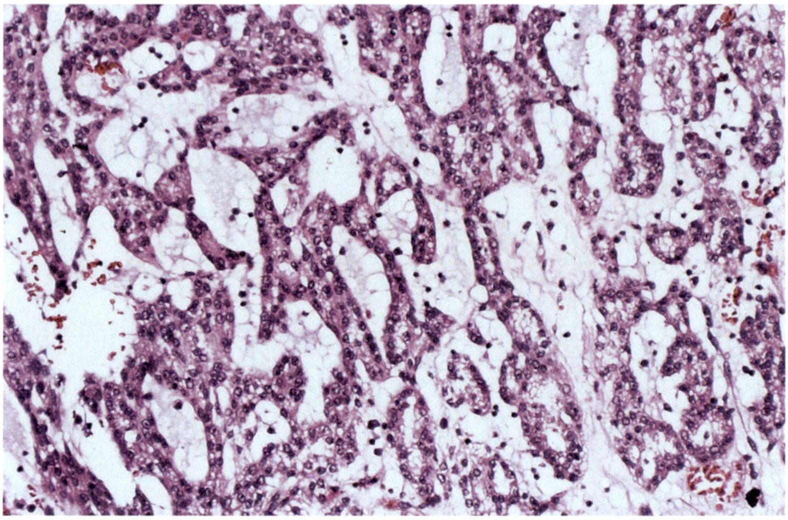

Fig. 1.25 Microscopic features of mucinous, spindle and tubular tumor (mucinous)

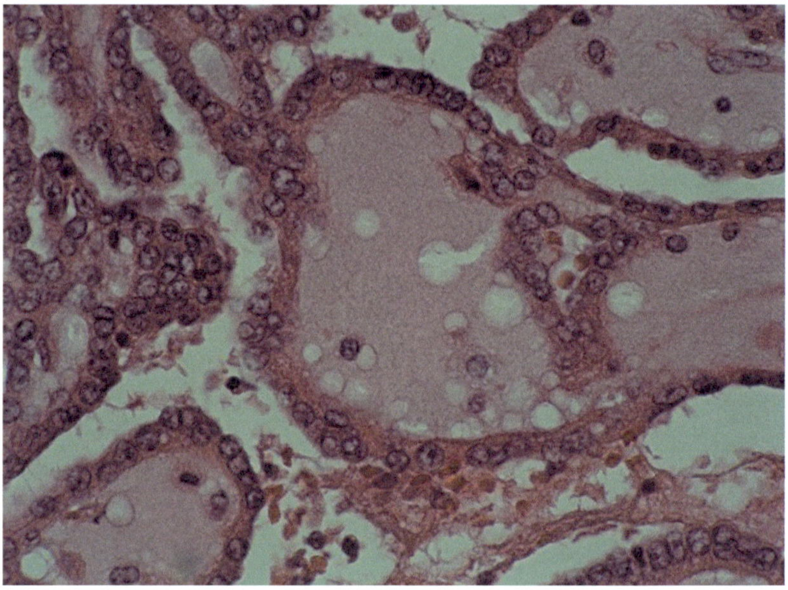

Fig. 1.26 Microscopic features of mucinous, spindle and tubular tumor (tubular)

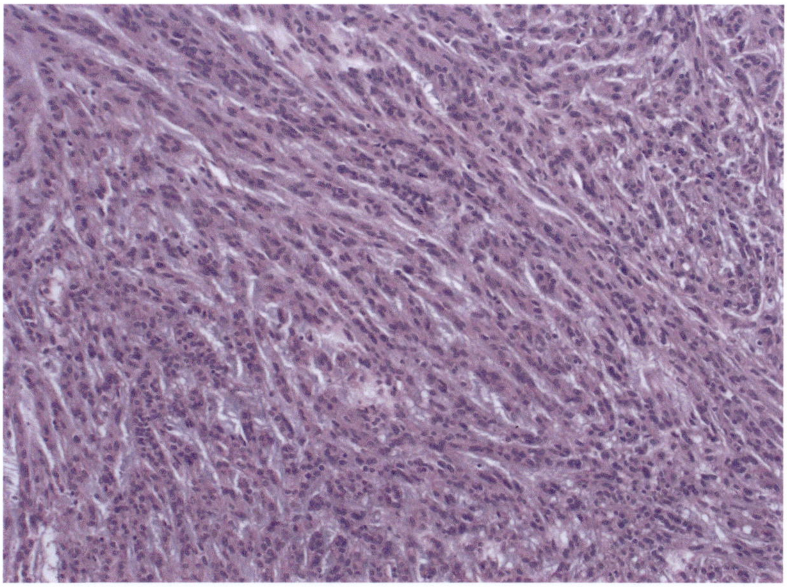

Fig. 1.27 Microscopic features of mucinous, spindle and tubular tumor (spindle)

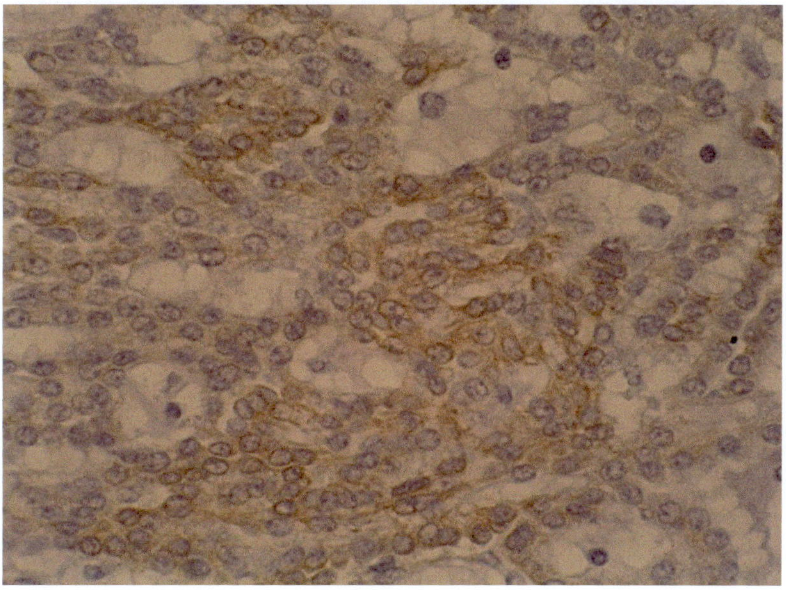

Fig. 1.28 Focal positivity of mucinous, spindle and tubular tumor with 34BE12

- There is a female predominance and the mean age is 50 years at diagnosis. One patient developed metastases on follow-up.

1.4.9 Renal Cell Carcinoma After Neuroblastoma

- A few cases of RCC arise in long term survivors of childhood neuroblastoma. This group is heterogeneous that shows oncocytoid features.
- Allelic imbalances occur at the 20q13 locus. The prognosis is similar to other RCC. Uni- or bilateral lesions develop at mean age of 13 years.

1.4.10 RCC with Sarcomatoid or Rhabdoid Differentiation

- Current WHO classification does not consider sarcomatoid RCC as an entity but rather as a progression of any RCC main type. Pure sarcomatoid morphology without recognizable epithelial elements falls into the unclassified RCC category (Figs. 1.29 and 1.30).
- RCC with sarcomatoid elements show higher proliferative activity than other renal cell carcinoma types and usually exhibit highly malignant behavior with a predilection for increased local invasiveness and a higher likelihood of distant metastasis.
- Sarcomatoid components may be seen in clear cell, papillary, chromophobe and collecting duct carcinomas. It is speculated that the sarcomatoid components of RCC represent areas of dedifferentiation or epithelial-mesenchymal transition.
- Patterns of allelic loss and of nonrandom X-chromosome inactivation in clear cell and sarcomatoid components of RCC from 22 patients and concluded that both clear cell and sarcomatoid components of RCC are derived from the same progenitor cell.
- The specific molecular mechanisms responsible for sarcomatoid transformation of a renal tumor are unknown, although some studies suggest a link with mutations of the TP53 tumor suppressor gene.
- RCC with rhabdoid differentiation is a rare and aggressive neoplasm with poor prognosis. Most patients are at high stage at diagnosis, develop metastases soon after and died of the disease within a year of diagnosis.

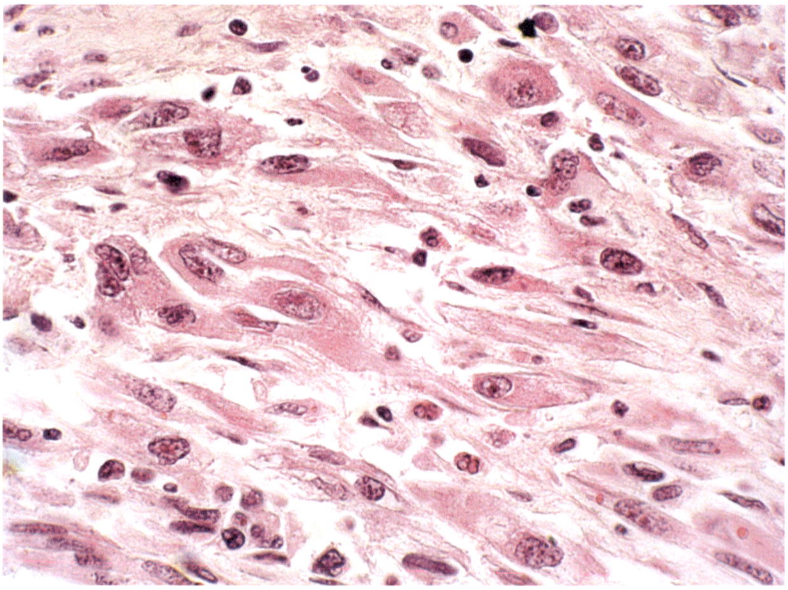

Fig. 1.29 Sarcomatoid renal cell carcinoma

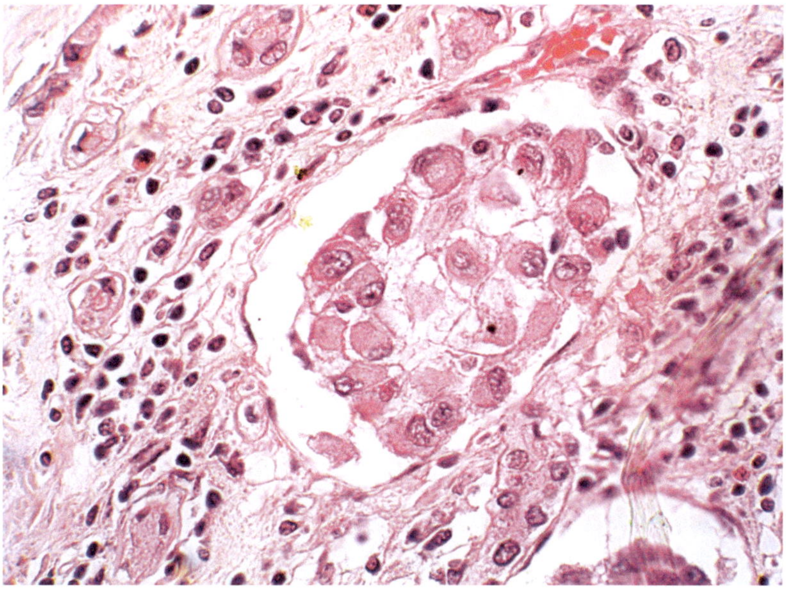

Fig. 1.30 Renal cell carcinoma with rhabdoid features

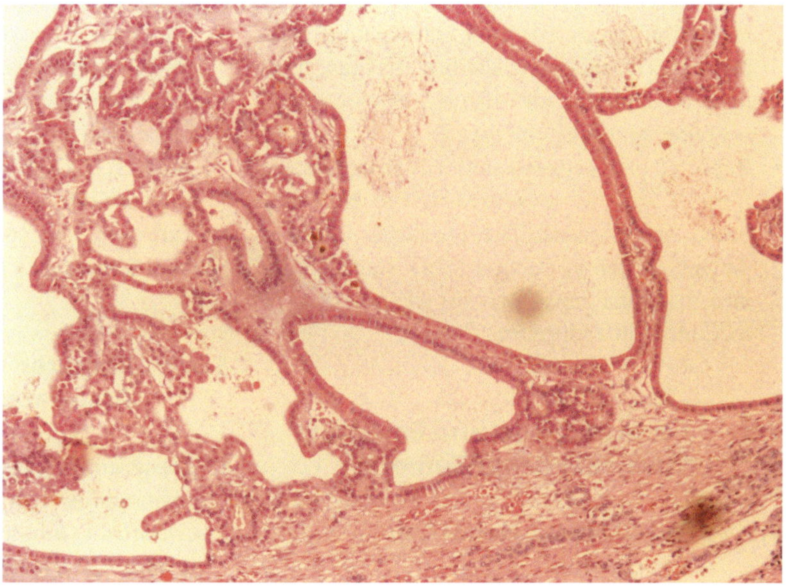

Fig. 1.31 Renal cell carcinoma unclassified with variable sized tubules

- Rhabdoid cells are large with eccentric atypical nucleus and eosinophilic intracytoplasmic inclusion that is positive for vimentin, EMA, and cytokeratin. Sarcomatoid change and rhabdoid features may coexist. Rhabdoid cells show loss of nuclear expression of the transcriptional regulator INI1/SMARCB1

1.4.11 Renal Cell Carcinoma, Unclassified

- It represents 4–6 % of renal tumors. At diagnosis, most are of high grade and stage with poor survival (Figs. 1.31 and 1.32).

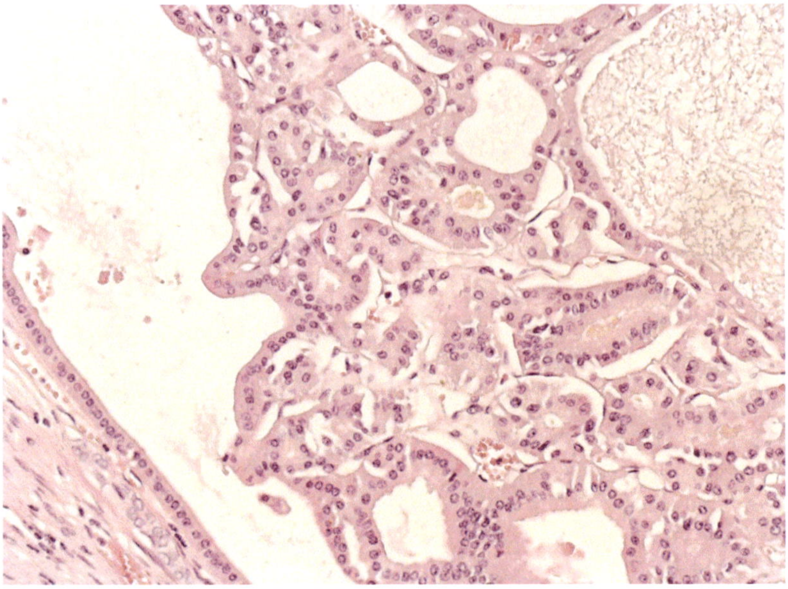

Fig. 1.32 Renal cell carcinoma unclassified with small sized tubules

- The WHO criteria include: (i) composites of recognised types, (ii) pure sarcomatoid morphology, (iii) mucin production, (iv) rare mixtures of epithelial and stromal elements, and (v) unrecognisable cell types.
- Reported data suggests that it is an aggressive form of RCC as confirmed in a recent study based on 56 cases. The prognosis of these patients is mainly related to pT stage, tumor size, vascular invasion, tumor necrosis or recurrence after surgery.

1.5 Proposed New and Emerging Epithelial Renal Tumors

1.5.1 Tubulocystic Renal Cell Carcinoma

- Is a rare renal tumor composed of tubular and cystic structures. The genomic alterations of tubulocystic carcinoma are alike but not identical to those of papillary RCC (Fig. 1.33).
- Like papillary RCC, it often exhibits trisomy of chromosome 17, but it does not show trisomy 7. It does not exhibit monosomy of chromosomes 1, 6, 14, 15, and 22 and frequent allelic loss on chromosomal arms 1q, 6p, 8p, 13q, and 21q, which are frequently seen in collecting duct cancer.
- Immunohistochemistry showed variable expression of CD10, AMACR, parvalbumin, 34βE12, PAX-2, CAIX, CK8, 18, CK19 and occasionally for CK7 and 34βE12.
- Rare cases may present with lymph node metastasis. Some may coexist with papillary RCC.

1.5.2 Acquired Cystic Disease-Associated RCC

- These are composed of cells with abundant eosinophilic cytoplasm and variably solid, cribriform, tubulocystic and papillary architecture. It shows no VHL gene deletions, although gains of chromosomes 7 and 17 are present in some cases.
- Deposits of calcium oxalate crystals are frequent finding in each tumor. One study based on FISH analysis showed no losses or gains of chromosomes 1, 2, 6, 10, or 17 in one tumor; gains of chromosomes 1, 2, and 6 were noted in two tumors, one of these also showed gains of chromosome 10 (Fig. 1.34).

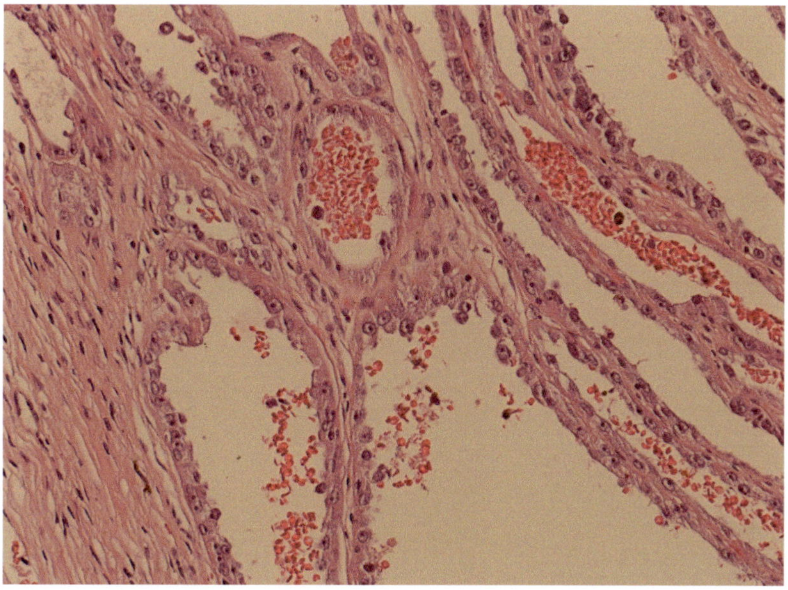

Fig. 1.33 Tubulocystic renal cell carcinoma

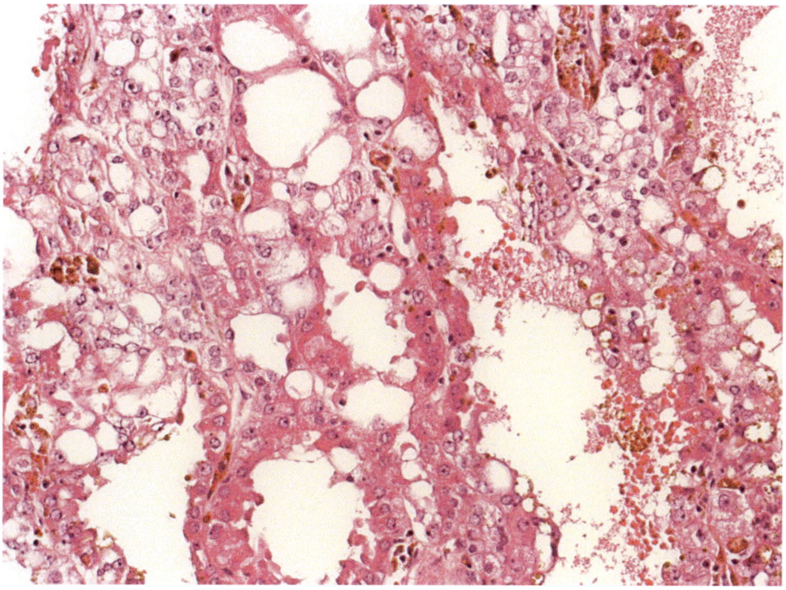

Fig. 1.34 Acquired cystic disease related renal cell carcinoma

1.5.3 Clear Cell Papillary (Tubulo-Papillary) RCC

- These are renal carcinomas composed mainly of papillary structures proliferating within cystic spaces, lined by cells with clear cytoplasm.
- All tumors lacked the gains of chromosome 7 and loss of Y that are typical for papillary renal cell carcinoma and furthermore lack the 3p deletion which is typical of clear cell RCC (Figs. 1.35 and 1.36).
- These tumors also occur in patients unrelated to end-stage renal disease.

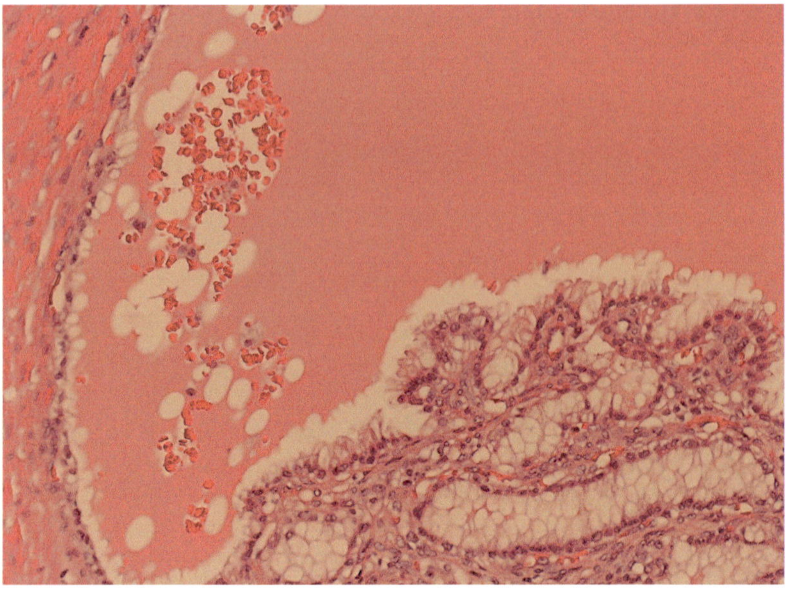

Fig. 1.35 Clear cell papillary renal cell carcinoma, cystic form

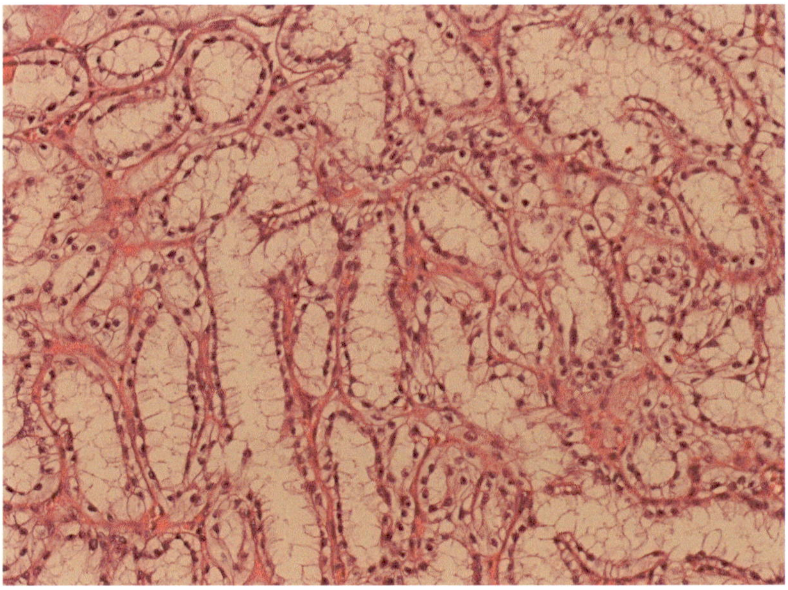

Fig. 1.36 Non-cystic clear cell papillary renal cell carcinoma

1.5.4 MiT Family Translocation RCC

- This type of RCC is defined by different translocations involving chromosome Xp11.2, all resulting in gene fusions involving the TFE3 gene. This carcinoma predominantly affects children and young adults, but may be seen in adults.
- The ASPL-TFE3 translocation carcinomas characteristically present at an advanced stage associated with lymph node metastases. RCC associated with Xp11.2 translocations resemble clear cell RCC on gross examination and seems to have an indolent evolution, even with metastasis (Figs. 1.37 and 1.38).
- The histopathologic appearance is that of a papillary carcinoma with clear cells and cells with granular eosinophilic cytoplasm with foci of calcifications regardless of the type of translocation.
- TFE3 immunostainings were positive in only 82 % of TFE3 translocation carcinomas. Both TFE3 and TFEB renal translocation carcinomas expressed CD10 and alpha-methylacyl-coenzyme-A racemase.
- Another subset of renal tumors are associated with a translocation t(6;11)(p21;q12) involving the transcription factor EB (TFEB). Translocation involving TFE3 and TFEB can be specifically identified by immunohistochemistry, but diagnosis may also be performed by FISH analysis (Fig. 1.39).
- Labeling for PAX8 distinguishes the t(6;11) RCC from epithelioid angiomyolipoma, which otherwise shares a similar immunoprofile.

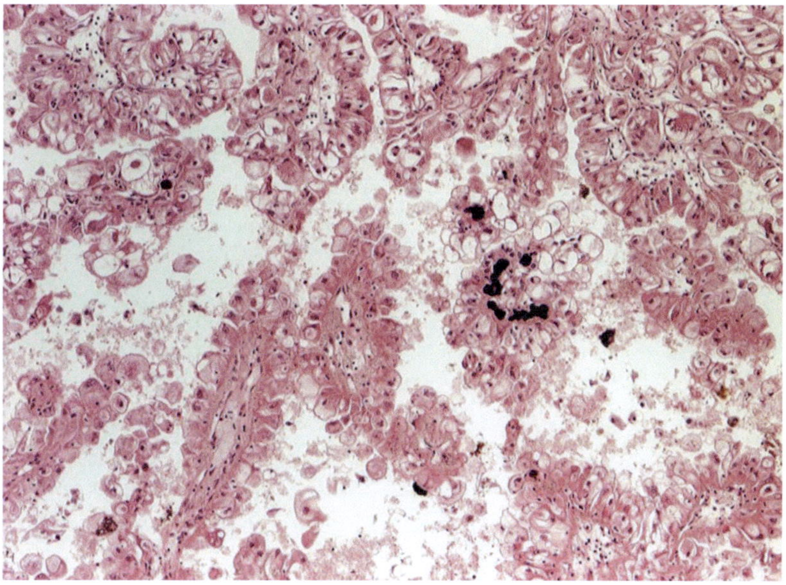

Fig. 1.37 TFE3 translocation carcinoma with papillary architecture and calcification

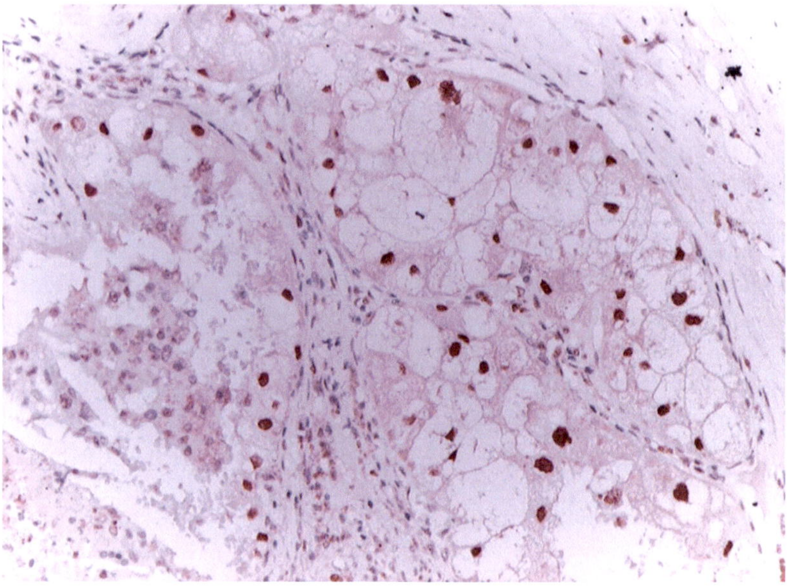

Fig. 1.38 TFE3 positive immunohistochemistry in translocation carcinoma

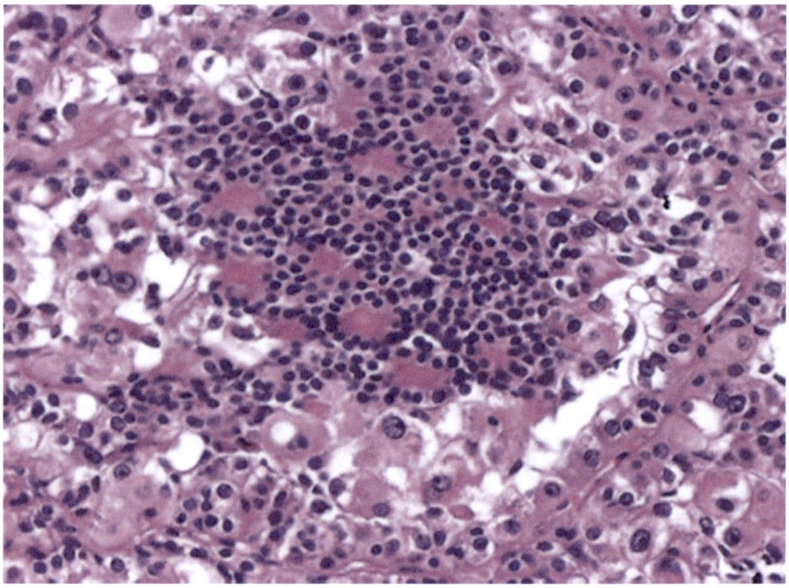

Fig. 1.39 TFEB associated translocation carcinoma

1.5.5 Thyroid-Like Follicular Renal Cell Carcinoma

- It is a rare variant of RCC resembling well differentiated follicular carcinoma of the thyroid gland. These tumors are well circumscribed, tan brown and homogenous.
- Microscopically they consist of tumor follicles of varying size containing dense eosinophilic colloid-like material (Fig. 1.40). The genetics and immunohistochemical expression of these tumors are, as yet, not fully characterized although thyroid follicular cell markers, thyroglobulin and TTF-1 are negative.
- The majority of cases reported to date have shown an indolent behavior, although metastases to lymph nodes in two cases and a single case with pulmonary metastases have been reported.

1.5.6 Succinic Dehydrogenase B Deficiency Associated Renal Cell Carcinoma

- These tumors are seen in patients within germline Succinate Dehydrogenase B mutation, which is associated with a syndrome characterized by pheochromocytoma, paraganglioma and type 2 gastrointestinal stromal tumors.
- Microscopically these tumors are characterized by the presence of compact nests of eosinophilic polygonal cells. Cytoplasmic vacuoles and pale eosinophilic cytoplasmic inclusions are commonly seen and these represent giant mitochondria.
- Less than ten cases have been reported to date and follow-up is limited. Of note, sarcomatoid change was identified in two patients with metastatic disease, one of whom died of tumor related causes.

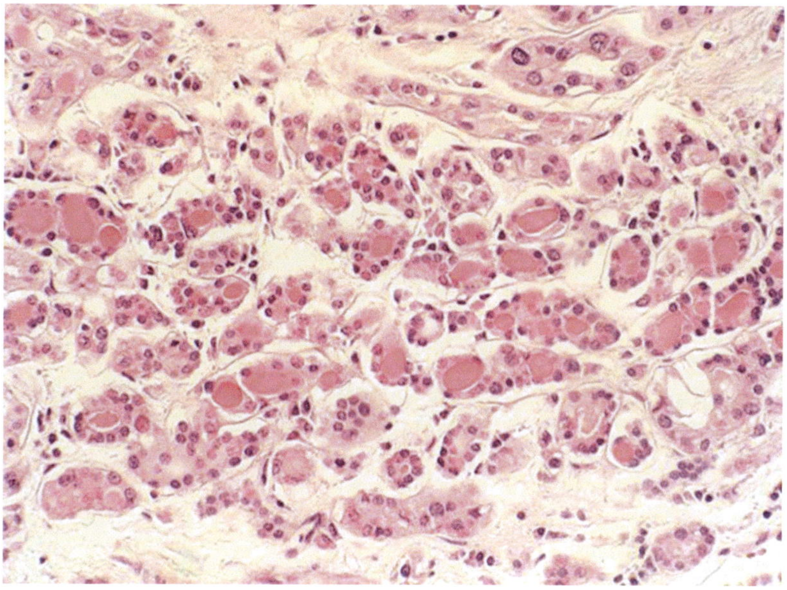

Fig. 1.40 Thyroid-like follicular renal cell carcinoma

1.5.7 ALK-Translocation Renal Cell Carcinoma

- A fusion of the anaplastic lymphoma kinase (*ALK*) gene with the gene for the cytoskeletal protein vinculin (*VCL*) resulting from the translocation t(2:10)(p23;q22) has been reported in two tumors observed in young patients.
- *VCL-ALK* translocation RCC appear to have a characteristic appearance, consisting of cells with a polygonal to spindled morphology with abundant eosinophilic cytoplasm and frequent intracytoplasmic lumina.
- While these two cases were associated with sickle cell trait, two further RCCs showing *ALK* fusion with different partner genes have been described in older patients, although neither of these showed a sickle cell association.
- Two additional cases of RCC demonstrating *ALK* fusion (fusion partner unknown) have been reported in adult patients that behave aggressively.
- A recent case showing *VCL-ALK* RCC in a child with sickle-cell trait has been recently reported.

1.5.8 Renal Cell Carcinoma with Smooth Muscle Stroma

- The stroma of clear cell tubulo-papillary RCC not infrequently demonstrates smooth muscle metaplasia. The extreme end of this spectrum includes tumors reported as renal angiomyoadenomatous tumor (RAT) to reflect the prominence of smooth muscle (Fig. 1.41).
- RATs appear to have the same clinic pathologic and immunohistochemical characteristics as clear cell tubulo-papillary RCC.

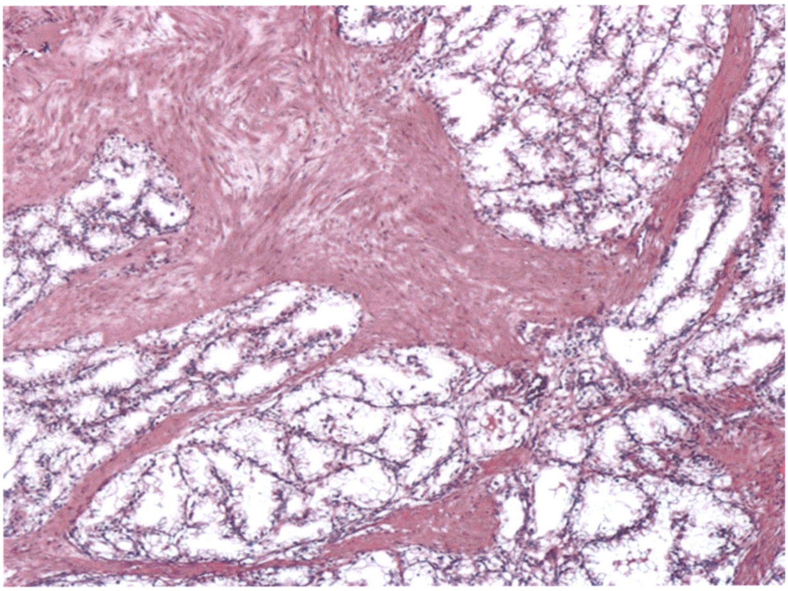

Fig. 1.41 Leiomyomatous renal cell carcinoma

- Smooth muscle stromal metaplasia has also been reported in association with clear cell RCC and Xp11 translocation RCC. Hence, it is suggested that smooth muscle metaplasia in the kidney may be a nonspecific common reaction to a variety of stimuli.
- A recent molecular study demonstrated that clear cell RCC with smooth muscle stroma lacks chromosome 3p and VHL alterations, thus suggesting that clear cell RCC with smooth muscle stroma should be considered an entity distinct from clear cell RCC.

1.5.9 Tuberous Sclerosis-Associated Renal Cell Carcinoma

- Tuberous sclerosis complex (TSC) is an autosomal dominant disorder with characteristic tumors involving multiple organ systems. Whereas renal angiomyolipoma (AML) is common in TSC, renal cell carcinoma (RCC) is rarely reported with a recent study on 57 RCCs from 13 female and 5 male TSC patients (Fig. 1.42).
- Mean age at surgery was 42 years. 50 % had multiple synchronous and/or metachronous RCCs (range of 2–20 RCCs) and 5 had bilateral RCCs (28 %). Ninety-four percent had histologically confirmed concurrent renal AMLs, including AMLs with epithelial cysts. None of the 15 patients with available clinical follow-up information had evidence of distant metastatic disease from 6 to 198 months after their initial surgery (mean: 52 months).
- Three major distinct morphologies were seen in TSC-associated RCC: (i) 17 RCCs (30 %) had features similar to tumors previously described as RCC with smooth muscle stroma; (ii) 34 RCCs (59 %) showed features similar to chromophobe RCC; and (iii) 6 RCCs (11 %) showed a granular eosinophilic-macrocystic morphology.
- Distinct histologic changes were also commonly present in the background kidney parenchyma and included cysts or renal tubules lined by epithelial cells with prominent eosinophilic cytoplasm, nucleomegaly, and nucleoli.
- Immunohistochemically, all RCCs tested showed strong nuclear reactivity for PAX8 and HMB45 negativity. Compared with sporadic RCCs, TSC-associated RCCs have unique clinicopathologic features including female predominance, younger age at diagnosis, multiplicity, association with AMLs, 3 distinctive histologic patterns, and an indolent clinical course.

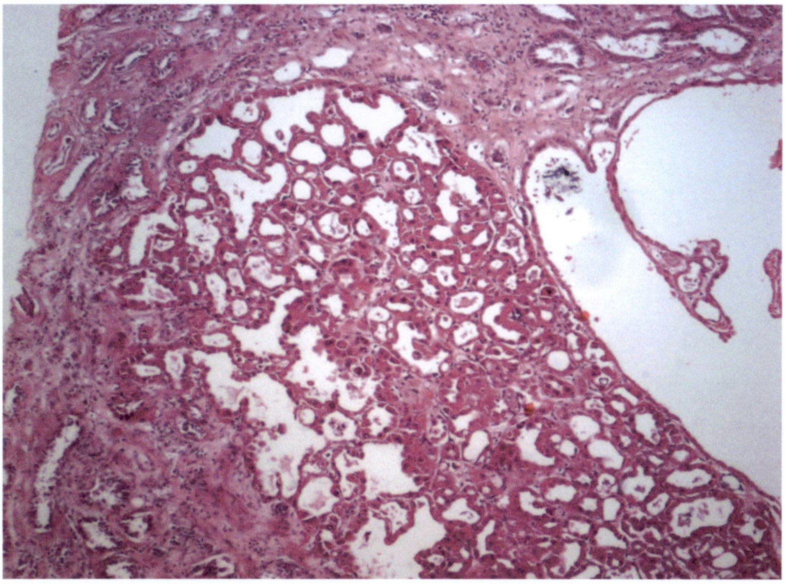

Fig. 1.42 Tuberous sclerosis associated renal cell carcinoma

1.6 Benign Tumors

1.6.1 Papillary Adenoma

- Papillary adenoma is usually solitary, 0.5 cm or smaller, well circumscribed, greyish or white lesion in the renal cortex that shows a tubulo-papillary architecture similar to cellular types 1 and 2 in papillary RCC.
- Papillary adenoma is the most common neoplasm of the epithelium of the renal tubules (Fig. 1.43). It is found in 10–40 % of specimens and shows genetic alterations similar to papillary RCC but less extensive. "Renal adenomatosis" refers to the occasional occurrence of multiple and/or bilateral papillary adenomas.

1.6.2 Metanephric Tumors

- This group includes metanephric adenoma, metanephric adenofibroma and metanephric stromal tumor.
- Metanephric adenoma is an epithelial neoplasm that occurs in children and adults with female preponderance; half are incidental. An exceptional case with metastasis has been reported, and therefore, appropriated follow-up is advised (Figs. 1.44 and 1.45).
- Rarely, it may coexist with Wilms' tumor or RCC. A case of high grade sarcoma arising in association with metanephric adenoma (metanephric adenosarcoma) has been described. Metanephric adenomas are 3–6 cm, usually solitary and not encapsulated. Metanephric adenoma has a normal karyotype.
- Metanephric adenofibroma shows an epithelial component similar to metanephric adenoma which is embedded in a fibroblast-like stroma.
- Rare cases of metanephric stromal tumor, entirely composed of stromal elements showing entrapped glomerulus with juxtaglomerular cell hyperplasia have been described.

1.6.3 Renal Oncocytoma

- Oncocytoma is a benign renal epithelial neoplasm that derives from the intercalated cells. It is well circumscribed, non-encapsulated, mahogany-brown or pale yellow with a central stellate scar. Tumor architecture may be nested, organoid (classic), tubulocytic, or mixed (Figs. 1.46, 1.47 and 1.48).
- The "oncocyte" has densely granular eosinophilic cytoplasm and round and regular nuclei. Mitotic activity and necrosis are

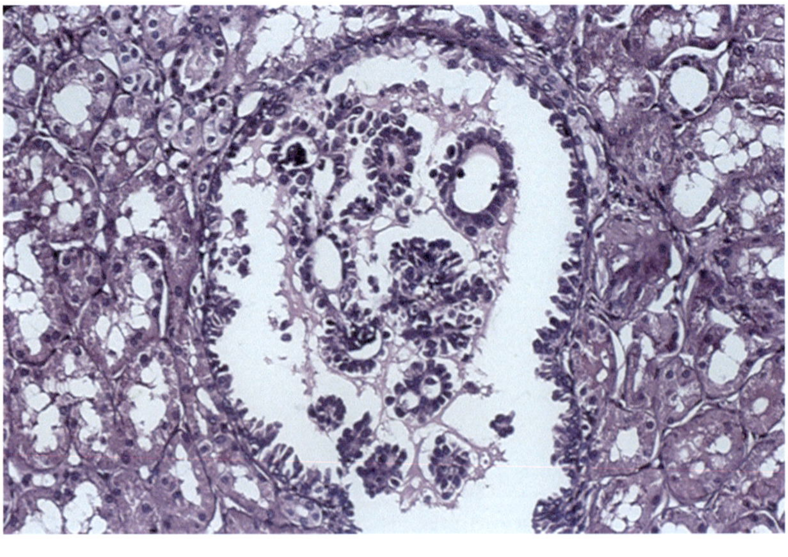

Fig. 1.43 Cortical papillary adenoma

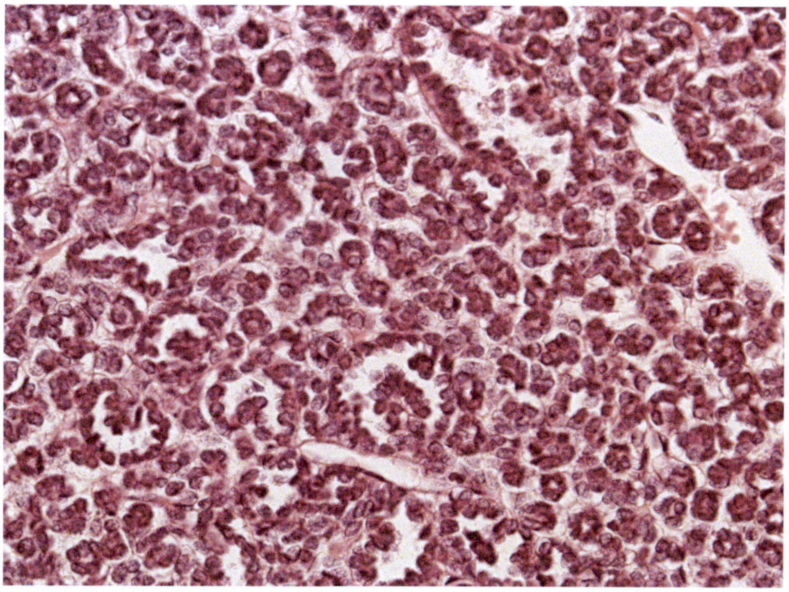

Fig. 1.44 Metanephric adenoma, tubular type

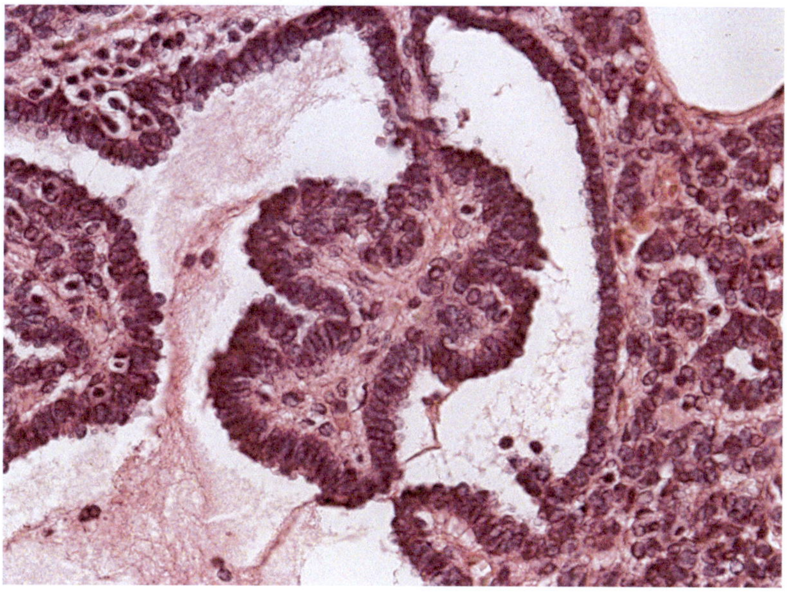

Fig. 1.45 Metanephric adenoma with focal papillary configuration

uncommon. Degenerative type nuclear atypia (endocrine-type), occasional clear cells embedded in hyalinized stroma, dilated tubules, minute papillary projections, focal extension into perinephric fat, or scattered binucleated cells may be focally present is some cases.

- Findings not permissible in the diagnosis of oncocytoma include areas of clear cell or spindle cell carcinoma, prominent papillary architecture, macroscopic or conspicuous microscopic necrosis, and significant mitotic activity (including atypical mitosis).

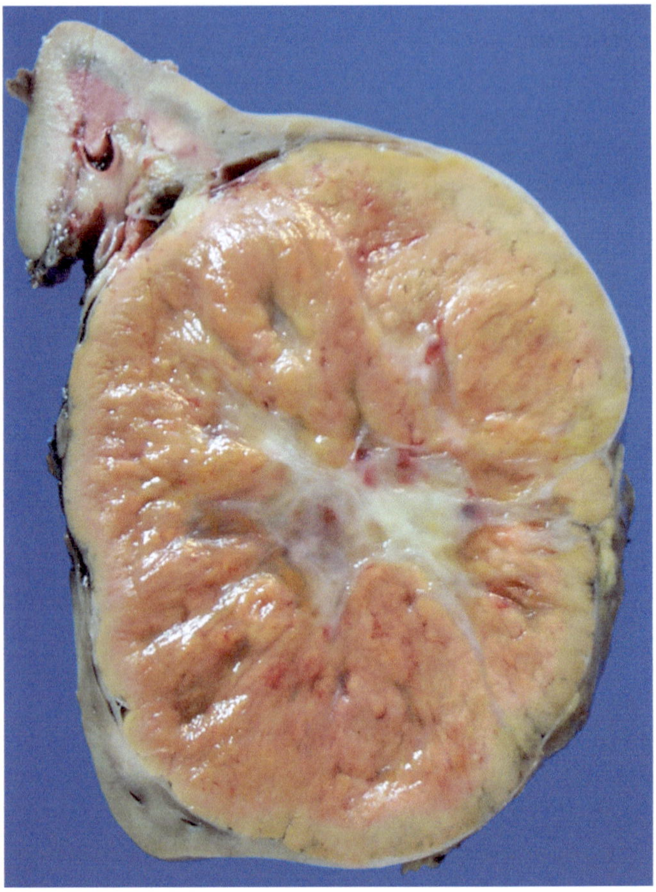

Fig. 1.46 Gross features of oncoytoma

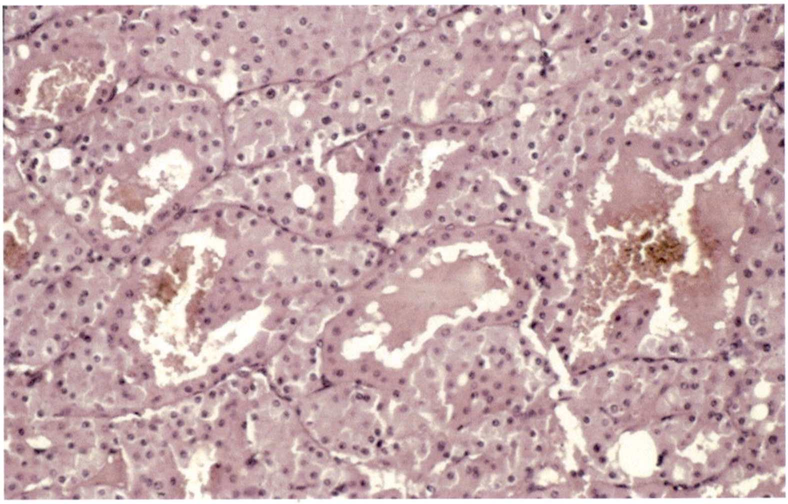

Fig. 1.47 Microscopic features of oncocytoma (low power)

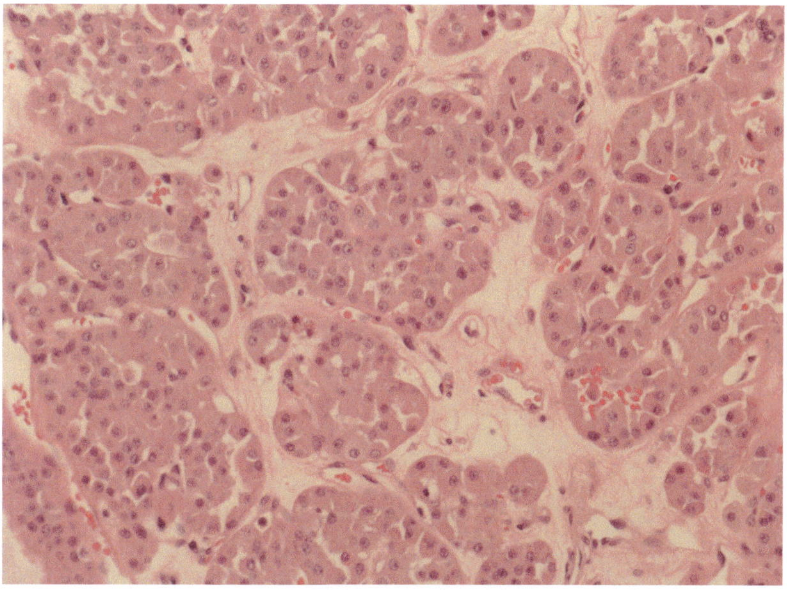

Fig. 1.48 Microscopic features of oncocytoma (high power)

- Oncocytoma comprises 3–9 % of all primary renal neoplasms. Most are incidental and sporadic but few are symptomatic.
- The eosinophilic variants of chromophobe RCC are difficult to distinguish from renal oncocytomas on hematoxylin and eosin stained sections. The distinction is important, as chromophobe renal cell carcinoma is a malignant tumor while oncocytoma is benign. Hale's colloidal iron stain shows a diffuse and strong reticular pattern in almost 100 % of chromophobe RCC, and it is frequently patchy and focal in oncocytoma. Immunohistochemistry is of help in distinction of oncocytoma from chromophobe RCC, mainly the eosinophilic variant (Table 1.6). Most oncocytomas are positive for kidney specific-cadherin, CD117, parvalbumin, and S100A1, and negative for CK7 (or focal positive), Moc31, EpCam, and CD82.
- Reports of "malignant" or "metastatic" oncocytomas are postulated to actually represent misdiagnosed chromophobe renal cell carcinomas. Chromosomes 1 and/or 14 loss and alterations of mitochondrial DNA are frequent.
- The term oncocytosis (oncocytomatosis) refers to a small subset of oncocytic tumors removed surgically because of a dominant mass that microscopically has the features of oncocytoma, although some may have either chromophobe RCC or hybrid features.

1.7 Percutaneous Biopsy of Renal Tumours

- Renal tumour biopsy today has limited morbidity and allows histologic diagnosis in the majority of cases.
- The increasing incidence of small renal masses, the development of conservative and minimally invasive treatments for low-risk RCC and benign renal tumors, and the discovery of targeted treatments for metastatic disease have provided the rationale for indications of percutaneous renal tumour biopsy.
- Renal tumor biopsy can avoid unnecessary surgeries, can confirm success after thermal ablation of small renal masses and support the selection of the appropriate systemic therapy for metastatic RCC.

- Current diagnostic yield of biopsies ranges from 78 to 100 %, with sensitivity and specificity for the diagnosis of 86–100 % and 100 %, respectively. Diagnostic accuracy for tumour subtyping ranges from 86 to 98 %.
- An immunohistochemical panel, including parvalbumin, CD10, a-methylacyl-coenzyme A racemase, cathepsin K, S100A1, cytokeratin 7, and carbonic anhydrase IX, seems to be the most promising.

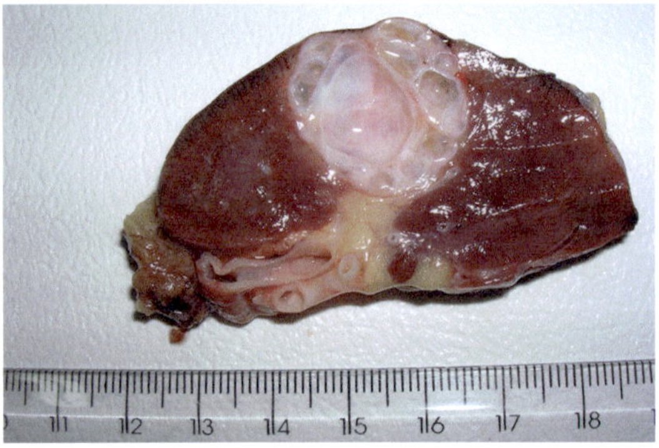

Fig. 1.49 Cystic Nephroma, gross features

1.8 Cystic Nephroma and Mixed Epithelial and Stromal Tumors

- Cystic Nephroma is a benign mixed epithelial and stromal neoplasm frequently unilateral, encapsulated, solitary and multilocular with no solid areas or necrosis (Figs. 1.49 and 1.50).
- Adult cases present after age of 30 with female predominance. Some are associated with pleuropulmonary blastoma. Clonal analysis supports its neoplastic nature.

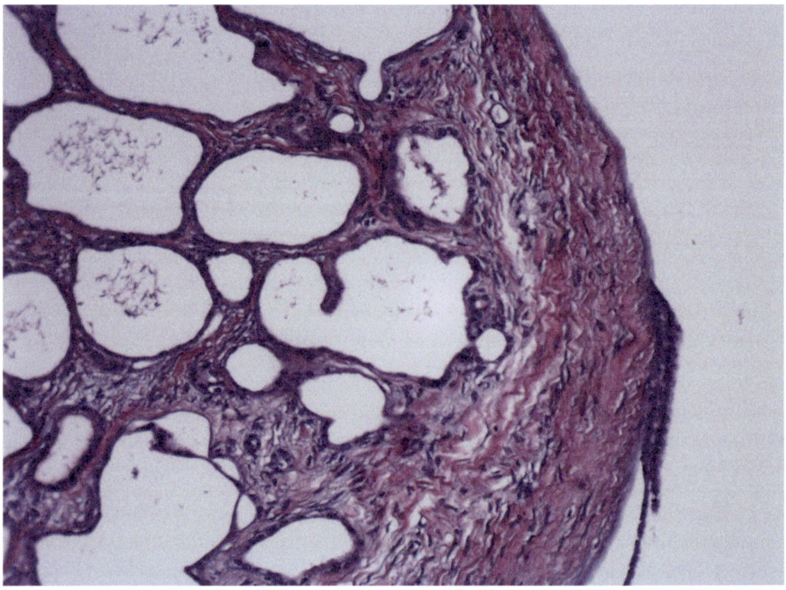

Fig. 1.50 Cystic Nephroma, microscopic features

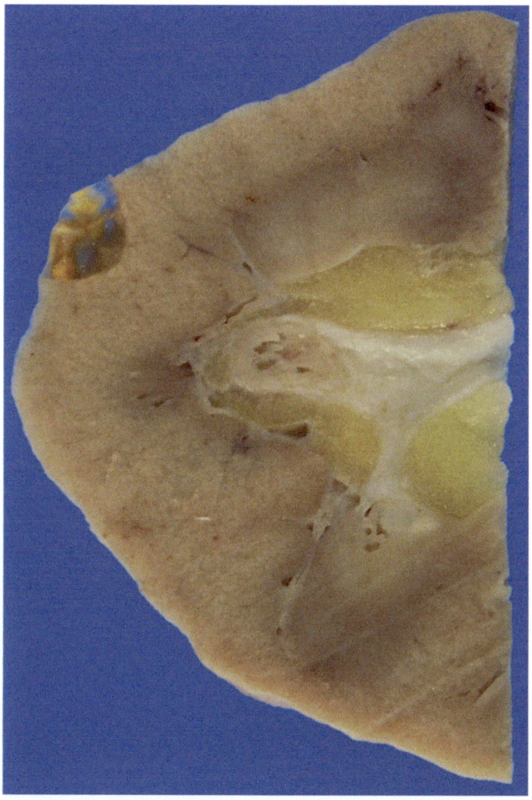

Fig. 1.51 Gross features of a benign mixed epithelial-stromal tumor

- Mixed epithelial and stromal tumor of kidney is a rare renal neoplasm composed of a mixture of stromal solid areas and epithelial (mostly cystic) elements previously reported as cystic hamartoma of renal pelvis or adult mesoblastic nephroma. Some stromal cells react with antibodies to estrogen and progesterone (Figs. 1.51 and 1.52).
- There is a female predominance with history of estrogen therapy. All cases have been seen in adults. Some may experience malignant sarcomatous transformation of the stromal component (Figs. 1.53, 1.54, 1.55 and 1.56).
- Some authors suggest that cystic nephroma and mixed epithelial and stromal tumors are part of the same spectrum of lesions, and therefore, they should be named as "renal epithelial and stromal tumor".

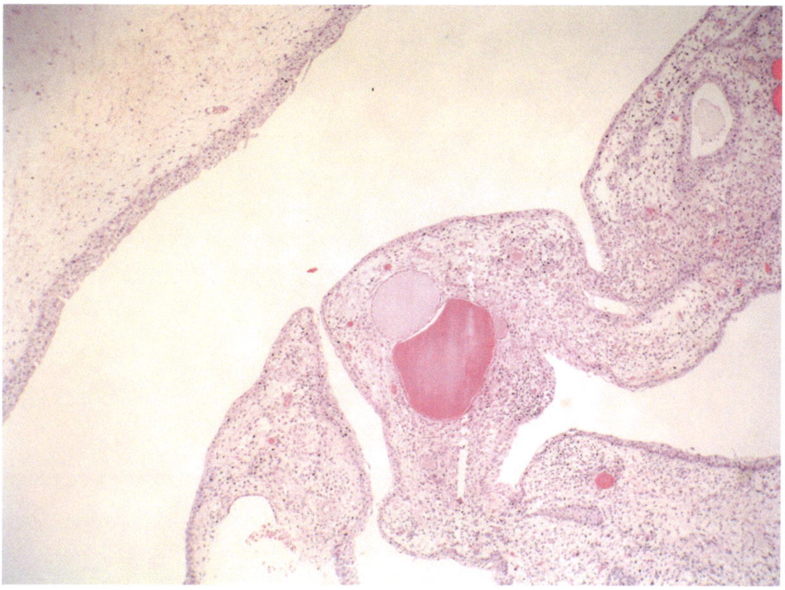

Fig. 1.52 Microscopic features suggest benign lesion

Fig. 1.53 Gross features of mixed epithelial-stromal with malignant transformation

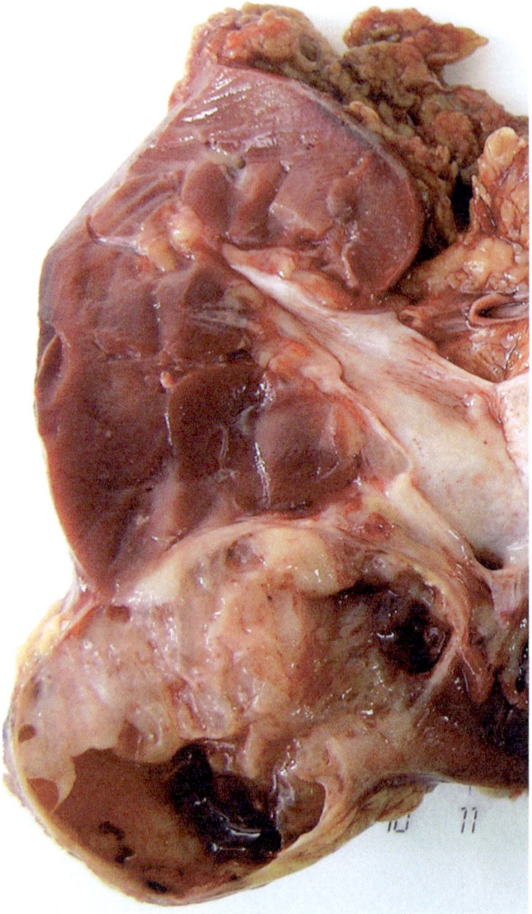

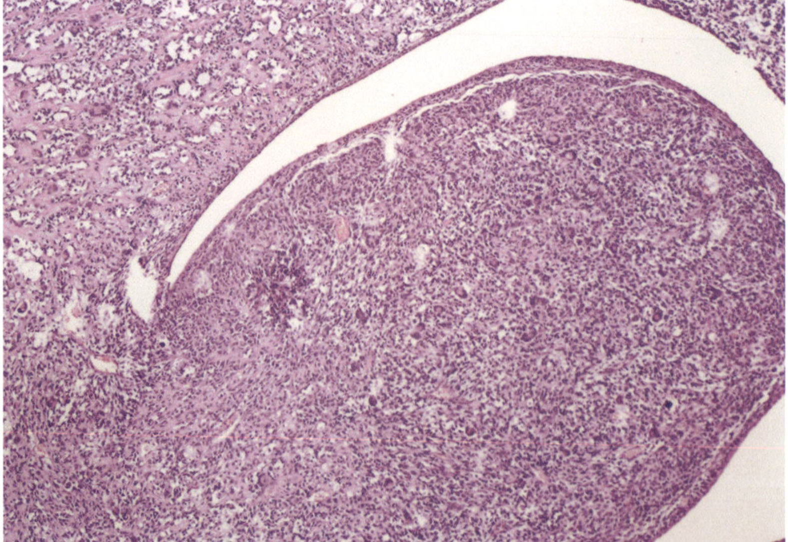

Fig. 1.54 Microscopic features of mixed epithelial-stromal tumor with rhabdomyosarcoma

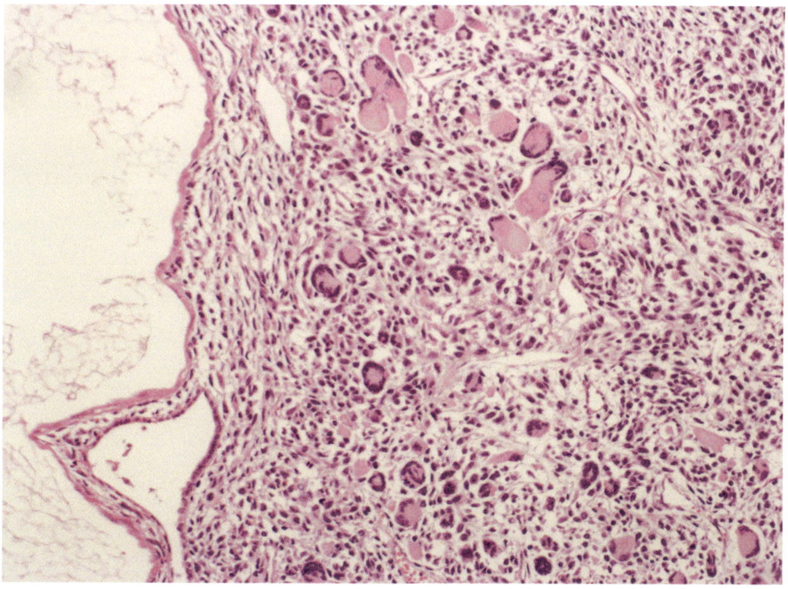

Fig. 1.55 High power view of image Fig. 1.54

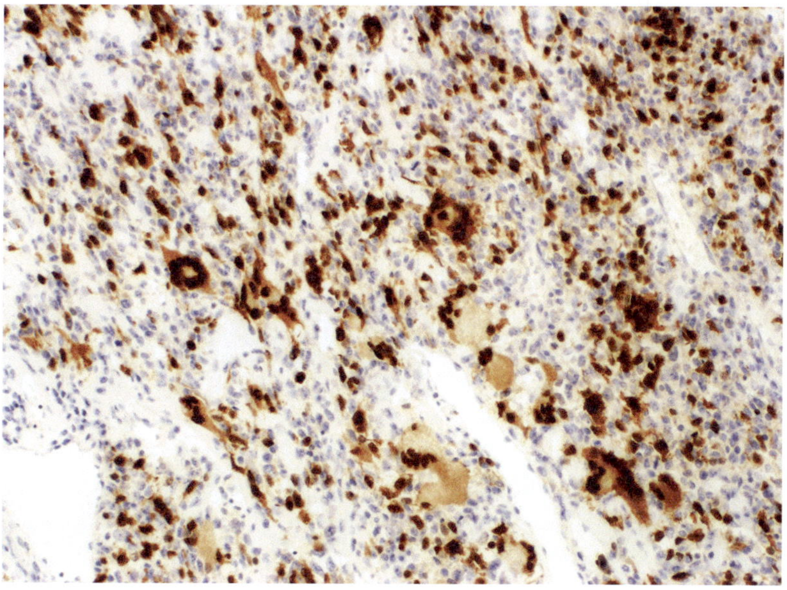

Fig. 1.56 Myogenin highlight muscle differentiation

1.9 Soft Tissue Tumors

1.9.1 Medullary Fibroma

- Also known as renomedullary interstitial cell tumor. These tumors are frequently multiple and found incidentally at autopsy or surgery for another condition. Tumors are un-encapsulated, circumscribed, white or grey, and paucicellular, measuring 0.1–0.5 cm (Fig. 1.57).
- The cells are small stellate, spindle or polygonal in a loose basophilic stroma and seems to originate from prostaglandin-producing interstitial cells in renal medulla. Tubules maybe entrapped at the periphery. Amyloid deposits may be present.

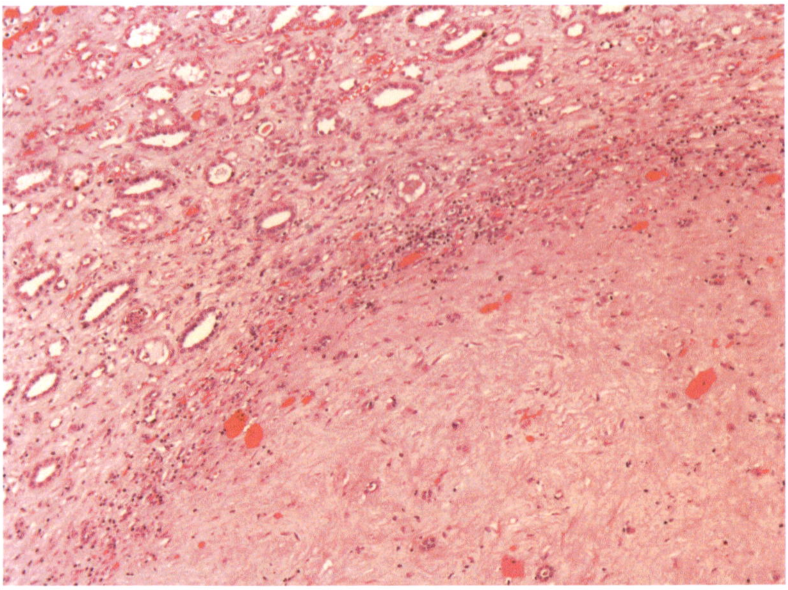

Fig. 1.57 Medullary fibroma

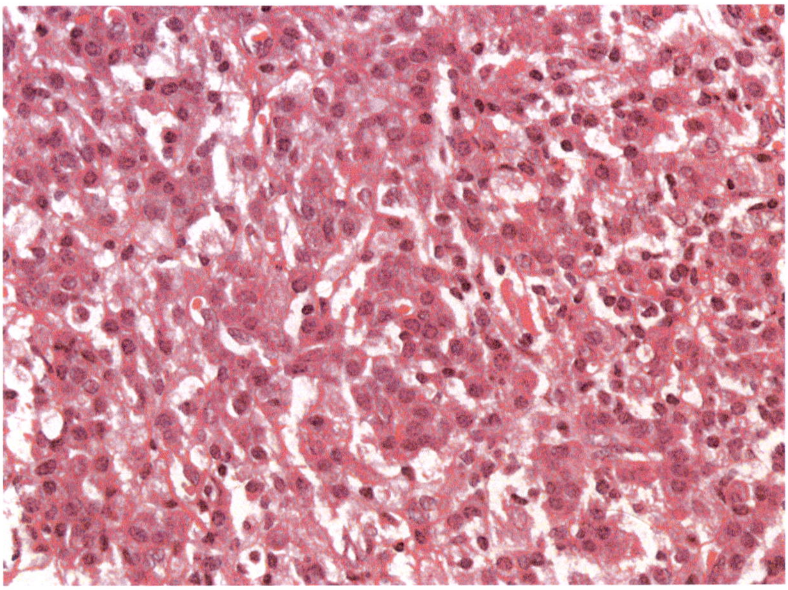

Fig. 1.58 Microscopic features of juxtaglomerular cell tumor

1.9.2 Juxtaglomerular Cell Tumor

- A benign renin-secreting tumor derived from modified smooth muscle cells of the juxtaglomerular apparatus in patients with refractory hypertension and high plasma rennin activity (Fig. 1.58).
- Most tumors are <4 cm unilateral, encapsulated, solitary, cortical and occur in females (mean age of 27 years). Histologically, sheets of uniform round, polygonal or spindled cells are present with uniform, round to oval nuclei with scattered mitotic figures.
- Thin and thick-walled blood vessels are often prominent. Immunoreactivity for renin, actin, vimentin, and CD34 is characteristic. Ultrastructurally, cells contain rhomboid renin-specific crystals.

1.9.3 Glomus Tumor

- A few cases of primary renal glomus tumor have been reported. There has been male predominance with a wide age range (17–80 years). Most cases are incidental and benign.
- The cut surface is frequently gelatinous and tumors size reach up to 8 cm in diameter. Microscopic features include cells that are usually small, round to oval, with eosinophilic to amphophilic cytoplasm with a delicate fibrovascular stroma.
- There may present solid, myxoid or glomangioma architectural patterns. Tumor cells react with smooth muscle actin, laminin (pericellular) an focally with CD34. Epithelial markers are not present.

1.9.4 Angiomyolipoma

- Angiomyolipoma (AML) is a benign tumor associated with several hereditary disorders including von Recklinghausen disease, von Hippel–Lindau syndrome, Autosomal dominant (adult) polycystic kidney disease or Tuberous sclerosis.
- It occurs in 80 % of patients with tuberous sclerosis. The mean age of patients with "sporadic" AML ranges 45–55 years but drops to 25–35 years of age in patients with tuberous sclerosis.
- AML is thought to be derived from perivascular epithelioid cell. AML frequently exhibits loss of heterozygosity in portions of the *TSC2* gene locus on chromosome 16p13 (in both sporadic and tuberous sclerosis cases), and less often in the *TSC1* gene on chromosome 9q34.
- It may occur in renal cortex, medulla or in perirenal soft tissues and may coexist with other renal neoplasms (RCC, oncocytoma) or being associated with lymphangioleiomyomatosis of lung.
- AML is typically unencapsulated, yellow to tan-pink, range from 3 to 20 cm and is composed of variable admixtures of mature adipose tissue, smooth muscle and abnormally formed blood vessels. Smooth muscle proliferations often appear to spin off perpendicularly from the outer layers of blood vessel walls (Figs. 1.59, 1.60 and 1.61).
- Smooth muscle cells may be spindled with mild degrees of nuclear atypia. Involvement of intrarenal veins, renal vein, vena cava, and regional lymph nodes are indicative of multifocal growth, rather than invasion or metastasis.

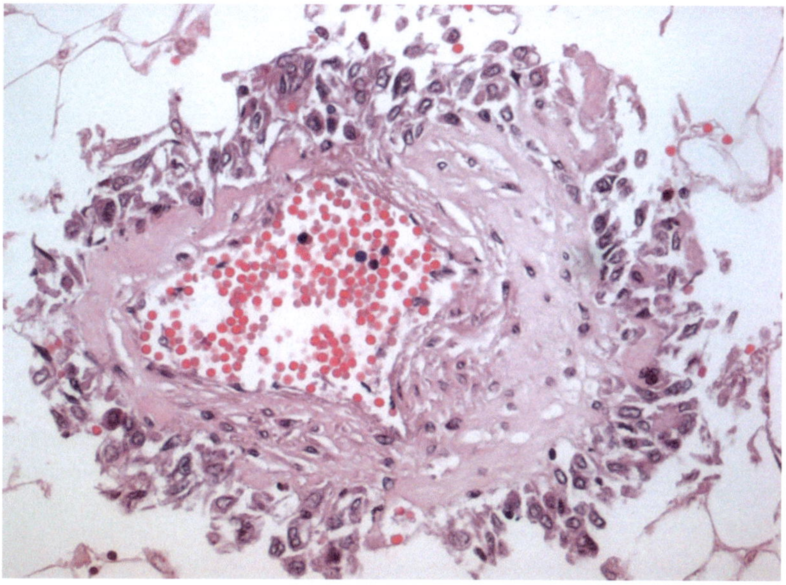

Fig. 1.59 Angiomyolipoma with perivascular arrangement of cells

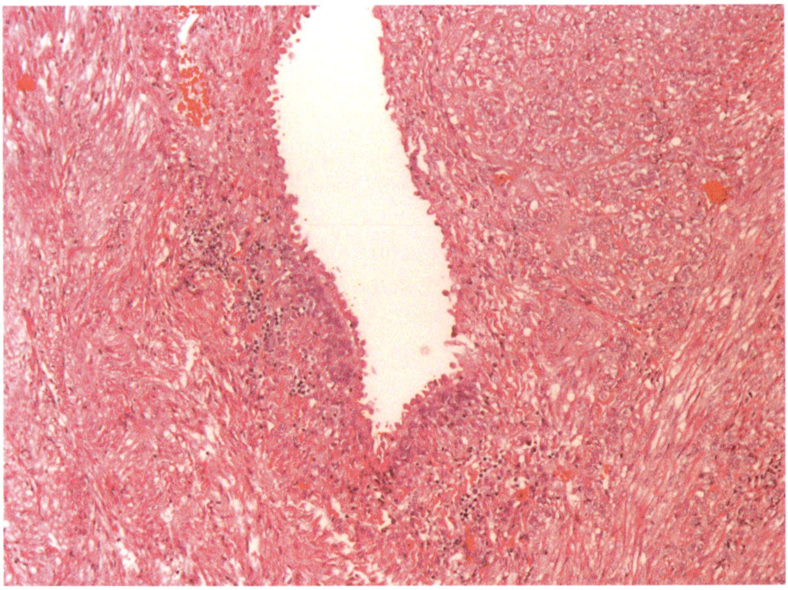

Fig. 1.60 Angiomyolipoma with epithelial cyst

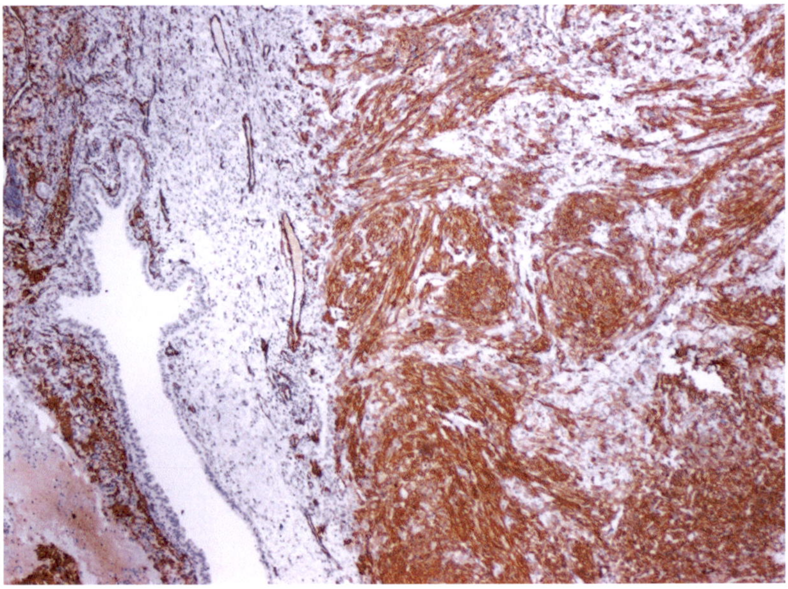

Fig. 1.61 Melan-A is positive in leiomyomatous cells

- AML is characterized by coexpression of melanocytic markers (HMB-45, CD63, MART-1/Melan A, microphthalmia transcription factor) and smooth muscle markers (muscle-specific actin, smooth-muscle actin, desmin) (Table 1.7).

1.9.5 Epithelioid Angiomyolipoma

- A potentially malignant mesenchymal neoplasm closely related to classic AML. Half of recorded cases have a history of tuberous sclerosis. Tumors exhibit allelic loss of the *TS2-containing* region.

Table 1.7 Immunohistochemical markers useful in differential diagnosis of renal tumors

Tumor histotype	Positive	Negative
Clear cell RCC	vimentin, keratin, EMA, CD10, Pax 2/8, RCCm, CAIX (membrane), CD15	CK7, parvalbumin, Kidney specific -cadherin
Papillary RCC	Keratin, CK7, AMACR, RCCm	CD117, Kidney specific -cadherin, parvalbumin, WT1
Chromophobe RCC	E-cadherin, Kidney specific -cadherin, CD117, EMA, CK AE1/AE3, CK7	vimentin, CAIX, and AMACR
Oncocytoma	Kidney specific-cadherin, CD117, parvalbumin, S100A1	CK7 (or focal positive), Moc31, EpCam, CD82
Collecting duct carcinoma	EMA, p63, CK7, HMWCK, Pax 2, Pax 8	CD10, RCCm, and CK20
Metanephric adenoma	S100, WT1, CD57	AMACR, RCCm
Translocation RCC	TFE3, TFEB, CD10, RCCm	CK (or weak positive)
Clear cell papillary RCC	CK7, Pax 2, Pax 8, CAIX (basolateral)	AMACR, RCCm
RCC with sarcomatoid features	CK7, Pax 2/Pax 8, CD10, vimentin, and AMACR	
Angiomyolipoma	HMB45, melan-A, and SMA	CK, CD10, RCCm, Pax 2, Pax 8
Urothelial carcinoma	CK, CK7, CK20, p63, thrombomodulin, uroplakin III, uroplakin II	RCCm, CD10, Pax 2, Pax 8

- Most are large, hemorrhagic, and locally infiltrative with sheets of cytologically malignant epithelioid cells, and is easy to misdiagnose as high grade carcinoma. The immunohistochemical profile is similar to that of classic AML. Some patients had metastasis and/or tumor related death.

1.9.6 Leiomyoma

- Rare benign smooth muscle tumors morphologically similar to those seen in other parts of the body. Smooth muscle predominant AML is more common. Therefore to accept a tumor as leiomyoma it must have convincing immunohistochemical evidence that the tumor is not an AML.
- Leiomyoma seems to arise from the capsule or renal parenchyma. As in other parts are solid, circumscribed rubbery masses. Microscopically, consist of bundles of smooth muscle fibers without nuclear pleomorphism. The finding of necrosis, nuclear atypia and atypical mitoses suggest leiomyosarcoma.

1.9.7 Lipoma

- A few lipomas arising in the kidney are on record. These are yellow, lobulated masses of variable size. As confounding factor, large tumors may have focal necrosis and hemorrhage.
- Histologic features of mature fat tissue without nuclear atypia is the hallmark of this tumor.
- The differential diagnosis includes AML, retroperitoneal lipoma and liposarcoma. Before a tumor can be accepted as renal lipoma rather than AML with predominant fat tissue, it must be widely sampled and a panel of immunohistochemical markers should be applied.
- Antibodies to HMB45, Melan-A, Catepsine K, SMA, desmin, estrogen receptor and progesterone receptor should give negative results before sign out the case as renal lipoma. Retroperitoneal lipoma how no vascular attachment to the kidney, and liposarcoma may be differentiated by pathologic investigation.

1.9.8 Hemangioma

- More frequently are solitary lesions seen in adults but about 10 % of patients may develop multiple and bilateral tumors. Hemangioma may be associated with Klippel-Trenaunay and Sturge-Weber syndromes.
- Most frequently occur in the medulla and papilla with a wise range in size (<1 cm to 21 cm). Microscopically, these lesions are composed of vascular spaces with large variation in size, some of which may have smooth muscle in their walls.

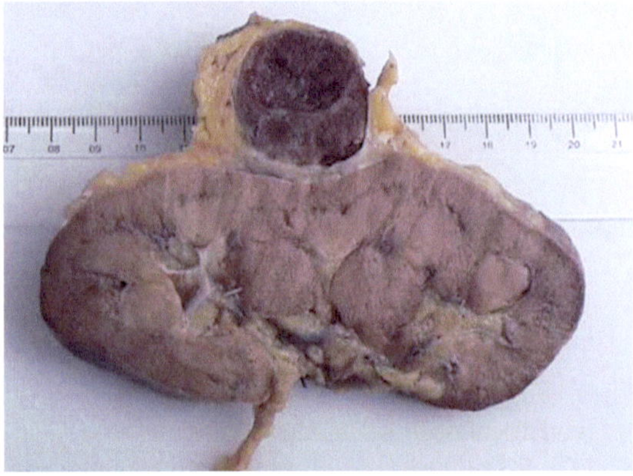

Fig. 1.62 Gross features of a renal hemangiona

- Thrombosis and organization is common, as well as extramedulary hematopoiesis. Capillary, cavernous or mixed types are most common but other types may be recognized. These lesions often have endothelium with a hobnail appearance and zones of sclerosis within the vessels.
- Hemangioma lack capsule and have irregular border. The lack of mitosis and cellular atypia supports its benign nature (Figs. 1.62 and 1.63).

1.9.9 Lymphangioma

- Presents as unilateral or bilateral tumor mass seen in both adults and children. May arise in the renal parenchyma, renal capsule, renal sinus or peripelvic tissues.
- Grossly are encapsulated masses of small cysts containing clear fluid, localized to the subcapsular cortex or may diffusely involve the kidney.
- Microscopically, lymphangioma consist of spaces lined by bland endothelial cells with fibrous septa that may contain smooth muscle.
- Main differential diagnosis is cystic nephroma. Lymphangioma does not have the ovarian-

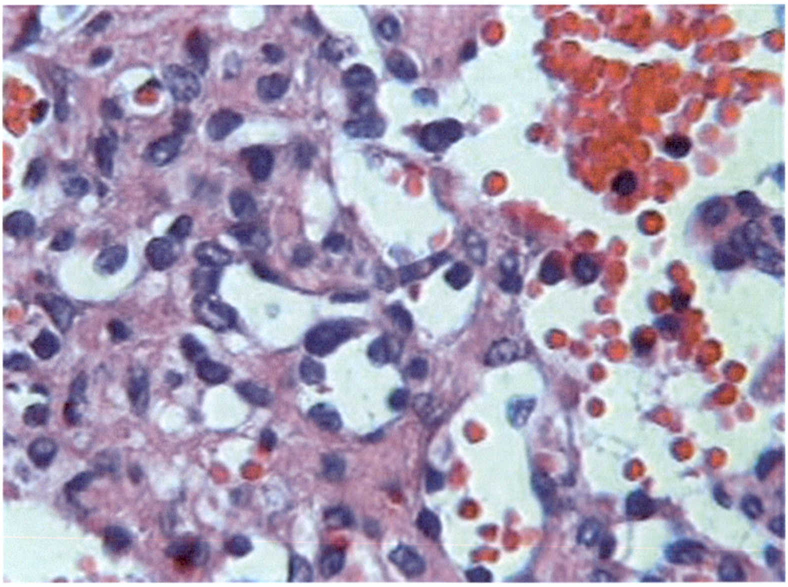

Fig. 1.63 Microscopic features of hemangioma

type stroma typical of cystic nephroma, and the endothelial cells are positive for CD31 and D2-40 (podoplanin).
- It is a benign neoplasia occasionally related to VHL gene mutation and abnormalities of chromosome 7 and X. May coexist with hemangioma in the same kidney.

1.9.10 Schwannoma

- This is a rare occurrence in the kidney with patients range 12–90 years of age and about equal gender distribution. Seems to be a benign tumor. Most frequently occurs with the renal sinus but may occur intrarenal or arise from the renal capsule.
- The size is variable and microscopically resemble peripheral nerve schwannoma from elsewhere devoid of atypia, necrosis and mitosis. Variable positivity with S100 protein is typical in this tumor.

1.9.11 Solitary Fibrous Tumor

- Spindle cell neoplasm that is most common in the pleura. It is rare, with equal gender distribution and age range from childhood to middle-age. May be incidentally detected.
- Most tumors present with size of about 10 cm of diameter. May originate from renal parenchyma or the capsule, and are usually circumscribed.
- Microscopically, the tumor consists of spindle cells exhibiting minimal nuclear pleomorphism. Storiform or fascicular architecture may be seen as well as hypocellular collagenous areas. Dilated vessels with hemangiopericytoma patter may be seen.
- Rare cases may behave as malignant, and those cases show grossly visible tumor necrosis, high mitotic count (2-7/10HPF), and extrarenal extension.
- Differential diagnosis include sarcomatoid carcinoma and spindle cell tumor of neural or smooth muscle origin, and immunohistochemistry is helpful.
- Strong diffuse positive reaction for CD34, bcl-2 and CD99 is the hallmark of this tumor. Sarcomatoid carcinoma is frequently positive for pancytokeratin and neural and smooth muscle neoplasm are positive for S100 or smooth muscle, respectively Table 1.7.

1.9.12 Leiomyosarcoma

- Is the most common renal sarcoma, constitutes 0.1 % of invasive renal tumors and 50 % of primary renal sarcomas. The age of presentation is largely variable with most cases within the fifth to sixth decade. The tumors usually arise in the renal sinus and originate from renal vasculature or the wall of the renal pelvis. May also originate from renal capsule.
- Usually are large tumors (mean 14 cm) showing a gray-white firm whorled cut surface. They are often well circumscribed and may have a pseudocapsule.
- Microscopically consist of sheets and fascicles of spindled cells with evident nuclear pleomorphism, and mitotic rate ranging 0–50 per 10 HPF. Tumor necrosis and vascular invasion are frequently seen. Some tumors may appear myxoid on histologic evaluation (Figs. 1.64, 1.65 and 1.66).
- Main differential diagnosis includes epithelioid AML, leiomyoma, and sarcomatoid carcinoma. Sarcomatoid carcinoma may be positive for CKAE1/AE3 and PAX8, although frequently focal. A wide sampling of these specimens might be necessary to achieve the correct pathologic diagnosis.
- AML may have a smooth-muscle predominant morphology and therefore is positive for smooth-muscle markers in addition to Melan A and HMB45, and therefore should be negative before the diagnosis of leiomyosarcoma is made.
- Metastases are frequent at diagnosis.

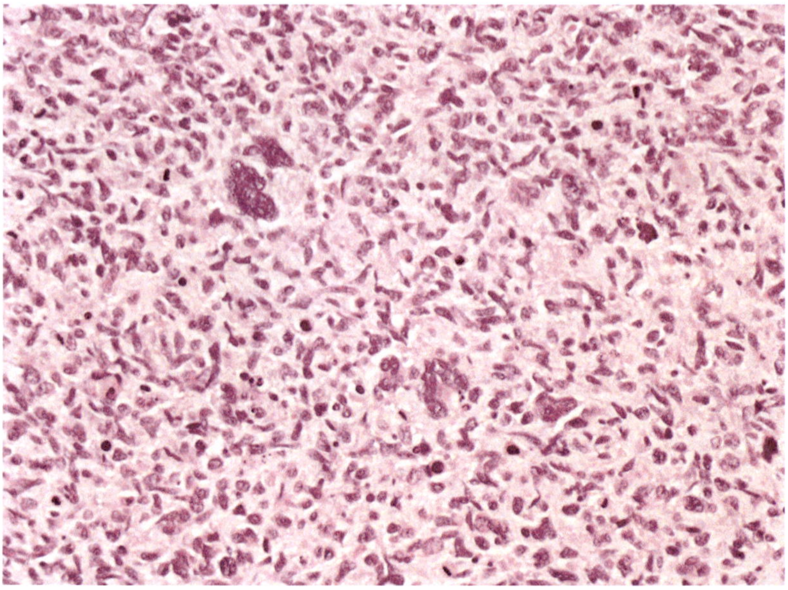

Fig. 1.64 Leiomyosarcoma of the kidney with myxoid appearance

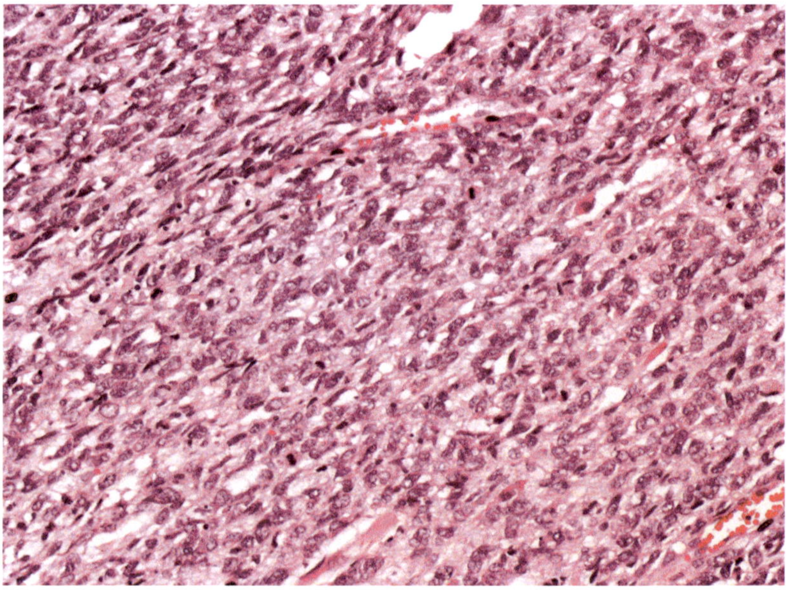

Fig. 1.65 Leiomyosarcoma of the kidney with high mitotic count

1.9.13 Angiosarcoma

- When primary, it is an uncommon neoplasia seen adult patients with male predominance. Grossly are ill defined, hemorrhagic, and may be multifocal. Microscopically, there is variable cellularity with interdigitating vascular spaces.
- Nuclear pleomorphism and high mitotic rate are characteristic of this tumor. Angiosarcoma show positive expression of CD31 and CD34. Metastases to the lungs, bone, and liver are common, frequently at time of presentation.

1.9.14 Liposarcoma

- Primary renal liposarcoma is rare with most cases involving the kidney of perirenal origin. Most described cases arise from the renal sinus in adults 50–60 years old.

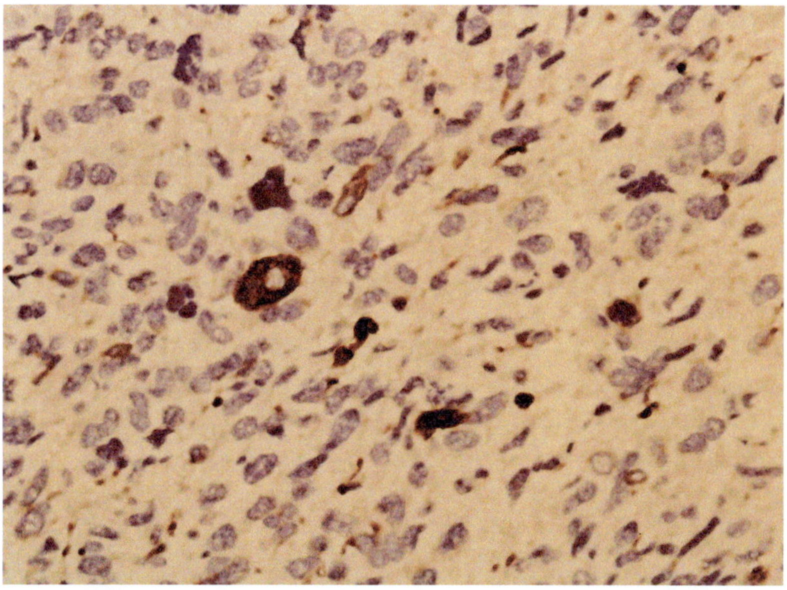

Fig. 1.66 Leiomyosarcoma of the kidney is focally positive for smooth muscle actin

- Grossly are large, frequently lobulated and yellow. These tumors show the same histologic patterns seen elsewhere in the body. Myxoid type seems to be the most frequent. Main differential diagnosis is AML and immunohistochemistry is of great value in these cases.

1.9.15 Rhabdomyosarcoma

- Rare tumors with equal gender distribution observed from early childhood to elderly patients. Tumors are typically large with histologic features of embryonal or pleomorphic rhabdomyosarcoma.
- As in other renal sarcomas, it is necessary to exclude sarcoma elsewhere and sarcomatoid carcinoma that may mimic virtually all types of sarcoma. A positive WT1 stain would indicate Willms tumor, an important differential diagnosis in childhood cases.

1.9.16 Malignant Fibrous Histiocytoma

- Primary tumors are rare with only a few reported cases are well documented. It is always difficult to ascertain whether the kidney is involved primarily or by extension from retroperitoneal primary.
- Patients are middle aged or older and tumors are usually large exhibiting haemorrhage and necrosis. The storiform and pleomorphic histology is characteristic of this tumor.

1.9.17 Hemangiopericytoma

- It is a neoplasm originating from pericytes. Most cases arise in the kidney capsule or perirrenal soft tissues. Patient's age ranges 15–70 years. Tumors range 1.5–24 cm, are well circumscribed but un-encapsulated.
- Histologically hemangiopericytoma is composed of sheets of tightly packed round to spindle shaped cells with elongated nuclei, separated by numerous slitlike and occasionally staghorn-shaped vascular spaces lines by endothelial cells.
- Tumor cells lack hyperchromasia or pleomorphism. Tumor cells show positive immunostaining for CD34, and negative immunostaining for CD31, actin, and CD99. No pathologic feature is predictive of outcome. About 50 % of patients die of their disease.
- Hemangioperocytoma may be difficult to distinguish from solitary fibrous tumor owing to their common expression of CD34.

- Some authorities consider that cases of hemangiopericytoma in the past should be considered to be solitary fibrous tumor.

1.9.18 Hemangioblastoma

- Hemangioblastoma is a benign, morphologically distinctive neoplasm that typically occurs in the central nervous system either in the setting of von Hippel-Lindau disease or more often sporadically. Extraneural hemangioblastoma is exceptional and raises a challenging differential diagnosis.
- Primary renal hemangioblastoma is exceedingly rare with less than 10 reported cases. Histologically, the tumor presents sheets of polygonal epithelioid stromal cells with ample pale or eosinophilic, vacuolated cytoplasm in an arborizing capillary network. It is considered a vascular tumor of borderline malignancy.
- Tumor cells showed variable nuclear pleomorphism, intranuclear cytoplasmic invaginations, scattered hyaline globules, and psammoma-like calcifications. Some areas showed branching hemangiopericytoma-like vessels with tumor cells radiating from the wall, while other areas were edematous and hyalinized with sparse stromal cells and abundant reticular vessels.
- Immunohistochemically, the tumor cells reacted strongly and diffusely with antibodies to PAX8, CD10, α-inhibin, S100 protein, neuron-specific enolase, and vimentin, and they showed focal positivity with antibodies to epithelial membrane antigen and AE1/AE3.
- A case of clear cell renal cell carcinoma with hemangioblastoma-like features has been recently described. The tumor expressed PAX8 and α-inhibin. The patient was 49-year-old man without stigmata of von Hippel-Lindau disease.

1.9.19 Osteosarcoma

- Extraosseous osteogenic sarcoma can occur anywhere in the body, but its location in renal tissue is exceedingly rare. Twenty-four cases of primary osteosarcoma of the kidney have been reported.
- Most frequently, these tumors are stage III or IV at diagnosis. Surgery, chemotherapy, and radiotherapy are often palliative treatments for this tumor, and the prognosis is poor. The diagnosis is based on radiologic and histologic findings.
- Grossly osteosarcoma of the kidney is gray-white, with hemorrhage, necrosis, and bony hard areas. Microscopically, the tumor are composed of pleomorphic polygonal to spindled cells with associated fibrous stroma and osteoid formation with lacelike ossification.
- Osteoclastic cells may be present. Abundant mitotic activity is frequently seen. And atypical cartilage formation is usually present. Histologic features of low-grade, chondroblastic, and osteoblastic osteosarcoma may be seen. Tumor size ranged from 3 to 27 cm (Figs. 1.67, 1.68 and 1.69).

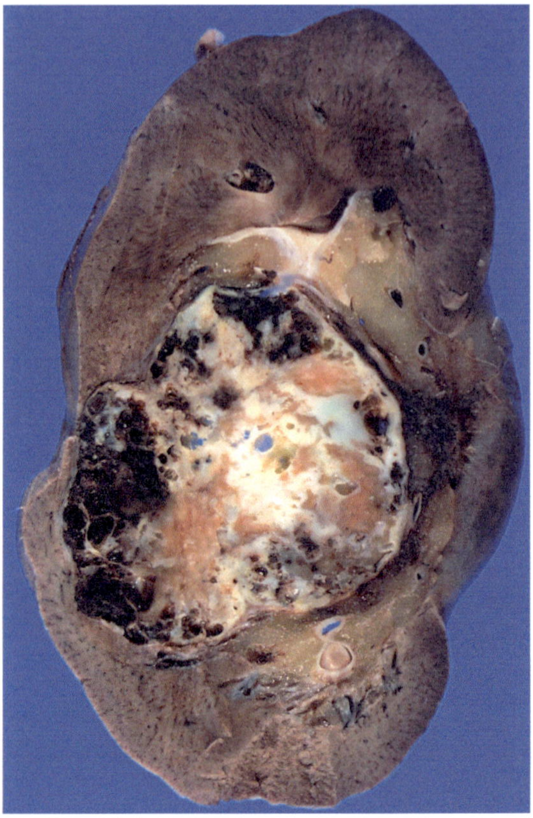

Fig. 1.67 Gross appearance of primary renal osteosarcoma

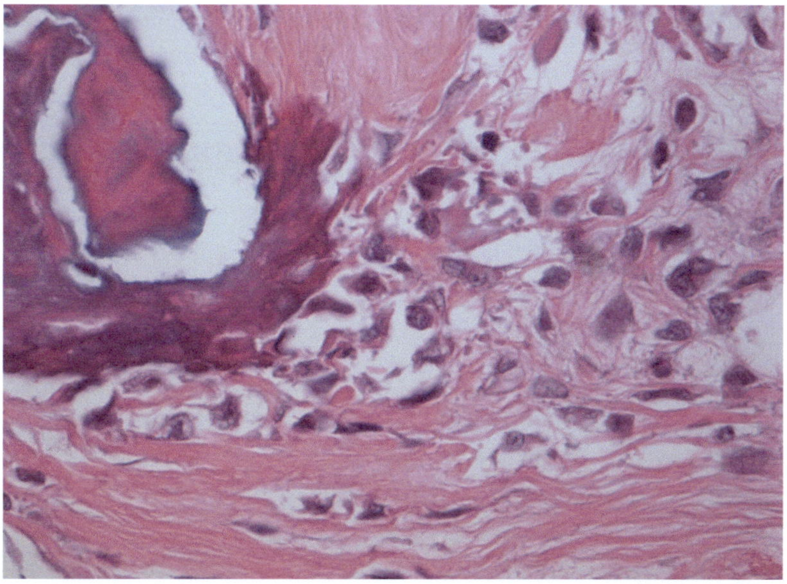

Fig. 1.68 Microscopic features of primary low grade renal osteosarcoma

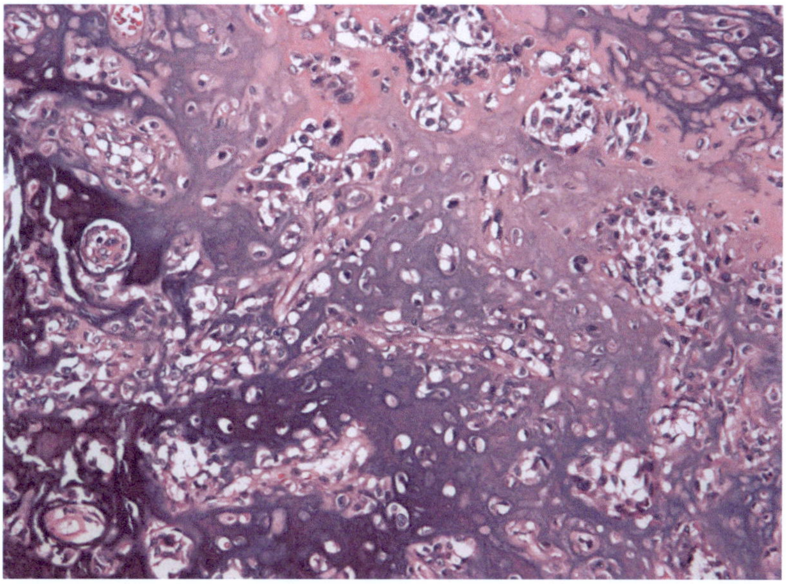

Fig. 1.69 Microscopic features of primary high grade renal osteosarcoma

- Immunohistochemistry gave focal positive results with PAX2 and CD10 in one case and S100 in another one. A summary of clinicopathologic features of reported cases is presented in Table 1.8.
- Osteosarcoma-like areas occurring in sarcomatoid carcinoma are more frequent than primary renal osteosarcoma, and therefore, sarcomatoid carcinoma should always been excluded.

1.9.20 Other Soft Tissue Tumors

- Extremely rare examples of chondrosarcoma, mesenchymal chondrosarcoma, malignant schwannoma, malignant mesenchymoma, clear cell sarcoma of the soft parts, low-grade fibromyxoid sarcoma of the renal capsule, and cystic embrional sarcoma, originating in the kidney have been reported.

Table 1.8 Clinicopathological characteristics of primary renal osteosarcoma

Characteristic	Value
Age, range (mean; median), year	47–81 (67; 65)
Sex	
Male	17 (63)
Female	10 (37)
Initial symptoms	
Weight loss	5 (19)
Palpable mass	8 (30)
Flank pain, weight loss	6 (22)
Flank pain, palpable mass	2 (7)
Pelvic and back pain	1 (4)
Back pain	1 (4)
Flank pain	3 (10)
Flank pain, gross hematuria	1 (4)
Histotype	
Classic (NOS)	10 (37)
Pleomorphic	11 (41)
Osteoblastic	3 (11)
Chondroblastic	2 (7)
Low grade	1 (4)
TNM stage	
pT1a N0M0	1 (4)
pT1b N0M0	1 (4)
pT3a N0M1	1 (4)
pT3aN1M1	9 (33)
pT4N1M1	15 (55)
Treatment	
RN	14 (52)
RN + ChT	9 (33)
RN + RT	4 (15)
Side	
Left	16 (59)
Right	11 (41)
Follow-up, month	
DOD (range, 2 weeks to 32 months; mean, 15 months)	21 (79)
AWD (both at 6-months follow-up)	2 (7)
NED (range, 25–68 months; mean, 46 months)	2 (7)
DOC (range, 9–10 months; mean, 9.5 months)	2 (7)

- A case of lipoblastoma has been reported in a child and a case of hibernoma has been reported in an adult.
- Before accepting a renal sarcoma as primary is always necessary to exclude sarcoma elsewhere and sarcomatoid carcinoma since sarcomatoid carcinoma may morphologically mimic virtually all sarcoma histotypes.

1.10 Wilms' Tumor and Other Renal Neoplasms in Children

1.10.1 Nephrogenic Rests and Nephroblastomatosis

- Nephrogenic rests are abnormally persistent foci of embryonal cells identifiable in 1 % of postmortem kidneys in infants and considered capable of developing into nephroblastoma. May be present in 25–40 % of kidneys harbouring Nephroblastoma.
- If diffuse and multifocal, the term "nephroblastomatosis" is applicable. Nephrogenic rests are sub-classified into perilobar (more common and multifocal) and intralobar (unifocal) types. The later is at higher risk of development of nephroblastoma.

1.10.2 Nephroblastoma (Wilms' Tumor)

- Usually occurs between 6 months and 3 years of age; rare after 3 years of age. It comprises 85 % of pediatric renal neoplasms and 5 % of childhood cancers.
- 5 % are multicentric, 5 % are bilateral, and 5 % are anaplastic. Lung metastasis is common and is frequently associated with cryptorchidism, hypospadias, hemihypertrophy, aniridia, renal ectopia, and horseshoe kidney (Figs. 1.70 and 1.71).
- Known risk factors include Beckwith–Wiedemann (hemihypertrophy) associated with the WT2 gene, Wilms–aniridia–genital anomaly–retardation syndrome: associated with the WT1 gene, Denys–Drash syndrome (glomerulonephritis, pseudohermaphroditism, and nephroblastoma) associated with the WT1 gene, Trisomy 18, and multicystic dysplastic kidney. Putative tumor suppressor genes are WT1 (chromosome 11p13), WT2 (chromosome 11p15.5), and WT3 (chromosome 16q).

- Most are circumscribed large tumors (>5 cm) that may be cystic or multicentric. Typical histology is triphasic tumor including blastema, epithelial component (abortive tubules and glomeruli) and stroma (skeletal muscle (most common), spindle cells, or cartilage). Positive WT1, Vimentin, Neuron-specific enolase (focal), (focal), and Desmin (focal) is the diagnostic signature.
- Anaplasia is one of the criteria for placing Wilms' tumor under unfavorable histology category; the other is the development of a high-grade sarcoma or carcinoma within nephroblastoma. Anaplasia indicates increased resistance to therapy rather than increased aggressiveness.

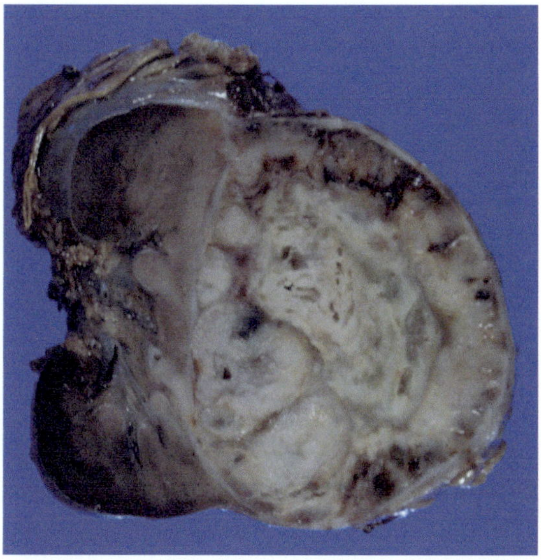

Fig. 1.70 Gross features of Wilms tumor showing the "cerebroid" appearance

- Definition of anaplasia include multipolar polyploid mitotic figures and each component of the abnormal metaphase must be as large as or larger than a normal metaphase, markedly enlarged and hyperchromatic nuclei (at least three times larger than adjacent non-neoplastic nuclei). Anaplasia is confined to renal parenchyma. Table 1.9 shows current staging.
- Main differential diagnosis include clear cell sarcoma, rhabdoid tumor, neuroblastoma, synovial sarcoma, and primitive neuroectodermal tumor (PNET) of the kidney.

1.10.3 Cystic Partially Differentiated Nephroblastoma

- Most are detected as palpable masses in children <4 years old with benign clinical course. Usually are 5–10 cm in diameter with fibrous pseudocapsule. Tumor is entirely composed of variably sized cysts, some of those may have papillary excrescences.
- Cysts are separated by septa of variable thickness and lined by flat, cuboidal, or hobnail

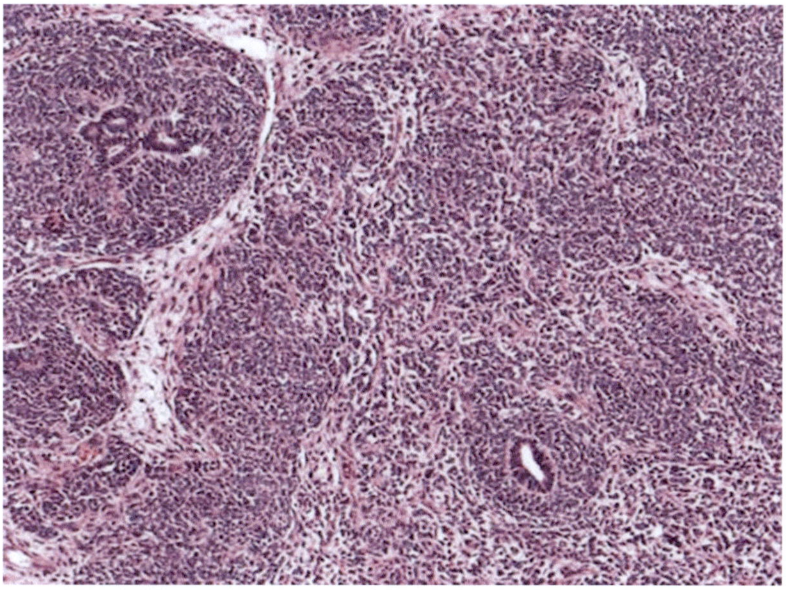

Fig. 1.71 Microscopic features of Wilms tumor showing the three components

Table 1.9 Staging nephroblastoma (Fifth Protocol, National Wilms' Tumor Study Group)

Stage I	Limited to kidney and completely resected. Renal capsule is intact. Renal sinus soft tissue may be minimally infiltrated
Stage II	Tumor infiltrates beyond kidney, but is completely resected. Tumor extends beyond renal capsule. Tumor infiltrates vessels within the renal sinus. Tumor with prior open or large core needle biopsies. Tumor with local spillage confined to flank
Stage III	Residual nonhematogenous tumor confined to abdomen. Tumor in abdominal lymph nodes. Diffuse peritoneal contamination: direct tumor growth, tumor implants, and spillage into peritoneum before or during surgery. Gross or microscopic involvement of specimen margins. Residual tumor in abdomen. Tumor removed noncontiguously (piece-meal resection)
Stage IV	Hematogenous metastases
Stage V	Bilateral renal involvement at diagnosis (tumor in each kidney should be separately substaged)

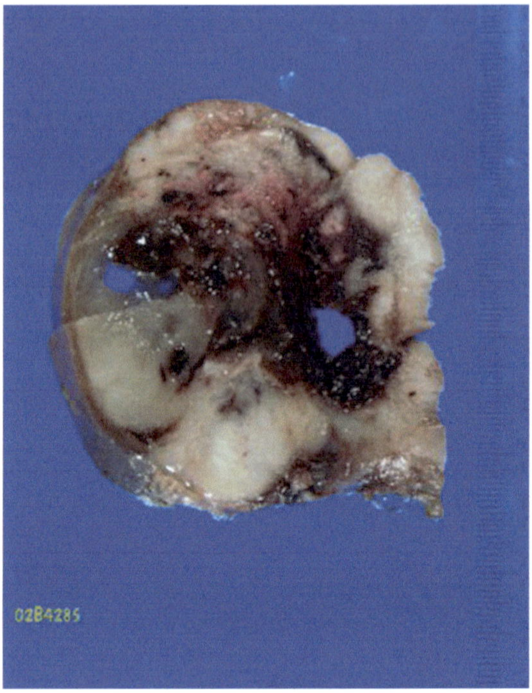

Fig. 1.72 Gross aspect of mesoblastic nephroma

epithelium. Septa contain blastema, nephroblastomatous epithelial elements, and differentiated and/or undifferentiated mesenchymal elements (skeletal muscle, cartilage, fat or myxoid mesenchyme).

- Solid expansile nodules warrant a diagnosis of cystic nephroblastoma. If no nephroblastomatous elements are seen in the fibrous septa, some apply the diagnostic term "cystic nephroma"; however, these lesions are viewed as being different from similar lesions in adults.

1.10.4 Congenital Mesoblastic Nephroma (CMN)

- Most common congenital renal neoplasm and 90 % of patients are <1 year old. It accounts for 2 % of all pediatric renal tumors and presents as a palpable mass. Metastasis and tumor-related death is rare; recurrences are attributable to incomplete initial resection.
- Two morphologic patterns: "classic congenital mesoblastic nephroma" and "cellular congenital mesoblastic nephroma (translocation t(12;15))" which confirms that it is an infantile fibrosarcoma of the kidney. Classic CMN is viewed as infantile fibromatosis (no translocation identified) (Figs. 1.72, 1.73 and 1.74).
- Usually are unilateral (mean diameter is 6 cm), solitary tumors that may have cysts, hemorrhage, and necrosis. The classic form shows intersecting bundles of spindle cells resembling fibroblasts and prominent irregular vascular spaces. Cellular form shows plump spindle cells, arranged in poorly formed fascicles. Mitotic figures are present.
- Mixed congenital mesoblastic nephroma shows features of both types. On immunohistochemistry, positive vimentin, Actin, Desmin (rare), and negative CD34, cytokeratins, and S100 protein are the characteristic signature.

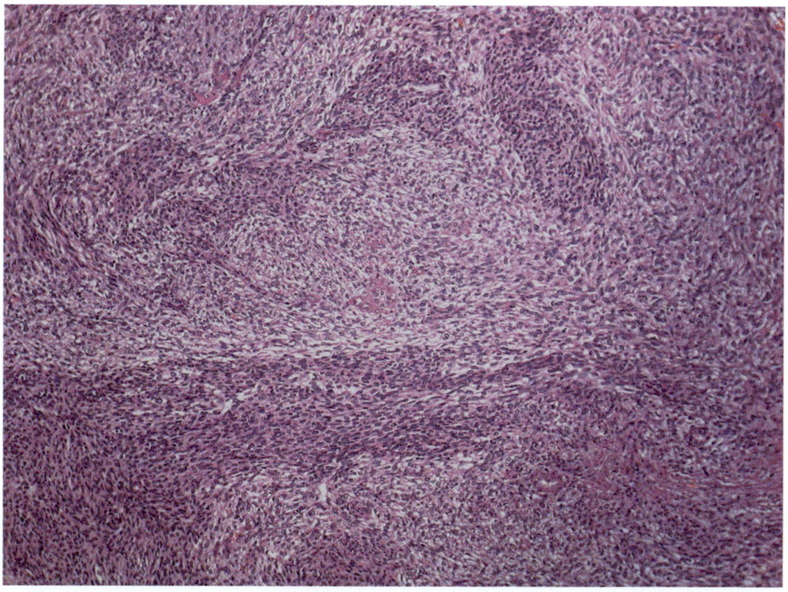

Fig. 1.73 Microscopic aspect of mesoblastic nephroma, cellular type

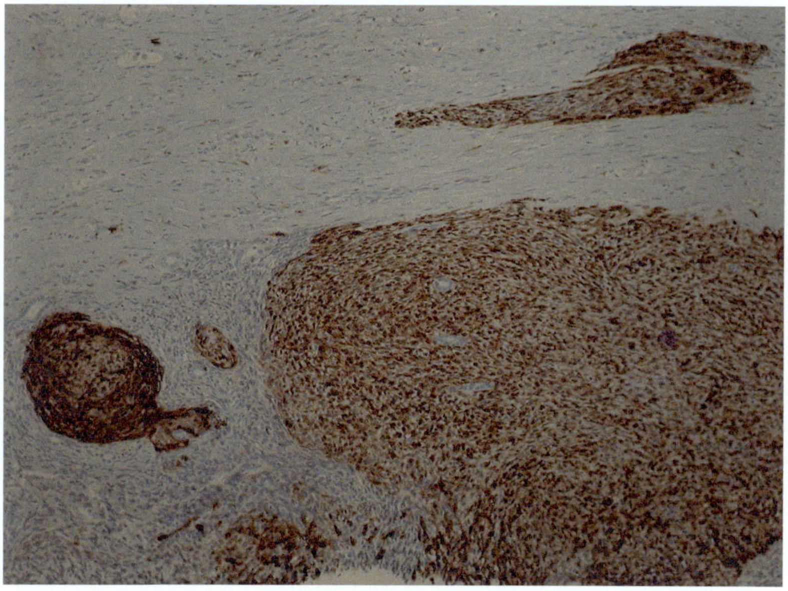

Fig. 1.74 Smooth muscle actin is positive in many cells of mesoblastic nephroma

1.10.5 Clear Cell Sarcoma of Kidney

- Accounts for about 3 % of all malignant pediatric renal neoplasms, it is twice as common in males ranging from 2 months–54 years. It is typically large (mean diameter 11 cm), has propensity for bone metastasis, unilateral, unicentric, soft to firm, homogeneous, light brown or gray and encapsulated. Five percent involve the renal vein.
- The classic pattern includes epithelioid or spindled cells arranged in nests or cords separated by fibrovascular septa of variable thickness. Cells are separated by myxoid extracellular matrix material that mimics clear cytoplasm. Cell nuclei are round to oval, with dispersed chromatin and inconspicuous or no nucleoli
- Mitotic activity is low. Many pattern variations have been described: myxoid, sclerosing, cellular, epithelioid, spindle cell, and palisading. Differential diagnosis from nephroblastoma may be difficult, likewise, pale H&E staining and negative immunostaining for all markers except vimentin and bcl-2 suggests clear cell sarcoma.

1.10.6 Rhabdoid Tumor of Kidney

- Accounts for about 2 % of all pediatric renal tumors and 80 % of patients have metastases at the time of diagnosis. Most patients die within 1 year. Almost all patients are <3 years old.
- Identical tumors involve other sites; especially central nervous system. The typical case is unilateral, large, unencapsulated, with hemorrhage and necrosis, sometimes with satellite intrarenal metastases.
- Histologically, rhabdoid tumor is composed of sheets of monotonous discohesive large cells with vesicular nuclei, prominent nucleoli and hyaline eosinophilic cytoplasmic inclusions of intermediate filaments. Usually there is extensive vascular invasion.
- Rhabdoid tumors in all sites are characterized by mutation or deletion of the INI1 tumor suppressor gene on the long arm of chromosome 22q11. Consequently, show loss of nuclear expression of the transcriptional regulator INI1/SMARCB1, thus reflecting the prevalent mutation of the gene.

1.10.7 Neuroblastoma

- Tumors are unencapsulated, hemorrhagic and poorly circumscribed with tipical organoid arrangement of cells, "salt and pepper" nuclear chromatin, and Homer-Wright rosettes.
- Cells are usually positive for neuron-specific enolase, synaptophysin, S100 protein, and chromogranin supportive of neuronal differentiation.

1.10.8 Primitive Neuroectodermal Tumor (PNET)

- Most patients are adolescent or young adults (range 1 month–72 years) showing poorly circumscribed tumors composed of primitive round cells with varying degrees of rosette formation (Fig. 1.75).
- The nuclei shows coarse nuclear chromatin and nuclei do not overlap. Typically, cells are CD99 (membranous) and FLI1 positive and WT1 negative (Fig. 1.76). Characteristic translocations include especially t(11;22)(q24;q12).

1.10.9 Desmoplastic Small Round Cell Tumor

- Rare cases of this tumor have been reported to occur in the kidney, both in adults and children. The typical histology of the tumor include small cells with hyperchromatic nuclei and scanty cytoplasm. Mitotic figures are frequent and necrosis is common. Focal dystrophic calcification and stromal desmoplasia are usually present.
- Tumors react with antibodies to vimentin and desmin (paranuclear dot-like expression). Frequently tumors also express NSE, CD56, FLI1, CAM5.2, WT1, CD56, CK AE1/AE3, EMA, and CD99 (cytoplasmic).
- All cases show EWS-WT1 gene fusion t(11;22)(p13;q12) characteristic of desmoplastic small round cell tumor.

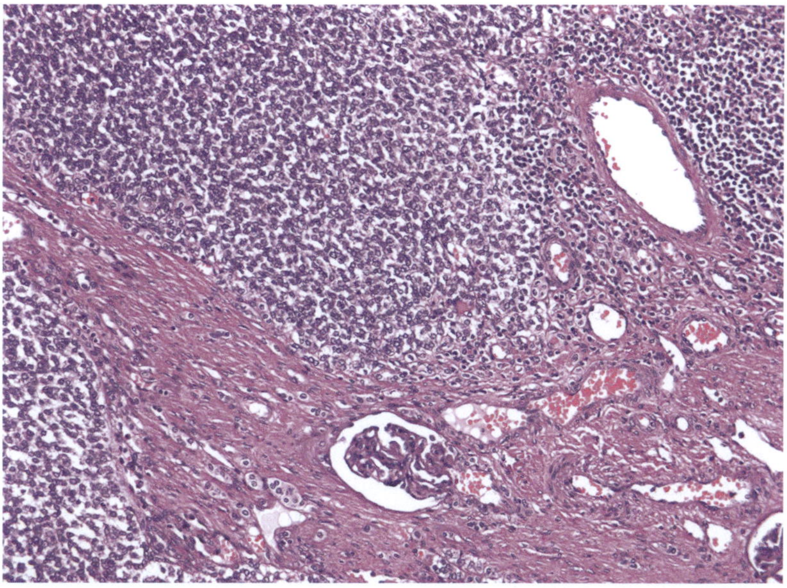

Fig. 1.75 Peripheral neuroectodermic tumor of the kidney

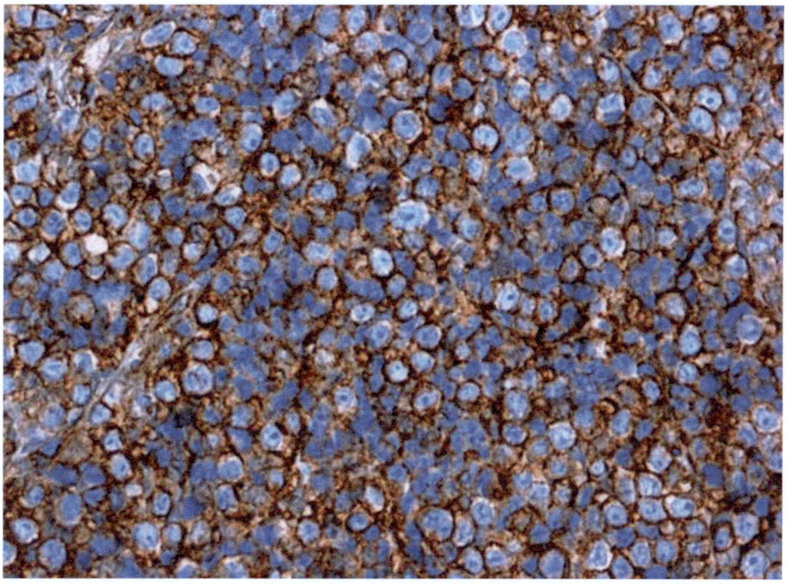

Fig. 1.76 CD99 is positive in neoplastic cells of peripheral neuroectodermic tumor

1.10.10 Synovial Sarcoma

- Large variably cystic tumors (mean diameter 11 cm) composed of primitive spindle cells with overlapping ovoid nuclei and scant cytoplasm admixed with variably sized cystic spaces that represent trapped dilated native renal tubules and ducts. Most renal examples are associated with monophasic histology.
- Variable expression of bcl-2, EMA, CD99, CD56, vimentin, calponin, and CD34 is present in most cases. CK is rarely positive except in cyst-lining epithelial cells. Expression of desmin, SMA, or S100 protein is not seen.
- Proliferating cells are typically WT1 negative but show t(X;18)(p11.2;q11.2) translocation. This results in fusion of the SS18 gene to one of the SSX genes.

- Most cases of synovial sarcoma demonstrate SYT-SSX2 gene fusion.

1.10.11 Ossifying Renal Tumor of Infancy

- This rare benign tumor is most frequently seen in males. The age at time of diagnosis ranges 6–17 months. Gross examination reveals a polypoid tumor growing into the pelvi-calyceal system.
- Most are single 2–6 cm. At histology it is composed of spindle cells admixed with partially calcified osteoid matrix. Trisomy 4 may be considered a characteristic genetic finding in this tumor.

1.11 Other Rare Tumors and Tumor-Like Conditions

1.11.1 Neuroendocrine Tumors

- Although neuroendocrine cells have not been documented in the normal renal parenchyma, a few neuroendocrine neoplasms have been reported to arise in the kidney. These rare tumors include carcinoids and small cell neuroendocrine carcinomas, whereas pure intrarenal neuroblastoma and paraganglioma/phaechromocytoma are exceedingly rare findings
- Carcinoids are well-differentiated neuroendocrine tumors frequently associated with horseshoe kidney. They occur in patients over 40 years of age as solitary, solid, well-circumscribed yellowish nodules. About one third of these tumors metastasize.
- Small cell neuroendocrine carcinomas are large, whitish, invasive masses arising in patients with an average age of 60 years and their prognosis is extremely poor. Both carcinoids and small cell neuroendocrine carcinomas are morphologically similar to those located at other sites.
- Renal paraganglioma is exceedingly rare and may be intrarenal or capsular measuring 2–17 cm. May present through evaluation for hypertension or with hematuria, flank pain, or abdominal mass.
- Histologically, may be solid or cystic composed of organoid clusters of cells surrounded by delicate fibrovascular stroma and sustentacular cells. Tumor cells show positivity for vimentin, chromogranin and synaptophysin. And negative or focally positive for CKs. Sustentacular cells show positive immunostaining for S100 protein.

1.11.2 Hematopoietic and Lymphoid Tumors

- Both primary and secondary lymphoma and involvement by plasmacytoma and leukemia can be observed in the kidney. The patterns of renal involvement can be either diffuse or with the formation of masses or as intravascular lymphomatosis of the kidney.
- Primary lymphoma represents 0.7 % of all extra-nodal lymphoma. Virtually all types of lymphoma may be encountered. Diffuse large B-cell lymphoma is the most common form of renal lymphoma.
- Renal leukemia frequently takes the form of myeloid sarcoma. Microscopically, renal tissue shows dense interstitial infiltration by mature granulocytic cells. A panel including CD20, CD43, CD68, and myeloperoxidase, can successfully identify most myeloid sarcomas.
- Plasmacytoma arising in the kidney is a rarity most frequently diagnosed after renal resection for clinical diagnosis of RCC. Most patients are male range 20–65 years. Microscopically, tumors are composed of sheets of plasma cells with varying degrees of cytologic atypia and mitotic activity.

1.11.3 Germ Cell Tumors

- Germs cell tumors are rare in the kidney with most cases showing characteristics of teratoma seen both in children and adults. Some may be associated to renal dysplasia or horseshoe kidney. Tumors may be single or multiple. A case of intrarenal mixed germ cell tumor, composed of YST and teratoma has been reported.

- Some reported cases of choriocarcinoma both primary and metastatic to the kidney are on record.

1.11.4 Other Rare Epithelial Tumors and Renal Cell Carcinoma in Children

- Anecdotal examples labeled as spiradenocylindroma or salivary-gland pleomorphic-adenoma-like tumor are on record.
- Renal cell carcinoma in children are rare and account for less than 0.3 % of all tumors and less than 1 % of all resected RCC cases. The median age at presentation ranges 10–14 years. Bilaterality is uncommon.
- Morphologically, RCC in the pediatric age group is diverse, including unclassified RCC, Papillary RCC, MiT family translocation RCC or clear cell RCC, with anecdotal examples of chromophobe RCC, CDC, postneuroblasotma RCC, and carcinoma combined with nephroblastoma.
- Rare examples of inflammatory myofibrobastic tumor has been reported to occur in the kidney parenchima, perirenal fat or in the renal capsula.

1.11.5 Tumor-Like Conditions

- The lesions that most frequently simulate neoplasms clinically and radiologically are xanthogranulomatous pyelonephritis, perirenal and intrarenal hemorrhagic cysts, malakoplakia, and pseudotumor due to Tamm–Horsfall extravasation.
- Xanthogranulomatous pyelonephritis is a tumor-forming subacute or chronic inflammation which can be associated with nephrolithiasis to a variable degree, ranging from 20 to 70 % of the cases. Grossly it appears as golden yellow nodules which are histologically composed of lipid-laden macrophages (xantoma cells) (Figs. 1.77 and 1.78).
- However, these cells immonostain for CD68, but not for cytokeratin, and may mimic the neoplastic cells of clear cell renal cell carcinoma. Multinucleated giant cells and spindled fibroblast and inflammatory cells, in particular granulocytes, are frequently present.
- Perirenal and intrarenal hemorrhagic cysts can radiologically mimic a solid mass or a complicated cyst. The morphologic hallmark of this cyst, frequently without identifiable epithelium, is the presence of numerous round laminated bodies called Liesegang rings in the inflammatory wall.
- Malakoplakia can present as a renal solid mass which is composed of eosinophilic macrophages with intracytoplasmic Michaelis–Gutman PAS-positive bodies
- Tamm–Horsfall protein is a kidney-specific protein which is produced in the Henle's loop. The extravasation of large amounts of this protein in the interstitium or in the adipose tissue of the sinus form the Tamm–Horsfall pseudotumor due to extravasation. The lesion can be clinically and radiologically misdiagnosed for a tumor.
- Localized cystic disease of the kidney may be challenging in differentiating from cystic tumors. Microscopically, cystic lesions involve renal papillae. Cysts are lined with cuboidal or flat epithelial cells identical to those lining the collecting ducts. Significant inflammation is absent. The surrounding renal parenchyma was normal.

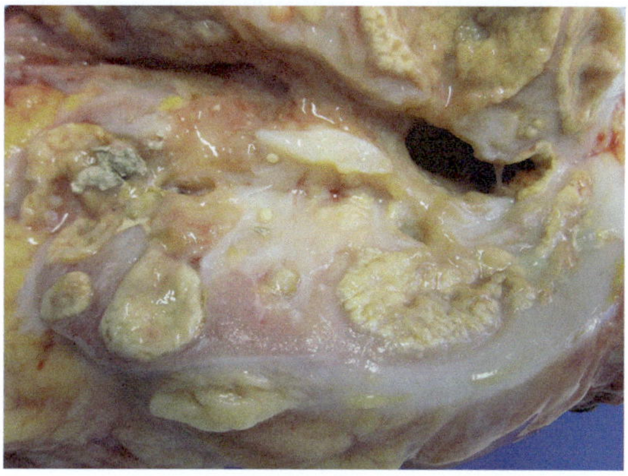

Fig. 1.77 Gross picture of xanthogranulomatous pyelonephritis

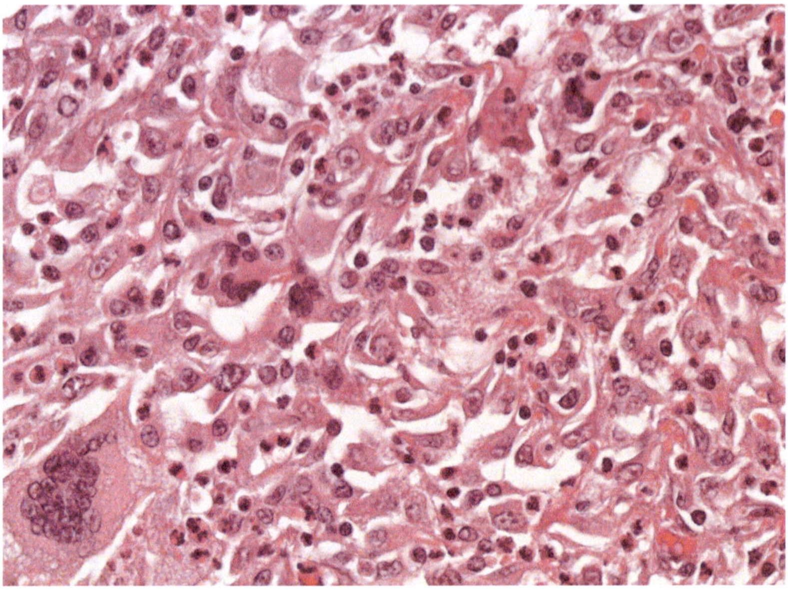

Fig. 1.78 Microscopic picture of xanthogranulomatous pyelonephritis

- Rare cases of IgG4 sclerosing tumor-like lesions have been described in the kidney, more frequently in association with the capsule or sinus fat.
- Other tumor-like conditions include rare cases of sarcoidosis, tuberculosis, fungal and parasitic infections described in the kidney causing tubulointerstitial nephritis that rarely presents as a tumor-like condition.

1.12 Secondary Tumors

- Secondary tumours to the kidney usually occur as part of a widespread dissemination. Renal involvement is frequently bilateral and in a multinodular fashion. Primary sources include lung, thyroid, skin (melanoma), contralateral kidney and gastro-intestinal tract.
- Renal cell carcinoma immunohistochemical markers, such as RCC marker and CD10, and urothelial carcinoma markers, such as uroplakin and thrombomodulin, can be of some utility when combined with other specific markers, including thyroid transcription factor-1 (lung and thyroid) and melanoma markers (HMB45 and MelanA) (Table 1.7).
- There are some primary tumours from the thyroid that very closely mimic primary kidney tumours i.e., follicular thyroid-like RCC, a poorly defined primary RCC negative with thyroglobulin and thyroid transcription factor 1 (both positive in thyroid carcinoma).
- PAX2 and/or PAX8 are considered most useful for the diagnosis of primary renal tumor metastasis in other organ.

Suggested Reading

Adley BP, Smith ND, Nayar R, Yang XJ. Birt-Hogg-Dube syndrome: clinicopathologic findings and genetic alterations. Arch Pathol Lab Med. 2006;130:1865–70.

Adsay NV, Eble JN, Srigley JR, Jones EC, Grignon DJ. Mixed epithelial and stromal tumor of the kidney. Am J Surg Pathol. 2000;24:958–70.

Akhtar M, Tulbah A, Kardar AH, Ali MA. Sarcomatoid renal cell carcinoma: the chromophobe connection. Am J Surg Pathol. 1997;21:1188–95.

Algaba F, Akaza H, Lopez-Beltran A, et al. Current pathology keys of renal cell carcinoma. Eur Urol. 2011;60:634–43.

Amin MB, Crotty TB, Tickoo SK, Farrow GM. Renal oncocytoma: a reappraisal of morphologic features with clinicopathologic findings in 80 cases. Am J Surg Pathol. 1997;21:1–12.

Angel JR, Alfred A, Sakhuja A, Sells RE, Zechlinski JJ. Ewing's sarcoma of the kidney. Int J Clin Oncol. 2010;15(3):314–8.

Argani P. Metanephric neoplasms: the hyperdifferentiated, benign end of the Wilms tumor spectrum? Clin Lab Med. 2005;25:379–92.

Argani P, Beckwith JB. Metanephric stromal tumor: report of 31 cases of a distinctive pediatric renal; neoplasm. Am J Surg Pathol. 2000;24:917–26.

Argani P, Ladanyi M. Translocation carcinomas of the kidney. Clin Lab Med. 2005;25:363–78.

Argani P, Antonescu CR, Illei PB, Lui MY, Timmons CF, Newbury R, Reuter VE, Garvin AJ, Perez-Atayde AR, Fletcher JA, Beckwith JB, Bridge JA, Ladanyi M. Primary renal neoplasms with the ASPL-TFE3 gene fusion of alveolar soft part sarcoma: a distinctive tumor entity previously included among renal cell carcinomas of children and adolescents. Am J Pathol. 2001;159:179–92.

Argani P, Antonescu CR, Couturier J, Fournet JC, Sciot R, Debiec-Rychter M, Hutchinson B, Reuter VE, Boccon-Gibod L, Timmons C, Hafez N, Ladanyi M. PRCC-TFE3 renal carcinomas: morphologic, immunohistochemical, ultrastructural, and molecular analysis of an entity associated with the t(X;1)(p11.2;q21). Am J Surg Pathol. 2002;26:1553–66.

Argani P, Lal P, Hutchinson B, Lui MY, Reuter VE, Ladanyi M. Aberrant nuclear immunoreactivity for TFE3 in neoplasms with TFE3 gene fusions: a sensitive and specific immunohistochemical assay. Am J Surg Pathol. 2003;27:750–61.

Argani P, Lae M, Hutchinson B, Reuter VE, Collins MH, Perentesis J, Tomaszewski JE, Brooks JS, Acs G, Bridge JA, Vargas SO, Davis IJ, Fisher DE, Ladanyi M. Renal carcinomas with the t(6;11)(p21;q12): clinicopathologic features and demonstration of the specific alpha-TFEB gene fusion by immunohistochemistry, RT-PCR, and DNA PCR. Am J Surg Pathol. 2005;29:230–40.

Argani P, Olgac S, Tickoo SK, Goldfischer M, Moch H, Chan DY, Eble JN, Bonsib SM, Jimeno M, Lloreta J, Billis A, Hicks J, De Marzo AM, Reuter VE, Ladanyi M. Xp11 translocation renal cell carcinoma in adults: expanded clinical, pathologic, and genetic spectrum. Am J Surg Pathol. 2007;31:1149–60.

Argani P, Yonescu R, Morsberger L, et al. Molecular confirmation of the t(6;11)(p21;q12) renal cell carcinomas in archival paraffin-embedded material using a break-apart TFEB FISH assay expands its clinicopathologic spectrum. Am J Surg Pathol. 2012;36:1516–26.

Arroyo MR, Green DM, Perlman EJ, et al. The spectrum of metanephric adenofibroma and related lesions. Am J Surg Pathol. 2001;25:433–44.

Beckwith JB, Kiviat NB, Bonadio JF. Nephrogenic rests, nephroblastomatosis, and the pathogenesis of Wilms' tumor. Pediatr Pathol. 1990;10(1–2):1–36.

Bruder E, Passera O, Harms D, Leuschner I, Ladanyi M, Argani P, Eble JN, Struckmann K, Schraml P, Moch H. Morphologic and molecular characterization of renal cell carcinoma in children and young adults. Am J Surg Pathol. 2004;28:1117–32.

Brunelli M, Eble JN, Zhang S, Martignoni G, Cheng L. Metanephric adenoma lacks the gains of chromosomes 7 and 17 and loss of Y that are typical of papillary renal cell carcinoma and papillary adenoma. Mod Pathol. 2003a;16:1060–3.

Brunelli M, Eble JN, Zhang S, Martignoni G, Cheng L. Gains of chromosomes 7, 17, 12, 16, and 20 and loss of Y occur early in the evolution of papillary renal cell neoplasia: a fluorescent in situ hybridization study. Mod Pathol. 2003b;16:1053–9.

Brunelli M, Eble JN, Zhang S, Martignoni G, Delahunt B, Cheng L. Eosinophilic and classic chromophobe renal cell carcinomas have similar frequent losses of multiple chromosomes from among chromosomes 1, 2, 6, 10, and 17, and this pattern of genetic abnormality is not present in renal oncocytoma. Mod Pathol. 2005;18:161–9.

Brunelli M, Gobbo S, Cossu-Rocca P, Cheng L, Hes O, Delahunt B, Pea M, Bonetti F, Mina MM, Ficarra V, Chilosi M, Eble JN, Menestrina F, Martignoni G. Chromosomal gains in the sarcomatoid transformation of chromophobe renal cell carcinoma. Mod Pathol. 2007;20:303–9.

Brunelli M, Eccher A, Gobbo S, Ficarra V, Novara G, Cossu-Rocca P, Bonetti F, Menestrina F, Cheng L, Eble JN, Martignoni G. Loss of chromosome 9p is an independent prognostic factor in patients with clear cell renal cell carcinoma. Mod Pathol. 2008;21:1–6.

Chen Y-B, Brannon AR, Toubaji A, Dudas ME, Won HH, Al-Ahmadie HA, Fine SW, Gopalan A, Frizzell N, Voss MH, Russo P, Berger MF, Tickoo SK, Reuter VE. Hereditary leiomyomatosis and renal cell carcinoma syndrome–associated renal cancer: recognition of the syndrome by pathologic features and the utility of detecting aberrant succination by immunohistochemistry. Am J Surg Pathol. 2014;38:627–37.

Cheng L, Williamson SR, Zhang S, MacLennan GT, Montironi R, Lopez-Beltran A. Understanding the molecular genetics of renal cell neoplasia: implications for diagnosis, prognosis and therapy. Expert Rev Anticancer Ther. 2010;10:843–64.

Chevarie-Davis M, Riazalhosseini Y, Arseneault M, et al. The morphologic and immunohistochemical spectrum of papillary renal cell carcinoma: study including 132 cases with pure type 1 and type 2 morphology as well as tumors with overlapping features. Am J Surg Pathol. 2014;38(7):887–94.

Cheville JC, Lohse CM, Zincke H, Weaver AL, Leibovich BC, Frank I, Blute ML. Sarcomatoid renal cell carcinoma: an examination of underlying histologic subtype and an analysis of associations with patient outcome. Am J Surg Pathol. 2004;28:435–41.

Cossu-Rocca P, Eble JN, Delahunt B, Zhang S, Martignoni G, Brunelli M, Cheng L. Renal mucinous tubular and spindle carcinoma lacks the gains of chromosomes 7 and 17 and losses of chromosome Y that are prevalent in papillary renal cell carcinoma. Mod Pathol. 2006a;19:488–93.

Cossu-Rocca P, Eble JN, Zhang S, Martignoni G, Brunelli M, Cheng L. Acquired cystic disease-associated renal tumors: an immunohistochemical and fluorescence in situ hybridization study. Mod Pathol. 2006b;19:780–7.

Cossu-Rocca P, Eble JN, Zhang S, Bonsib SM, Martignoni G, Brunelli M, Cheng L. Interphase cytogenetic analysis with centromeric probes for chromosomes 1, 2, 6, 10, and 17 in 11 tumors from a patient with bilateral renal oncocytosis. Mod Pathol. 2008;21:498–504.

Davenport KP, Blanco FC, Sandler AD. Pediatric malignancies: neuroblastoma, Wilm's tumor, hepatoblastoma, rhabdomyosarcoma, and sacroccygeal teratoma. Surg Clin North Am. 2012;92(3):745–67.

Davidoff AM. Wilms's tumor. Curr Opin Pediatr. 2009;21:357–64.

Davis Jr CJ, Barton JH, Sesterhenn IA, Mostofi FK. Metanephric adenoma. Clinicopathological study of fifty patients. Am J Surg Pathol. 1995a;19:1101–14.

Davis Jr CJ, Mostofi FK, Sesterhenn IA. Renal medullary carcinoma. The seventh sickle cell nephropathy. Am J Surg Pathol. 1995b;19:1–11.

de Peralta-Venturina M, Moch H, Amin M, Tamboli P, Hailemariam S, Mihatsch M, Javidan J, Stricker H, Ro JY, Amin MB. Sarcomatoid differentiation in renal cell carcinoma: a study of 101 cases. Am J Surg Pathol. 2001;25:275–84.

Debelenko LV, Raimondi SC, Daw N, et al. Renal cell carcinoma with novel *VCL-ALK* fusion: new representative of ALK-associated tumor spectrum. Mod Pathol. 2011;24:430–42.

Delahunt B, Eble JN. Papillary renal cell carcinoma: a clinicopathologic and immunohistochemical study of 105 tumors. Mod Pathol. 1997;10:537–44.

Delahunt B, Sika-Paotonu D, Bethwaite PB, McCredie MR, Martignoni G, Eble JN, Jordan TW. Fuhrman grading is not appropriate for chromophobe renal cell carcinoma. Am J Surg Pathol. 2007;31:957–60.

Delahunt B, Sika-Paotonu D, Bethwaite PB, et al. Grading of clear cell renal cell carcinoma should be based on nucleolar prominence. Am J Surg Pathol. 2011;35(8):1134–9.

Delahunt B, Cheville JC, Martignoni G, et al. The International Society of Urological Pathology (ISUP) grading classification for renal cell carcinoma and other prognostic parameters. Am J Surg Pathol. 2013;37:1490–504.

Drut R, Drut RM, Ortolani C. Metastatic metanephric adenoma with foci of papillary carcinoma in a child: a combined histologic, immunohistochemical, and FISH study. Int J Surg Pathol. 2001;9:241–7.

Eble JN. Mucinous tubular and spindle cell carcinoma and post-neuroblastoma carcinoma: newly recognised entities in the renal cell carcinoma family. Pathology. 2003;35:499–504.

Eble JN, Amin MB, Young RH. Epithelioid angiomyolipoma of the kidney: a report of five cases with a prominent and diagnostically confusing epithelioid smooth muscle component. Am J Surg Pathol. 1997;21:1123–30.

Eble JN, Sauter G, Epstein JI, Sesterhenn IA. Pathology and genetics. Tumors of the urinary system and male genital organs. Lyon: IARC Press; 2004.

Fan R. Primary renal neuroblastoma–a clinical pathologic study of 8 cases. Am J Surg Pathol. 2012;36(1):94–100.

Ficarra V, Brunelli M, Cheng L, et al. Prognostic and therapeutic impact of the histopathologic definition of parenchymal epithelial renal tumors. Eur Urol. 2010;58:655–68.

Filosa A, Fabiani A. From biopsy to active surveillance in small renal masses: is it feasible? Anal Quant Cytol Histol. 2012;34:109–10.

Gill AJ, Pachter NS, Chou A, et al. Renal tumors associated with germline SDHB mutations show distinctive morphology. Am J Surg Pathol. 2011;35:1578–85.

Gobbo S, Eble JN, Grignon DJ, Martignoni G, MacLennan GT, Shah RB, Zhang S, Brunelli M, Cheng L. Clear cell papillary renal cell carcinoma. A distinct histopathologic and molecular genetic entity. Am J Surg Pathol. 2008;32:1239–45.

Granter SR, Fletcher JA, Renshaw AA. Cytologic and cytogenetic analysis of metanephric adenoma of the kidney: a report of two cases. Am J Clin Pathol. 1997;108:544–9.

Grignon DJ, Che M. Clear cell renal cell carcinoma. Clin Lab Med. 2005;25:305–16.

Grignon DJ, Eble JN. Papillary and metanephric adenomas of the kidney. Semin Diagn Pathol. 1998;15:41–53.

Guo J, Tretiakova MS; Troxell ML, Osunkoya AO, Fadare O, Sangoi AR, Shen SS, Lopez-Beltran A, Mehra R, Heider A, Higgins JP, Harik LR, Leroy X, Gill AJ, Trpkov K, Campbell SC, Przybycin C, Magi-Galluzzi C, McKenney JKL. Tuberous sclerosis-associated renal cell carcinoma: a clinicopathologic study of 57 separate carcinomas in 18 patients. Am J Surg Pathol (in press).

Gupta R, Viswanathan S, D'Cruz A, Kane SV. Metastatic papillary carcinoma of thyroid masquerading as a renal tumour. J Clin Pathol. 2008;61:143–6.

Gupta R, Billis A, Rajal B, et al. Carcinoma of the collecting ducts of Bellini and renal medullary carcinoma clinicopathologic analysis of 52 cases of rare aggressive subtypes of renal cell carcinoma with a focus on their interrelationship. Am J Surg Pathol. 2012;36:1265–78.

Hes O, Brunelli M, Michal M, Cossu Rocca P, Hora M, Chilosi M, Mina M, Boudova L, Menestrina F, Martignoni G. Oncocytic papillary renal cell carcinoma: a clinicopathologic, immunohistochemical, ultrastructural, and interphase cytogenetic study of 12 cases. Ann Diagn Pathol. 2006;10:133–9.

Honda H, Coffman CE, Berbaum KS, Barloon TJ, Masuda K. CT analysis of metastatic neoplasms of the kidney. Comparison with primary renal cell carcinoma. Acta Radiol. 1992;33:39–44.

Hu Y, Hartmann A, Stoehr C, Zhang S, Wang M, Tacha D, Montironi R, Lopez-Beltran A, Cheng L. PAX8 is expressed in the majority of renal epithelial neoplasms: an immunohistochemical study of 223 cases using a mouse monoclonal antibody. J Clin Pathol. 2012;65(3):254–6. Epub 2011 Dec 1.

Ishida Y, Kato K, Kigasawa H, Ohama Y, Ijiri R, Tanaka Y. Synchronous occurrence of pleuropulmonary blastoma and cystic nephroma: possible genetic link in cystic lesions of the lung and the kidney. Med Pediatr Oncol. 2000;35:85–7.

Jockle GA, Toker C, Shamsuddin AM. Metastatic renal oncocytic neoplasm with benign histologic appearance. Urology. 1987;30:79–81.

Jones EC, Pins M, Dickersin GR, Young RH. Metanephric adenoma of the kidney. A clinicopathological, immunohistochemical, flow cytometric, cytogenetic, and electron microscopic study of seven cases. Am J Surg Pathol. 1995;19:615–26.

Jones TD, Eble JN, Wang M, MacLennan GT, Delahunt B, Brunelli M, Martignoni G, Lopez-Beltran A, Bonsib SM, Ulbright TM, Zhang S, Nigro K, Cheng L. Molecular genetic evidence for the independent origin of multifocal papillary tumors in patients with papillary renal cell carcinomas. Clin Cancer Res. 2005a;11:7226–33.

Jones TD, Eble JN, Wang M, Maclennan GT, Jain S, Cheng L. Clonal divergence and genetic heterogeneity in clear cell renal cell carcinomas with sarcomatoid transformation. Cancer. 2005b;104:1195–203.

Jung SJ, Chung JI, Park SH, Ayala AG, Ro JY. Thyroid follicular carcinoma-like tumor of kidney: a case report with morphologic, immunohistochemical, and genetic analysis. Am J Surg Pathol. 2006;30: 411–5.

Kapusta LR, Weiss MA, Ramsay J, et al. Inflammatory myofibroblastic tumors of the kidney: a clinicopathologic and immunohistochemical study of 12 cases. Am J Surg Pathol. 2003;27:658–66.

Kovacs A, Kovacs G. Low chromosome number in chromophobe renal cell carcinomas. Genes Chromosomes Cancer. 1992;4:267–8.

Kovacs G, Akhtar M, Beckwith BJ, Bugert P, Cooper CS, Delahunt B, Eble JN, Fleming S, Ljungberg B, Medeiros LJ, Moch H, Reuter VE, Ritz E, Roos G, Schmidt D, Srigley JR, Storkel S, van den Berg E, Zbar B. The Heidelberg classification of renal cell tumours. J Pathol. 1997;183:131–3.

Koyle MA, Hatch DA, Furness 3rd PD, Lovell MA, Odom LF, Kurzrock EA. Long-term urological complications in survivors younger than 15 months of advanced stage abdominal neuroblastoma. J Urol. 2001;166:1455–8.

Kuhn E, De Anda J, Manoni S, Netto G, Rosai J. Renal cell carcinoma associated with prominent angioleiomyoma-like proliferation: Report of 5 cases and review of the literature. Am J Surg Pathol. 2006;30:1372–81.

Latif F, Duh FM, Gnarra J, Tory K, Kuzmin I, Yao M, Stackhouse T, Modi W, Geil L, Schmidt L, et al. von Hippel-Lindau syndrome: cloning and identification of the plasma membrane Ca(++)-transporting ATPase isoform 2 gene that resides in the von Hippel-Lindau gene region. Cancer Res. 1993;53:861–7.

Lendvay TS, Marshall FF. The tuberous sclerosis complex and its highly variable manifestations. J Urol. 2003;169:1635–42.

Lhermitte B, Leval L. Interpretation of needle biopsies of the kidney for investigation of renal masses. Virchows Arch. 2012;461:13–26.

Liu Q, Galli S, Srinivasan R, Linehan WM, Tsokos M, Merino MJ. Renal medullary carcinoma: molecular, immunohistochemistry, and morphologic correlation. Am J Surg Pathol. 2013;37(3):368–74.

Lopez-Beltran A, Scarpelli M, Montironi R, Kirkali Z. WHO classification of the renal tumors of the adults. Eur Urol. 2004;2006(49):798–805.

Lopez-Beltran A, Suzigan S, Montironi R, Drut R, Romero A, Hayashi T, Gentili AL, Fonseca PS, de Torres I, Billis A, Japp LC, Bollito E, Algaba F, Requena-Tapias MJ. Multilocular cystic renal cell carcinoma: a report of 45 cases of a kidney tumor of low malignant potential. Am J Clin Pathol. 2006;125:217–22.

Lopez-Beltran A, Kirkali Z, Cheng L, et al. Targeted therapies and biological modifiers in urologic tumors: pathobiology and clinical implications. Semin Diagn Pathol. 2008;25:232–44.

Lopez-Beltran A, Carrasco JC, Cheng L, Scarpelli M, Kirkali Z, Montironi R. 2009 update on the classification of renal epithelial tumors in adults. Int J Urol. 2009;16:432–43.

Lopez-Beltran A, Montironi R, Egevad L, et al. Genetic profiles in renal tumors. Int J Urol. 2010;17:6–19.

Lopez-Beltran A, Kirkali Z, Montironi R, et al. Unclassified renal cell carcinoma: a report of 56 cases. BJU Int. 2012;110:786–93.

Lopez-Beltran A, Cheng VA, Scarpelli M, Kirkali Z, Blanca A, Montironi R. Pathology of renal cell carcinoma. Un update. Anal Quant Cytopathol Histopathol. 2013;35:61–76.

Martignoni G, Brunelli M, Gobbo S, Remo A, Ficarra V, Cossu-Rocca P, Pea M, Chilosi M, Menestrina F, Cheng L. Role of molecular markers in diagnosis and prognosis of renal cell carcinoma. Anal Quant Cytol Histol. 2007;29:41–9.

Martin SA, Mynderse LA, Lager DJ, et al. Juxtaglomerular cell tumor: a clinicopathologic study of four cases and review of the literature. Am J Clin Pathol. 2001;116:854–63.

Mazzucchelli R, Galosi AB, Scarpelli M, Lopez-Beltran A, Cheng L, Montironi R. Contemporary update on pathology related issues of the adults renal neoplasms. Anal Quant Cytopathol Histopathol. 2014;36:1–8.

Merino MJ, Torres-Cabala C, Pinto P, Linehan WM. The morphologic spectrum of kidney tumors in hereditary leiomyomatosis and renal cell carcinoma (HLRCC) syndrome. Am J Surg Pathol. 2007;31:1578–85.

Montironi R, Mazzucchelli R, Lopez-Beltran A, Martignoni G, Cheng L, Montorsi F, Scarpelli M. Cystic nephroma and mixed epithelial and stromal tumour of the kidney: opposite ends of the spectrum of the same entity? Eur Urol. 2008a;54:1237–46.

Montironi R, Scarpelli M, Martignoni G, Cheng L, Lopez-Beltran A. Splitting and lumping adult renal epithelial tumours: is that what the urologists want? Eur Urol. 2008b;53:673–5; discussion 676–80.

Montironi R, Scarpelli M, Cheng L, Lopez-Beltran A, Burattini M, Kirkali Z, Montorsi F. Immunoglobulin G4-related disease in genitourinary organs: an emerging fibroinflammatory entity often misdiagnosed preoperatively as cancer. Eur Urol. 2012. doi:10.1016/j.eururo.2012.11.056. pii: S0302-2838(12)01462-5.

Montironi R, Mazzucchelli R, Scarpelli M, Lopez-Beltran A, Cheng L. Update on selected renal cell tumors with clear cell features. With emphasis on multilocular cystic clear cell renal cell carcinoma. Histol Histopathol. 2013;28:1555–66.
Morichetti D, Mazzucchelli R, Lopez-Beltran A, et al. Secondary neoplasms of the urinary system and male genital organs. BJU Int. 2009;104:770–6.
Muir TE, Cheville JC, Lager DJ. Metanephric adenoma, nephrogenic rests, and Wilms' tumor. Am J Surg Pathol. 2001;25:1290–6.
Nickerson ML, Warren MB, Toro JR, Matrosova V, Glenn G, Turner ML, Duray P, Merino M, Choyke P, Pavlovich CP, Sharma N, Walther M, Munroe D, Hill R, Maher E, Greenberg C, Lerman MI, Linehan WM, Zbar B, Schmidt LS. Mutations in a novel gene lead to kidney tumors, lung wall defects, and benign tumors of the hair follicle in patients with the Birt-Hogg-Dube syndrome. Cancer Cell. 2002;2:157–64.
Paner GP, Srigley JR, Radhakrishnan A, Cohen C, Skinnider BF, Tickoo SK, Young AN, Amin MB. Immunohistochemical analysis of mucinous tubular and spindle cell carcinoma and papillary renal cell carcinoma of the kidney: significant immunophenotypic overlap warrants diagnostic caution. Am J Surg Pathol. 2006;30:13–9.
Patard JJ, Pouessel D, Bensalah K, Culine S. Targeted therapy in renal cell carcinoma. World J Urol. 2008;26:135–40.
Presti Jr JC, Moch H, Reuter VE, Huynh D, Waldman FM. Comparative genomic hybridization for genetic analysis of renal oncocytomas. Genes Chromosomes Cancer. 1996;17:199–204.
Rakozy C, Schmahl GE, Bogner S, Storkel S. Low-grade tubular-mucinous renal neoplasms: morphologic, immunohistochemical, and genetic features. Mod Pathol. 2002;15:1162–71.
Rao Q, Liu B, Cheng L, et al. A clinicopathologic study emphasizing unusual morphology, novel alpha-TFEB gene fusion point, immunobiomarkers, and ultrastructural features, as well as detection of the gene fusion by fluorescence in situ hybridization. Am J Surg Pathol. 2012;36:1327–38.
Ro JY, Ayala AG, Sella A, Samuels ML, Swanson DA. Sarcomatoid renal cell carcinoma: clinicopathologic. A study of 42 cases. Cancer. 1987;59: 516–26.
Sanders ME, Mick R, Tomaszewski JE, Barr FG. Unique patterns of allelic imbalance distinguish type 1 from type 2 sporadic papillary renal cell carcinoma. Am J Pathol. 2002;161:997–1005.
Sanz-Ortega J, Vocke C, Stratton P, Linehan WM, Merino MJ. Morphologic and molecular characteristics of uterine leiomyomas in hereditary leiomyomatosis and renal cancer (HLRCC) syndrome. Am J Surg Pathol. 2013;37(1):74–80.
Schmidt L, Duh FM, Chen F, Kishida T, Glenn G, Choyke P, Scherer SW, Zhuang Z, Lubensky I, Dean M, Allikmets R, Chidambaram A, Bergerheim UR, Feltis JT, Casadevall C, Zamarron A, Bernues M, Richard S, Lips CJ, Walther MM, Tsui LC, Geil L, Orcutt ML, Stackhouse T, Lipan J, Slife L, Brauch H, Decker J, Niehans G, Hughson MD, Moch H, Storkel S, Lerman MI, Linehan WM, Zbar B. Germline and somatic mutations in the tyrosine kinase domain of the MET proto-oncogene in papillary renal carcinomas. Nat Genet. 1997;16:68–73.
Schoolmeester JK, Cheville JC, Folpe AL. Synovial sarcoma of the kidney: a clinicopathologic, immunohistochemical, and molecular genetic study of 16 cases. Am J Surg Pathol. 2014;38:60–5.
Sebire NJ, Vujanic GM. Paediatric renal tumours: recent developments, new entities and pathological features. Histopathology. 2009;54(5):516–28.
Shen SS, Truong LD, Scarpelli M, Lopez-Beltran A. Role of immunohistochemistry in diagnosing renal neoplasms: when is it really useful? Arch Pathol Lab Med. 2012;136:410–7.
Sika-Paotonu D, Bethwaite PB, McCredie MR, William Jordan T, Delahunt B. Nucleolar grade but not Fuhrman grade is applicable to papillary renal cell carcinoma. Am J Surg Pathol. 2006;30:1091–6.
Speicher MR, Schoell B, du Manoir S, Schrock E, Ried T, Cremer T, Storkel S, Kovacs A, Kovacs G. Specific loss of chromosomes 1, 2, 6, 10, 13, 17, and 21 in chromophobe renal cell carcinomas revealed by comparative genomic hybridization. Am J Pathol. 1994;145:356–64.
Srigley JR, Delahunt B. Uncommon and recently described renal Carcinomas. Mod Pathol. 2009;22:S2–23.
Srigley JR, Eble JN. Collecting duct carcinoma of kidney. Semin Diagn Pathol. 1998;15:54–67.
Srigley JR, Delahunt B, Eble JN, et al. The International Society of Urological Pathology (ISUP) Vancouver classification of renal neoplasia. Am J Surg Pathol. 2013;37:1469–89.
Sterlacci W, Verdorfer I, Gabriel M, Mikuz G. Thyroid follicular carcinoma-like renal tumor: a case report with morphologic, immunophenotypic, cytogenetic, and scintigraphic studies. Virchows Arch. 2008;452:91–5.
Tan PH, Cheng L, Rioux-Leclercq N, et al. Renal tumors: diagnostic and prognostic markers. Am J Surg Pathol. 2013;37:1518–31.
Thoenes W, Storkel S, Rumpelt HJ, Moll R, Baum HP, Werner S. Chromophobe cell renal carcinoma and its variants–a report on 32 cases. J Pathol. 1988;155:277–87.
Thoenes W, Storkel S, Rumpelt HJ, Moll R. Cytomorphological typing of renal cell carcinoma–a new approach. Eur Urol. 1990;18 Suppl 2:6–9.
Tickoo SK, Reuter VE, Amin MB, Srigley JR, Epstein JI, Min KW, Rubin MA, Ro JY. Renal oncocytosis: a morphologic study of fourteen cases. Am J Surg Pathol. 1999;23:1094–101.
Tickoo SK, de Peralta-Venturina MN, Harik LR, Worcester HD, Salama ME, Young AN, Moch H, Amin MB. Spectrum of epithelial neoplasms in end-stage renal disease: an experience from 66 tumor-bearing kidneys with emphasis on histologic patterns distinct from those in sporadic adult renal neoplasia. Am J Surg Pathol. 2006;30:141–53.

Tomlinson IP, Alam NA, Rowan AJ, Barclay E, Jaeger EE, Kelsell D, Leigh I, Gorman P, Lamlum H, Rahman S, Roylance RR, Olpin S, Bevan S, Barker K, Hearle N, Houlston RS, Kiuru M, Lehtonen R, Karhu A, Vilkki S, Laiho P, Eklund C, Vierimaa O, Aittomaki K, Hietala M, Sistonen P, Paetau A, Salovaara R, Herva R, Launonen V, Aaltonen LA. Germline mutations in FH predispose to dominantly inherited uterine fibroids, skin leiomyomata and papillary renal cell cancer. Nat Genet. 2002;30:406–10.

Toro JR, Wei MH, Glenn GM, Weinreich M, Toure O, Vocke C, Turner M, Choyke P, Merino MJ, Pinto PA, Steinberg SM, Schmidt LS, Linehan WM. BHD mutations, clinical and molecular genetic investigations of Birt-Hogg-Dube syndrome: a new series of 50 families and a review of published reports. J Med Genet. 2008;45:321–31.

Trpkov K, Grignon DJ, Bonsib SM, et al. Handing and staging of renal cell carcinoma: the International Society of Urological Pathology (ISUP) Consensus Conference recommendations. Am J Surg Pathol. 2013;37:1505–17.

Turbiner J, Amin MB, Humphrey PA, Srigley JR, De Leval L, Radhakrishnan A, Oliva E. Cystic nephroma and mixed epithelial and stromal tumor of kidney: a detailed clinicopathologic analysis of 34 cases and proposal for renal epithelial and stromal tumor (REST) as a unifying term. Am J Surg Pathol. 2007;31:489–500.

Van den Hoek J. Cystic nephroma, cystic partially differentiated nephrobastoma and cystic Wilm's tumor in children: a spectrum with therapeutic dilemmas. Urol Int. 2009;82:65–70.

Venneti S, Le P, Martinez D, et al. Malignant rhabdoid tumors express stem cell factors, which relate to the expression of EZH2 and Id proteins. Am J Surg Pathol. 2011;35(10):1463–72.

Volpe A, Finelli A, Gill IS, Jewett MAS, Martignoni G, Polascik TJ, Remzi M, Uzzo RG. Rationale for percutaneous biopsy and histologic characterisation of renal tumours. Eur Urol. 2012;62:491–504.

Vujanić GM, Sandstedt B. The pathology of Wilms' tumour (nephroblastoma): the International Society of Paediatric Oncology approach. J Clin Pathol. 2010;63(2):102–9.

Weirich G, Glenn G, Junker K, Merino M, Storkel S, Lubensky I, Choyke P, Pack S, Amin M, Walther MM, Linehan WM, Zbar B. Familial renal oncocytoma: clinicopathological study of 5 families. J Urol. 1998;160:335–40.

Williamson SR, Zhang S, Eble JN, Grignon DJ, Martignoni G, Brunelli M, Wang M, Gobbo S, Baldridge LA, Cheng L. Clear cell papillary renal cell carcinoma–like tumors in patients with Von Hippel-Lindau disease are unrelated to sporadic clear cell papillary renal cell carcinoma. Am J Surg Pathol. 2013;37(8): 1131–9.

Woodward ER. Familial non-syndromic clear cell renal cell carcinoma. Curr Mol Med. 2004;4:843–8.

Yang XJ, Zhou M, Hes O, Shen S, Li R, Lopez J, Shah RB, Yang Y, Chuang ST, Lin F, Tretiakova MM, Kort EJ, Teh BT. Tubulocystic carcinoma of the kidney: clinicopathologic and molecular characterization. Am J Surg Pathol. 2008;32:177–87.

Zisman A, Chao DH, Pantuck AJ, Kim HJ, Wieder JA, Figlin RA, Said JW, Belldegrun AS. Unclassified renal cell carcinoma: clinical features and prognostic impact of a new histological subtype. J Urol. 2002;168: 950–5.

2 Tumors and Tumor-Like Conditions of Urinary Bladder, Renal Pelvis, Ureter and Urethra

Contents

2.1	**Introduction**	63
2.1.1	Basic Anatomy and Histology	63
2.2	**Urinary Bladder**	68
2.2.1	Urothelial Carcinoma	68
2.2.2	Flat Intraepithelial Lesions	68
2.2.3	Urothelial Carcinoma	84
2.2.4	Benign Urothelial Neoplasms	122
2.2.5	Glandular Neoplasms	128
2.2.6	Squamous Cell Neoplasms	135
2.2.7	Neuroendocrine Tumors	139
2.2.8	Soft Tissue Tumors	148
2.2.9	Malignant Melanoma	166
2.2.10	Germ Cell Tumors	167
2.2.11	Hematologic Malignancies	167
2.2.12	Tumor-Like Conditions	168
2.2.13	Metastatic Tumors and Secondary Extension	176
2.2.14	Metastatic Urothelial Carcinoma	176
2.3	**The Renal Pelvis and Ureter**	177
2.4	**The Urethra**	181
Suggested Reading		187

2.1 Introduction

2.1.1 Basic Anatomy and Histology

Urinary bladder

- The bladder is a hollow muscular organ whose main function is that of a reservoir. When empty, the adult bladder lies behind the symphysis pubis, and is largely a pelvic organ. When full, the bladder rises above the symphysis and can readily be palpated.
- The empty bladder has an apex (superior surface), two infralateral or anterolateral surfaces, a base (posterior surface), and a neck. The apex extends a short distance above the pubic bone and ends as a fibrous cord derivative of the urachus. This fibrous cord extends from the apex of the bladder to the umbilicus between the peritoneum and the transversalis fascia.
- The apex of the bladder is apposed to the uterus and ileum in the female, and the ileum and pelvic portion of the colon in the male.
- The base of the bladder faces posteriorly and is separated from the rectum by the uterus and vagina in the female, and by the vasa deferentia, seminal vesicles, and ureters in the male.
- The anterolateral surface on each side of the bladder is apposed to the pubic bone, levator ani, and obturator internus muscles, but the central anterior bladder is separated from the pubic bone by the retropubic space, that contains abundant fat and venous plexuses.

A. Lopez-Beltran et al., *Rare Tumors and Tumor-like Conditions in Urological Pathology*,
DOI 10.1007/978-3-319-10253-5_2,

- The neck of the bladder, its most inferior part, connects with the urethra. When the bladder is distended with urine, the neck remains fixed and stationary, whereas the dome rises above the pelvic cavity into the lower abdomen, touching the posterior aspect of the lower anterior abdominal wall and the small and large bowel.
- Beneath the urothelial lining of the inner bladder, there is loose connective tissue that permits considerable stretching of the mucosa. As a result, the urothelial mucosal lining is wrinkled when the bladder is empty but smooth and flat when distended.
- This arrangement exists throughout the bladder except at the trigone, where the mucous membrane adheres firmly to the underlying muscle; consequently, the trigone is always smooth, regardless of the level of distension.
- The bladder is supplied by the superior, middle, and inferior vesical arteries, all of which are branches of the anterior division of the hypogastric artery.
- Between the bladder wall proper and the outer adventitial layer, there is a rich plexus of veins that ultimately terminate in the hypogastric veins after converging in several main trunks.
- The bladder lymphatics drain into the external iliac, hypogastric, and common iliac lymph nodes. There are rich lymphatic anastomoses between the pelvic and genital organs.
- The bladder is richly innervated by divisions of the autonomic nervous system. Sympathetic nerves originate from the lower thoracic and upper lumbar segments, mainly T11-T12 and L1-L2.
- These sympathetic fibers descend into the sympathetic trunk and the lumbar splanchnic nerves, connecting with the superior hypogastric plexus, an inferior extension of the aortic plexus.
- Parasympathetic nerves arise from sacral segments S2-S4, and these form the rich pelvic parasympathetic plexus. This plexus joins the sympathetic hypogastric plexus, and vesical branches emerge from this plexus toward the bladder base, innervating the bladder and urethra.
- Paraganglia are rarely found in routine sections of the urinary bladder. Paraganglionic tissue typically demonstrates immunoreactivity with Neuroendocrine markers such as chromogranin, synaptophysin, and neuron specific enolase. The sustentacular cells exhibit immunostaining for S-100 protein.
- The urothelium is a unique stratified epithelium of variable thickness. The number of cell layers depends on the degree of distension of the bladder, usually varying from three to seven layers. When distended, the bladder is three to six cell layers thick, although the typical biopsy contains about five layers; in the contracted state, it consists of six to eight layers (Figs. 2.1, 2.2, and 2.3)
- The normal urothelium contains a layer of large superficial (umbrella cells) cells that are frequently multinucleated. These cells have abundant eosinophilic cytoplasm, with large nuclei whose long axes are perpendicular to those of the smaller cells of the underlying basal and intermediate cell layers. Superficial umbrella cells express uroplakins and CK 20 on immunohistochemistry.
- Basal and intermediate cells are located between the basal lamina and the superficial cells. These cells are morphologically identical to each other, and are distinguished only by their position in the mucosa. They are regularly arranged, with distinct cell boundaries and oval, round, or fusiform nuclei with occasional prominent nuclear grooves.
- The basal layer of epithelial cells expresses Bcl-2 while the intermediate cells express RB1 and PTEN at varying intensities. HER2/neu and p53 are not expressed by normal urothelial cells. Ki67, indicating proliferation, may not be expressed in a single field.
- The long axis of the basal and intermediate cells is perpendicular to the basement membrane. Basement membrane markers such as laminin and type IV collagen may be useful diagnostically in select cases to define the basement membrane, but are not routinely employed.
- The lamina propria, located beneath the basement membrane, consists of a compact layer of fibrovascular connective tissue. It contains an incomplete muscularis mucosa

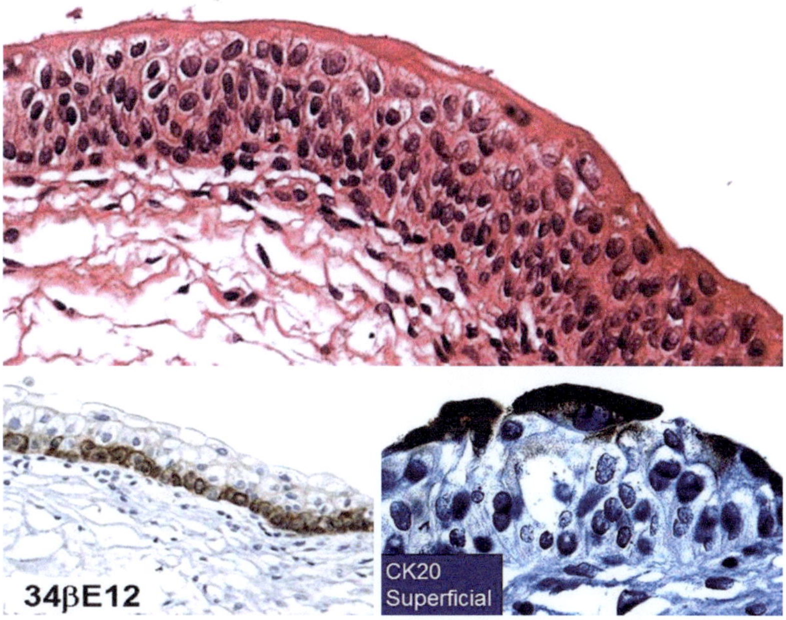

Fig. 2.1 Microscopic appearance of normal uothelium (*upper*). 34BE12 highlights basal cell layer (*lower left*) and CK 20 highlights superficial cells (*lower right*)

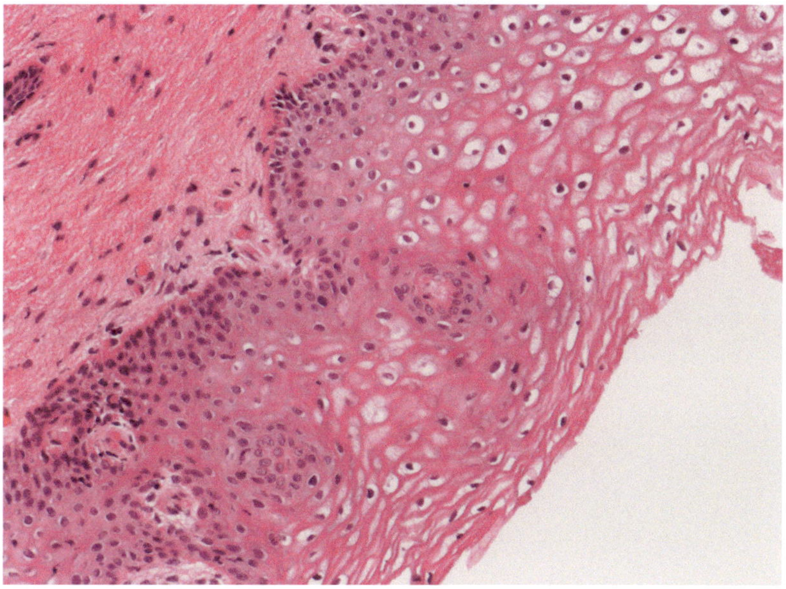

Fig. 2.2 Non-keratinized squamous epithelium in the trigone

composed of thin delicate smooth muscle fibers that may be mistaken for muscularis propria in biopsy specimens.

- In biopsy specimens, these smooth muscle fibers may appear as a continuous layer, a discontinuous or interrupted layer, or as scattered thin bundles of smooth muscle fibers that do not form an obvious layer. The muscle fibers lie parallel to the mucosal surface, midway between the epithelium and the underlying muscularis propria (Figs. 2.4 and 2.5)
- Moderate size or large thick-walled blood vessels are a constant feature of the lamina propria, running parallel to the surface urothelium in close association with the smooth muscle fibers of the muscularis mucosa.
- The muscle proper of the bladder, the muscularis propria, is moderately thick and consists of an

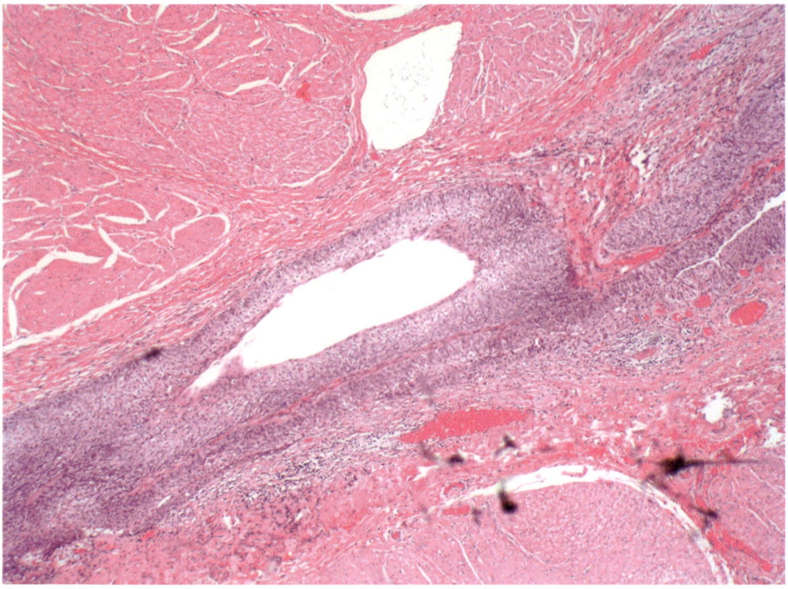

Fig. 2.3 Urothelial lined urachus

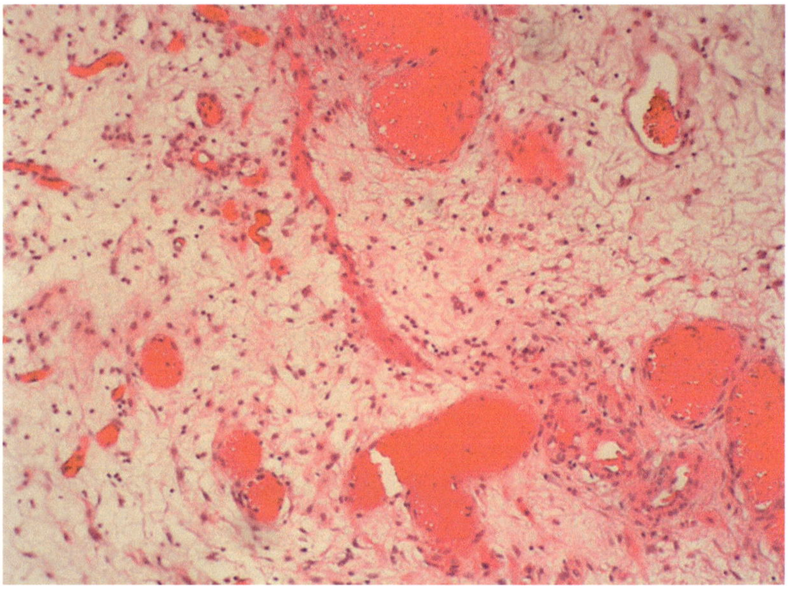

Fig. 2.4 Incomplete muscularis mucosae

inner longitudinal layer, middle circular layer, and outer longitudinal layer. It spirals around each ureteral orifice and increases in thickness around the internal urethral orifice, forming the internal sphincter of the bladder. The muscularis is surrounded by a coat of fibroelastic connective tissue, the adventitia, and perivesical fat.

The Urachus

- The urachus is an intra-abdominal embryonic remnant. It contains the allantois, connecting the apex of the urinary bladder to the body wall at the umbilicus.
- At birth, the dome of the bladder and the umbilicus are closely apposed, and the urachus is only 2.5–3 mm long, with a diameter of 1 mm throughout most of its course and 3 mm where it joins the bladder.
- The urachus lies in a space anterior to the peritoneum, bounded anteriorly and posteriorly by the umbilicovesical fascia. Laterally, it is bounded by the two umbilical arteries

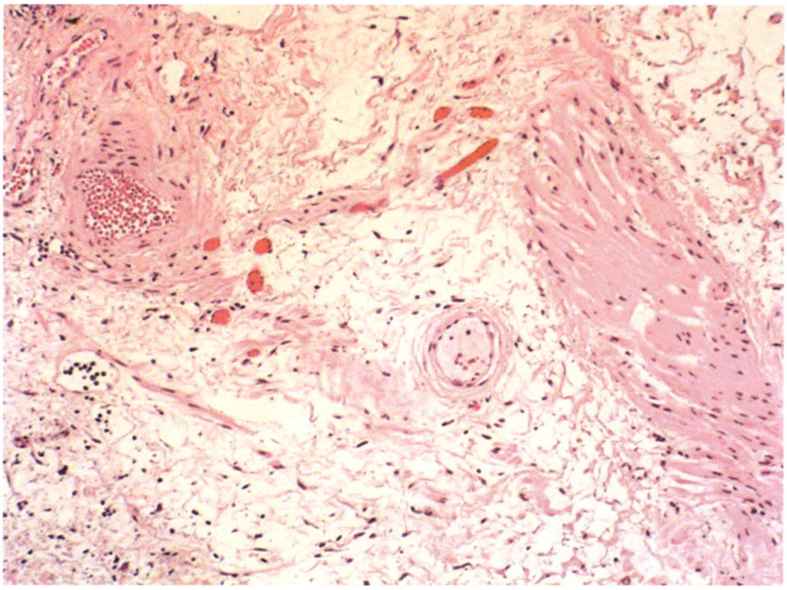

Fig. 2.5 Occasionally, smooth muscle fibers of muscularis mucosae have an hypertrophic appearance

that, in turn, are surrounded by umbilicovesical fascia.

- Inferiorly, the umbilicovesical fascial layers cover the surface of the dome of the bladder. This space, the space of Retzius, is roughly pyramidal, and fascial planes separate it from the peritoneum and other structures. At the junction with the urinary bladder, the adult urachus is 4–8 mm wide, narrowing to about 2 mm at its superior end.
- The urachus has three segments, including the supravesical, intramural, and intramucosal segments. Tubular urachal remnants are found within the wall of the urinary bladder in approximately one-third of adults and are evenly distributed between men and women.
- There are three architectural patterns of intramural urachal canals varying from simple tubular canals to complex branching canals.
- The mucosal portion of the urachus may have a wide diverticular opening, papilla, or a small opening flush with the mucosal surface. The majority (70 %) of intramural urachal remnants are lined by urothelium; the remainder are lined by columnar epithelium, occasionally with small papillae or, rarely, mucous goblet cells or mucus-secreting columnar epithelium.

The Renal Pelvis and Ureters

- The lumen of the renal pelvis and ureter is lined by urothelium that rests on a basement membrane. The urothelium is composed of 3–5 layers of cells in the pelvis and 4–7 layers of cells in the ureter.
- The pelvis and ureter have a continuous muscular wall that originates in the fornices of the minor calyces as small interlacing fascicles of the smooth muscle cells. The muscularis propria is not divided into distinct layers.

The Urethra

- The epithelium of the urethra is derived from the urogenital sinus. In females, the epithelium of the urethra is derived from endoderm of the urogenital sinus, while the surrounding connective tissue and smooth muscle arise from splanchnic mesenchyme.
- In males the epithelium also is derived from the urogenital sinus except in the fossa navicularis, where it is derived from ectodermal cells migrating from the glans penis. As in females, the connective tissue and smooth muscle surrounding the male urethra is derived from splanchnic mesenchyme.
- The male urethra is 15–20 cm long and is divided in three anatomical segments. The prostatic urethra begins at the internal urethral

orifice at the bladder neck and extends through the prostate to the prostatic apex. In the central part of the urethral crest is an eminence called the verumontanum.

- The verumontanum contains a slitlike opening that leads to an epithelium-lined sac called the prostatic utricle, a Mullerian vestige. The ejaculatory ducts empty into the urethra on either side of the prostatic utricle. The membranous urethra extends from the prostatic apex to the bulb of penis.
- Cowper's glands are located on the left and right sides of the membranous urethra and their ducts empty into it. Bulbourethral glands are located in the proximal (bulbous) portion of the penile urethra. In addition, scattered mucus-secreting periurethral glands (Littre's glands) are present at the periphery of the penile urethra except anteriorly.
- The female urethra is approximately 4 cm long, and, at its periphery, contains paraurethral Skene's glands.
- The type of epithelium lining the urethra varies along its length. In general, urothelium lines the prostatic urethra, pseudostratified columnar epithelium lines the membranous segment and most of the penile urethra, and nonkeratinized stratified squamous epithelium lines the fossa navicularis and external urethral orifice.
- In females, the proximal one-third of the urethra is lined by urothelium and the distal two-thirds by nonkeratinized stratified squamous epithelium.
- The urothelium has a characteristic immunophenotype. It expresses cytokeratins of both low and high molecular weights, including keratins 7, 8, 13, and 19; cytockeratin 18 and 20 are present in the superficial cells.
- This pattern of expression differs from that of normal stratified squamous epithelium, that shows predominantly high molecular weight keratin immunoreactivity, and from endometrium, endocervix, colorectum, and prostate, that demonstrate a preponderance of low molecular weight keratin.
- High molecular weight keratin immunoreactivity is restricted to the basal cell layer of the urothelium and squamous mucosa of the trigone.

2.2 Urinary Bladder

2.2.1 Urothelial Carcinoma

Overview

- Carcinoma of the urinary bladder is the fourth most common malignancy in men, and more than 90 % of bladder cancer cases are urothelial (transitional cell) carcinoma, whereas primary squamous cell carcinoma, adenocarcinoma, small cell carcinoma, and other tumors are less common.
- Bladder cancer is morphologically heterogeneous disease. The classification of urinary bladder neoplasia used in this chapter follows the most recent World Health Organization (WHO) classification of tumors of the urinary system.

2.2.2 Flat Intraepithelial Lesions

- The classification of nonpapillary (flat) intraepithelial lesions and conditions of the urothelium has evolved over the years (Table 2.1). This classification includes epithelial abnormalities (reactive urothelial atypia and flat urothelial hyperplasia), presumed preneoplastic lesions and conditions (keratinizing squamous and glandular metaplasia, and malignancy associated cellular changes) as well as preneoplastic (dysplasia) and neoplastic noninvasive (carcinoma in situ) lesions (Figs. 2.6, 2.7, 2.8, 2.9, 2.10, 2.11, 2.12, 2.13, 2.14, 2.15, 2.16, 2.17, 2.18, 2.19, and 2.20)
- Recent studies have shown that 50 % of the histologically normal urothelium adjacent to superficial urothelial carcinoma harbors genetic anomalies on chromosome 9, similar to the anomalies found in the coexisting carcinoma. In addition, non-diploid nuclear DNA histograms occur in 4–54 % of histological normal urothelium adjacent to bladder tumors. These genetic alterations suggest a neoplastic potential for flat urothelial lesions, regardless of whether cytologic atypia is present or not.

Table 2.1 Classification of flat urothelial lesions of the urinary bladder based on the Ancona International Consultation

Flat urothelial hyperplasia
Reactive urothelial atypia
Presumed preneoplastic lesions and conditions
Keratinizing squamous metaplasia
Intestinal metaplasia
Malignancy associated cellular changes
Preneoplastic lesions
Dysplasia
Neoplastic non-invasive lesion
Urothelial carcinoma in situ

Flat urothelial hyperplasia (simple hyperplasia)

- Urothelial hyperplasia is characterized by markedly thickened mucosa with an increase in the number of cell layers, usually 10 or more. However, it is not necessary to count the number of cell layers for the diagnosis (Table 2.2). The cells in urothelial hyperplasia do not show any significant cytologic abnormalities, although slight nuclear enlargement may be focally present.

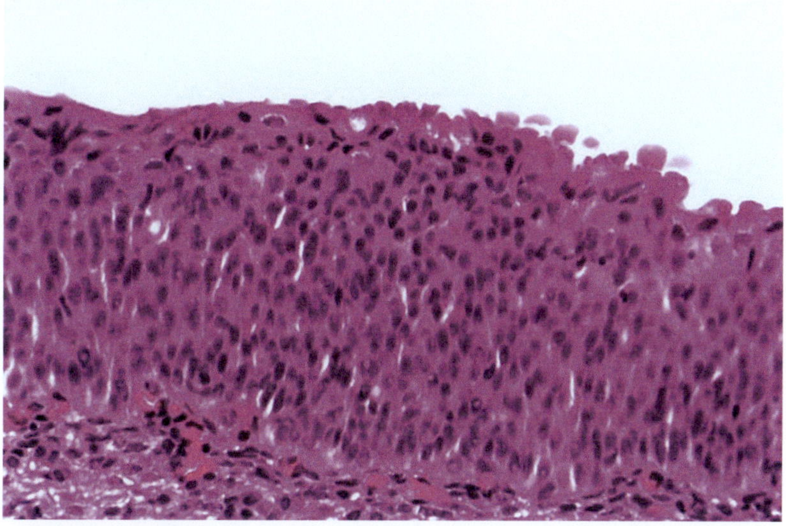

Fig. 2.6 Microscopic appearance of flat urothelial hyperplasia

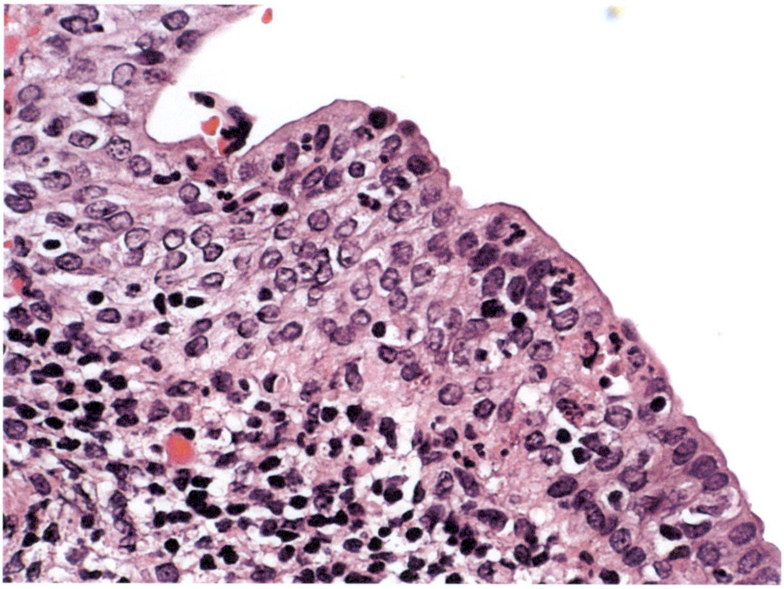

Fig. 2.7 Microscopic changes of reactive urothelium

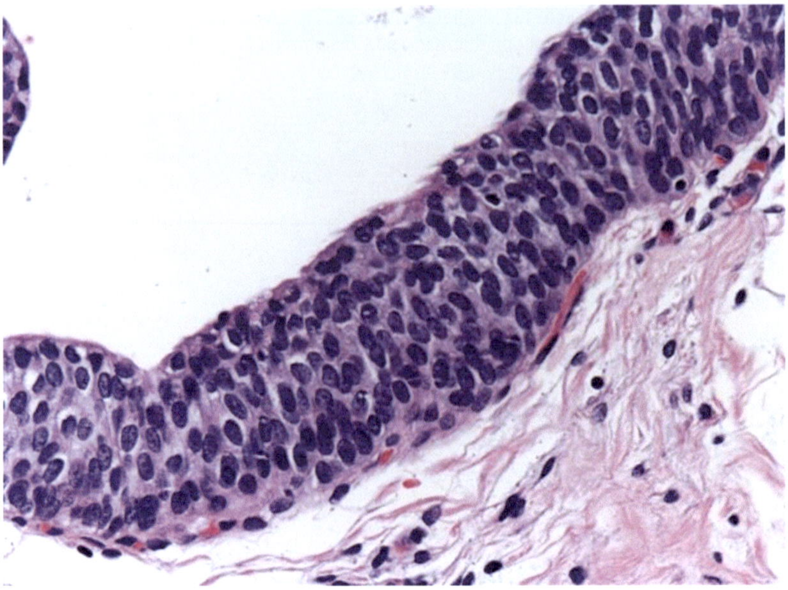

Fig. 2.8 Microscopic appearance of urothelial dysplasia

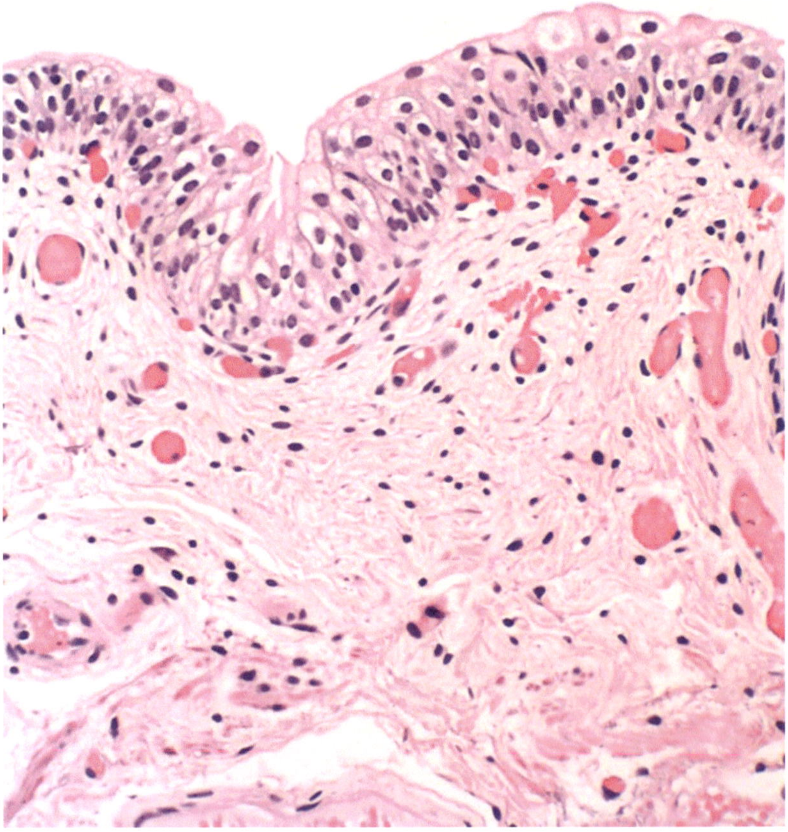

Fig. 2.9 A comparison with normal urothelium is helpful in diagnosing flat urothelial lesions

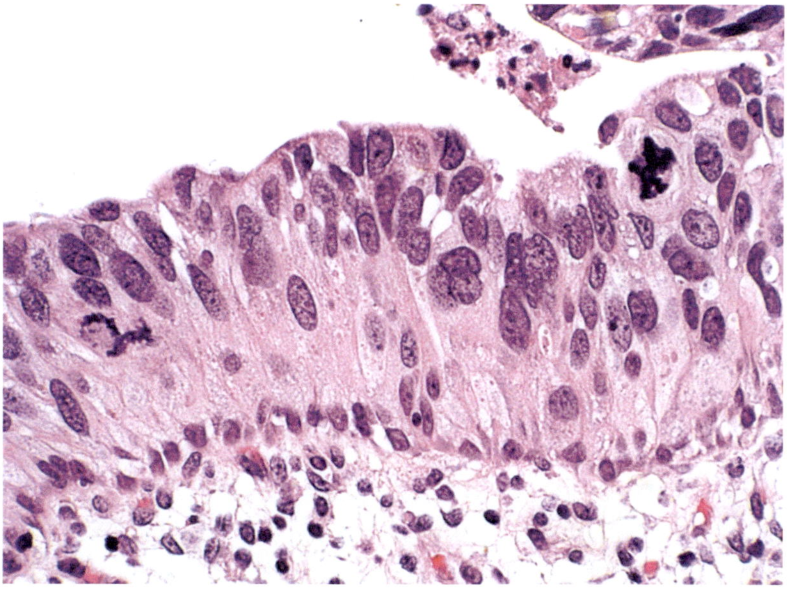

Fig. 2.10 Urothelial carcinoma in situ

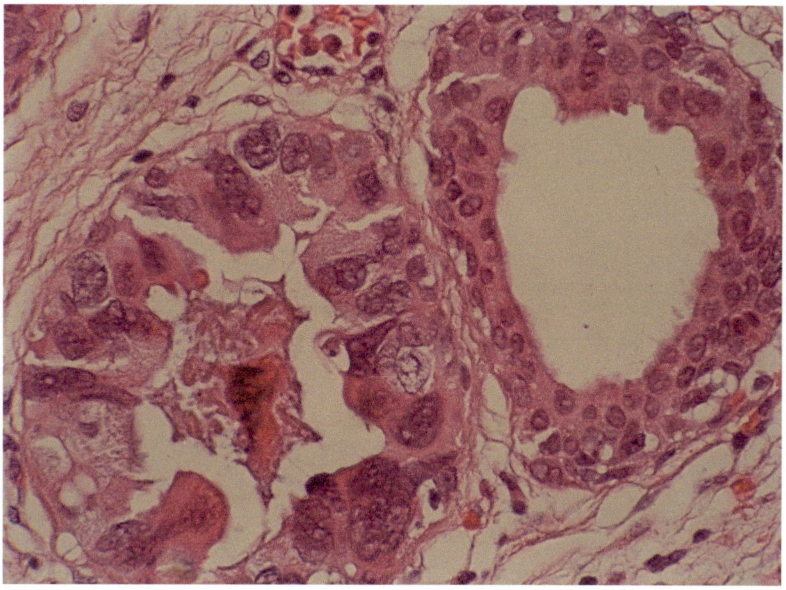

Fig. 2.11 Urothelial carcinoma in situ in von Brunn nest showing marked pleomorphism

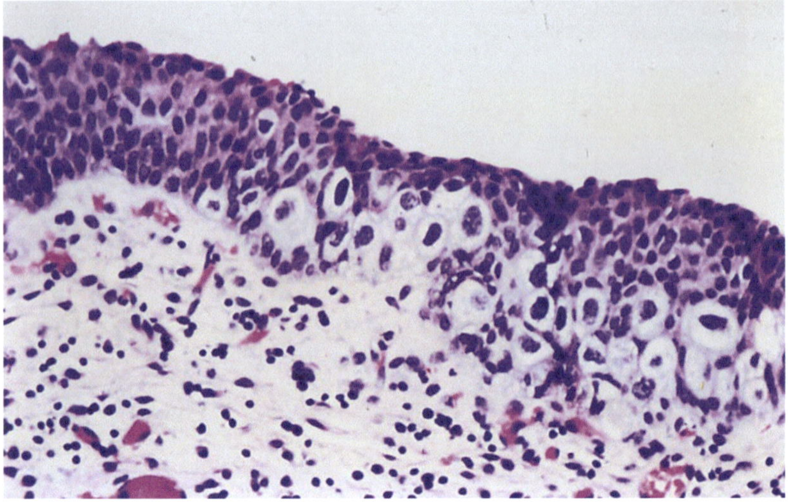

Fig. 2.12 Pagetoid urothelial carcinoma in situ

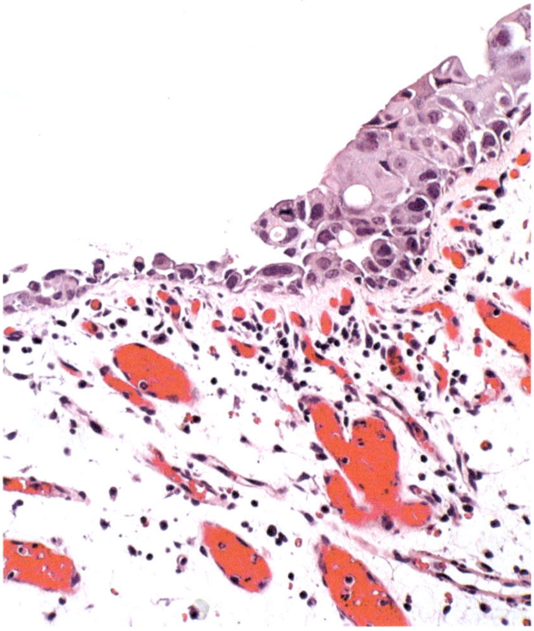

Fig. 2.13 Urothelial carcinoma in situ with squamous features (*right*)

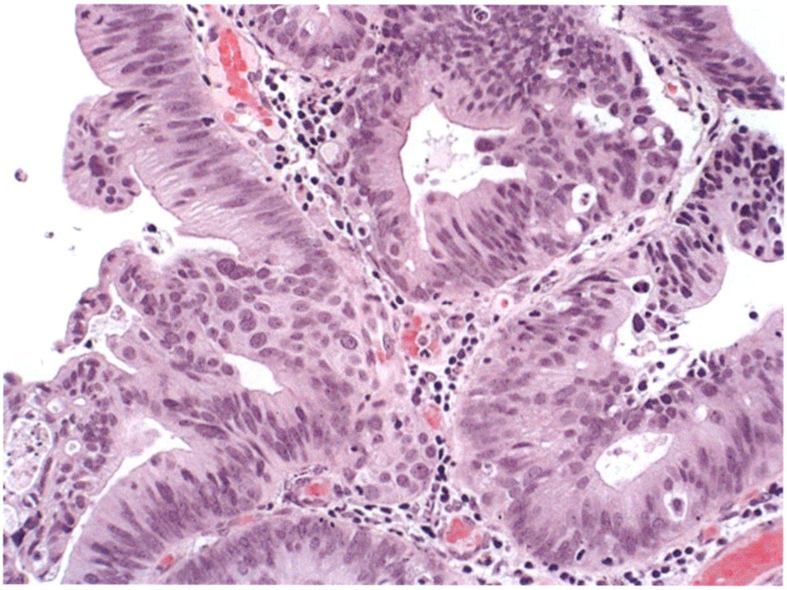

Fig. 2.14 Urothelial carcinoma in situ with glandular differentiation

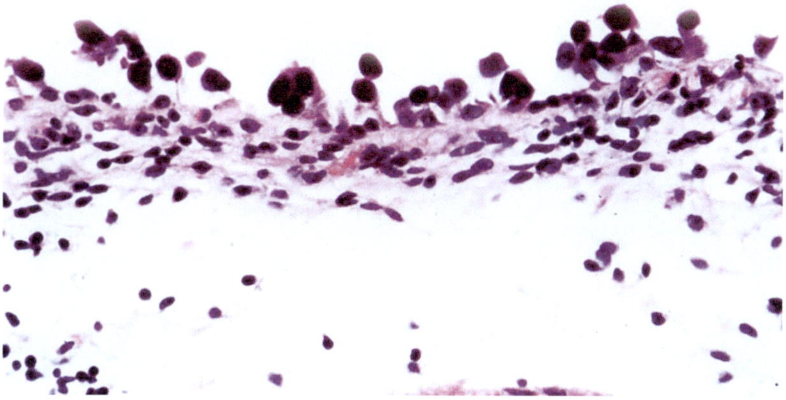

Fig. 2.15 Urothelial carcinoma in situ, clinging type

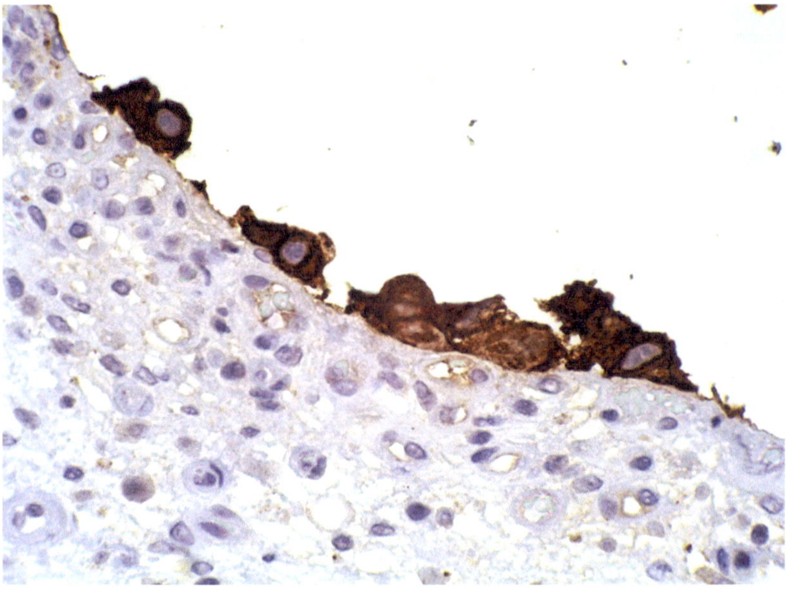

Fig. 2.16 Urothelial carcinoma in situ, clinging type. Keratin staining highlights residual cells

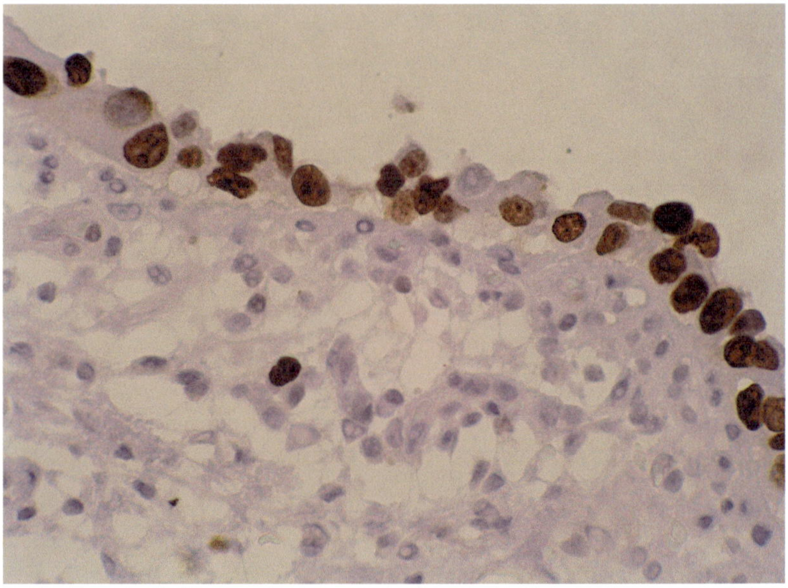

Fig. 2.17 P53 nuclear accumulation in urothelial carcinoma in situ

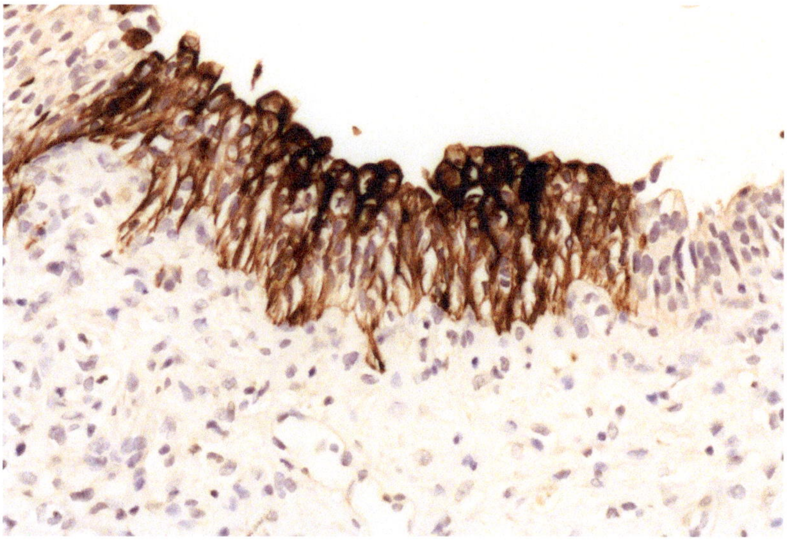

Fig. 2.18 Aberrant CK20 expression in urothelial carcinoma in situ

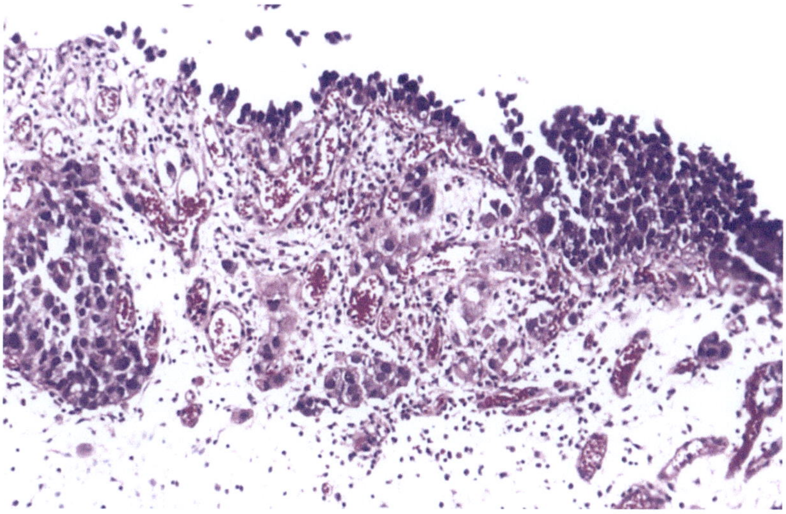

Fig. 2.19 Urothelial carcinoma in situ with microinvasion

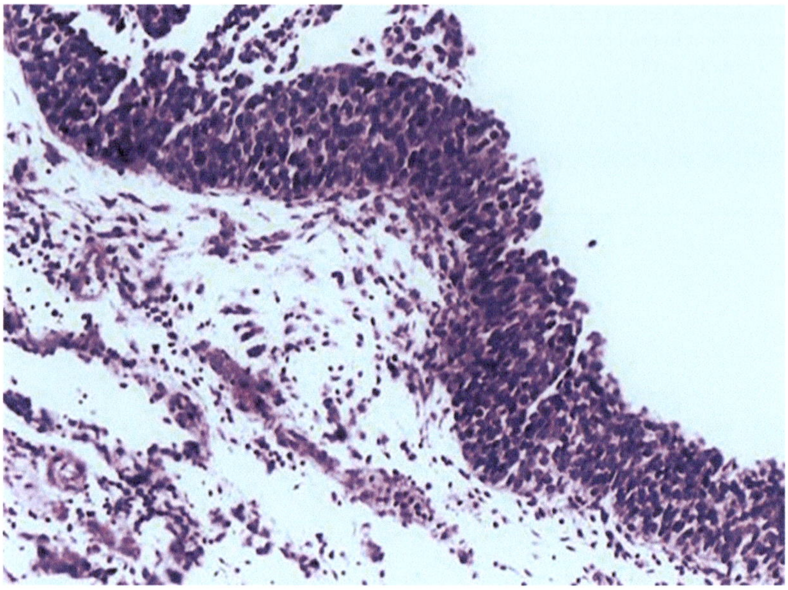

Fig. 2.20 Small cell type of urothelial carcinoma in situ

- Morphologic evidence of maturation from base to surface is generally evident. Urothelial compression artifact or tangential sectioning of mucosa with pseudopapillary growth (lacking a true vascular core) may resemble flat urothelial hyperplasia.
- Flat urothelial hyperplasia has been observed in association with a variety of conditions including inflammatory disorders, urolithiasis, papillary urothelial hyperplasia, dysplasia, carcinoma in situ and low grade papillary tumors. Flat urothelial hyperplasia has been considered by some authors to be the source of low grade papillary neoplasia.
- When seen as an isolated phenomenon, there is no evidence to suggest that primary urothelial hyperplasia has a pre-malignant potential. Likewise, molecular analyses showing chromosome 9q deletions and mutations in the Fibroblast Growth Factor Receptor 3 (FGFR3) gene in both urothelial hyperplasia and low grade papillary neoplasia suggest that this lesion may be clonally related to the papillary tumors in bladder cancer patients.

Urothelial reactive atypia

- Urothelial abnormalities whose architectural and cytologic changes are of lesser degree than those of dysplasia have often been termed atypia. The term atypia is, by its very nature, non-specific. Two similar categories of atypia have been recently recognized, namely reactive atypia and atypia of unknown significance. Both of them are placed among the "benign" urothelial abnormalities.
- Reactive atypia is characterized by mild nuclear abnormalities occurring in acutely or chronically inflamed urothelium. In most cases, there is a history of cystitis, instrumentation, infection, stones, or previous therapy. The epithelium may or may not be thickened in reactive atypia. The cells are often larger than normal, with more abundant cytoplasm (squamoid appearance) than normal urothelial cells.
- Nuclei are uniformly enlarged, vesicular, and may have prominent centrally located nucleoli. Mitotic figures may be frequent but occur in the lower epithelial layers. Inflammatory cells occupying the lamina propria and infiltrating into the urothelium are present. CD44 is positive in reactive atypia, and CK20 or p53 are negative.
- The term "atypia of unknown significance" was introduced to describe lesions in which the pathologist was uncertain whether the changes were reactive or preneoplastic

Table 2.2 Comparison of flat intraepithelial lesions

	Reactive atypia	Hyperplasia	Dysplasia	Carcinoma in situ
Cell layers	Variable	>7 cells	Variable	Variable
Polarization	Slightly abnormal	Normal	Slightly abnormal	Abnormal
Cytoplasm	Vacuolated	Homogeneous	Homogeneous	Homogeneous
N:C ratio	Normal or slightly increased	Normal or slightly increased	Slightly increased	Increased
Nuclei				
Anisonucleosis	Normal	Normal	Mild	Moderate to severe
Borders	Regular/smooth	Regular/smooth	Notches/creases	Pleomorphic
Chromatin	Fine/dusty	Fine	Slight hyperchromasia	Coarse/hyperchromatic
Chromatin distribution	Even	Even	Even	Uneven
Nucleoli	Large	Small/absent	Small/absent	Large/prominent
Mitotic figures	Variable	Absent	Rare and rare	Often
Denudation	Variable	No	No	Variable
Cytokeratin 20	Surface	Surface	Variable	Variable
Stromal microvascular proliferation	Variable	Variable	Less prominent	Often prominent

(dysplasia). Atypia of unknown significance is characterized by nuclear changes similar to those seen in reactive atypia. However, the degree of nuclear pleomorphism and hyperchromasia is greater than in reactive atypia and dysplasia cannot be definitely ruled out.
- Inflammation in the lamina propria with urothelial infiltration is often present. However, the cellular changes seem to be disproportionate to the degree of inflammation.
- The clinical outcome of patients with atypia of unknown significance is identical to that of patients with reactive atypia. The use of the designation "atypia of unknown significance" is discouraged.

Urothelial dysplasia (low grade intraurothelial neoplasia)
- Urothelial dysplasia is defined as abnormal urothelium with cytologic and architectural changes that do not meet all the criteria for an unequivocal diagnosis of urothelial carcinoma in situ. The overall appearance is that of the urothelium in low grade papillary urothelial carcinoma (Table 2.2).
- The cytologic abnormalities in urothelial dysplasia, characterized by cellular crowding, loss of orderly maturation, and loss of cellular polarity, are not present in the full thickness of the urothelium. Occasionally, there may be an increased number of cell layers. The superficial umbrella cells are usually present. Most cellular abnormalities in dysplasia are restricted to the basal and intermediate cell layers.
- Individual dysplastic cells show enlarged nuclei and nucleoli with irregular contours and coarsening of the chromatin. Multiple nucleoli and nuclear overlapping may be seen. The cells often show cytoplasmic clearing. Mitotic figures, when present, are generally basally located. The transition from normal to abnormal urothelium is subtle Non-dysplastic urothelial cells are often dispersed among the dysplastic cells.
- Nuclear and architectural features are the primary criteria for distinguishing dysplasia from reactive atypia and urothelial carcinoma in situ.
- Grading of urothelial dysplasia and the use of the term "atypia" as a synonym for urothelial dysplasia is discouraged.
- Primary dysplasia occurs in the absence of urothelial tumors. In one autopsy study, primary dysplasia was present in up to 6.8 % of males and 5.7 % of females. These patients are predominantly middle-aged men with irritative symptoms with or without hematuria. Dysplasia is not cystoscopically visible. It is estimated that de novo (primary) dysplasia progresses to bladder neoplasia in 14–19 % of cases.
- Secondary dysplasia is seen in patients with a history of bladder neoplasia. The incidence of dysplasia in patients with established bladder neoplasia varies from 22 to 86 % and approaches 100 % in patients with invasive carcinoma. The presence of urothelial dysplasia indicates urothelial instability. Recurrence rate was 73 % of patients with superficial neoplasia and concomitant dysplasia compared with 43 % without coexisting dysplasia.

Immunohistochemistry
- CK20 immunostaining is limited to the superficial cell layers in normal urothelium; in contrast, CK20 immunostaining is usually present in the superficial and intermediate cell layers of dysplastic urothelium (aberrant CK20 exoression). Positive CD44 immunostaining is observed only in the basal cells in normal urothelium, and is either absent entirely or present only in scattered cells in urothelial dysplasia, whereas full-thickness positive membranous CD44 staining is typical of reactive urothelium (Table 2.3).
- Dysplastic cells show increased p53 expression, whereas p53 nuclear accumulation is predominantly undetectable or only weakly evident in the basal and parabasal cells in reactive urothelium. P16 has been reported variable positive in urothelial dysplasia and weak/patchy in reactive urothelium.

Table 2.3 Immunohistochemical features of flat-related lesions

	Normal	Flat urothelial hyperplasia	Reactive Atypia	Atypia of unknown significance	Dysplasia
CK20	Limited to umbrella cells	Limited to umbrella cells	Limited to umbrella cells	Limited to umbrella cells	Deep layers
CD44	Limited to basal cells	Limited to basal cells	Increased reactivity in all cell layers	Increased reactivity in all cell layers	Absent
p53	Absent	Absent	Absent	Absent	Positive

Urothelial carcinoma in situ (high grade intraurothelial neoplasia)

- Urothelial carcinoma in situ is a flat non-invasive lesion in which the urothelium is entirely composed of cytologically malignant cells. The patient's age at diagnosis ranged from 32 to 90 years (mean, 66 years). The male-to-female ratio in patients with carcinoma in situ is approximately 7:1.
- Clinical presentations include gross and microscopic hematuria, irritative symptoms (dysuria, pain, and frequency), nocturia, and sterile pyuria. Approximately 25 % of patients are asymptomatic. Carcinoma in situ usually is multifocal, with a predilection for the trigone, lateral wall, and dome of the bladder. Cystoscopically, it may appear as erythematous velvety or granular patches, although it may also be visually undetectable. Erythematous changes are often apparent at gross examination.
- De novo or isolated carcinoma in situ (often referred to as primary carcinoma in situ) accounts for 1–3 % of bladder neoplasms. Mapping studies of cystectomy specimens show involvement of the prostatic urethra and of the ureter in as many as 67 and 57 % of cases, respectively.
- Urothelial carcinoma in situ has a high likelihood of progressing to invasive carcinoma if left untreated. The mean interval between a diagnosis of carcinoma in situ and the detection of cancer progression is 5 years. The actuarial progression-free survival, cancer-specific survival, and all-cause survival rates are 63, 79, and 55 %, respectively, at 10 years.
- Factors predictive of progression include multifocality, coexistent bladder neoplasia, DNA aneuploidy, CCND3 gene amplification, prostatic urethral involvement, and recurrence after treatment. Urothelia carcinoma in situ is often associated with invasive carcinoma elsewhere in the bladder (referred as secondary carcinoma in situ).
- Microscopically, urothelial carcinoma in situ is characterized by flat, disordered proliferation of urothelial cells with marked cytologic abnormalities. The morphological diagnosis of carcinoma in situ requires severe cytological atypia (anaplasia).
- Full thickness-change is not required, and it ranges from one cell layer to the thickness of hyperplasia (greater than 7 cells). Superficial (umbrella) cells may or may not be present. Marked disorganization of cells is characteristic, with loss of cellular polarity and decreased cellular cohesiveness.
- The tumor cells tend to be large and pleomorphic, with moderate to abundant cytoplasm. Nevertheless, the cells of carcinoma in situ are sometimes small with a high nucleus to cytoplasmic ratio. The chromatin tends to be coarse and clumped. Nucleoli may be multiple and they are large and prominent in at least some of the cells. Mitotic figures, which are often atypical, are seen in the uppermost layers of the urothelium.
- Tissue edema, vascular ectasia and proliferation of small capillaries are frequently observed in the lamina propria.

Immunohistochemistry

- Carcinoma in situ shows intense CK 20 and p53 positivity in the majority of malignant

Table 2.4 Morphologic patterns of urothelial carcinoma in situ (CIS)

Large cell CIS
Small cell CIS
Denuding and "clinging pattern" of CIS
Pagetoid and undermining (lepedic) of CIS
CIS with squamous or glandular differentiation
CIS with microinvasion (CISmic)

cells. Increased Ki-67 labeling is noted in carcinoma in situ but this can be seen also in reactive atypia of the urothelium thus limiting its usefulness in practice. P16 is typically positive in carcinoma in situ (about 90 % of cases) and Racemase is positive in 50–80 % of cases of carcinoma in situ.

- The neoplastic cells are uniformly negative for CD44 immunostaining. In contrast, cytokeratin 20 stainings show patchy cytoplasmic immunoreactivity only in the superficial umbrella cell layer and CD44 stains only the basal cells in the adjacent normal or reactive urothelium. Reactive urothelium is negative for p16 and Racemase, findings that need to be validated in larger cohorts.
- Other markers of potential interest include HER-2neu diffuse expression in carcinoma in situ with few positive cells in reactive urothelium.

Histological variants of urothelial carcinoma in situ

- Awareness of the histologic diversity of carcinoma in situ may aid in the diagnosis of this important lesion. In practice, it is not necessary to mention these specific growth patterns or morphologic variants in the surgical pathology report (Table 2.4)

Large cell carcinoma in situ

- Large cell carcinoma in situ constitutes the most common morphologic form of this entity. Cytologic findings include nuclear pleomorphism, variably abundant cytoplasm and anaplastic nuclear features. In rare cases, large cell carcinoma in situ may have minor nuclear pleomorphism but still exhibits architectural disarray. Rarely, it may focally exhibit high pleomorphism with bizarre giant cells (pleomorphic/giant cell carcinoma in situ).

Small cell carcinoma in situ

- The small cell pattern refers to the size of the cells and may or may not coexist with small cell carcinoma and is unrelated to neuroendocrine differentiation. In such cases, the pleomorphism is minimal, the cytoplasm is scant and nuclei are enlarged and hyperchromatic, with coarse unevenly distributed chromatin.
- The scattered prominent nucleoli are distorted and angulated. Recognition of the small cell pattern of carcinoma in situ is important to avoid misdiagnosis of basal cell hyperplasia which has been observed in patients treated with bacille Calmette-Guérin (BCG). This shows a small cell pattern but lack nuclear atypia or loss of polarity.

Denuding and clinging carcinoma in situ

- In some cases, the neoplastic urothelial cells are strikingly dyscohesive and undergo extensive exfoliation, with the result that biopsies may show only a few residual carcinoma cells on the surface ("clinging carcinoma in situ") or no recognizable epithelial cells on the surface, a condition referred to as "denuding cystitis".
- In the clinging pattern of carcinoma in situ there is a patchy, usually single layer of atypical cells. In mucosal biopsies entirely lacking surface epithelium, carcinoma in situ may be present only in von Brunn's nests. A careful search for carcinoma in situ in deeper sections or in other submitted biopsy fragments is important, and a recommendation for evaluation of urine cytology for carcinoma cells is warranted.

Pagetoid carcinoma in situ

- Cancerization of the urothelium, shows either pagetoid spread (clusters or isolated single cells) or undermining or overriding of the normal urothelium (lepidic growth). Carcinoma in situ exhibiting pagetoid growth is characterized by large single cells or small clusters of cells within otherwise normal urothelium of ureter, urethra, prostatic ducts or in areas of squamous metaplasia. Individual cells showing pagetoid spread have enlarged nuclei with coarse chromatin; frequently, the cytoplasm is clear.

- Pagetoid growth patterns can be found in up to 15 % of carcinoma in situ cases. Most patients are male and their ages range from 31 years to 78 years (mean, 64 years). Pagetoid carcinoma in situ is usually a focal lesion and is easily overlooked; it occurs in a clinical and histological setting of conventional carcinoma in situ with coexisting invasive urothelial carcinoma, and such patients essentially have the same progression and survival rates as patients without pagetoid changes.
- In cases with extensive urothelial denudation, pagetoid carcinoma in situ may be focally present in adjacent otherwise normal-looking urothelium, thus alerting the pathologist to search for additional carcinoma in situ elsewhere in the bladder.
- Since primary extramammary Paget's disease of the external genitalia and of the anal canal may extend to the bladder, and conversely, some cases of pagetoid carcinoma in situ of the bladder may extend to the urethra, ureter, and external genitalia, differentiating between these two entities represents an important diagnostic and therapeutic challenge.
- A panel of immunostains including cytokeratin 7, cytokeratin 20, and thrombomodulin may assist in differentiating pagetoid urothelial carcinoma in situ from extramammary Paget's disease, which is known to be cytokeratin 7 positive and cytokeratin 20 negative.

Carcinoma in situ with squamous or glandular differentiation.

- Rare cases of carcinoma in situ may exhibit squamous differentiation characterized by intercellular bridges. Carcinoma in situ with squamous features is most often observed in association with urothelial carcinoma showing extensive squamous differentiation elsewhere in the bladder.
- A much less frequently encountered pattern is carcinoma in situ with morphological and immunohistochemical evidence of glandular differentiation. Some authors refer to this as adenocarcinoma in situ; such lesions may show papillary, cribriform, or flat morphology. Carcinoma in situ involving von Brunn's nests, cystitis glandularis or cystitis cystica may be difficult to distinguish from adenocarcinoma in situ in the absence of concurrent invasive adenocarcinoma.
- A recent report based on 25 cases of urothelial carcinoma in situ with glandular differentiation showed high ki-67 index and p53 accumulation, high nuclear and cytoplasmic p16 expression and diffuse PTEN expression, a phenotype that also characterized concurrent conventional carcinoma in situ. MUC5A, MUC2, CK20 and c-erbB2 were positive in all 25 cases of urothelial carcinoma in situ with glandular differentiation and CDX-2 was present in 19 cases; MUC1, CK7 or 34ßE12 was focally present in 21, 19 and 18 cases, respectively.
- The authors concluded that urothelial carcinoma in situ with glandular differentiation is a variant of carcinoma in situ that follows the natural history of conventional urothelial carcinoma in situ. The immunophenotype suggests urothelial origin with the expression of MUC5A and CDX2 as signature for glandular differentiation.

Carcinoma in situ with microinvasion

- Carcinoma in situ with microinvasion was initially defined as invasion into the lamina propria to a depth of 5 mm or less from the basement membrane. Recent consensus conference suggested that cases with more than 20 cells measured from the stromal-epithelial interface should be classified as fully invasive. Microinvasion appears as direct extension in cords (tentacular), single cells, or single cells and clusters of cells.
- The clusters of cells may have retraction artifact that mimics vascular invasion. Stromal response may be present, but in most cases is absent. In cases with a prominent stromal inflammatory response the invasive

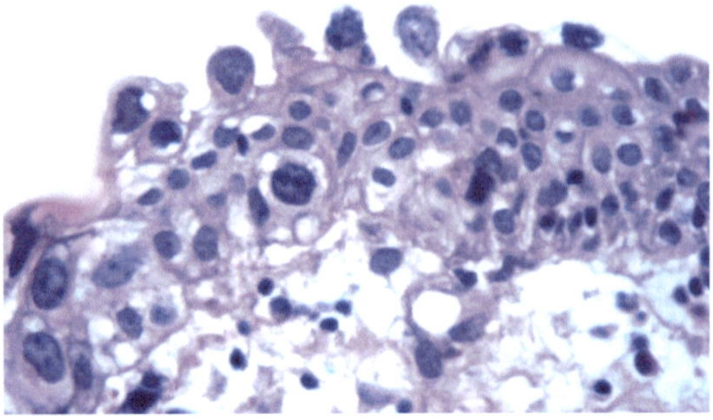

Fig. 2.21 Reactive urothelial atypia following mitomycin C therapy

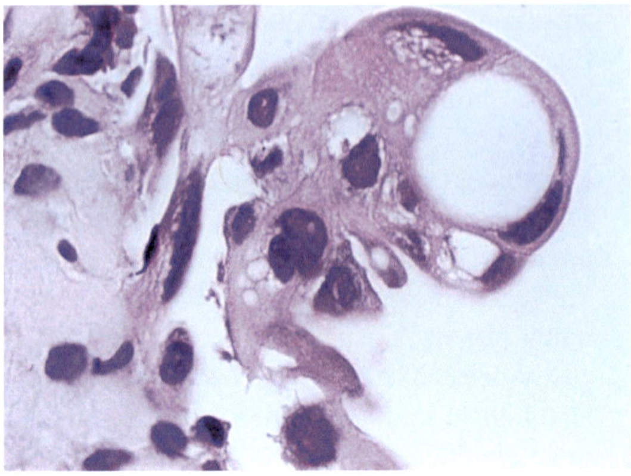

Fig. 2.22 Reactive urothelial atypia following thiotepa therapy

neoplastic cells may be interspersed among lymphocytes, making them inconspicuous. In these circumstances, immunohistochemical staining with antibodies against cytokeratins (such as AE1/AE3) exposes the invading cells.

- A potential pitfall to be avoided is the known positivity of myofibroblastas present in bladder's lamina propria with antibodys against keratins.

Therapy-induced changes in the urothelium and mimics of urothelial flat neoplasia

- Antineoplastic agents used in the bladder or systemically, such as thiotepa (triethylenethiophosphoramide), mitomycin C, cyclophosphamide, bacille Calmette-Guérin (BCG), and radiation therapy produce urothelial changes that can mimic cancer histologically (Figs. 2.21, 2.22, 2.23, and 2.24)
- Pathologists must be aware of the diagnostic pitfalls and exercise caution when evaluating urothelial atypia following treatment with chemotherapy or irradiation. In most cases, knowledge of the prior treatment is crucial to correctly diagnosing the epithelial and stromal changes present.
- If the distinction between treatment-induced atypia and dysplasia/carcinoma-in-situ is uncertain, a conservative approach with repeat cystoscopy and biopsy is indicated, preferably after the inflammation has subsided.
- Cyclophosphamide therapy may induce stromal fibrosis, vascular intimal thickening, mural fibrin deposition in vessels, and vascular ectasia. It also induces epithelial necrosis followed by rapid atypical regeneration. The metabolic effects of cyclophosphamide including arrest of cell and nuclear division produce bi- and multi-nucleated cells, often with large bizarre nuclei resembling radiation injury changes that can be mistaken for malignancy.
- Cyclophosphamide may also induce reactivation of polyomavirus infection causing marked nuclear atypia in the surface urothelium. In rare cases, polyomavirus infection (BK virus) infection mimics flat intraepithelial lesions.
- In BCG treated bladders, residual carcinoma in situ might only be present in von Brunn nests. Loss of intercellular cohesion in carcinoma in situ may result in the so-called "denuding cystitis" or in residual neoplastic cells loosely attached to the surface ("clinging" pattern). Also of importance are the reactive changes associated with BCG therapy, which include both acute and chronic inflammation. There may also be a pattern of reactive epithelial atypia and granulomatous reaction in the bladder wall.
- Mitomycin C and thiotepa, when used as topical chemotherapeutic agents in the bladder,

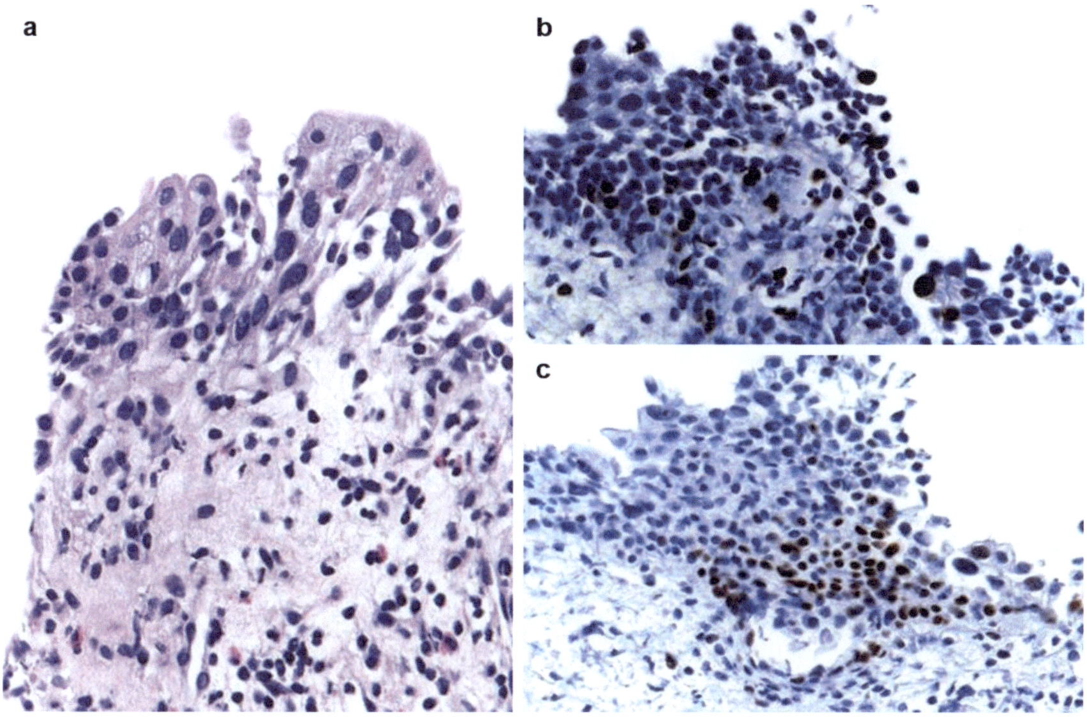

Fig. 2.23 Reactive urothelial atypia following cyclophosphamide therapy (**a**), showing low ki67 proliferation (**b**), and low p53 nuclear accumulation (**c**)

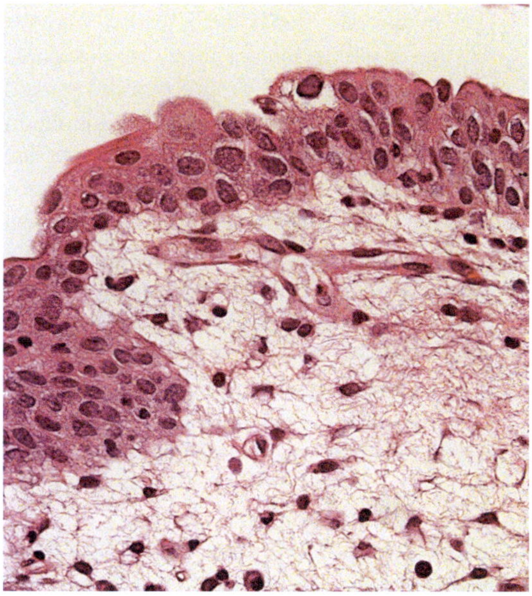

Fig. 2.24 Polyomavirus infection in urothelium following renal transplant

produce identical histologic changes. These include exfoliation, epithelial denudation, multinucleation, cytoplasmic vacuolization, and the appearance of bizarre, non-malignant nuclei in the superficial layer of the urothelium.

- A marked necro-inflammatory process follows administration of topical mitomycin C. There is a histiocytic response extending deep into the bladder wall. Mitomicin C may also initiate eosinophilic cystitis, a useful clue for the surgical pathologist when evaluating small bladder biopsies in this setting. These agents are not metabolic inhibitors of DNA replication and thus do not produce full-thickness urothelial atypia, as is seen after cyclophosphamide therapy.
- Patients receiving ketamine may present reactive urothelial changes that can mimic urothelial CIS.

- Radiation therapy produces a variety of bladder lesions associated with a progression of pathologic findings. The earliest change, usually seen after 3–6 weeks, consists of acute cystitis with desquamation of urothelial cells and hyperemia with edema of the lamina propria. The urothelium shows varying degrees of atypia, including cytoplasmic and nuclear vacuolization, karyorrhexis, stromal hyalinization, thrombosis of blood vessels, and mesenchymal cell atypia similar to that seen in giant cell cystitis.
- Enlarged nuclei may have large nucleoli, and degenerative nuclear features are usually present. Surface ulceration with fibrin deposition, or a reactive, tumor-like epithelial proliferation associated with fibrosis of the lamina propria and/or muscularis propria, arteriolar mural thickening and hyalinization, and atypical and sometimes multinucleated stromal cells are features seen in late cases of radiation cystitis, usually becoming evident months or years after radiation therapy.
- An important long term effect of radiotherapy is the development of de novo radiation induced bladder cancer which usually is a urothelial carcinoma; occasionally it is a squamous cell neoplasm. Rare examples of sarcomatoid carcinoma (or carcinosarcoma) and sarcoma of the urinary bladder have been reported.
- In addition, the damaged mucosa may become ulcerated, with adjacent atypical regenerating urothelium showing pseudoepitheliomatous hyperplasia. This change is more common after ulceration related to radiation therapy.

2.2.3 Urothelial Carcinoma

General features

- Bladder cancer is the 7th most common cancer worldwide, accounting for approximately 336,000 new cases each year. There are significant variations in incidence, morbidity, and mortality rates of bladder cancer in different countries and ethnicity groups.
- African American men have a much lower incidence of bladder cancer, but their mortality rates are similar to white Caucasians. Bladder cancer occurs two to five times more frequently in men than women. This has been attributed to different smoking and occupational exposure between men and women.
- The majority of bladder cancer patients present with hematuria. Approximately 20 % of patients being evaluated for gross hematuria will subsequently be diagnosed with bladder cancer. Similarly, of patients presenting with microscopic hematuria, up to 10 % will be diagnosed with bladder cancer.
- A significant proportion of patients also have irritative voiding symptoms, including urgency, frequency and dysuria, their symptoms are mistakenly attributed to urinary tract infection.

Field cancerization and tumor multicentricity

- Development of multifocal tumors in the same patient, either synchronous or metachronous, is a common characteristic of urothelial malignancy. Multiple coexisting tumors have often arisen before clinical symptoms are apparent. The separate tumors may or may not share a similar histology. Two theories have been proposed to explain the frequency of urothelial tumor multifocality.
- One theory, the monoclonal theory, suggests that the multiple tumors arise from a single transformed cell which proliferates and spreads throughout the urothelium either by intraluminal implantation or by intraepithelial migration.
- The second theory, the field-effect theory, explains tumor multifocality as a development secondary to field cancerization effect.

Histologic grading (1998 International Society of Urological Pathology (ISUP)/2004 World Health Organization (WHO) Classification)

- In 1998, a revised system of classifying noninvasive papillary urothelial neoplasms of the urinary bladder was proposed. This system was subsequently formally adopted by the World Health Organization (2004).
- This new system separates noninvasive papillary urothelial neoplasms into 4 categories, designated papilloma, papillary urothelial neoplasm of low malignant potential (PUNLMP), low grade carcinoma, and high grade carcinoma.

Table 2.5 Proposals to histological grading of urothelial carcinoma of the urinary bladder

1973 WHO	1998 WHO/ISUP	1999 WHO	2004 WHO	Current Proposal
Papilloma	Papilloma	Papilloma	Papilloma	Papilloma
Grade 1	PUNLMP	PUNLMP	PUNLMP	Grade 1 (low grade)
Grade 2	Low grade	Grade 1	Low grade	Grade 2 (low grade)
		Grade 2		Grade 3 (high grade)
Grade 3	High grade	Grade 3	High grade	Grade 4 (high grade)

Note: All the grading schemes have substantial inter and intraobserver variabilities. There is no exact correlation between different grading systems. Some 1973 WHO grade 2 tumors are "low grade" and some are classified as "high grade." The 1998 WHO/ISUP system is the same as the 2004 WHO system

Abbreviations: *WHO* World Health Organization, *IUSP* International Society of Urological Pathology, *PUNLMP* papillary urothelial neoplasm of low malignant potential

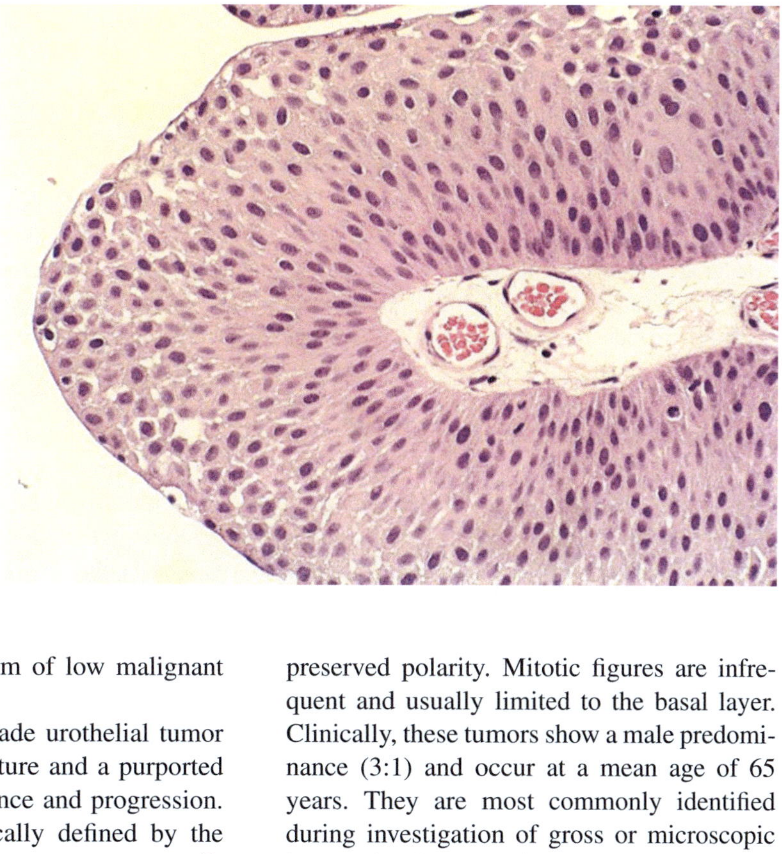

Fig. 2.25 Microscopic appearance of papillary urothelial neoplasia of low malignant potential

Papillary urothelial neoplasm of low malignant potential (PUNLMP)

- A PUNLMP is a low-grade urothelial tumor with a papillary architecture and a purported low incidence of recurrence and progression. This lesion is histologically defined by the WHO (2004) classification system as a papillary urothelial tumor which resembles the exophytic urothelial papilloma, but with increased cellular proliferation exceeding the thickness of normal urothelium. All such tumors would have been considered grade 1 urothelial carcinomas by the WHO 1973 grading system (Table 2.5).
- Cytologic atypia is minimal or absent and architectural abnormalities are minimal with preserved polarity. Mitotic figures are infrequent and usually limited to the basal layer. Clinically, these tumors show a male predominance (3:1) and occur at a mean age of 65 years. They are most commonly identified during investigation of gross or microscopic hematuria. Cystoscopically, these lesions are typically 1–2 cm in greatest dimension, and located on the lateral wall of the bladder or near the ureteric orifices (Fig. 2.25)
- The published recurrence and progression rates show about 30 % recurrence and about 3 % progression rate. Reproducibility between observers in diagnosis of PUNLMP is low, and therefore, it remains a controversial category.

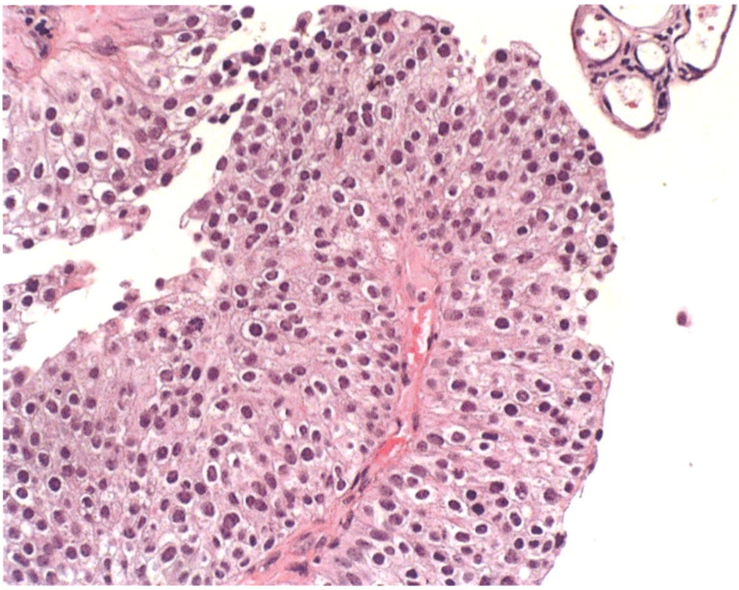

Fig. 2.26 Microscopic appearance of low grade urothelial carcinoma

Low grade urothelial carcinoma

- A low grade papillary urothelial carcinoma shows fronds with recognizable variation in architecture and cytology. The tumor shows slender papillae with frequent branching and variation in nuclear polarity; nuclei show enlargement and irregularity; chromatin is vesicular and nucleoli are often present (Fig. 2.26)
- Mitotic figures may occur at any level in low grade papillary urothelial carcinoma. Such cases would have been considered as grade 1 or grade 2 in the WHO (1973) classification scheme. Altered expression of cytokeratin 20, CD44, p53 and p63 is frequent. Some tumors are diploid, but aneuploidy is the rule.
- FGFR3 mutations are seen with about the same frequency as in PUNLMP. The male: female ratio is 2.9:1 and the mean age is 70 years (range 28–90 years). Most patients present with hematuria and have a single tumor in the posterior or lateral bladder wall.
- However, 22 % of patients with low grade papillary urothelial carcinoma have two or more tumors. Tumor recurrence, stage progression and tumor-related mortality are 50, 10 and 5 %, respectively.

High grade urothelial carcinoma

- In high grade papillary urothelial carcinoma, the cells lining papillary fronds show obviously disordered arrangement with cytologic atypia (Fig. 2.27) All tumors classified as grade 3 in the 1973 WHO scheme, as well as some tumors assigned grade 2 in that classification, would be considered high grade carcinoma in the 2004 WHO classification.
- The papillae are frequently fused. Both architectural and cytologic abnormality are recognizable at scanning power. The nuclei are pleomorphic with prominent nucleoli and altered polarity. Mitotic figures are frequent. The thickness of the urothelium varies considerably.
- Carcinoma-in-situ is frequently evident in the adjacent mucosa. Changes in cytokeratin 20, p53 and p63 expression, as well as aneuploidy are more frequent than in low grade lesions. Molecular alterations in these tumors include over-expression of p53, HER2 or EGFR, and loss of p21Waf1 or p27kip1 as seen with invasive cancers.
- Genetically, high-grade non-invasive lesions (pTa G3) resemble invasive tumors. A comparative genomic hybridization-based study showed deletions at 2q, 5q, 10q, and 18q as well as gains at 5p and 20q.

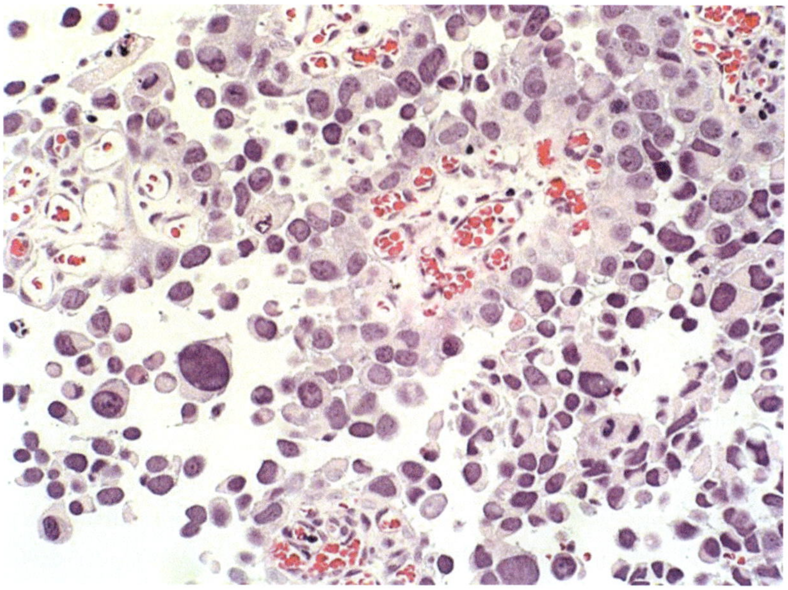

Fig. 2.27 Microscopic appearance of high grade urothelial carcinoma

- Hematuria is common and the endoscopic appearance varies from papillary to nodular or solid. There may be single or multiple tumors. Stage progression and death due to disease are observed in as many as 65 % of patients.

Histologic grading (1973 World Health Organization (WHO) Classification)

- Histologic grading is one of the most important prognostic factors in bladder cancer. The first widely accepted grading system for papillary urothelial neoplasms, that is still in use in many institutions, was the WHO (1973) classification system.
- It has four categories: papilloma, grade 1 carcinoma, grade 2 carcinoma, and grade 3 carcinoma. Histologic grading is based on the degree of cellular anaplasia with grade 1 tumors having the least degree of anaplasia compatible with a diagnosis of malignancy, grade 3 tumors have the most severe degree of anaplasia, and grade 2 tumors have an intermediate degree of cellular anaplasia.
- Anaplasia is further defined by the authors of the WHO (1973) classification as increased cellularity, nuclear crowding, disturbed cellular polarity, failure of differentiation from the base to the surface, nuclear polymorphism, irregularity cell size, variations in nuclear shape and chromatin pattern, displaced or abnormal mitotic figures, and giant cells. Urothelial papilloma will be discussed later under benign tumors.

Grade 1 urothelial carcinoma

- Grade 1 papillary carcinoma consists of an orderly arrangement of normal urothelial cells lining delicate papillae with minimal architectural abnormality and minimal nuclear atypia. Nuclear grooves are usually present. There may be some complexity and fusion of the papillae, but this is usually not prominent. The urothelium is often thickened to more than 7 cell layers.
- The urothelium displays normal maturation and cohesiveness, with an intact superficial cell layer. The nuclei tend to be uniform in shape and spacing, although there may be some enlargement and elongation. The chromatin texture is finely granular, without significant nucleolar enlargement. Mitotic figures are rare or absent, and basally located. Grade 1 tumor should be distinguished from urothelial papilloma which is a benign lesion.

Grade 2 urothelial carcinoma

- Grade 2 carcinoma represents a broad group of tumors encompassing a spectrum of cytologic atypia and some variability in the relative proportions of cells with atypical features. Grade 2 carcinomas retain some of the orderly architectural appearance and maturation of grade 1 carcinoma, but display at least focal moderate variation in orderliness, nuclear appearance, and chromatin texture apparent at low magnification.

- Cytologic abnormalities are invariably present in grade 2 carcinoma, with moderate nuclear crowding, moderate loss of cell polarity, moderate nuclear hyperchromasia, moderate anisonucleosis, and mild nucleolar enlargement. Mitotic figures are usually limited to the lower half of the urothelium, but this is an inconstant feature. Superficial cells are usually present, and the urothelial cells are predominantly cohesive, although variation in cohesion may be present.
- Some tumors may be extremely orderly, reminiscent of grade 1 carcinoma, with only a small focus of obvious disorder or irregularity. These are considered grade 2 cancer, recognizing that tumor grade is based on the highest level of abnormality present.
- The prognosis for patients with grade 2 urothelial carcinoma is significantly worse than for those with lower grade papillary cancer. Recurrence risk for patients with non-invasive grade 2 cancer is 45–67 %. Invasion occurs in up to 20 %.

Grade 3 urothelial carcinoma

- Grade 3 carcinoma displays the most extreme nuclear abnormality of any papillary urothelial cancer, similar to changes observed in urothelial carcinoma in situ. The obvious urothelial disorder and loss of polarity is present at scanning magnification. The superficial cell layer is partially or completely absent with grade 3 carcinoma, accompanied by prominent cellular dyscohesion.
- There is obvious loss of normal architecture and cell polarity, and frequent atypical mitotic figures. Cellular anaplasia, characteristic of grade 3 carcinoma, is defined as increased cellularity, nuclear crowding, random cellular polarity, absence of normal mucosal differentiation, nuclear pleomorphism, irregularity in cell size, variation in nuclear shape, capricious chromatin pattern, increased frequency of mitotic figures and occasional neoplastic giant cells.
- Recurrence risk for patients with non-invasive grade 3 cancer is 65–85 %, with invasion occurring in 20–52 % and cancer-specific death in up to 35 % following surgical treatment. Of surgically treated patients with grade 3 cancer and lamina propria invasion, 46–71 % develop recurrences, 24–48 % develop muscle-invasive cancer, and 25–71 % suffer cancer-specific death, emphasizing a need for appropriated treatment of these patients.

Histologic Grading of Urothelial Carcinoma: The Four-tier Proposal

- Recently, a four-tier proposal has been reported. In this proposal, noninvasive papillary urothelial carcinomas are separated into four categories: grade 1 urothelial carcinoma (low grade), grade 2 urothelial carcinoma (low grade), grade 3 urothelial carcinoma (high grade), and grade 4 urothelial carcinoma (high grade) (Table 2.6). PUNLMP is classified as "grade 1 urothelial carcinoma (low grade)" in the four-tier grading scheme. Urothelial papilloma remains as a benign urothelial tumor following identical diagnostic criteria and terminology to those defined in the 1973 and 2004 WHO classification.

Grade 1 Urothelial Carcinoma (Low Grade)

- The diagnostic criteria are identical to those defined in the 1998 WHO/ISUP and 2004 WHO classification for PUNLMP. We propose to change the terminology of PUNLMP to "grade 1 urothelial carcinoma (low grade)." In these tumors, cytologic atypia is minimal or absent and architectural abnormalities are slight with preserved polarity. Mitotic figures are infrequent and usually limited to the basal layer. Grade 1 tumor should be distinguished from urothelial papilloma, which is a benign lesion without invasive potential or risk of progression. The key difference between papilloma and grade 1 urothelial carcinoma (low grade) is the number of epithelial layers covering the papillae.

Grade 2 Urothelial Carcinoma (Low Grade)

- The diagnostic criteria are identical to those defined in the 1998 WHO/ISUP and 2004 WHO classification for low grade urothelial carcinomas. These tumors are characterized

Table 2.6 Histological criteria for the proposed grading system of urothelial carcinoma of the bladder (4-tier system)

Characteristics	Grade 1 (low grade)	Grade 2 (low grade)	Grade 3 (high grade)	Grade 4 (high grade)
Increased cell layers (>7)	Yes	Variable	Variable	Variable, usually <7 layers
Superficial umbrella cells	Present	Often present	Usually absent	Usually absent
Polarity/overall architecture	Normal	Mildly distorted	Moderately distorted	Severely distorted
Discohesiveness	Normal	Normal	Mild to moderate	Severe
Clear cytoplasm	May be present	May be present	Usually absent	Usually absent
Nuclear size	Normal or slightly increased	Mildly increased	Moderately increased	Markedly increased
Nuclear pleomorphism	Uniform, slightly elongated to oval	Mild, round to oval with slight variation in shape and contour	Moderate	Marked
Nuclear polarization	Normal to slightly abnormal	Abnormal	Abnormal	Absent
Nuclear hyperchromasia	Slight or minimal	Mild	Moderate	Severe
Nuclear grooves	Present	Present	Absent	Absent
Nucleoli	Absent or inconspicuous	Inconspicuous	Enlarged, often prominent	Multiple prominent nucleoli
Mitotic figures	None/rare, basal location	May be present, at any level	Often present	Prominent and frequent, atypical forms
Stromal invasion	Rare	Uncommon	May be present	Often present

Note: In current proposal, grade 1 (low grade) tumors are classified as "papillary urothelial neoplasm of low malignant potential" (PUNLMP) in the 2004 WHO classification system; grade 2 (low grade) tumor are classified as "low grade urothelial carcinoma" (2004 WHO/ISUP); grade 3 (high grade) and grade 4 (high grade) tumors are both classified as "high grade urothelial carcinoma" (2004 WHO/ISUP)

by an overall orderly appearance but with areas of variation in architectural and cytologic features recognizable at scanning power. They are differentiated from grade 1 urothelial carcinoma (low grade) by the presence of easily recognizable cytologic atypia including variation of polarity and nuclear size, shape, and chromatin texture. Mitotic figures are infrequent and may be seen at any level of the urothelium.

Grade 3 Urothelial Carcinoma (High Grade)

- We feel that the spectrum of high grade urothelial carcinomas under the 2004 WHO classification scheme is quite broad and there is a need to separate these tumors for further investigation. Grade 3 urothelial carcinomas (high grade) display an intermediate degree of architectural and cytologic abnormality between grade 2 urothelial carcinomas (low grade) and grade 4 urothelial carcinomas (high grade). Architectural disorder in these tumors is obvious, with branching and bridging of papillary projections. Nevertheless, a certain degree of polarity and nuclear uniformity are still discernible. Severe anaplasia is not seen in these tumors. All grade 3 urothelial carcinomas would be classified as high grade urothelial carcinoma using the 2004 WHO classification scheme.

Grade 4 Urothelial Carcinoma (High Grade)

- Cases with severe nuclear anaplasia are considered grade 4 urothelial carcinoma in the current proposal. These tumors present an overall impression of complete architectural disorder with absence of polarity, loss of superficial umbrella cells, and marked variation of all nuclear parameters. Numerous irregularly distributed mitotic figures are frequently noted. Severe cytologic atypia is usually uniformly present in all fields or all histologic sections examined. Unlike grade 1 or grade 2 urothelial carcinoma (low grade),

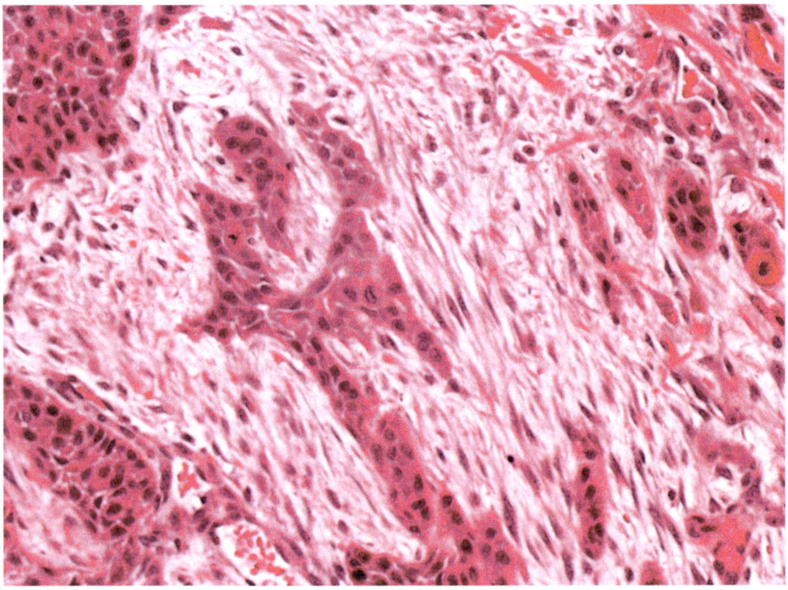

Fig. 2.28 High grade urothelial carcinoma infiltrating múscularis propria and desmoplastic stroma

these tumors often have less than seven layers in thickness. There is remarkable cellular discohesiveness. These cases are typically associated with stromal invasion and advanced stage bladder cancer.

- Aggressive variants of urothelial carcinoma, including nested variant, micropapillary variant, plasmacytoid variant, sarcomatoid carcinoma, small cell carcinoma, large cell undifferentiated carcinoma, pleomorphic giant cell carcinoma, should also be graded as grade 4 tumor in the current grading scheme.

Tumor heterogeneity

- The WHO (2004)/ISUP system provides clearly defined histologic criteria for each of its diagnostic categories; however, urothelial neoplasms frequently demonstrate features of more than one grade (grade heterogeneity). The grading of papillary urothelial tumors is typically based on the worst grade present.

Invasive urothelial carcinoma

General features

- At gross examination, most tumors present as a single, solid, polypoid mass with or without ulceration, and may also appear sessile and extensively infiltrate the bladder wall.
- Histologically, the neoplastic cells invade the bladder wall as nests, cords, trabeculae, small clusters, or single cells that are often separated by a desmoplastic stroma. The tumor sometimes grows in a more diffuse, sheet-like pattern, but even in these cases, focal nests and clusters are generally present.
- The cells show moderate to abundant amphophilic or eosinophilic cytoplasm and large hyperchromatic nuclei. In larger nests, palisading of nuclei may be seen at the edges of the nests. The nuclei are typically pleomorphic and have irregular contours with angular profiles. Nuclear grooves may be identified in some cells. Nucleoli are highly variable in number and appearance (Fig. 2.28)
- Some cells contain single or multiple small nucleoli and others have large eosinophilic nucleoli. Foci of marked pleomorphism may be seen, with bizarre and multinuclear tumor cells present. Mitotic figures are common, including many abnormal forms. Invasive tumors are most commonly high grade, usually showing marked anaplasia with focal giant cell formation.
- Pathologic stage is most critical for assessing patient prognosis. The 2010 TNM (tumor, lymph node, and metastasis) staging information should be provided in the pathology report.

Table 2.7 Histologic features that are useful for the diagnosis of stromal invasion

Histologic grade:
Invasive cells are usually higher nuclear grade
Invading epithelium
Irregularly shaped nests
Single cell infiltration
Irregular or absent basement membrane
Tentacular finger-like projections
Paradoxical differentiation
Angiolymphatic invasion
Stromal response
Desmoplasia or fibrotic stroma
Retraction artifact
Inflammation
Myxoid stroma
Pseudosarcomatous stroma

Table 2.8 Pitfalls in the diagnosis of stage pT1 urothelial carcinoma

Tangential sectioning and poor orientation
Obscuring inflammation
Thermal injury
Urothelial carcinoma in situ involving von Brunn's nests
Muscle invasion indeterminate for type of muscle (muscularis propria versus muscularis mucosae)
Variants of urothelial carcinoma with deceptively bland cytology
Pseudoinvasive nests of benign proliferative urothelial lesions

Nonmuscleinvasive bladder carcinoma (T1 tumor)

- Infiltrating urothelial carcinoma is defined by the World Health Organization (WHO) as a urothelial tumor that invades beyond the basement membrane. The 2010 TNM staging system defines T1 tumors of the bladder as those invading the lamina propria/submucosa, but not the muscularis propria.
- The recognition of lamina propria invasion by urothelial carcinoma is one of the most challenging fields in surgical pathology, and the pathologist should follow strict criteria in its assessment (Tables 2.7 and 2.8), as follows:
- Histologic grade:
- While invasion may be present in low-grade tumors, it is much more commonly encountered in high grade lesions, reaching 70–96 % in some series (Figs. 2.29, 2.30, 2.31, 2.32, and 2.33)
- Stroma-epithelial interface: Tangentially sectioned, densely packed non-invasive papillary tumors exhibit a stroma-epithelial interface that is smooth and regular. In instances of true invasion, one is likely to see variable sized and irregularly shaped nests or individual tumor cells insinuating through the stroma.
- When the specimen includes tangential sections through non-invasive tumor or when urothelial carcinoma involves von Brunn's nests, the basement membrane preserves a regular contour, whereas it is frequently absent or disrupted in cases of true invasion.
- The smoothness of the epithelial-stromal interface may be assessed on H&E stains. In some cases, however, additional findings may be helpful; for example, there is a parallel array of thin-walled vessels that evenly line the basement membrane of non-invasive nests. These are absent in patients with invasive tumors.
- Invading epithelium:
- The invasive front of the neoplasm may show one of several features. Most commonly, tumors invade the underlying stroma as single cells or irregularly shaped nests of tumor cells. Sometimes tentacular or finger-like extensions can be seen arising from the base of the papillary tumor.
- Frequently, the invading nests appear cytologically different from cells at the base of the non-invasive component. Invasive tumor cells often have more abundant cytoplasm and a higher degree of nuclear pleomorphism. In some cases, particularly in microinvasive disease, the invasive tumor cells may acquire abundant eosinophilic cytoplasm.
- At low to medium power magnification, these microinvasive cells seem to be more differentiated than the overlying non-invasive disease, a feature known as paradoxical differentiation.
- Stromal response:
- The stromal response to invading carcinoma is not always uniformly present in invasive urothelial carcinoma, and the diagnosis of invasion may rely on identification of the typical characteristics of the invading epithelium. The stromal reaction in the lamina propria associated with invasive tumor may be inflammatory, myxoid, or fibrous.

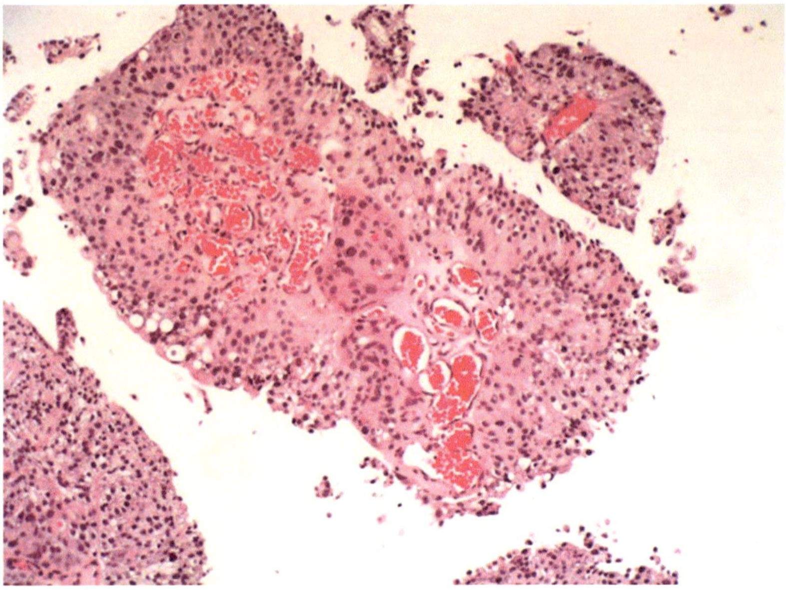

Fig. 2.29 High grade urothelial carcinoma with invasion into stalk and paradoxical differentiation of the invasive nest

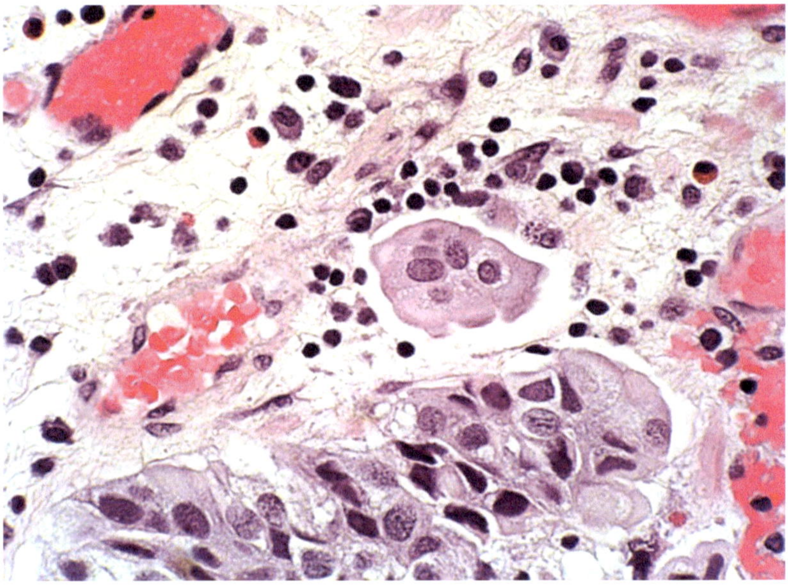

Fig. 2.30 Infiltrating tumor nests with retraction artefact

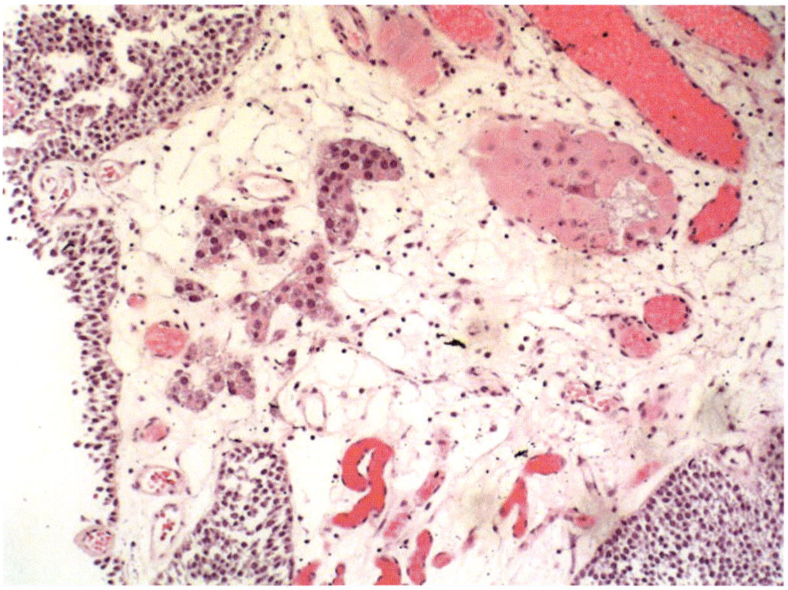

Fig. 2.31 Low grade urothelial carcinoma with early invasion into stalk

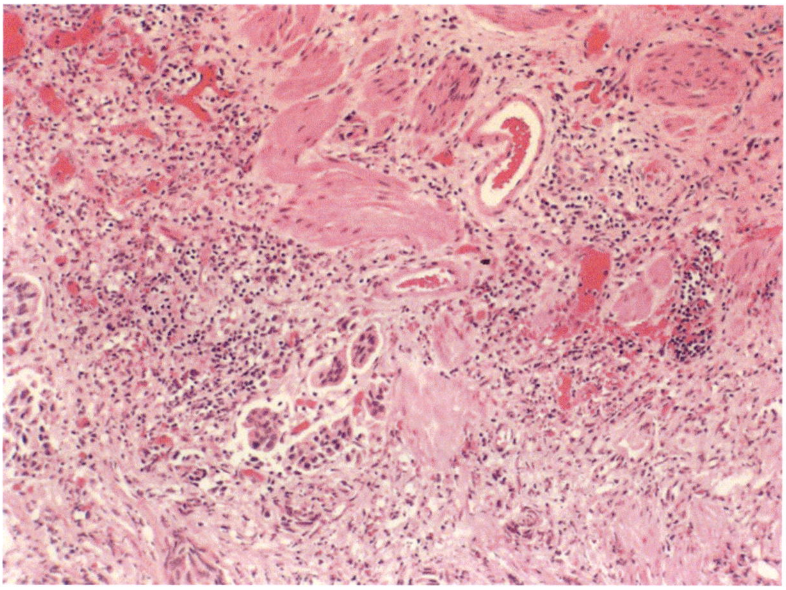

Fig. 2.32 Relationship of invading nests with múscularis mucosae

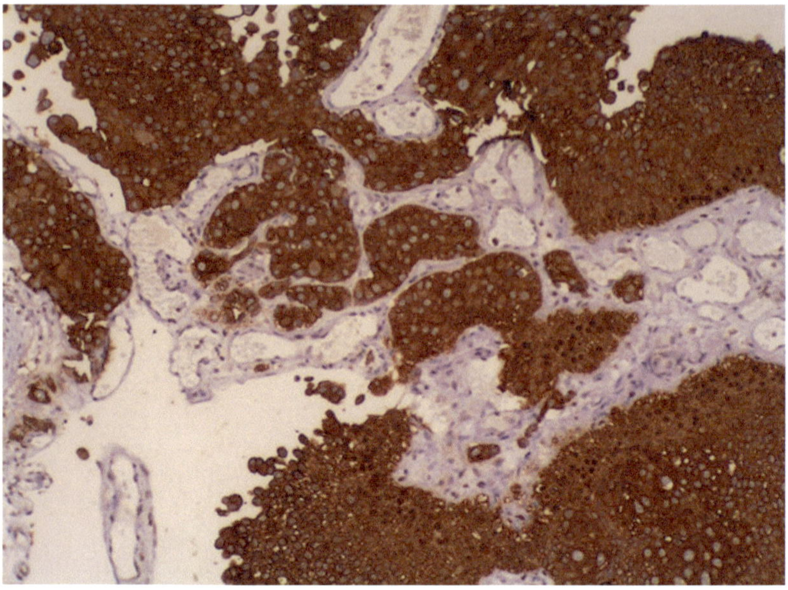

Fig. 2.33 Keratin staining highlights invading carcinoma nests

- Assessment of differences in stromal growth pattern provides an important diagnostic clue. Although the majority of bladder tumors with unquestionable lamina propria invasion exhibit some sort of stromal reaction, microinvasive disease usually does not, making its identification even more difficult. In some cases, retraction artifact around superficially invasive individual tumor cells may mimic angiolymphatic invasion.
- Often, this finding is focal, and may itself be one of the early signs of invasion into the lamina propria. Lamina propria invasion may elicit a brisk inflammatory response. Numerous inflammatory cells in the lamina propria often obscure the interface between epithelium and stroma. This makes small nest or single cell invasion difficult to recognize. Cytokeratin immunostaining is useful in difficult cases.
- Invasive urothelial carcinoma may have a cellular stroma with spindled fibroblasts and variable collagenization, or a hypocellular stroma with myxoid background.
- Rarely, the tumor induces an exuberant proliferation of fibroblasts, which may display alarming cellular atypia similar to giant cell cystitis. This feature, although a helpful clue to invasion, should not be mistaken for the spindle cell component of sarcomatoid urothelial carcinoma.
- Immunostains for cytokeratin are helpful in difficult cases though some myofibroblasts may also be positive for keratin. The proliferating stroma is usually nonexpansile, being limited to areas around the neoplasm, and is composed of cells which have a degenerate or smudged appearance.
- Diagnostic pitfalls:
- Transuretheral resection specimens are excised in a piecemeal fashion. Submitted tissue fragments are of variable shape and size and are difficult if not impossible to orient properly (Table 2.8). Furthermore, due to their complex architecture, papillary tumors are inevitably tangentially sectioned in multiple planes, resulting in the presence of isolated nests of non-invasive tumor cells within connective tissue. Smooth, round, and regular contours favor tangential sectioning, whereas irregular, jagged nests with haphazard arrangement favor stromal invasion.
- Diagnosis of invasion in some of these cases can be facilitated by immunohistochemical study with anti-cytokeratin antibodies. Thermal injury or cautery artefact produces severely distorted morphology, rendering accurate diagnosis of invasion difficult.

- Tumor cells involving von Brunn's nests may also mimic lamina propria invasion. This is especially problematic when von Brunn's nests are prominent or when they have been distorted by inflammatory or cautery artifact.
- Substaging of T1 tumors:
- The recurrence and progression rates for T1 tumors are highly variable. There is need for an accurate, easy-to-use, reproducible substaging system to stratify pT1 patients into different prognostic groups.
- Muscularis mucosae consists of thin and wavy fascicles of smooth muscle frequently associated with large, thin walled blood vessels. Muscularis mucosae can be identified in 15–83 % of biopsy specimens,; however, 6 % of the radical resection specimens do not have discernable muscularis mucosae. Thus, the "large" vessels have been used as a surrogate marker of muscularis mucosae in all published studies that have proposed T1 substaging based on muscularis mucosae invasion. Some authors have raised concerns about the practicality and validity of substaging pT1 disease based on assessment of muscularis mucosa invasion, and currently this practice is not universally

Stage pT2 tumor

- The 2010 TNM staging system subclassifies pT2 tumor into two categories: cancer invading less than one-half of the depth of muscular propria (pT2a) and cancer invading greater than one-half of the depth of muscularis propria (Table 2.9). Tumors with an infiltrative growth pattern are associated with a worse prognosis than tumor displaying a non-infiltrative (nodular or trabecular) growth pattern.

Stage pT3 tumor

- Stage pT3 bladder carcinomas is defined as tumor invading into perivesical soft tissue. The subdivision of pT3 tumors into T3a (tumors with microscopic extravesical tumor extension) and pT3b (tumors with gross extravesical extension).Stage pT4 tumorStage pT4 bladder cancer is defined as tumor invading into adjacent organ including the uterus, vagina, prostate. pelvic wall or abdominal wall.

Table 2.9 TNM classification of bladder cancer (2010 revision)

Primary tumor	
TX	Primary tumor can not be assessed
T0	No evidence of primary tumor
Ta	Non-invasive papillary carcinoma
Tis	Carcinoma in situ: "flat tumor"
T1	Tumor invades subepithelial connective tissue (lamina propria)
T2	Tumor invades muscularis propria
T2a	Tumor invades superficial muscle (inner half)
T2b	Tumor invades deep muscle (outer half)
T3	Tumor invades perivesical tissue
T3a	Microscopically
T3b	Macroscopically (extra-vesical mass)
T4	Tumor invades any of the following: prostate, uterus, vagina, pelvic wall, and abdominal wall
T4a	Tumor invades prostate or uterus or vagina
4b	Tumor invades pelvic wall or abdominal wall
The suffix "m" should be added to the appropriate T category to indicate multiple tumors. The suffix "is" may be added to any T to indicate the presence of associated carcinoma in situ	
Regional Lymph Nodes (N)	
NX	Regional lymph nodes cannot be assessed
N0	No regional lymph node metastasis
N1	Single regional lymph node metastasis in the true pelvis (hypogastric, obturator, external iliac, or presacral lymph node)
N2	Multiple regional lymph node metastasis in the true pelvis (hypogastric, obturator, external iliac, or presacral lymph node)
N3	Lymph node metastasis to the common iliac lymph nodes
Distant Metastasis (M)	
M0	No distant metastasis
M1	Distant metastasis

- Cancers with prostatic involvement that penetrated the full thickness of bladder wall to involve the prostate vs. involved the prostate by extension from the prostatic urethra. Five-year overall survivals were 21 and 55 % for the former or later group of patients, respectively.

Histologic variants of invasive bladder cancer

- Urothelial carcinoma has a propensity for divergent differentiation. Virtually the whole spectrum of bladder cancer variants described below may be seen in variable proportions in otherwise typical urothelial carcinoma or in its pure forms (Table 2.10).

Table 2.10 Histologic variants of urothelial carcinoma

Urothelial carcinoma with mixed differentiation (specify type and percentage)
With squamous cell differentiation
With glandular differentiation
Other
Urothelial carcinoma, nested variant
With small tubules
Urothelial carcinoma, large nests variant
Urothelial carcinoma, inverted growth variant
Urothelial carcinoma, micropapillary variant
Urothelial carcinoma, microcystic variant
Lymphoepithelioma-like (urothelial) carcinoma
Plasmacytoid urothelial carcinoma
Urothelial carcinoma, clear cell (glycogen-rich) variant
Urothelial carcinoma, lipoid cell variant
Urothelial carcinoma with syncytiotrophoblastic giant cells
Sarcomatoid urothelial carcinoma
Small cell carcinoma
Large cell neuroendocrine carcinoma
Urothelial carcinoma with myxoid stroma
Urothelial carcinoma with rhabdoid features
Urothelial carcinoma in augmentation cystoplastia
Large cell undifferentiated carcinoma
Giant cell carcinoma
With osteclast-type giant cells
NOS (not otherwise specified)
Urothelial carcinoma with unusual stromal reactions
Pseudosarcomatous stroma
Stromal osseous or cartilaginous metaplasia
Osteoclast-type giant cells
Prominent lymphoid infiltrate

Urothelial carcinoma with squamous differentiation

- About 20 % of urothelial carcinomas contain areas of squamous or glandular differentiation. Squamous differentiation, defined by the presence of intercellular bridges or keratinization, occurs in 21 % of urothelial carcinomas of the bladder. Its frequency increases with grade and stage. Some cases have urothelial carcinoma in situ as the only urothelial component (Figs. 2.34 and 2.35).
- Cases with areas of squamous differentiation may have a less favorable response to therapy than pure urothelial carcinoma.
- Low-grade urothelial carcinoma with focal squamous differentiation has a higher recurrence rate than pure low grade urothelial carcinoma. Tumors with any identifiable urothelial element are classified as urothelial carcinoma with squamous differentiation, and an estimate of the percentage of squamous component should be provided.
- Urothelial carcinoma with squamous differentiation may express urothelial (S100P 83 %, GATA3 35 %, uroplakin III 13 %) and squamous associated markers CK14 87 % and desmoglein-3 70 %)

Urothelial carcinoma with glandular differentiation

- Glandular differentiation is less common than squamous differentiation and may be present in about 6 % of urothelial carcinomas of the bladder. Glandular differentiation is defined by the presence of true glandular spaces within the tumor. These may be tubular or enteric glands with mucin secretion.
- A colloid-mucinous pattern characterized by nests of cells "floating" in extracellular mucin, occasionally with signet ring cells, may be present. Cytoplasmic mucin-containing cells are present in 14–63 % of typical urothelial carcinoma and are not considered to represent glandular differentiation. The diagnosis of adenocarcinoma is reserved for pure tumors.
- A tumor with mixed glandular and urothelial differentiation is classified as urothelial carcinoma with glandular differentiation, and an estimate of the percentage of glandular component should be provided. A form of glandular differentiation with villous–like appearance has been described associated with papillary urothelial carcinoma (Figs. 2.36 and 2.37).
- The expression of MUC5AC-apomucin may be useful as immunohistochemical marker of glandular differentiation in urothelial tumors.
- When adenocarcinoma is present in association with urothelial carcinoma, even focally, it portends a poor prognosis.

Urothelial carcinoma, nested variant

- The nested variant of urothelial carcinoma is an aggressive neoplasm. There is a marked male predominance, and 70 % of patients die 4–40 months after diagnosis, in spite of therapy. This rare pattern of urothelial carcinoma was first described as a tumor with a

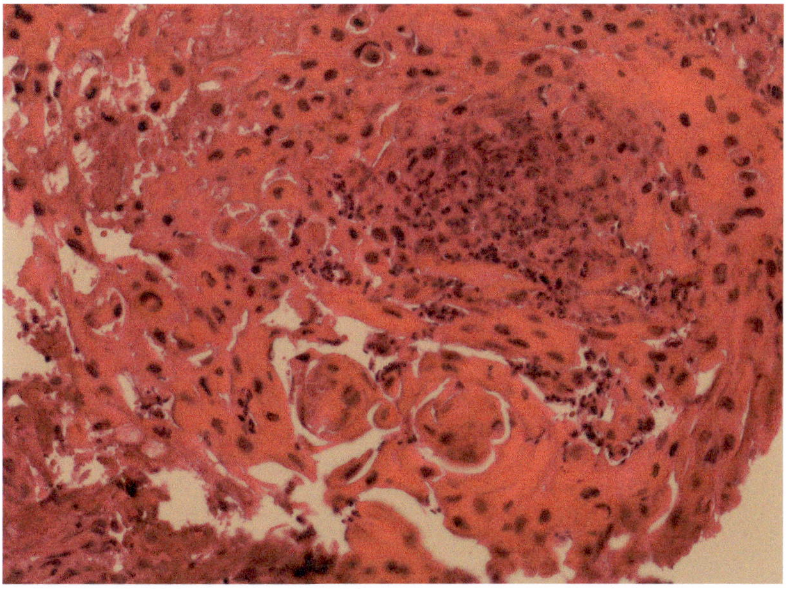

Fig. 2.34 Urothelial carcinoma with prominent keratinizing squamous cell differentiation

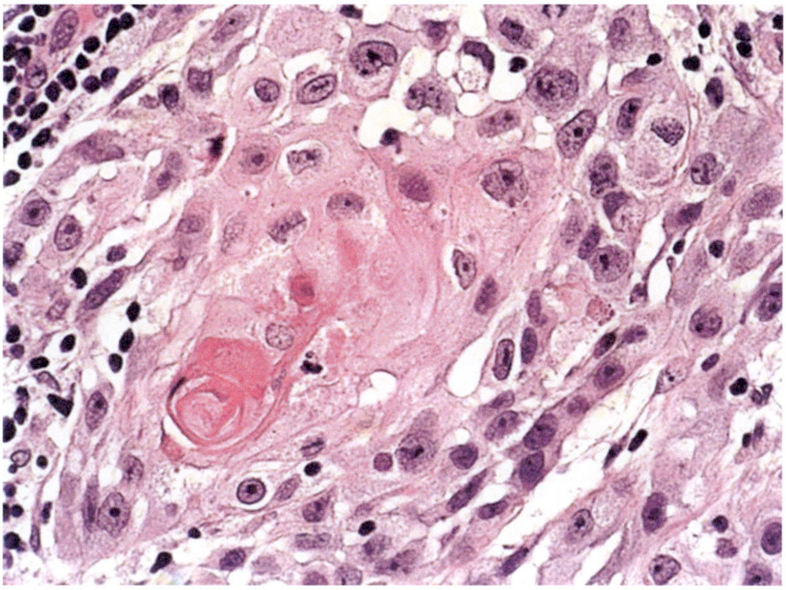

Fig. 2.35 Urothelial carcinoma with focal squamous cell differentiation

"deceptively benign" appearance that closely resembles von Brunn's nests infiltrating the lamina propria. A variable proportion of infiltrating cell nests may exhibit small tubular lumens (Tables 2.11, 2.12, and 2.13).

- A recent study based on 56 cases of the nested variant showed that architectural pattern of the tumor varied from solid expansile to infiltrative nests characterized by deceptively bland histologic features resembling von Brunn nests. Typical features of high grade conventional urothelial carcinoma were present in 32 cases. Most neoplastic cells had nuclei of low to intermediate nuclear grade with occasional nuclear enlargement, most frequently seen in deep areas of tumor (Figs. 2.38, 2.39, and 2.40).

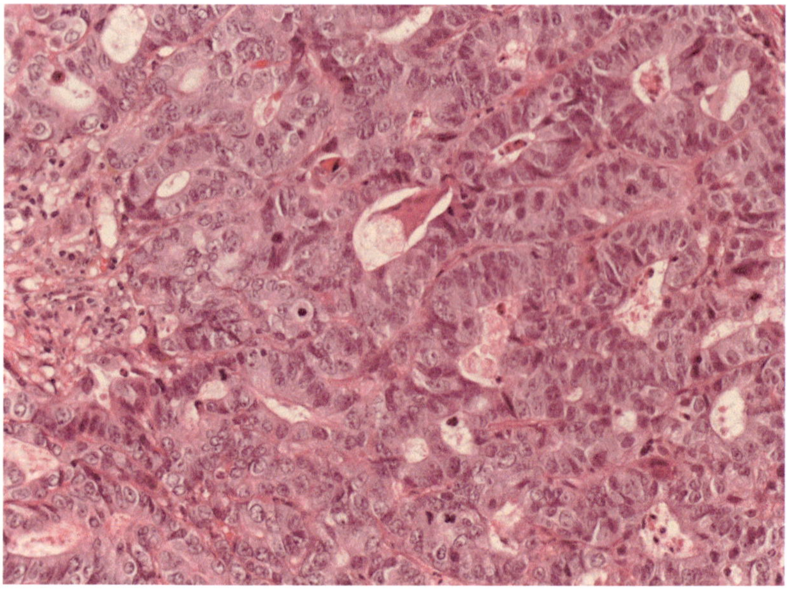

Fig. 2.36 Urothelial carcinoma with glandular differentiation

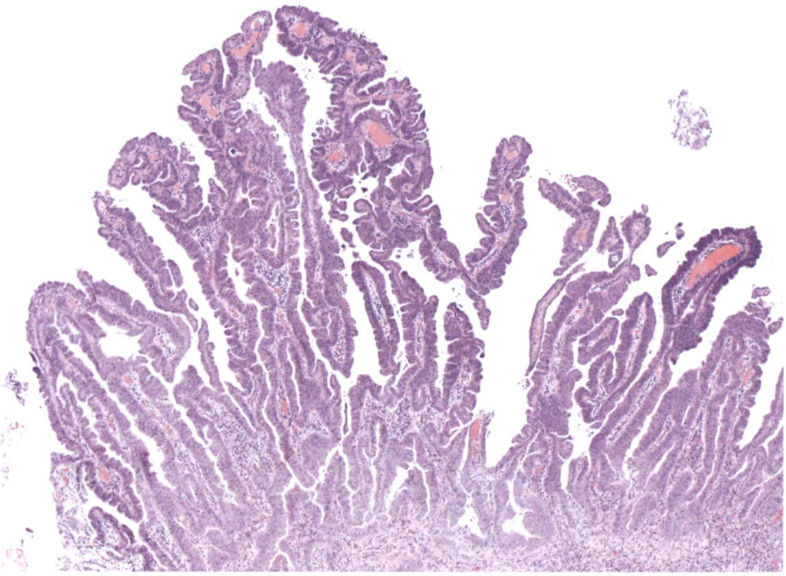

Fig. 2.37 Urothelial carcinoma with villous-like glandular differentiation

- Nuclei generally show little or no atypia, but invariably the tumor contains foci of unequivocal cancer with cells exhibiting enlarged nucleoli and coarse nuclear chromatin. Anaplastic features are often more apparent in the deeper aspects of the cancer. The nested urothelial carcinoma, seen either in pure form or with a component of usual urothelial carcinoma, had poor outcomes.
- The architectural pattern of nested carcinoma component ranged from a predominantly disorderly proliferation of discrete, small, variably sized nests to tubular growth pattern with focal random nuclear atypia centered within the base of the tumor. A component of usual urothelial carcinoma is frequently present.
- The differential diagnosis of the nested variant of urothelial carcinoma include lesions and

tumors with nested-like morphology as prominent von Brunn's nests, cystitis cystica, cystitis glandularis, inverted papilloma, nephrogenic metaplasia, carcinoid tumor, paraganglionic tissue, and paraganglioma.

- The immunohistochemical features of the nested variant of urothelial carcinoma are similar to those of aggressive urothelial carcinomas of the usual type, with frequent loss of p27 and a high MIB-1 labeling index. In the differential diagnosis between florid von Brunn nests and the nested variant of urothelial carcinoma, CK20 immunohistochemical evaluation does not appear to be useful, but significantly greater MIB-1 expression and p53 expression are seen in nested variant urothelial carcinoma when compared to florid von Brunn nests, with MIB-1 expression in >7 % of lesional cells and p53 expression in >3 % of lesional cells seen only in carcinoma.
- The nested component expressed cytokeratins 7, 20, CAM5.2, and high molecular weight (34ßE12), p63, Ki67, p53, p27, and GATA3. Tumor extension ranged T1 to T4a. On follow-up, 36 of patients died of or were alive with disease from 2 to 80 months (mean 21 months).
- Univariate survival analysis showed no differences for nested carcinoma compared with conventional urothelial carcinoma. As in conventional urothelial carcinoma, in nested carcinoma of the bladder pT category defined different survival groups.

Table 2.11 Diverse morphologic manifestations and pitfalls in the diagnosis of urothelial carcinoma variants

Feature of urothelial carcinoma	Benign lesion in differential diagnosis
Nests (including occasional small lumens)	Von Brunn's nests, cystitis glandularis
Small tubules	Nephogeneic metaplasia, von Brunn's nests, cystitis glandularis
Glands of medium size	Cystitis glandularis, cystitis cystica
Cysts (microcysts)	Cystitis cystica, cystitis cystica et glandularis
Inverted growth	Inverted papilloma

Table 2.12 Variants of urothelial carcinoma according to their differential diagnosis

Variants of urothelial carcinoma	Main differential diagnosis
Urothelial carcinoma with squamous and/or glandular differentiation	Squamous cell carcinoma, adenocarcinoma
Urothelial carcinoma, nested variant (including small tubules type)	Von Brunn's hyperplasia
Urothelial carcinoma, inverted variant	Inverted papilloma
Urothelial carcinoma, micropapillary variant	Adenocarcinoma, serous carcinoma of the ovary
Urothelial carcinoma, microcystic variant	Cystitis cystica and cystistis glandularis, rarely adenocarcinoma
Lymphoepithelioma-like (urothelial) carcinoma	Lymphoma
Urothelial carcinoma, plasmacytoid variant	Plasmacytoma
Urothelial carcinoma, clear cell (glycogen-rich) variant	Clear cell carcinomas from kidney and other sites
Urothelial carcinoma, lipoid cell variant	Carcinosarcoma/sarcomatoid carcinoma of hetorologous type (liposarcoma)
Urothelial carcinoma with syncitiotrophoblastic giant cells	Choriocarcinoma either primary or secondary
Large cell undifferentiated carcinoma	Metastasis from other sites
Urothelial carcinoma with rhabdoid feature	Plasmacytoma, inflammatory myofibroblastic tumor, metastasis from other sites
Urothelial carcinoma with peudosarcomatous stroma	Sarcomatoid carcinoma
Urothelial carcinoma with stromal osseous or cartilaginous metaplasia	Sarcomatoid carcinoma with hetorologous element
Urothelial carcinoma with osteoclast-type giant cells	Reactive granulomatous lesion
Urothelial carcinoma with prominent lymphoid infiltrate	Lymphoma, lymphoepithelial carcinoma

Table 2.13 Key features in the differential diagnosis of the nested variant of urothelial carcinoma

	Lumen formation	Marked cytologic atypia in deeper portion	Infiltrative base	Muscle invasion	Immunohistochemistry
Nested variant	Present, variable	Present, frequent	Present, frequent	Present, frequent	Low $p27^{kip1}$, high MIB1 proliferation index
Florid von Brunn nests	Present, variable	Absent	Absent	Absent	Variable
Nephrogenic metaplasia	Present	Absent	Present, frequent	Present, rare	Variable
Cystitis cystica, cystitis glandularis	Present	Absent	Absent	Absent	Variable
Paraganglionic tissue and paraganglioma	Absent, associated prominent vascular network	Absent	Absent	Present	Neuroendocrine markers positive

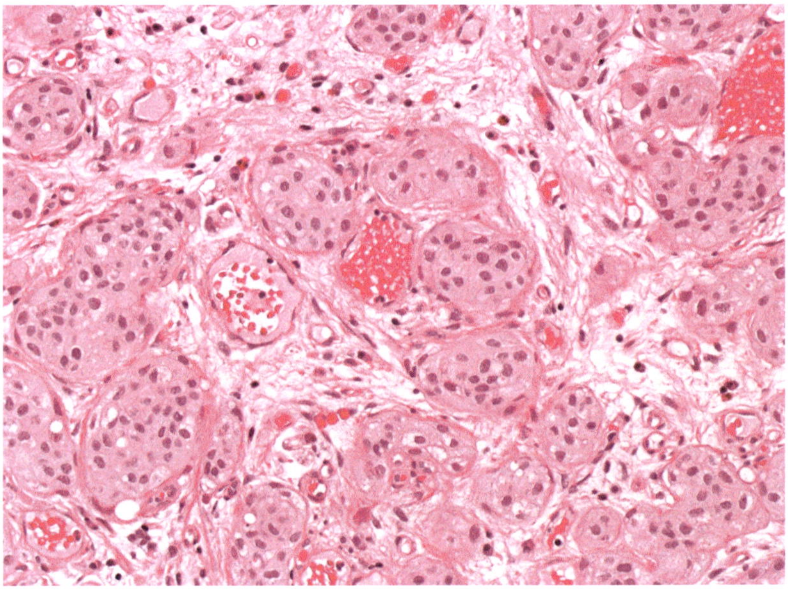

Fig. 2.38 Microscopic features of nested type of urothelial carcinoma

Urothelial carcinoma, inverted growth (endophytic) variant

- This variant also has been referred as urothelial carcinoma with endophytic (inverted papilloma-like) growth or inverted urothelial carcinoma. The potential for misinterpretation of urothelial carcinoma with inverted growth as benign inverted papilloma is high (Table 2.14).
- The inverted variant of urothelial carcinoma demonstrates significant nuclear pleomorphism, architectural abnormality and increased mitotic activity. In most cases, the surface of the neoplasm shows similar abnormalities and is readily recognized as typical urothelial carcinoma.
- An exophytic papillary or invasive component is often associated with the inverted element. However, in cases of inverted papilloma fragmented during transurethral resection, a pseudoexophytic pattern may result. Large papillary tumors with prominent endophytic growth may appear to "invade" the lamina propria with a pushing border. Unless this pattern is accompanied by true destructive stromal invasion the likelihood of metastasis is minimal, because the basement membrane is not truly breached.

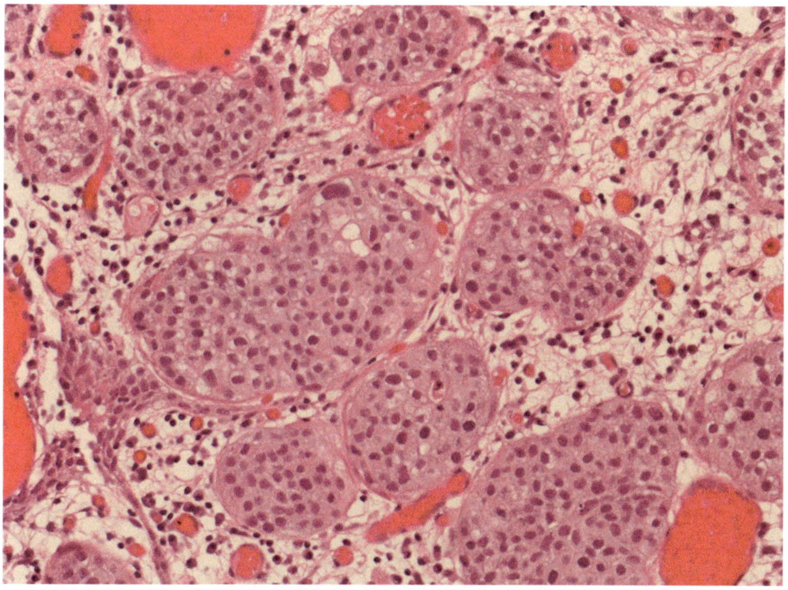

Fig. 2.39 Microscopic features of nested type of urothelial carcinoma, deeper aspect

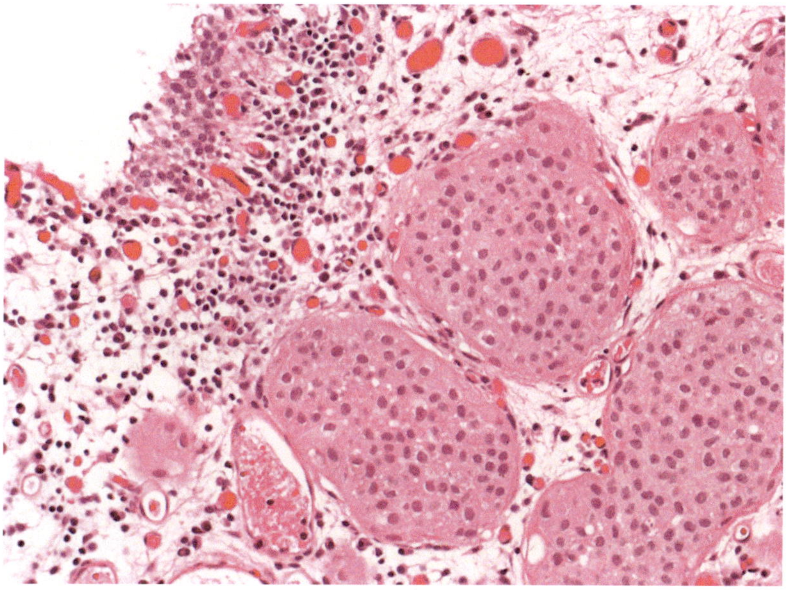

Fig. 2.40 Microscopic features of large nested urothelial carcinoma

- A recent proposal suggests grading these tumors following the same criteria as usual urothelial carcinoma (Figs. 2.41 and 2.42).
- Inverted papillomas of the urinary bladder and urothelial carcinomas with an inverted growth pattern may be distinguished using a combination of morphologic, immunohistochemical, and molecular genetic assessments.
- Whereas inverted papillomas usually do not demonstrate immunoreactivity for Ki-67, p53, or cytokeratin 20, urothelial carcinomas with inverted growth pattern frequently express one or more of these biomarkers. Similarly, inverted papillomas do not show the molecular features of urothelial carcinoma on UroVysion FISH analysis, whereas inverted-pattern urothelial carcinomas often demonstrated genetic alterations that are commonly seen in bladder cancer.

Table 2.14 Differences between urothelial carcinoma with inverted growth and inverted papilloma

Characteristics	Urothelial carcinoma, inverted growth	Inverted papilloma
Surface	Variable, usually exophytic papillary lesion present	Smooth, dome shaped, usually intact cytologically unremarkable surface urothelium
Growth pattern	Endophytic, thick trabeculae, circumscription variable	Endophytic, sharply delineated, anastomosing cords and trabeculae
Cytologic features	Cytologic atypia is invariably present, mitotic figures often present, less maturation or palisading	Orderly polarized cells, some spindling and palisading at periphery, absence of necrosis and diffuse severe cytologic atypia. Mitotic figures absent or rare
Biologic potential	Recurrences and progression may occur	Benign, no recurrences when completely resected[a]
Immunohistochemistry	Variable with grade; usually high p53 accumulation or Ki67-MIB1 counts	Low p53 accumulation and Ki-67-MIB1 counts. 45 % FGFR3 mutations. No TP53 mutations
UroVision FISH	Positive	Negative

[a]Rare recurrences related to incomplete surgical excision

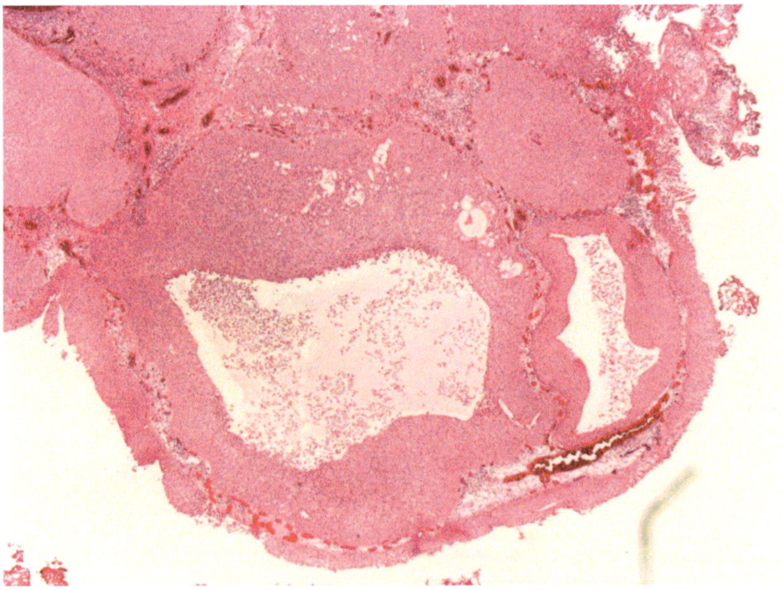

Fig. 2.41 Microscopic features of low grade urothelial carcinoma with inverted growth

Urothelial carcinoma, micropapillary variant

- Micropapillary carcinoma is a distinct variant of urothelial carcinoma that resembles papillary serous carcinoma of the ovary. Approximately 60 cases have been reported in the literature.
- There is a male predominance and the patient age ranges from the fifth to the ninth decade with a mean age of 66 years. Micropapillary carcinoma should be considered a variant of urothelial carcinoma with poor prognosis.
- As recently reported, 62 % of patients with invasive Micropapillary carcinoma had lymph node metastases, with 85 % of patients died of disease at a mean interval from the diagnosis of 6.2 months.
- A recent study by the MDACC suggested that high grade urothelial carcinoma stage pT1 has a high frequency of micropapillary carcinoma (so called superficial micropapillary carcinoma) and that patients in this category should be offered aggressive therapy instead of intravesical immunotherapy to improve long term survival.
- Some studies suggest that the prognosis is related to the proportion of the micropapillary

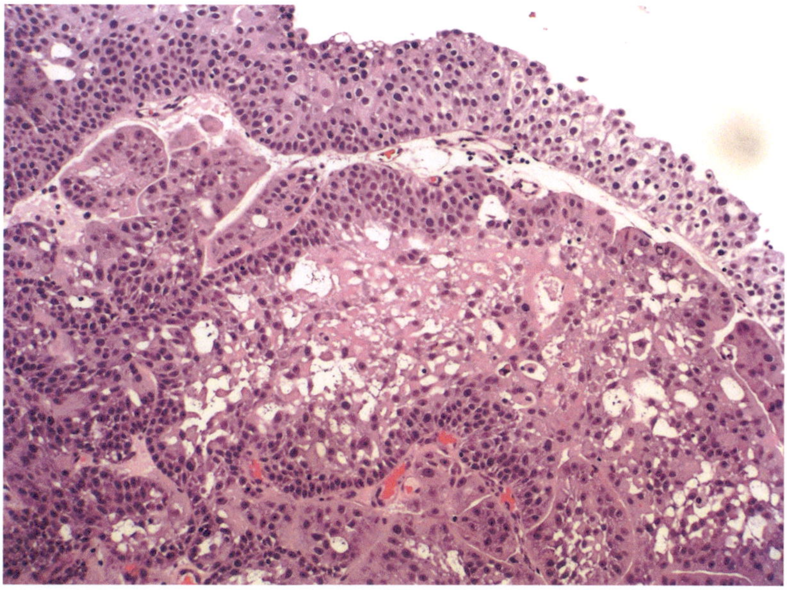

Fig. 2.42 Microscopic features of high grade urothelial carcinoma with inverted growth

component. Cases with a moderate or extensive micropapillary component are at high risk for having an advanced stage at presentation. Cases with less than 10 % micropapillary component and a surface micropapillary component have a high chance of detection at an early stage.

- Micropapillary carcinoma is accompanied by noninvasive papillary or invasive urothelial carcinoma in 80 % of reported cases. The presence of a micropapillary component at the surface in bladder biopsy specimens is an unfavorable prognostic feature. In such cases deeper biopsies may prove useful, since muscle invasion is a significant concern in these cases.
- Micropapillary carcinoma is composed of infiltrating slender delicate filiform processes or small tight papillary tumor cell clusters that lie within lacunae that resemble lymphovascular spaces; however, no lining endothelial cells are demonstrable by immunohistochemistry in these small lacunar spaces.
- Interobserver reproducibility for a diagnosis of IMPC remains moderate (kappa: 0.54). Although classification as IMPC among the 10 "classic" IMPC cases was relatively uniform (93 % agreement), the classification in the subset of 20 invasive urothelial carcinomas with extensive retraction and varying sized tumor nests was more variable. Multiple nests within the same lacunar space had the highest association with a diagnosis of classic IMPC (Figs. 2.43, 2.44, 2.45, and 2.46).
- Twenty-five percent of cases show glandular differentiation, and some authors consider it a variant of adenocarcinoma. Psammoma bodies are infrequent. True vascular and lymphatic invasion is commonly demonstrable, and most cases show invasion of the muscularis propria or deeper.
- Metastases are common at the time of initial diagnosis. The main differential consideration is metastatic serous micropapillary ovarian carcinoma in women or mesothelioma in either gender.
- Expression of keratins by tumor cells of micropapillary carcinoma is similar to that of typical urothelial carcinoma, but micropapillary carcinomas are much more likely to express CA-125, suggesting that the micropapillary phenotype is a form of glandular differentiation. Micropapillary carcinoma also show positive immunostaining for EMA, cytokeratins 7 and 20, and Leu M-1 (CD-15). MUC1 expression is seen in the stroma-facing aspect of the tumor cell groups, indicating a reversal of the normal cell orientation in these tumors.

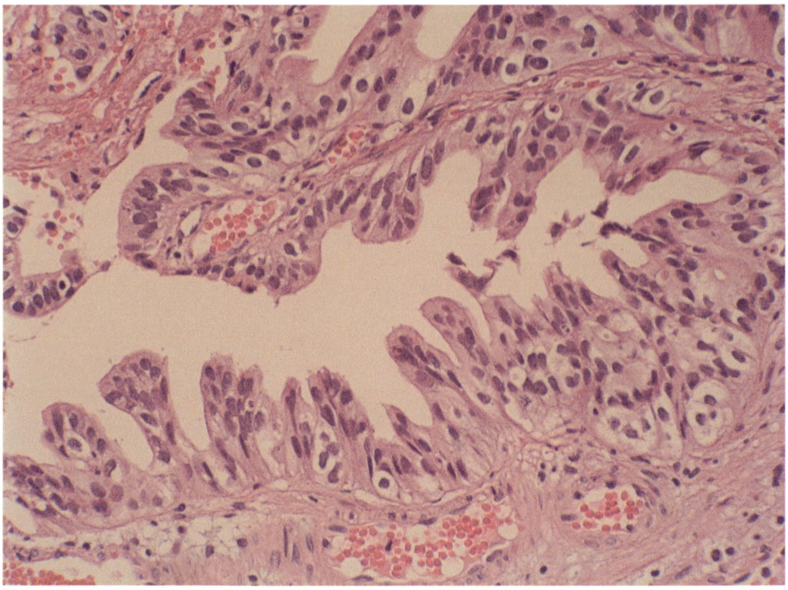

Fig. 2.43 Microscopic features of early micropapillary (superficial) urothelial carcinoma

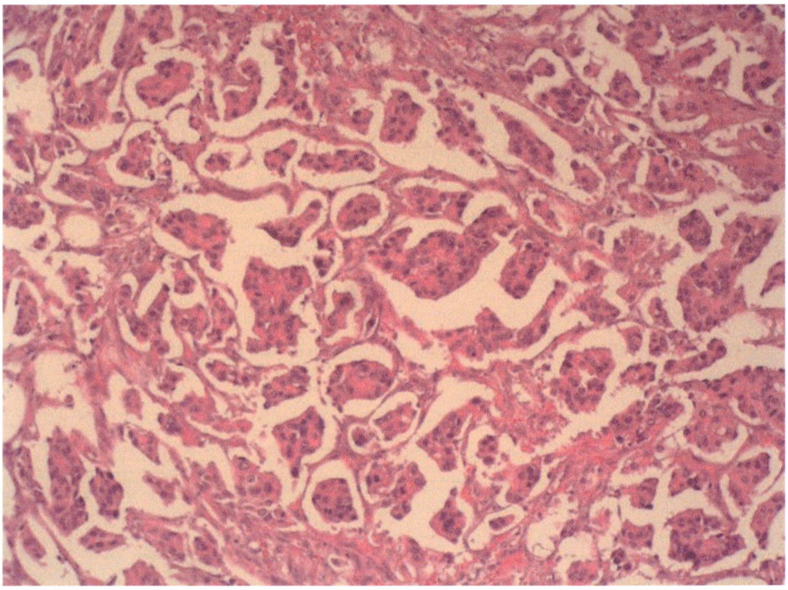

Fig. 2.44 Microscopic features of invasive micropapillary urothelial carcinoma (low power)

- ERBB2 amplification by FISH technology is more frequently observed in micropapillary urothelial carcinoma than in conventional urothelial carcinoma. These patients have worse cancer-specific survival. It also provides a role for ERBB2 targeted therapy.
- Carcinomas with micropapillary histology have also been reported in the lung, breast, pancreas, colo-rectum, and salivary glands. Clinical correlation is usually required, but the possibility of a bladder primary may be suggested if there is no obvious primary tumor at another anatomic site. Identification of an admixed urothelial carcinoma of more typical morphology or immunohistochemical support (CK7, CK20, and uroplakin III positivity) would be helpful.

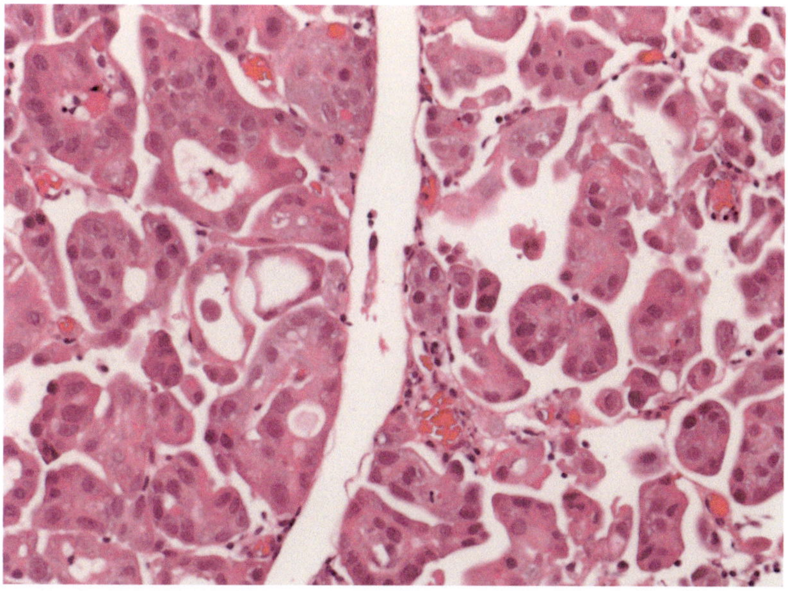

Fig. 2.45 Microscopic features of invasive micropapillary urothelial carcinoma with focal ring formation

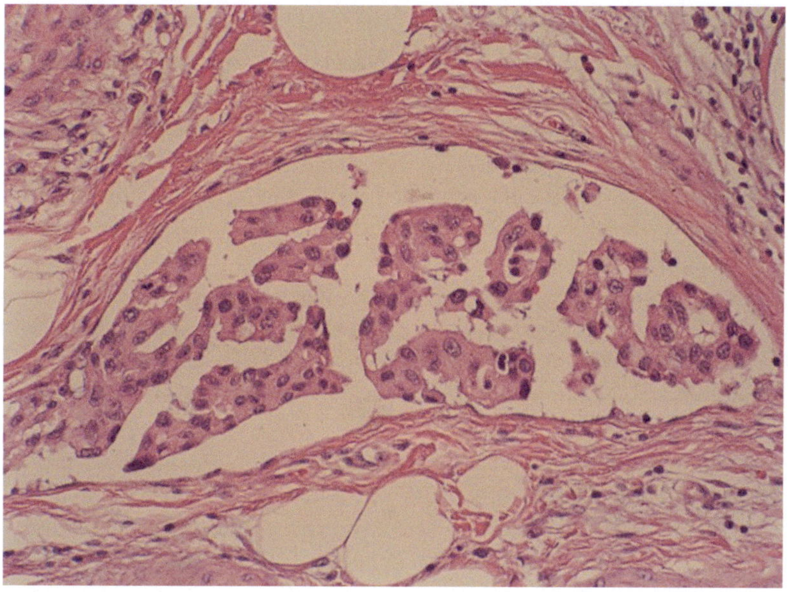

Fig. 2.46 Microscopic features of invasive micropapillary urothelial carcinoma with small papillae within lacunae

Urothelial carcinoma, microcystic variant

- The microcystic variant of invasive urothelial carcinoma is characterized by microcysts, macrocysts, or tubular structures with cysts ranging from microscopic up to 2 cm in diameter (Fig. 2.47).
- A recent report based on the clinicopathological features of 20 cases of microcystic urothelial bladder carcinoma showed the cysts were round–oval and of varying sizes; the periphery of large cysts was frequently punctuated by many smaller cysts. The cysts were lined by urothelial, low columnar cells or by a single layer of flattened epithelium of low–intermediate nuclear grade. Focal high-grade conventional urothelial carcinoma was present in eight cases.
- On follow-up, 60 % of patients died of disease at 11–56 months. Univariate survival analysis showed no differences for microcystic carcinoma versus conventional urothelial carcinoma.

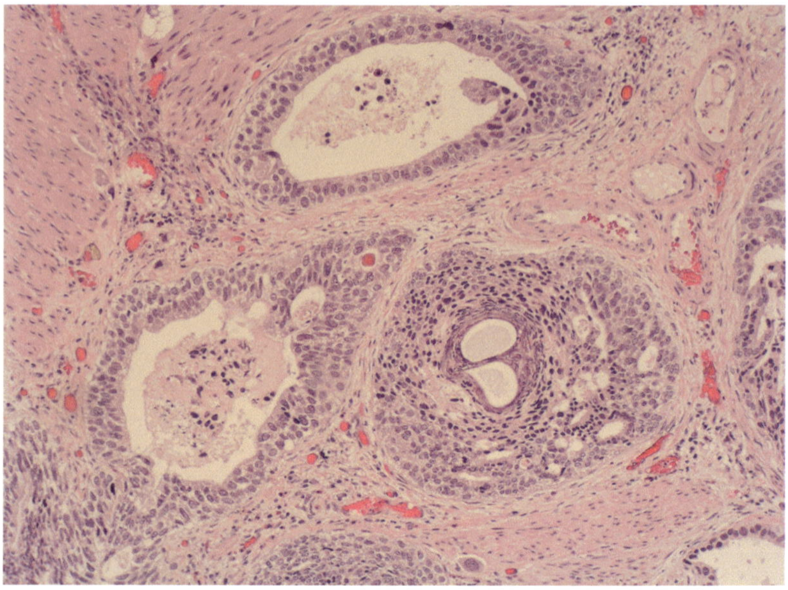

Fig. 2.47 Microscopic features of invasive microcystic carcinoma of the bladder

- This variant of urothelial carcinoma may be confused with benign proliferations such as florid polypoid cystitis cystica and glandularis and nephrogenic metaplasia.
- This pattern should be separated from the nested variant of urothelial carcinoma with tubular differentiation.
- Rarely, microcystic variant may simulate Gleason 3 + 3 prostatic adenocarcinoma showing negative prostate markers and positive for urothelial markers (CK7, CK20 and thrombomodulin).
- Immunohistochemistry demonstrated variable positivity for cytokeratins 7 and 20, MUC1, MUC5AC, p63 and GATA3. Extent of expression of Ki67, p53 and p27kip1 ranged from 20 to 60 %, 10–40 % and 10–30 % of cells, respectively.

Lymphoepithelioma-like (urothelial) carcinoma

- Carcinoma that histologically resembles lymphoepithelioma of the nasopharynx has been described in the urinary bladder, with fewer than 100 cases reported. It is more common in men than in women (3:1 ratio) and tends to occur in late adulthood (range: 52–81 years; mean: 69 years).
- Most patients present with hematuria. The tumor is solitary and usually involves the dome, posterior wall, or trigone, often with a sessile growth pattern. Histologically, it may be pure or mixed with typical urothelial carcinoma, the latter being focal and inconspicuous in some instances.
- Glandular and squamous differentiation may be seen. The epithelial component is composed of nests, sheets, and cords of undifferentiated cells with large pleomorphic nuclei and prominent nucleoli (Fig. 2.48). The cytoplasmic borders are poorly defined, imparting a syncytial appearance. The background consists of a prominent lymphoid stroma that includes T and B lymphocytes, plasma cells, histiocytes, and occasional neutrophils or eosinophils.
- Epstein-Barr virus or human papilloma virus infection have not been identified in lymphoepithelioma-like carcinoma of the bladder. Immunohistochemistry reveals cytokeratin immunoreactivity (cytokeratin AE1/3 and cytokeratin 7) in the malignant cells, confirming their epithelial nature. The epithelial cells are rarely positive or negative for cytokeratin 20. Lelc cases have common Urovysion probes alteration and frequent p53 accumulations supporting a similar pathogenesis to conventional urothelial carcinoma.

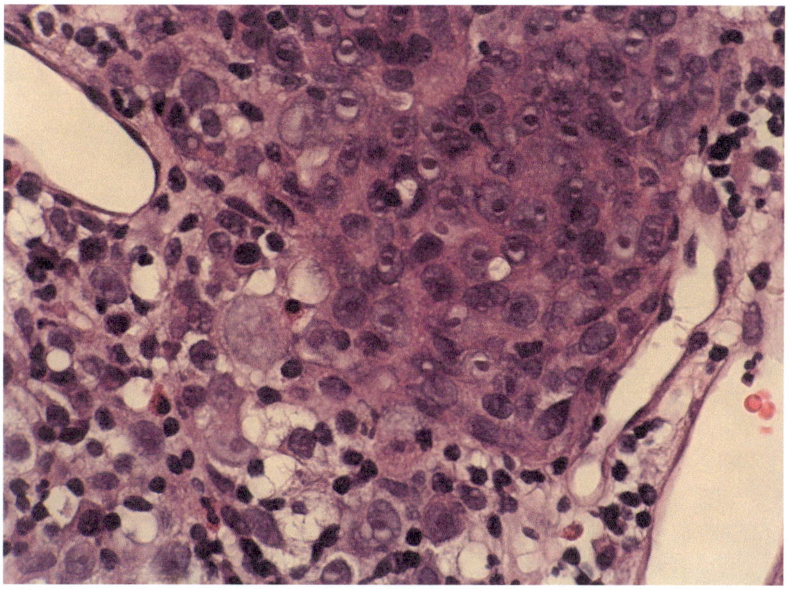

Fig. 2.48 Lymphoepithelioma-like carcinoma of the urinary bladder showing syncytial arrangement of the cells

- The major differential diagnostic considerations are poorly differentiated urothelial carcinoma with lymphoid inflammatory response, poorly differentiated squamous cell carcinoma, and lymphoma. Lymphoepithelioma-like bladder carcinoma has been found to be responsive to chemotherapy if the tumor is encountered in its pure form.
- Although most reported cases occurring in the urinary bladder are associated with a relatively favorable prognosis when pure or predominant, when lymphoepithelioma-like carcinoma is only focally present in an otherwise typical urothelial carcinoma, the prognosis is the same as that of patients with conventional urothelial carcinoma of the same grade and stage.

Urothelial carcinoma, plamacytoid variant

- It is composed of cells with a monotonous appearance mimicking lymphoma. The tumor cells were medium-sized, with eosinophilic cytoplasm and eccentric nuclei producing a plasmacytoid appearance. The differential diagnostic considerations include lymphoid reaction, lymphoma, multiple myeloma, urothelial carcinoma with rhabdoid feature, signet ring cell adenocarcinoma, paraganglioma, neuroendocrine carcinoma, melanoma, and rhabdomyosarcoma.
- Identification of an epithelial component by Immunohistochemistry confirms the diagnosis. A series report of 11 cases showed that the plasmacytoid component comprised greater than 50 % of the tumor in eight cases, with two additional cases showing pure plasmacytoid carcinoma (Figs. 2.49, 2.50, and 2.51).
- All patients had advanced-stage cancer (>pT3), and 73 % had lymph node metastases. On follow-up, 82 % of patients died of disease from 2 to 11 months, and two patients were alive with disease at 8 and 16 months.
- The architectural pattern of the tumor varied from solid expansile nests with discohesive cells to mixed solid and alveolar growth; a streaking discohesive architecture was additionally present in two cases (18 %).
- Rarely, a myxoid pattern can be present. Histologically, the individual tumor cells had an eccentrically placed nucleus and abundant eosinophilic cytoplasm reminiscent of plasma cells. Most neoplastic cells had nuclei of low to intermediate nuclear grade with occasional nuclear pleomorphism. Small intracytoplasmic vacuoles were variably present in all cases.

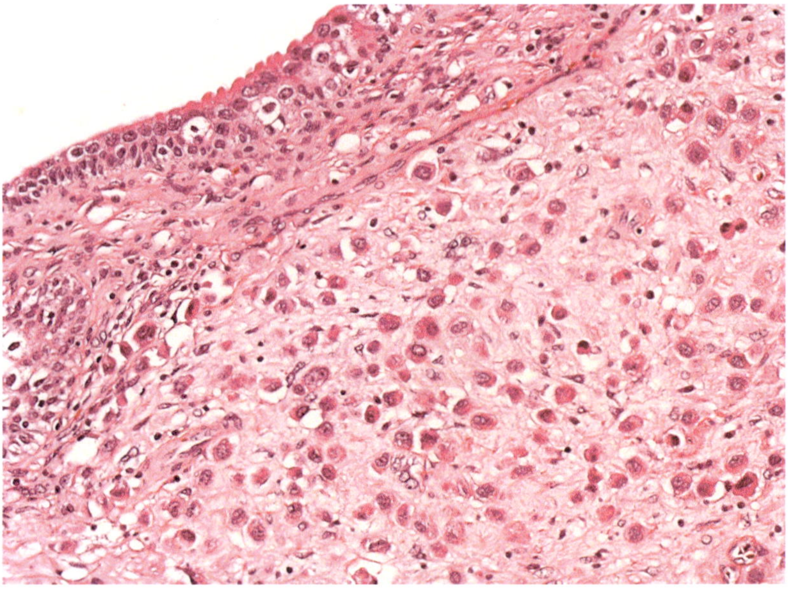

Fig. 2.49 Microscopic features of plasmacytoid urothelial carcinoma

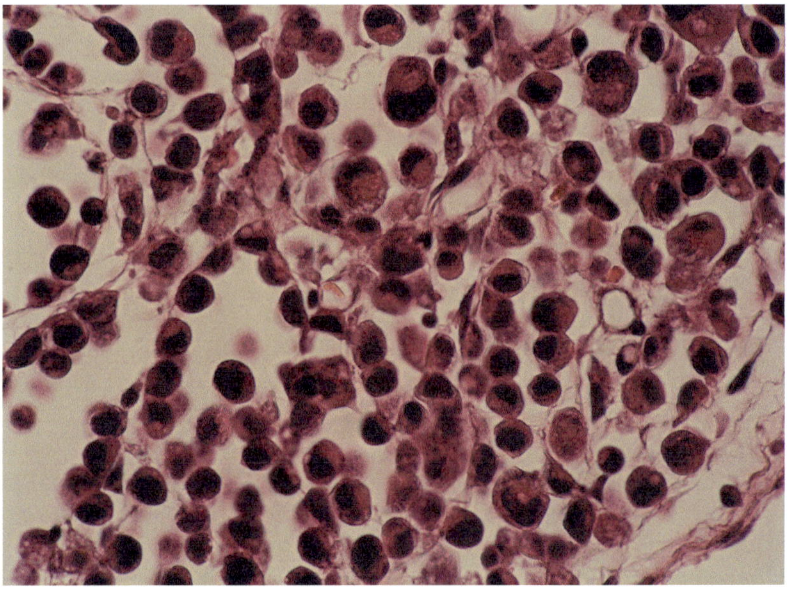

Fig. 2.50 High power view of plasmacytoid urothelial carcinoma

- Immunohistochemical staining demonstrated that both plasmacytoid and associated conventional urothelial carcinoma were positive for CK7, CK20, AE1/AE3, and EMA; CD138 (marker of plasma cells) was positive in three cases. Ring-like structures are most consistent features in diagnosis.
- Artefactual expression of kappa light chains have been seen focally is some cases, a further confounding factor.
- Dyscohesive growth pattern and morphological features mimicking infiltrating lobular carcinoma of the breast and diffuse carcinoma of the stomach have been described in some cases, more frequently male patients with the mean age of 67
- All the cases showed single-cell diffusely infiltrative growth pattern. In some areas the tumor cells were arranged in linear single-cell files (Indian-file pattern) and in other areas there

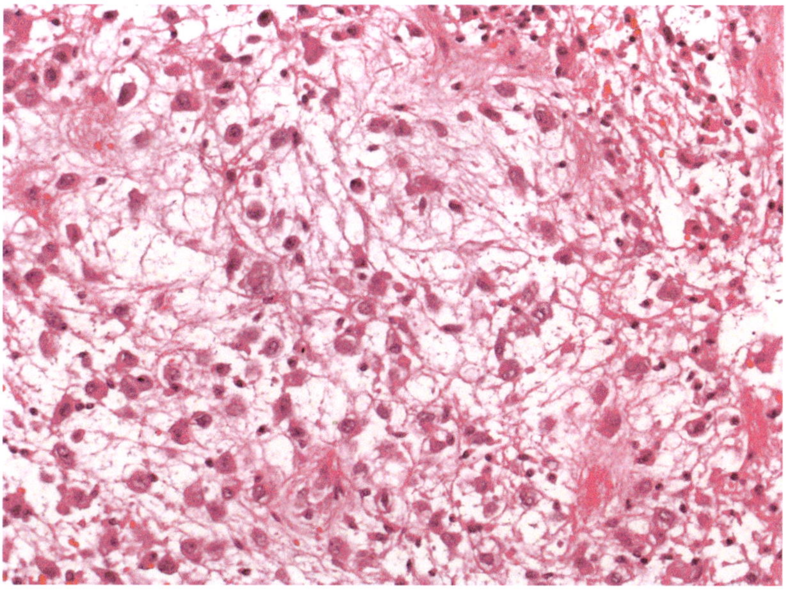

Fig. 2.51 Occasionally, plasmacytoid carcinoma shows myxoid stroma

were solid sheets of dyscohesive cells. In all cases there were tumor cells showing prominent intracytoplasmic vacuoles. Half of reported cases also showed typical transitional cell carcinoma or carcinoma in situ.

- The tumor cells expressed cytokeratin 20 but not estrogen receptor, and some were negative for E-Cadherin. Currently, most authorities place discohesive growth pattern as a form of plasmacytoid variant of bladder cancer.

Urothelial carcinoma, clear cell (glycogen-rich) variant

- Up to two-thirds of urothelial carcinoma cases have foci of clear cell change resulting from abundant glycogen. The glycogen-rich clear cell "variant" of urothelial carcinoma, recently described, appears to represent the extreme end of the morphologic spectrum.
- It consists predominantly or exclusively of cells with abundant clear cytoplasm (Fig. 2.52). Tumor cells show positive immunostaining for cytokeratin 7.
- Recognition of this pattern avoids confusion with clear cell adenocarcinoma of the bladder and metastatic clear cell carcinoma from the kidney or prostate. Cytoplasmic clearing as a result of thermal artifact in transurethral resections should not be mistaken for this variant of bladder cancer.

Urothelial carcinoma, lipid cell variant

- Lipid cell variant is a rare neoplasm defined as an urothelial carcinoma which exhibits transition to a cell type resembling signet-ring lipoblasts (Figs. 2.53 and 2.54).
- A recent report based on 27 cases showed that the lipid cell component varied from 10 to 50 % of the tumor specimen. Pathologic stage at diagnosis was Ta ($n=1$), T1 ($n=2$), T2, (at least $n=7$), T3a ($n=4$), T3b ($n=8$), and T4a ($n=5$). Sixteen of the patients died of disease from 16 to 58 months (mean, 33 months).
- The architectural pattern of the tumor varied from solid expansile to infiltrative nests. The large epithelial tumor cells had an eccentrically placed nucleus and abundant vacuolated cytoplasm resembling signet ring lipoblasts. Mucin stains were negative in all cases. Most neoplastic cells had nuclei of intermediate nuclear grade with occasional nuclear pleomorphism.
- Immunohistochemical staining demonstrated that the lipid cell component was positive for cytokeratins 7, 20, CAM5.2, high-molecular-weight (34βE12) and AE1/AE3, epithelial membrane antigen, and thrombomodulin; vimentin and S-100 protein were negative. The loss of heterozygosity (LOH) analysis was performed on eight cases. The LOH

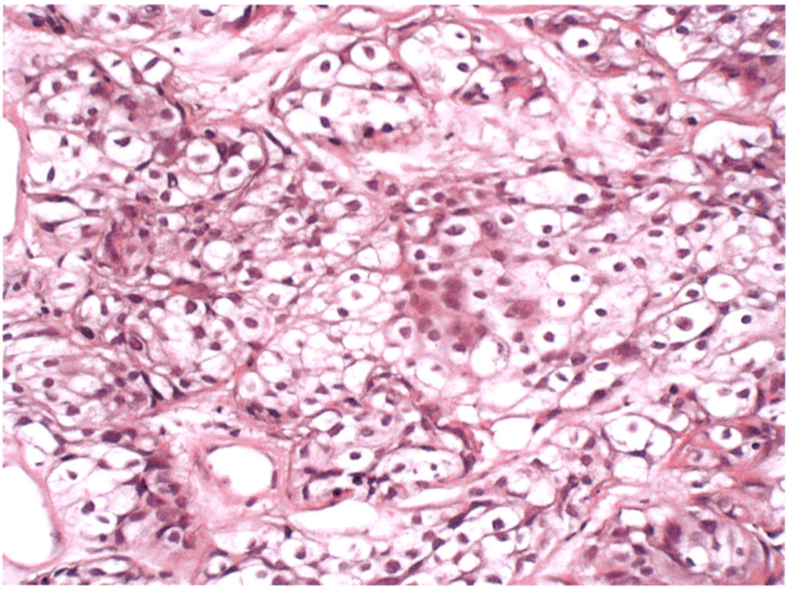

Fig. 2.52 Urothelial carcinoma with glycogen-type clear cells

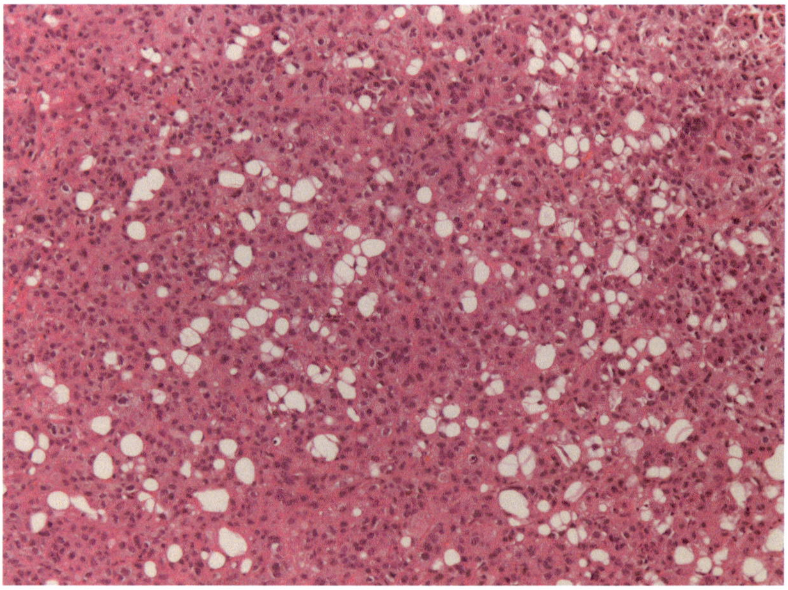

Fig. 2.53 Lipid variant of urothelial carcinoma (low power)

results were the same for lipid variant and concurrent conventional urothelial carcinoma.

- Electron microcopy analysis based on two cases supported lipid content in tumor cells. In limited samples, lipid cell variant urothelial carcinoma may be misdiagnosed as liposarcoma, sarcomatoid carcinoma (carcinosarcoma) with a liposarcomatous component, or signet ring cell carcinoma. The finding of lipid cells immunoreactive for epithelial markers can be very useful in this setting.

Urothelial carcinoma with syncytiotrophoblastic giant cells

- Syncytiotrophoblastic giant cells are present in up to 28 % of urothelial carcinoma cases, producing substantial amounts of immunoreactive beta-human chorionic gonadotropin (HCG) indicative of syncytiotrophoblastic differentiation (Fig. 2.55).

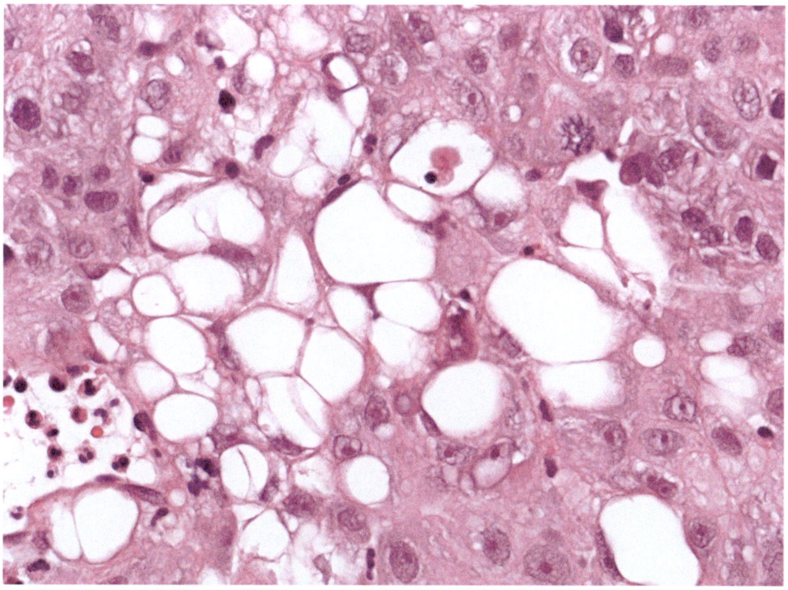

Fig. 2.54 Lipid variant of urothelial carcinoma (high power)

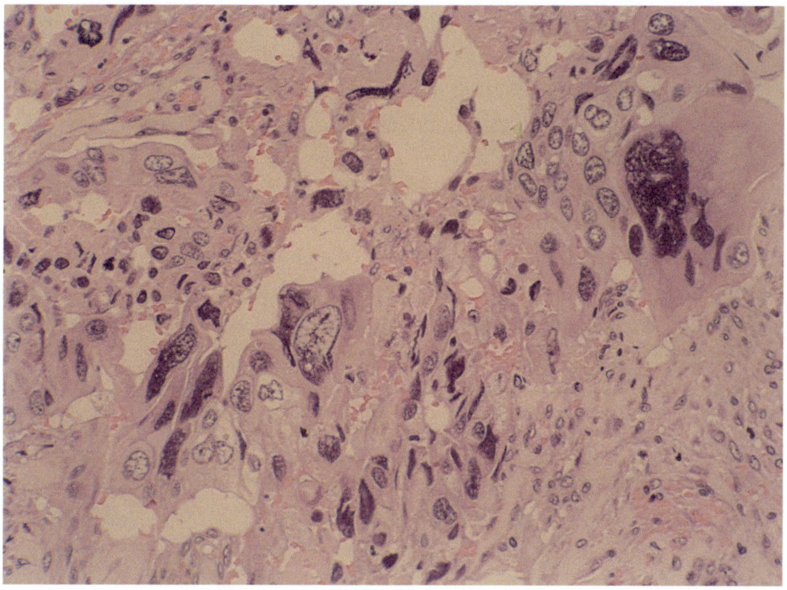

Fig. 2.55 Urothelial carcinoma with trophoblastic differentiation

- The number of HCG-immunoreactive cells is inversely associated with cancer grade. Secretion of HCG into the serum may be associated with a poor response to radiation therapy.
- The most important differential diagnostic consideration is choriocarcinoma whose diagnosis may require a high copy number of the isochromosome 12p as seen by FISH, thus supporting germ cell differentiation. HCG expression in poorly differentiated urothelial carcinoma without overt syncytiotrophoblastic differentiation probably represents a metaplastic phenomenon. It seems likely previously reported "primary choriocarcinomas of the bladder" represent urothelial carcinoma with syncytiotrophoblasts.

Urothelial Carcinoma with Small Tubules

- Although a prominent tubular component may accompany a nested carcinoma, some urothelial

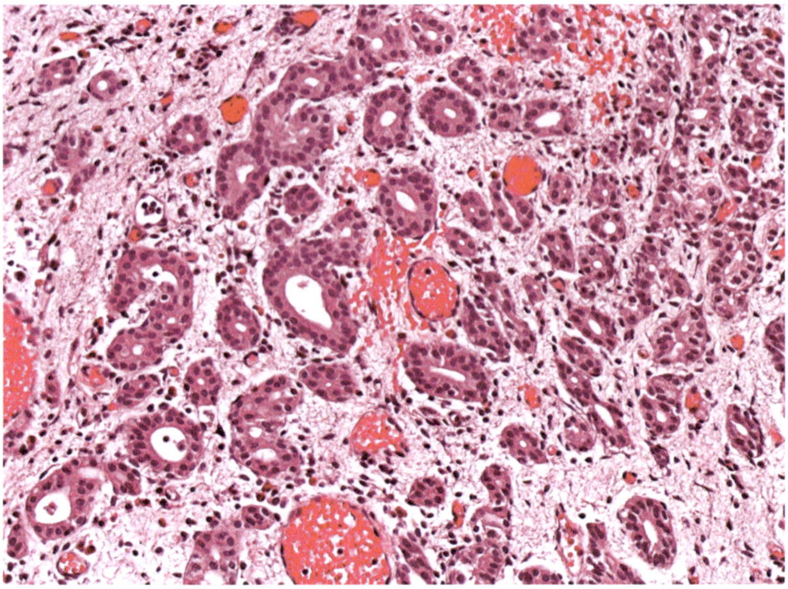

Fig. 2.56 Urothelial carcinoma with small tubules lined by attenuated urothelial cells

carcinomas may have an almost exclusive component of small- to medium-sized, round to elongated tubules that may be misdiagnosed as nephrogenic adenoma, adenocarcinoma, or cystitis glandularis (Fig. 2.56).

- Furthermore, the tubules of urothelial carcinoma are lined by attenuated urothelial cells, in contrast to the varying admixture of cuboidal, columnar, and occasionally flattened cells that line the tubules of nephrogenic adenoma. Urothelial carcinoma with small tubules may be widely invasive despite their deceptively bland histology.
- The significance of this pattern is unclear given the rarity of cases, but some of these cases occur in conjunction with the nested pattern and are widely invasive and have an aggressive outcome because of their high stage at presentation.
- Similar to the nested variant, the chief reason for the awareness of this morphological variant of urothelial carcinoma is not to mistake it in superficial biopsies as a benign glandular proliferative lesion. Some authors believe that urothelial carcinoma with small tubules should be considered within the spectrum of nested carcinoma.
- The differential diagnosis with an extension of a prostatic carcinoma is often also a consideration but is easily handled by immunohistochemistry prostate-specific antigen (PSA), prostatic-specific acid phosphatase (PSAP): positive in prostate cancer; CK20, high-molecular-weight cytokeratin; and p63: positive in more than half of urothelial carcinomas.

Urothelial Carcinoma with myxoid stroma

- This is a recently described entity with myxoid stroma and chordoid-like morphology characterized by prominent cellular cording and associated myxoid stromal matrix, a pattern that may resemble extraskeletal myxoid chondrosarcoma (Figs. 2.57 and 2.58).
- These carcinomas maintain an immunophenotype characteristic of urothelial carcinoma and usually present with high-stage disease. The patients' ages ranged from 50 to 85 years (mean: 68 years); there were eight males and four females. Morphologically, each case had at least focal areas in which acellular myxoid stroma was associated with the carcinoma cells.
- Occasionally, cells were arranged into cords closely mimicking extraskeletal myxoid chondrosarcoma, chordoma, mixed tumor/ myoepithelioma of soft tissue, and yolk sac tumor. All 12 cases had foci of typical urothelial carcinoma present at least focally.

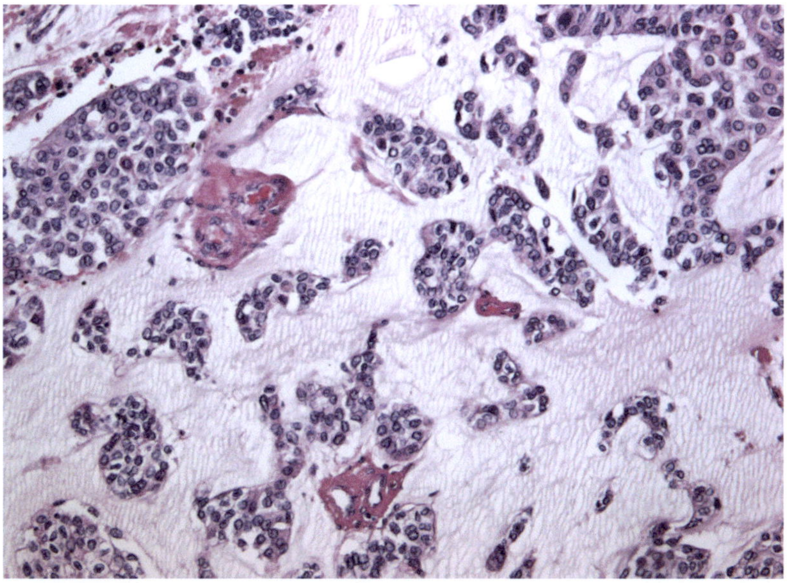

Fig. 2.57 Urothelial carcinoma with myxoid stroma showing a mucinous appearance

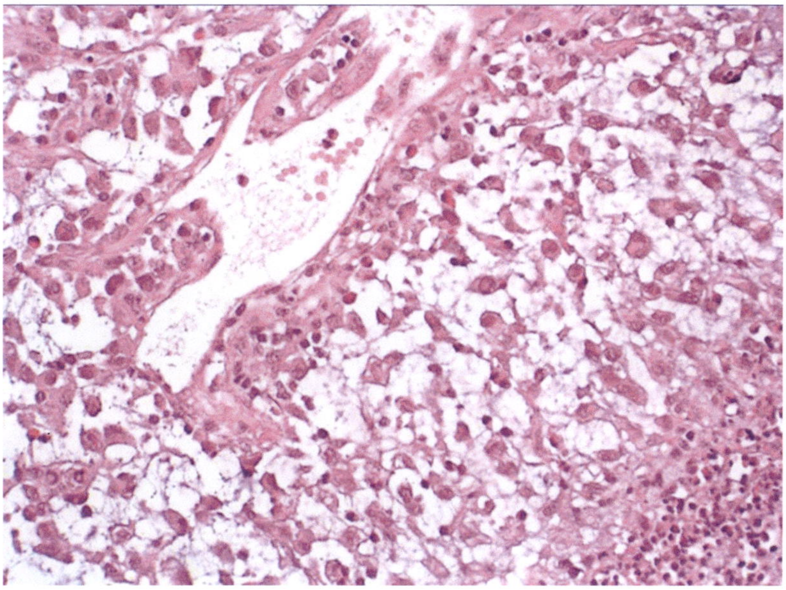

Fig. 2.58 Urothelial carcinoma with myxoid stroma showing a chordoid-like pattern

- Immunophenotypically, these tumors show strong immunoreactivity for p63 (nuclear) and CK34βE12 (cytoplasmic).
- Immunostains for CK20, calponin, glial fibrillary acidic protein, oncofetal protein glypican-3, and brachyury and were negative in the seven cases studied, whereas S-100 protein had focal staining (<5 %) in one case. The myxoid stromal component was diffusely colloidal iron and Alcian blue positive; periodic acid–Schiff was negative in all eight cases, whereas mucicarmine was focally positive in only two of eight cases. Most cases were high stage and 75 % with nodal sampling had metastatic disease.
- Nine of 12 patients had available follow-up: two were dead of disease (1 and 10 months), four were alive with disease (5–8 months) with distant metastasis in three, and three had no evidence of disease at last follow-up (2–120 months).

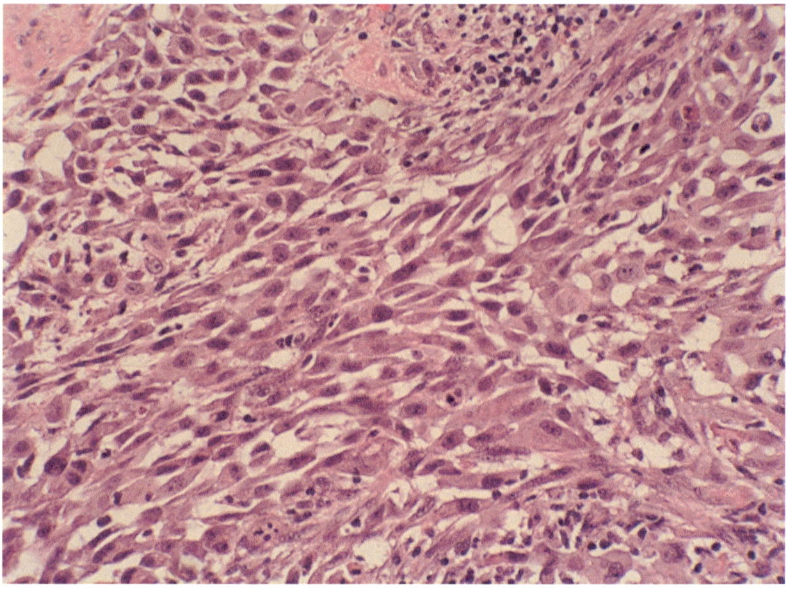

Fig. 2.59 Sarcomatoid carcinoma with atypical spindle cells

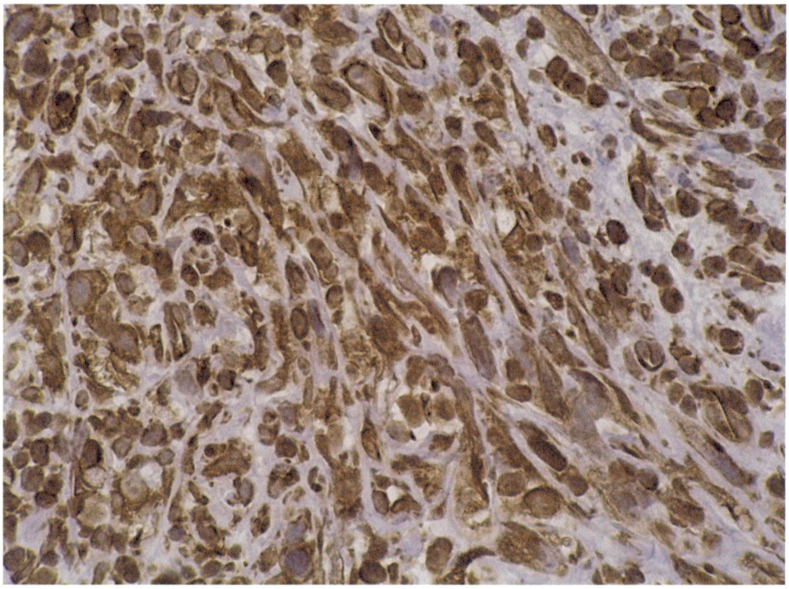

Fig. 2.60 Spindle cells in sarcomatoid carcinoma are positive for cytokeratin

Sarcomatoid carcinoma

- The term sarcomatoid carcinoma applies when a malignant neoplasm exhibits morphologic or immunohistochemical evidence of both epithelial and mesenchymal differentiation. Heterologous elements may be present and should be acknowledged in the pathology report. We postulate that sarcomatoid carcinoma is a common final pathway of all forms of epithelial bladder tumors, a hypothesis supported by molecular data and morphogic evidence (Figs. 2.59, 2.60, and 2.61).
- Sarcomatoid transformation has been observed in various epithelial tumor of the urinary bladder, including conventional urothelial carcinoma, small cell carcinoma, adenocarcinoma, squamous cell carcinoma, large cell neuroendocrine carcinoma.
- Various terms have been used for these neoplasms, including carcinosarcoma, sarcomatoid

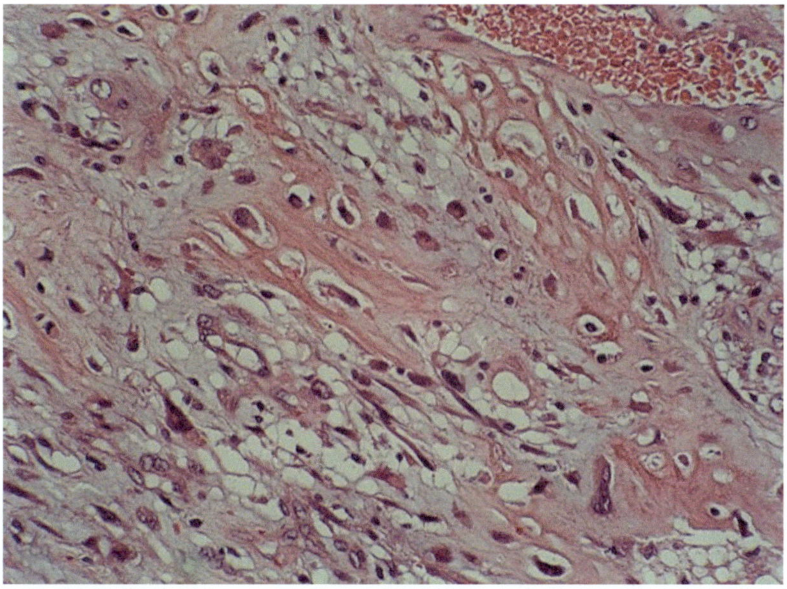

Fig. 2.61 Sarcomatoid carcinoma with heterologous (osteosarcoma) differentiation

carcinoma, pseudosarcomatous transitional cell carcinoma, malignant mesodermal mixed tumor, spindle cell carcinoma, giant cell carcinoma, and malignant teratoma.

- In some reports, both carcinosarcoma and sarcomatoid carcinoma are included under the term "sarcomatoid carcinoma". In others they are regarded as separate entities. There is widespread consensus that the most appropriate term for all of these neoplasms is sarcomatoid carcinoma. We prefer to use the term sarcomatoid carcinoma for the majority of cases in which there is a spindle cell component with positive vimentin staining. Some may use the term carcinosarcoma for cases with identifiable heterologous elements on hematoxylin and eosin stained sections or positive staining for markers of specific mesenchymal differentiation.
- Both diagnostic categories appear to be variations of the same neoplastic transformation process and have the same clinical features and prognosis.
- Sarcomatoid carcinoma represents approximately 0.3 % of bladder carcinomas. The most frequent presenting symptoms are hematuria, dysuria, nocturia, acute urinary retention, and lower abdominal pain. The mean patient age is 66 years (range 50–77 years). In some patients, there is a history of carcinoma treated by radiation, or exposure to cyclophosphamide therapy.
- The presence of specific types of differentiation of the spindle cell component does not influence the prognosis, but sarcomatoid carcinoma is usually high grade, biologically aggressive and associated with a poor prognosis. Pathological stage is the best predictor of survival in sarcomatoid carcinoma.

Pathology

- The gross appearance is characteristically "sarcoma-like," with a dull gray fleshy cut surface and infiltrative margins. The tumors are often polypoid and tend to form large intraluminal masses. Microscopically, sarcomatoid carcinoma is composed of a urothelial, glandular or small cell epithelial component showing variable degrees of differentiation.
- Carcinoma in situ is present in 30 % of cases and occasionally is the only apparent epithelial component. A small subset of sarcomatoid carcinomas may have a prominent myxoid stroma.
- The mesenchymal component most frequently observed is an undifferentiated high grade spindle cell neoplasm. The most common heterologous element is osteosarcoma, followed by chondrosarcoma, rhabdomyosarcoma,

leiomyosarcoma, liposarcoma, angiosarcoma or multiple types of mesenchymal differentiation.

Differential diagnosis and immunohistochemistry

- Sarcomatoid carcinoma is characterized by strong staining with keratins (AE1/AE3, CAM5.2) and/or epithelial membrane antigen with coexpression of vimentin in the majority of cases. In contrast to smooth muscle neoplasms, actin and desmin are typically negative. However, sarcomatoid carcinomas with heterologous differentiation may rarely be encountered and in this situation expression of other mesenchymal markers such as actin, desmin, S-100 protein may be observed.
- Sarcomatoid carcinoma of the urinary bladder is usually biphasic, composed of both epithelial and mesenchymal elements. In cases exclusively composed of spindle cells, the main differential diagnostic consideration is sarcoma, particularly leiomyosarcoma. In view of the rarity of primary bladder sarcoma, any malignant spindle cell tumor in the urinary bladder in an adult be considered sarcomatoid carcinoma until proven otherwise.
- Cytokeratin immunostaining may be helpful in this setting. One should also bear in mind that focal cytokeratin immunoreactivity may be seen in smooth muscle tumors and pseudosarcomatous myofibroblastic proliferations. Smooth muscle tumors are additionally immunoreactive for desmin and vimentin, even when they express cytokeratin antigens.
- Sarcomatoid carcinoma with prominent myxoid and sclerosing stroma may be mistaken for pseudosarcomatous myofibroblastic tumor, postoperative spindle cell nodule, or urothelial carcinoma with pseudosarcomatous stroma. The presence of slit-like vessels and the absence of mitotic figures and significant cytologic atypia favor the diagnosis of benign lesion.

Molecular genetics

- Recent molecular studies strongly argue for a monoclonal origin of both the epithelial and mesenchymal components in sarcomatoid carcinoma and carcinosarcoma. These two categories have similar clinical characteristics, including patient age, gender presentation and outcome.
- A recent analysis of 30 sarcomatoid urothelial carcinomas for X-chromosome inactivation status as well as loss of heterozygosity (LOH) has shed light on the pathogenesis of this tumor. Results of this study found identical patterns of allelic loss in the carcinomatous and in the sarcomatous components, identified at four of six polymorphic microsatellite markers where genetic alterations occur frequently in urothelial carcinomas, including D8S261 (86 %), D9S177 (75 %), IFNA (57 %), and D11S569 (78 %) loci.
- Furthermore, discordant allelic loss of microsatellite markers was also found at the various sites as the bladder tumors underwent malignant progression leading to genetic divergence of high grade anaplastic malignancies following the initial neoplastic transformation. Additionally, the study found the same pattern of nonrandom X-chromosome inactivation in both carcinomatous and sarcomatous components in 5 of 8 female patients.
- The identical X-chromosome inactivation and significant concordance of LOH support the contention that both carcinomatous and sarcomatous tumor components arise from a monoclonal primordial cell. Clonal divergence may occur during tumor progression and lead to differentiation into mesenchymal as well as epithelial phenotypes.

Small cell carcinoma

- Small cell carcinoma is a malignant neoplasm derived from the urothelium which mimics its pulmonary counterpart (discussed later in this chapter, page). It often co-exists with conventional urothelial carcinoma, squamous carcinoma, and adenocarcinoma or sarcomatoid carcinoma.

Urothelial carcinoma with rhabdoid features

- A variety of tumors with rhabdoid differentiation have been described in the literature. Very few cases have been described in the urinary tract, mainly in the bladder.
- In all cases, the rhabdoid component was admixed with other components, including conventional urothelial carcinoma, sarcomatoid carcinoma, and/or small cell carcinoma.

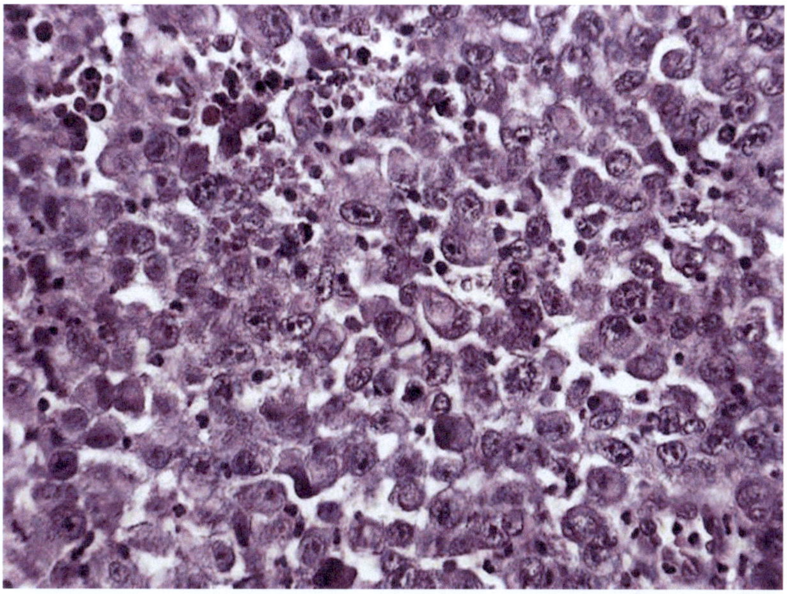

Fig. 2.62 Microscopic features of rhabdoid tumor of the urinary bladder

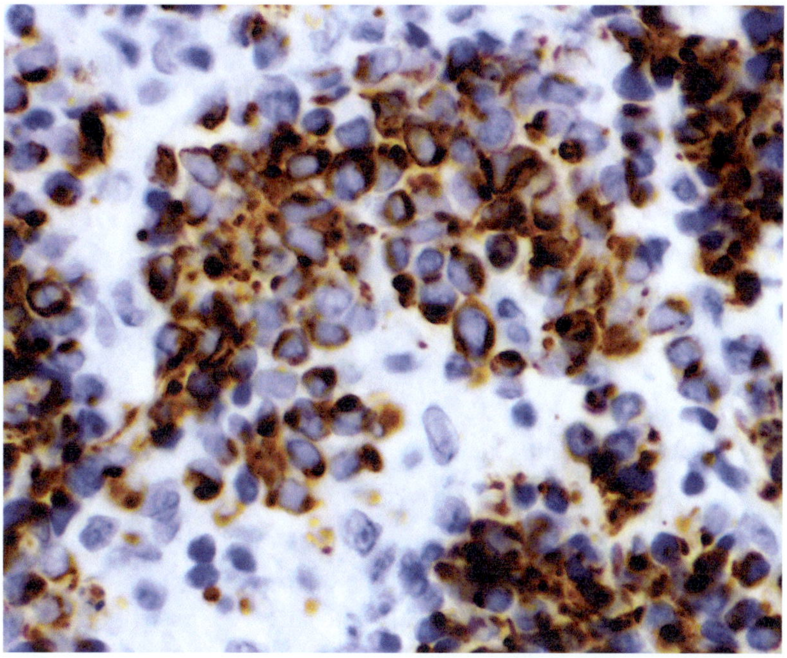

Fig. 2.63 Rhabdoid tumor cells express cytokeratin in a dot-like manner

- Rhabdoid cells have abundant eosinophilic cytoplasm, vesicular nuclei, and prominent nucleoli. they show positive immunostaining for cytokeratin markers (epithelial membrane antigen, CAM5.2, and AE1/3) (Figs. 2.62 and 2.63). These tumors are highly aggressive: 50 % of patients die of bladder cancer shortly after the diagnosis.
- Rhabdoid cells typically lack INI1 reactivity.

Large cell undifferentiated carcinoma

- Large cell undifferentiated carcinoma is more common in the lung but has been described in other organs as a rare and aggressive disease. Large cell undifferentiated carcinoma of the urinary bladder refers to carcinomas that are composed of sheets or isolated undifferentiated

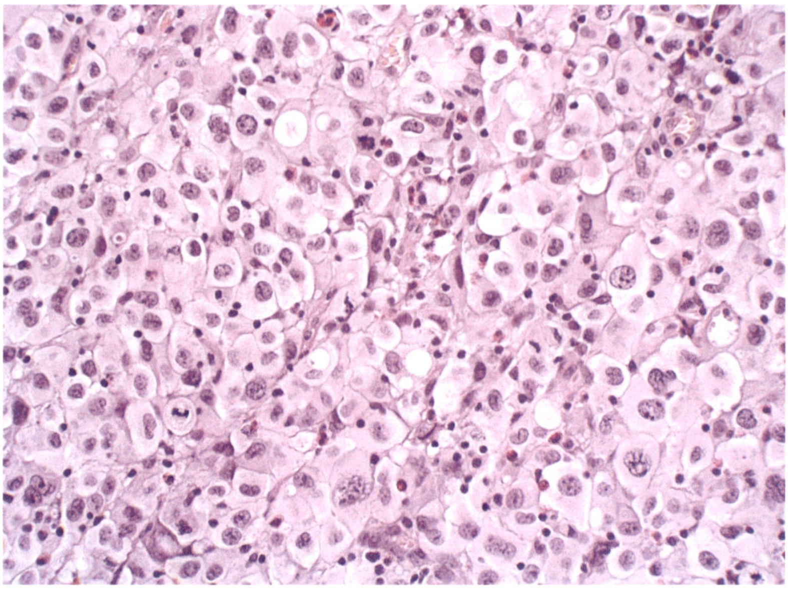

Fig. 2.64 Microscopic features of large cell undifferentiated bladder carcinoma with a solid growth

cells that do not fit into urothelial, squamous, adenocarcinoma, or any other recognized category of bladder carcinoma.

- These tumors are rare and if present in a metastatic site, the histology would not suggest a urothelial primary. A recent report presented the clinicopathologic features of eight cases of large cell undifferentiated bladder carcinoma. These tumors are characterized by sheets of large polygonal or round cells with moderate to abundant cytoplasm and distinct cell borders. The architectural pattern of the tumor varied from infiltrating tumor to solid expansile nests (Figs. 2.64, 2.65, and 2.66).
- Immunohistochemical staining demonstrated that large cell undifferentiated cases were positive for AE1/AE3 and CK7. CAM5.2, CK20, thrombomodulin, and uroplakin III were positive in some cases. Other immunohistochemical markers performed in the differential diagnosis context included α-fetoprotein, βhCG, PSA, vimentin, synaptophysin, and chromogranin, and all were negative.
- Large cell undifferentiated is an aggressive variant of urothelial carcinoma that presents at an advanced stage with poor prognosis. In a series of eight cases, all patients had advanced-stage cancer (≥pT3), and seven (88 %) had lymph node metastases.
- Six patients died of disease from 5 to 26 months and two patients were alive with metastases at 6 and 14 months. The prognosis of large cell undifferentiated carcinoma was compared with conventional urothelial carcinoma of similar stages showing survival differences ($p = 0.0004$).

Osteoclast-rich Undifferentiated Carcinoma

- Osteoclast-rich "giant cell tumors" or "osteoclastoma-like giant cell tumors" have been reported in many organs. Fewer than 20 cases of a similar spectrum have been reported in the bladder, most as case reports (Figs. 2.67 and 2.68).
- A large majority of patients reported in case reports that have adequate follow-up also had documented metastatic disease or cancer death. The tumors are composed of mononuclear cells (frequently positive for epithelial markers) with a spectrum of atypia, including marked pleomorphism, and osteoclast-like giant cells (positive CD68, CD51, and CD54), and recognizable usual urothelial neoplasia (CIS, papillary, or invasive carcinoma) in varying proportions.

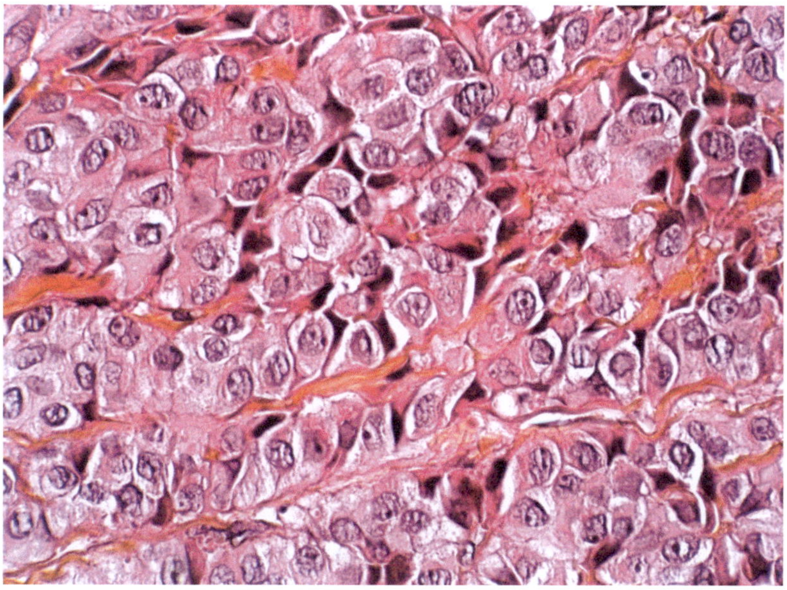

Fig. 2.65 Cellular features in large cell undifferentiated bladder carcinoma

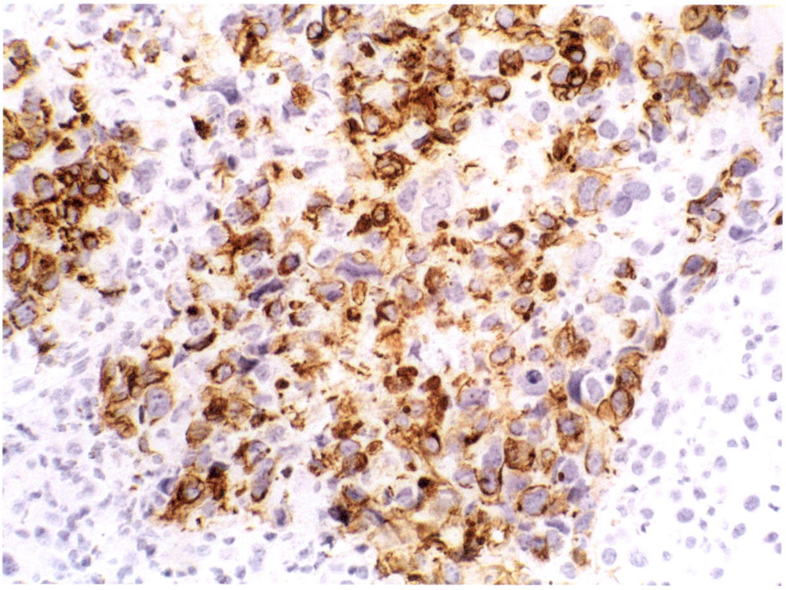

Fig. 2.66 CK 20 expression in large cell undifferentiated bladder carcinoma

- These mononuclear cells may stain for pancytokeratin, EMA, CAM5.2, and CK7; and rarely for S-100 protein, actin, desmin, and p53. These tumors should be distinguished from urothelial carcinoma with syncytiotrophoblastic giant cells and urothelial carcinoma with osteoclast-type giant cell reaction (see the discussion below).

Pleomorphic Giant Cell Carcinoma

- Pleomorphic giant cell carcinoma is a rare form of bladder cancer recognized by the current WHO classification of urologic tumors. It

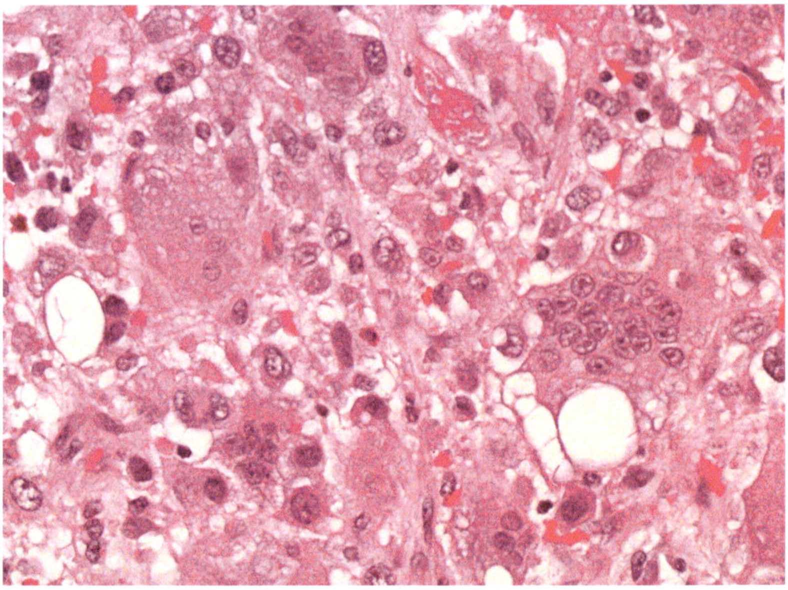

Fig. 2.67 Osteoclast-type of undifferentiated bladder carcinoma

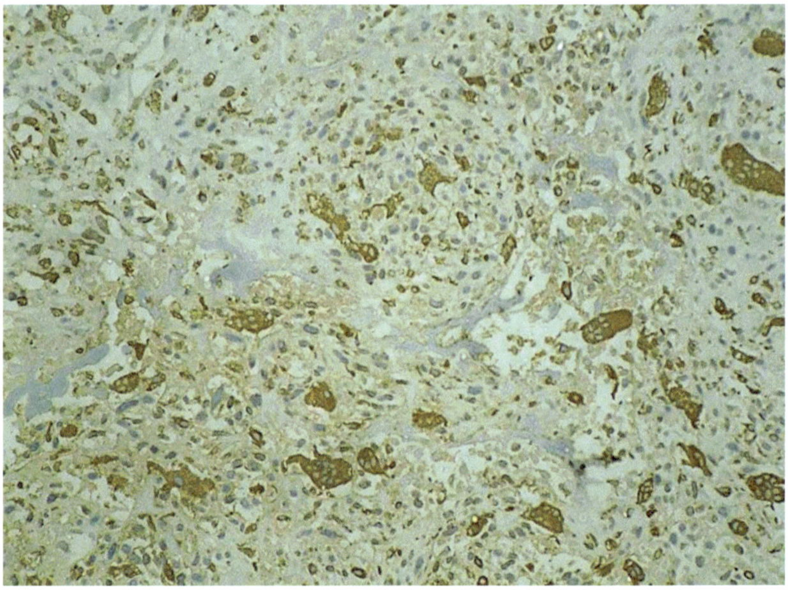

Fig. 2.68 CD68 is positive in osteoclast-cells in osteoclast-type of undifferentiated bladder carcinoma

is an aggressive variant of urothelial carcinoma associated with poor prognosis that presents at an advanced stage.

- A recent study based on eight cases showed that the The architectural pattern of the tumor varied from infiltrating pleomorphic tumor with bizarre giant cells to solid expansile nests with discohesive growth pattern; a hypocellular desmoplastic stromal response was present in 25 %, with single cells in sclerotic stroma.
- Histologically, giant, bizarre, anaplastic cells with frequent typical or atypical mitotic figures were present in all cases Seven mixed cases had concurrent conventional high-grade urothelial carcinoma. Variable sized intracytoplasmic vacuoles were present in two cases (Fig. 2.69).
- All patients had advanced-stage cancer (>pT3); and six (75 %) had lymph node metastases. Immunohistochemical staining demon-

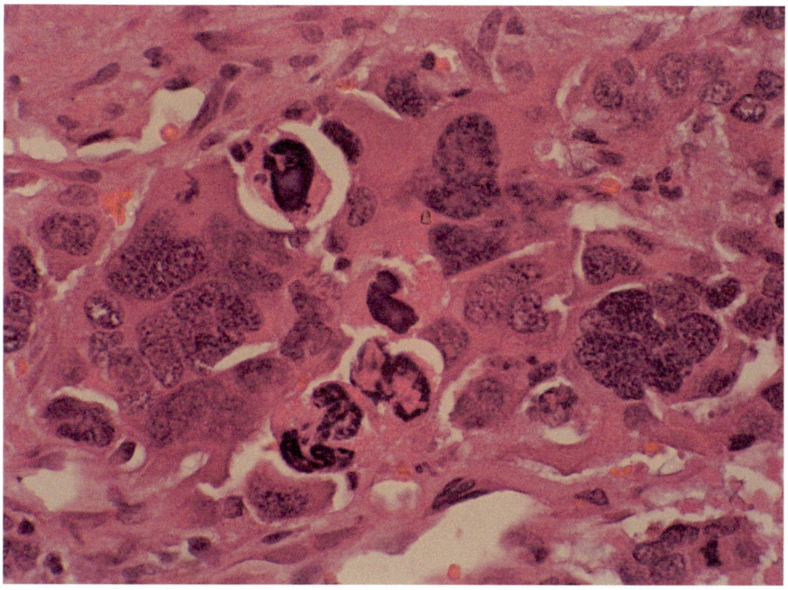

Fig. 2.69 Microscopic features of pleomorphic giant cell carcinoma

strated that both pleomorphic giant cell and associated conventional urothelial carcinoma were positive for CK7, CAM5.2, AE1/AE3, and EMA. P63, thrombomodulin, and uroplakin III were positive in six, three, and two cases, respectively.

- On follow-up, five patients died of disease from 6 to 17 months, and two patients were alive with metastases at 11 and 19 months. The main differential diagnosis includes giant cell carcinoma in the lung or from other uncommon anatomic locations, and this is currently based on clinical means. In limited samples, pleomorphic giant cell carcinoma may be misdiagnosed as sarcoma, a pitfall of paramount importance for its clinical management.

Pseudoangiosarcomatous Urothelial Carcinoma

- The pseudoangiosarcomatous pattern recently described in bladder cancer is unique for its striking morphologic resemblance to angiosarcoma. It is more frequently seen in males ranging in age from 47 to 87 years.
- Histologically, the pseudoangiosarcomatous carcinomas were characterized by tumor cell discohesion and lysis that created pseudolumina formations surrounded by attached residual tumor cells. Detached degenerating tumor cells variably admixed with inflammatory cells were common in the false lumina (Fig. 2.70).
- Partly intact urothelial carcinoma nests contained irregular or cleft-like spaces and disintegrating tumor cells with stretched intercellular bridges. The tumor was commonly associated with a dense collagenous matrix, often surrounding the lytic nests. Similar tumor cell discohesion and breakdown were observed in 3 tumors with foci of squamous cell differentiation, distinguished by the presence of dyskeratosis and keratin formation.
- Other associated non pseudoangiosarcomatous carcinoma components included conventional urothelial carcinoma, squamous differentiation, sarcomatoid spindle cell carcinoma, small cell carcinoma, micropapillary carcinoma, and glandular differentiation.
- The pseudoangiosarcomatous urothelial carcinomas were all diffusely CK7 positive, most were GATA3 positive, and none expressed vascular-associated markers. All tumors were high stage at cystectomy. Follow-up data available in 6 cases revealed a poor outcome with an overall median survival of 8.5 months.

Urothelial carcinoma with prominent stromal reaction

- Infiltrating urothelial carcinoma may be associated with a variety of stromal reactions. There may be a pseudosarcomatous stroma, which rarely displays sufficient cellularity,

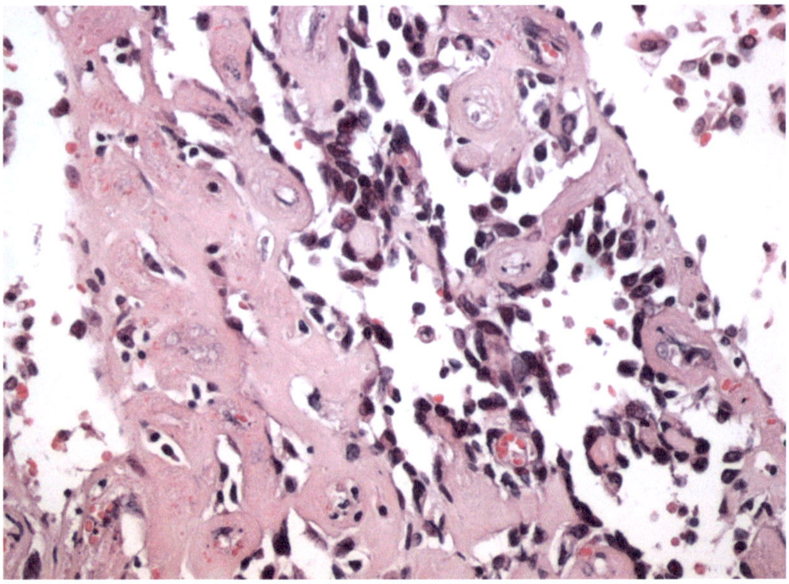

Fig. 2.70 The pseudoangiosarcomatous carcinoma shows tumor cell discohesion that creates pseudolumina

cytologic atypia, spindle cell proliferation or myxoid appearance to raise serious concern about sarcomatoid carcinoma.

- The stromal cells in these circumstances are invariably cytokeratin negative or only focally positive. Tumor-associated osseous or chondroid metaplasia is present in some cases of urothelial carcinoma and its metastases. This stromal reaction may be difficult to differentiate from osteosarcoma or chondrosarcoma.
- The metaplastic bone or cartilage is histologically benign, and the presence of osteoclast-like giant cells in cases of invasive high-grade urothelial carcinoma is uncommon. The giant cells had abundant eosinophilic cytoplasm and numerous small, round, regular nuclei. These giant cells displayed immunoreactivity for vimentin and CD68 but not for epithelial markers.
- The presence of osteoclast-like giant cells does not appear to influence prognosis. An inflammatory cell response in the stroma adjacent to invasive tumors is relatively common. This response usually takes the form of a lymphocytic infiltrate with a variable admixture of plasma cells. Generally, this cellular reaction is mild to moderate, but occasionally it may be intense. Sometimes, a neutrophilic response is observed, with or without extensive eosinophilic infiltration.
- There is evidence suggesting that carcinomas occurring in the absence of a cellular immune response are likely to behave more aggressively. In a recent study, intense inflammation in bladder carcinoma was indicative of a good prognosis. Exclusion of lymphoepithelioma-like carcinoma of the urinary bladder is important when there is extensive inflammation in the stroma.

2.2.4 Benign Urothelial Neoplasms

Urothelial papilloma

- Urothelial papilloma is a benign exophytic urothelial neoplasm that typically occurs in patients less than 50 years of age. The male to female ratio is 2:1. The most common symptom is hematuria. Most tumors are located near the ureteric orifices. Urothelial papilloma may recur. However, recurrent papilloma does not progress.
- Using the restrictive diagnostic criteria recommended by the WHO, urothelial papilloma represents less than 1 % of papillary urothelial neoplasms. Urothelial papilloma is composed of a delicate fibrovascular core covered by

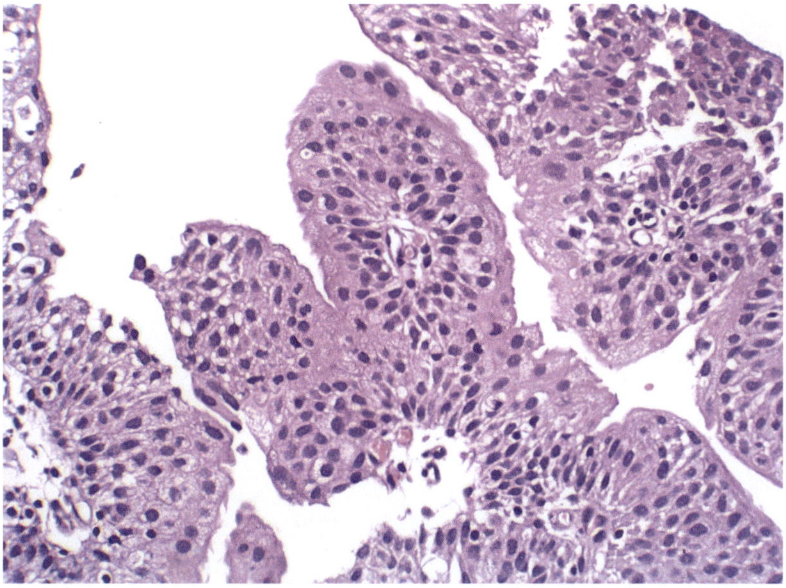

Fig. 2.71 Microscopic features of urothelial papilloma

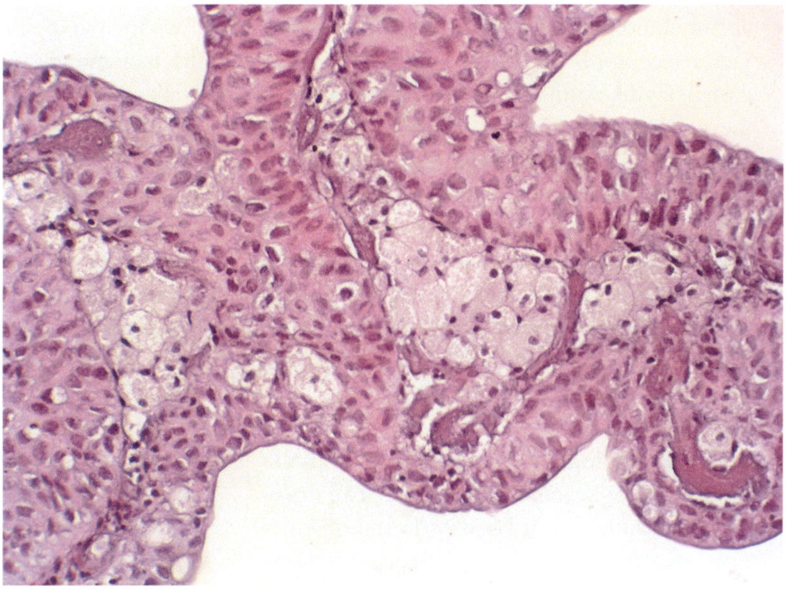

Fig. 2.72 Urothelial papilloma with xanthoma cells

cytologically and architecturally normal urothelium with no more than 7 layers of cells (Fig. 2.71).

- The superficial cells are often prominent and may have vacuolization of the cytoplasm, eosinophilic syncytial morphology, apocrine-like morphology, or may demonstrate mucinous metaplasia. Mitotic figures are absent to rare and, if present, are located in the basal cell layer (Fig. 2.71).
- The stroma may show edema and/or inflammatory cells. Rare cases show dilated lymphatics within the fibrovascular fronds. Occasionally, foamy histiocytes accumulate within the fibrovascular stalks (Xanthoma cells) (Fig. 2.72). Secondary budding of small fronds from larger simple primary papillary fronds is commonly observed.
- Papilloma is a diploid tumor with a low proliferation rate, undetectable or very limited p53

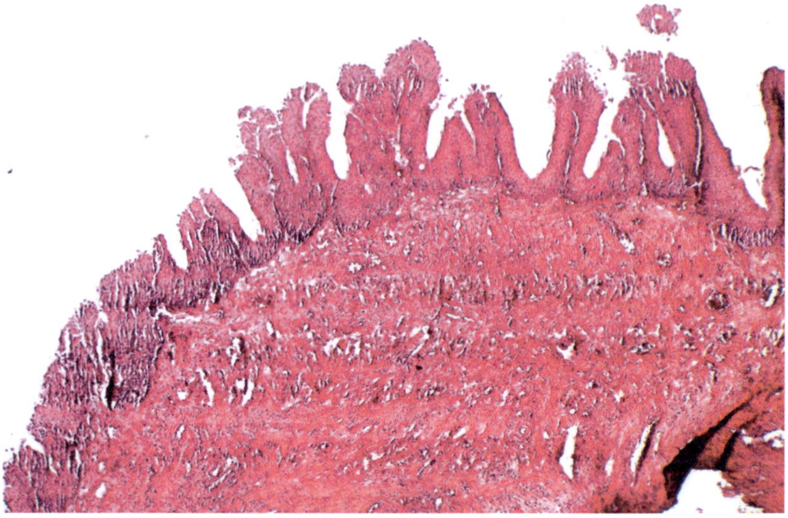

Fig. 2.73 Diffuse papillomatosis

accumulation, and frequent fibroblast growth factor receptor 3 (FGFR3) mutation (75 % of cases). Cytokeratin 20 expression is limited to the superficial (umbrella) cells.

- Diffuse papillomatosis is applicable when the mucosa is extensively involved by multiple small delicate papillary processes, creating a velvety cystoscopic appearance. These papillary structures are covered by normal urothelium with no cytological atypia It seems to be a florid variant of urothelial papilloma with potential for recurrence (Fig. 2.73).

Inverted papilloma

- Inverted papilloma is usually found in males in the sixth or seven decade of life. The male-to-female ratio is 7:1. Hematuria and obstructive symptoms are the most common symptoms at presentation. The majority of inverted papillomas develop in the region of the trigone and bladder neck. Some cases may be multifocal. The incidence of multiplicity ranges from 1.3 to 4.4 %.
- Histologically, inverted papilloma shows an inverted growth pattern, usually composed of anastomosing islands and trabeculae of histologically and cytologically normal urothelial cells invaginating from the surface urothelium into the subjacent lamina propria but not into the muscularis propria.
- Two main morphologically distinct variants, trabecular and glandular have been described. The trabecular variant is composed of anastomosing cords and trabeculae of urothelial cells invaginating the lamina propria at various angles.
- These invaginating structures demonstrate mature urothelium centrally, with darker and palisading basal cells peripherally, usually surrounded by fibrotic stroma without marked inflammation.
- The glandular variant, has considerable morphologic overlap with florid cystitis glandularis, and is not widely accepted as a diagnostic entity.
- Within the spectrum of findings in inverted papilloma, vacuolization and foamy xanthomatous cytoplasmic changes may be seen. These "clear cells" may be concentrated within distinct regions of the tumor, but more frequently are diffusely intermingled with usual inverted papilloma cells.
- Foci of non-keratinizing squamous metaplasia and neuroendocrine differentiation have been reported. Mitotic figures are either absent or rare. Some cases may demonstrate focal minor cytologic atypia that is likely degenerative in nature and has no clinical significance.
- Inverted papilloma may coexist with carcinoma, and it is most important to differentiate inverted papilloma from urothelial carcinoma

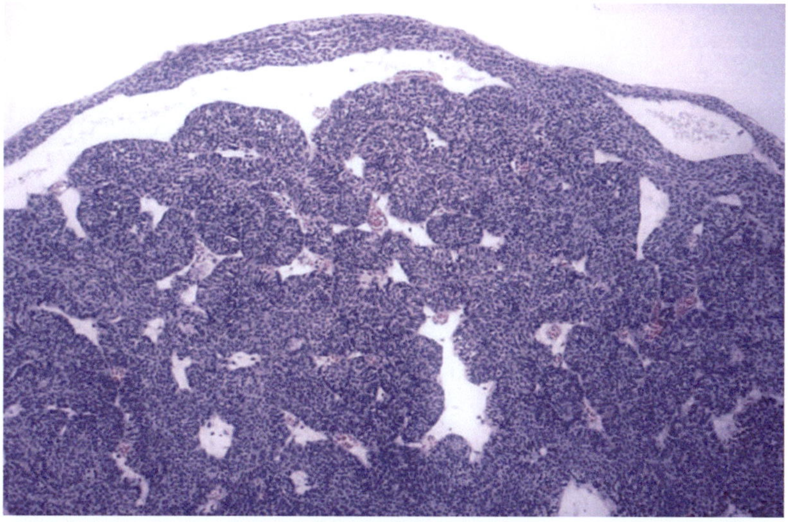

Fig. 2.74 Microscopic features of inverted papilloma covered by non-neoplastic urothelium

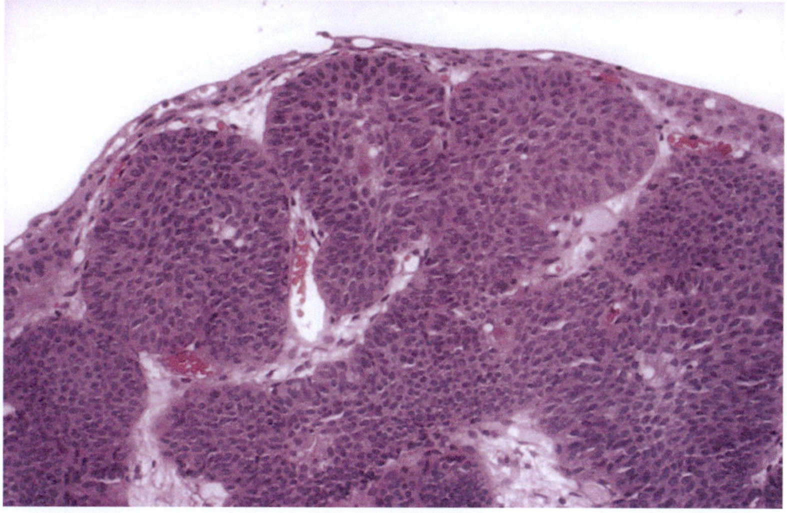

Fig. 2.75 Microscopic features of inverted papilloma with variable sized nests

with inverted growth pattern. Such distinction may be difficult, especially in limited biopsy specimens or when interpretation is confounded by crush artifact.

- Inverted papilloma usually exhibits orderly maturation of invaginated trabeculae and cords, composed of spindling and peripherally palisading cells. In contrast, urothelial carcinoma with inverted growth pattern often has thick and irregular tumor columns with transition to more solid nests (Figs. 2.74, 2.75, 2.76, 2.77, 2.78, and 2.79).
- Additionally, the presence of an exophytic papillary component and unequivocal tumor invasion in the lamina propria or muscularis propria justify a diagnosis of inverted urothelial carcinoma. Marked cytological atypia, including nuclear pleomorphism, nucleolar prominence, and abundant mitotic activity further support a diagnosis of malignancy.
- In a large series of 75 patients, all but one patient had an uneventful course without either tumor recurrence or progression to urothelial malignancy during a mean followup of 68 months. Consequently, transurethral resection of inverted papilloma is adequate treatment, and surveillance protocols as rigorous as those employed in the management of

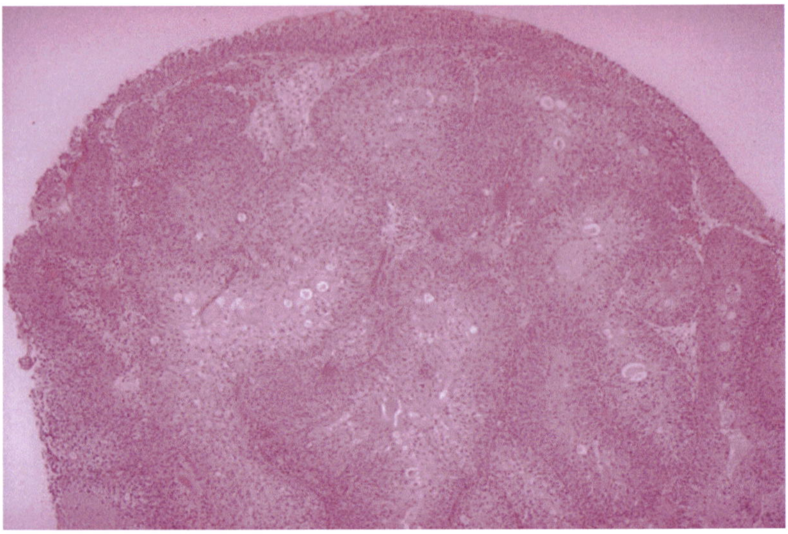

Fig. 2.76 Microscopic features of inverted papilloma hyperplastic type

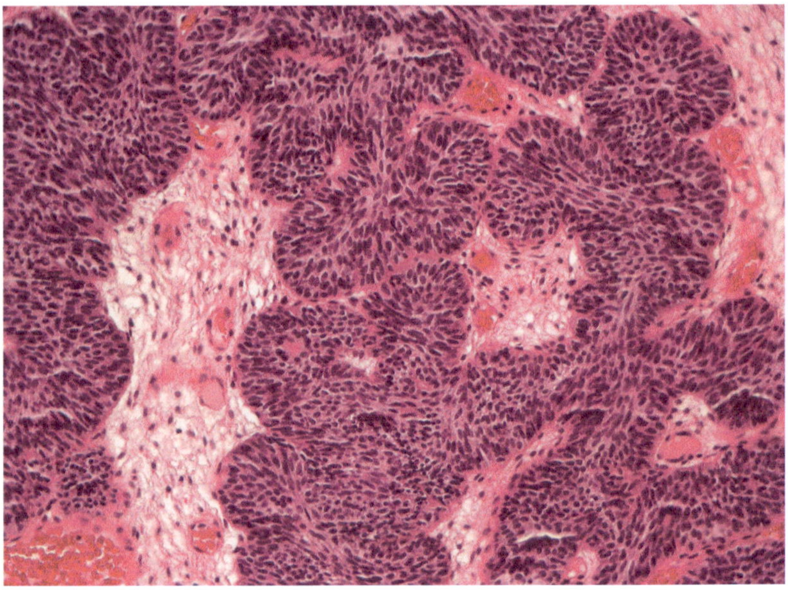

Fig. 2.77 Trabecular appearance of inverted papilloma

urothelial carcinoma seem unnecessary for this benign entity.

- It has been well documented by the finding of nonrandom inactivation of X-chromosomes that inverted papilloma is a clonal neoplasm that arises from a single progenitor cell. The incidence of loss of heterozygosity in inverted papilloma is low (8–10 %) and contrasts with the high frequency of loss of heterozygosity (29–80 %) in urothelial carcinoma and papillary urothelial neoplasm of low malignant potential. The low frequency of allelic loss in inverted papilloma is similar to that of normal urothelium.
- In addition, a recent study based on 20 cases of inverted papilloma in the urinary tract evaluated mutations of FGFR3 (exons 7, 10, and 15) and TP53 genes by DNA sequencing in these cases. Point mutations of the FGFR3 gene were identified in 45 % (9 of 20) of inverted papillomas with four cases exhibiting mutations at multiple exons. Seven cases had exon 7 mutations containing R248C, S249T, L259L, P260P, and V266M. Two cases had

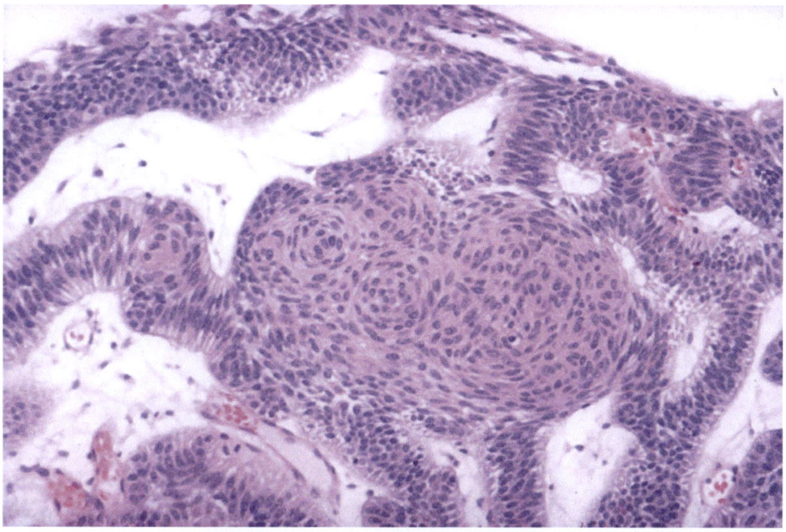

Fig. 2.78 Inverted papilloma with spindle cells nest

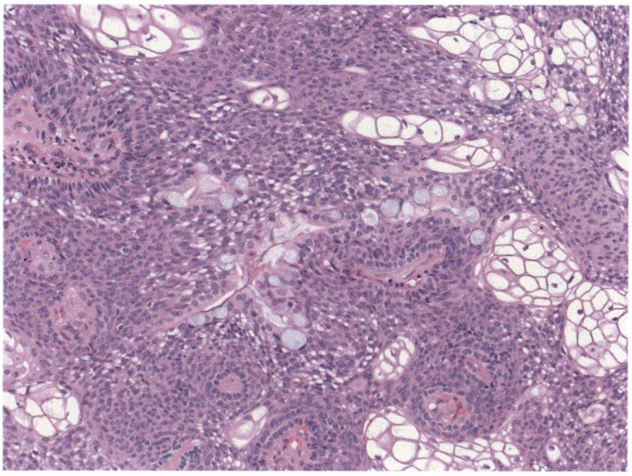

Fig. 2.79 Inverted papilloma with non-keratinizing squamous metaplasia and globlet cells

exon 10 and 15 mutations including A366D, H412H, E627D, D641N, and H643D; five cases had N653H.

- The most frequent mutation was identified at R248C. None of the inverted papillomas exhibited mutations in TP53. The markedly reduced frequency of loss of heterozygosity, the absence of TP53 mutations, and the pattern of FGFR3 mutations in inverted papilloma as compared to that of urothelial carcinoma suggest that inverted papilloma does not harbor the key genetic abnormalities that predispose to the development of urothelial carcinoma and may indicate that these entities arise through separate and distinct pathogenetic mechanisms.

Squamous papilloma

- Squamous papilloma is a rare benign neoplasm; it may represent the squamous counterpart of urothelial papilloma. It is unrelated to human papillomavirus infection. It usually occurs in elderly women and followed a benign clinical course.
- Histologically, it is composed of papillary cores with overlying benign squamous epithelium. These tumors are diploid with undetectable or very limited nuclear p53 accumulation.

Papillary Urothelial Hyperplasia

- Recent data suggest that papillary hyperplasia may be an early low-grade papillary neoplasm. Papillary urothelial hyperplasia typically occurs in patients with either a prior or

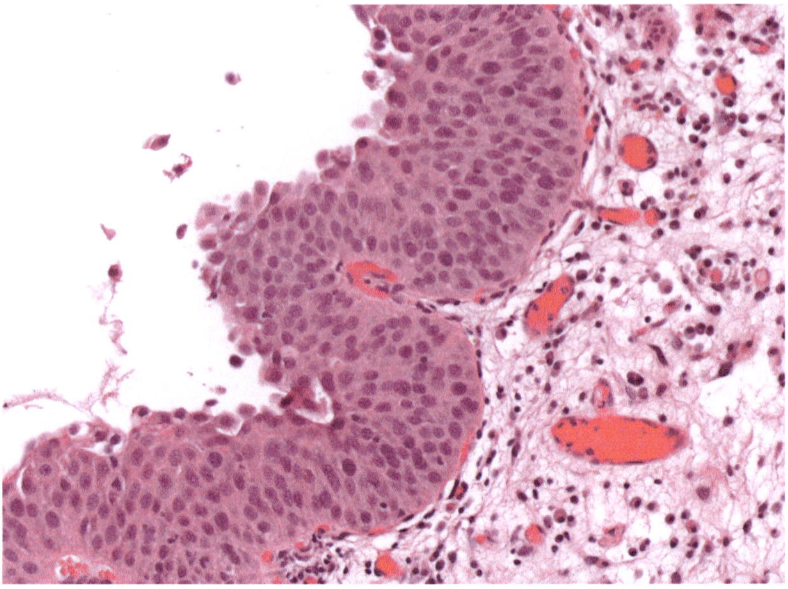

Fig. 2.80 Papillary hyperplasia of the urinary bladder is currently viewed as an early papillary carcinoma

concurrent low-grade papillary urothelial neoplasia. Most patients are men with a mean age of 67 years. These lesions are characterized by undulating folds of urothelium that lack cytologic atypia and fibrovascular cores.

- Cytologically, the cells in papillary hyperplasia lack atypia and maintain nuclear polarity. There may be increased vascularity in the stroma at the base of the papillary folds (Fig. 2.80).
- Papillary urothelial hyperplasia with varying degrees of atypia, ranging from dysplasia to flat carcinoma *in situ* (atypical papillary urothelial hyperplasia), have been reported. On follow up, most of these patients developed high-grade urothelial neoplasms. This lesion is best considered as an urothelial carcinoma in situ with papillary architecture or as non-invasive (Ta) high grade papillary urothelial carcinoma.

2.2.5 Glandular Neoplasms

Villous Adenoma

- Villous adenoma is an uncommon benign glandular epithelial neoplasm with exophytic growth that is often associated with urachal adenocarcinoma. Patients often present with hematuria and/or irritative symptoms. Mucusuria may be present in rare cases. There is no apparent gender predominance. The tumor usually occurs in elderly patients (mean age, 65 years; range, 23–94 years) with a predilection for the urachus, dome, and trigone of the urinary bladder. Its cystoscopic appearance is that of an exophytic tumor.
- Histologically, villous adenoma of the bladder is identical to villous adenoma of the colon, with columnar mucin-filled goblet cells lining delicate fibrovascular stalks (Fig. 2.81). Nuclear findings include pseudo-stratification, crowding, occasional prominent nucleoli and hyperchromasia, as in the colon.
- Villous adenomas of the bladder show positive immunostaining for cytokeratin 20 (100 % of cases), cytokeratin 7 (56 %) and carcinoembryonic antigen (89 %). Acid mucin is demonstrable in 78 % of cases with Alcian blue periodic acid-Schiff stain. Patients with an isolated villous adenoma have an excellent prognosis, but progression to adenocarcinoma appears to occur in 21–33 % of cases.
- The differential diagnosis includes adenocarcinoma of bladder. Villous adenomas of the bladder may coexist with in situ and invasive adenocarcinoma, a confounding diagnostic factor. On limited sampling there may be only changes of villous adenoma. Therefore, the entire specimen should be processed to

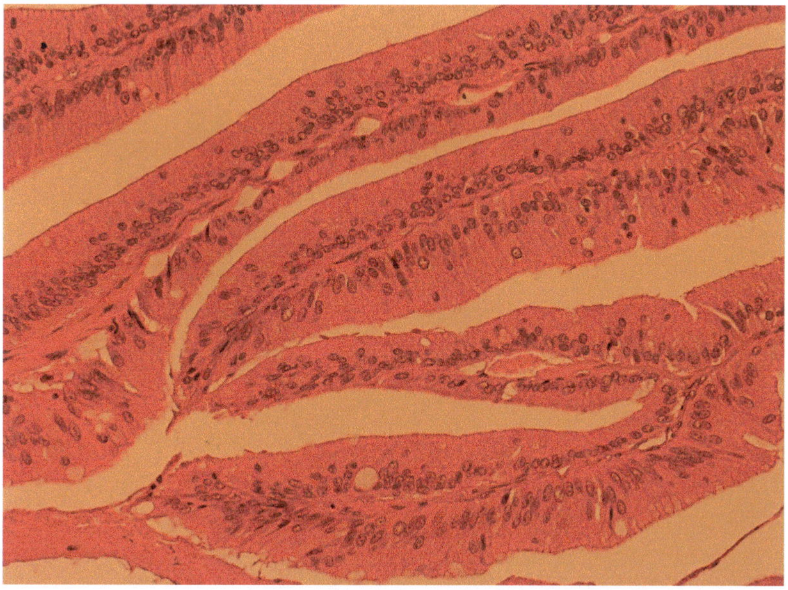

Fig. 2.81 Villous adenoma of the urachus

Table 2.15 Histologic variants of adenocarcinoma of the urinary bladder

Adenocarcinoma, not otherwise specified (NOS)
Enteric (colonic type)
Signet ring cell
Mucinous/colloid
Clear cell
Hepatoid
Mixed
Urachal

exclude invasive disease and a caution note added to the report.

Adenocarcinoma

- Adenocarcinoma is defined as a malignant neoplasm derived from the urothelium showing histologically pure glandular phenotype. It accounts for 0.5–2 % of all malignant bladder tumors. Adenocarcinoma of the urinary bladder occurs more commonly in males than in females with a peak incidence in the sixth decade of life. Patients typically present with hematuria (Table 2.15).
- Two major categories have been recognized: those arising in the bladder proper and those arising from urachal remnants. Approximately one-third arise in the urachus. Recent molecular evidence suggest that intestinal metaplasia is a putative precursor for adenocarcinoma.

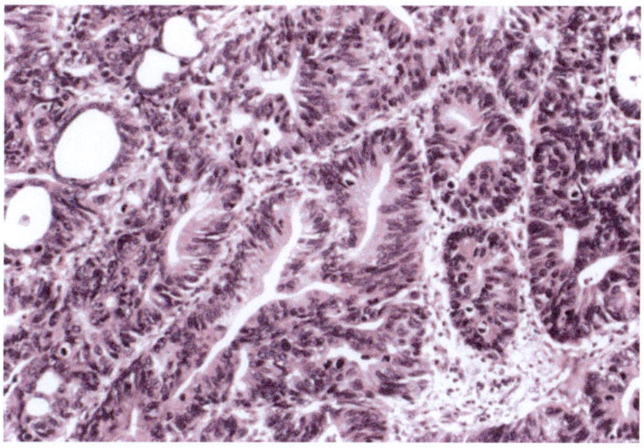

Fig. 2.82 Bladder adenocarcinoma of the enteric type

- Adenocarcinoma of the bladder may show different histologic growth patterns.: (i) enteric (colonic) type, (ii) adenocarcinoma not otherwise specified (NOS), (iii) mucinous (colloid) type, (iv) signet ring cell type, (v) clear cell type, (vi) hepatoid type and (vii) mixed forms (Figs. 2.82, 2.83, 2.84, 2.85, 2.86, and 2.87; Table 2.16).
- The enteric type closely resembles adenocarcinoma of the colon. The NOS type consists of adenocarcinoma with a nonspecific glandular growth pattern. Tumors that show abundant mucin and tumor cell clusters apparently floating in mucin are classified as mucinous (colloid) type.

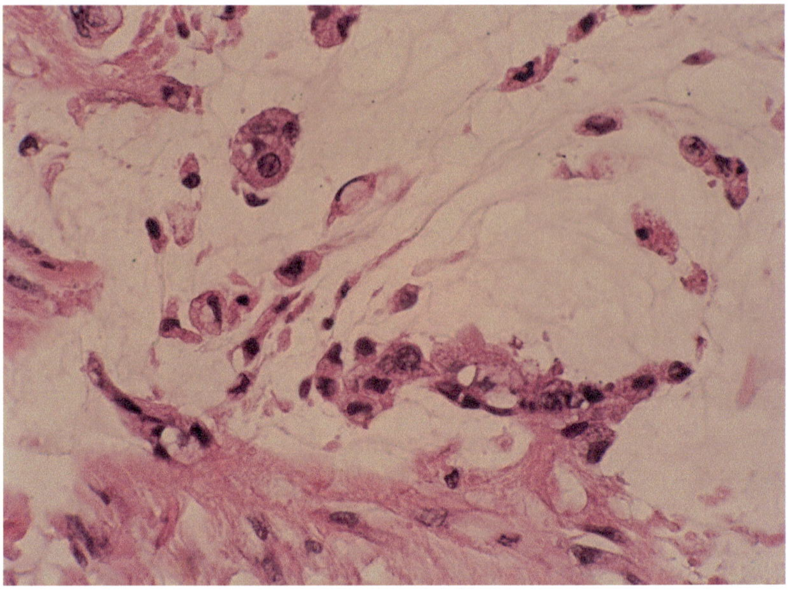

Fig. 2.83 Bladder adenocarcinoma of the colloid (mucinous) type

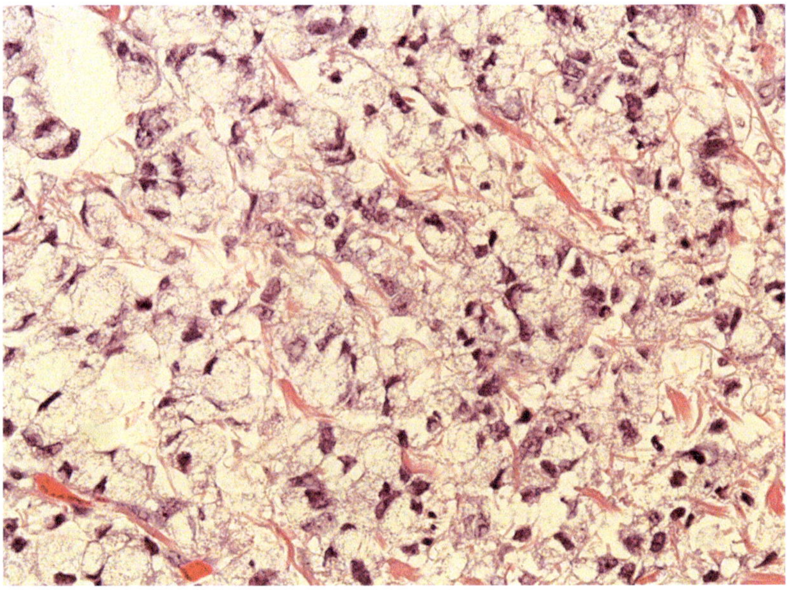

Fig. 2.84 Bladder adenocarcinoma of the signet ring cell type

- The signet ring cell variant may be diffuse or mixed, and may have a monocytoid or plasmacytoid phenotype. Pure signet ring cell carcinoma carries the worst prognosis among different histologic types of adenocarcinoma. It is not uncommon to find a mixture of these growth patterns. The grading system for adenocarcinoma of the bladder is based on degree of glandular differentiation and nuclear pleomorphism, categorized as well, moderately, and poorly differentiated.
- The reported immunohistochemical profile of bladder adenocarcinoma is variable but generally resembles that of colonic adenocarcinoma. Cytokeratin 7 positivity is variable, while cytokeratin 20 is positive in most bladder adenocarcinomas.
- The "intestinal marker" CDX2, a nuclear transcription factor, may be misleading in

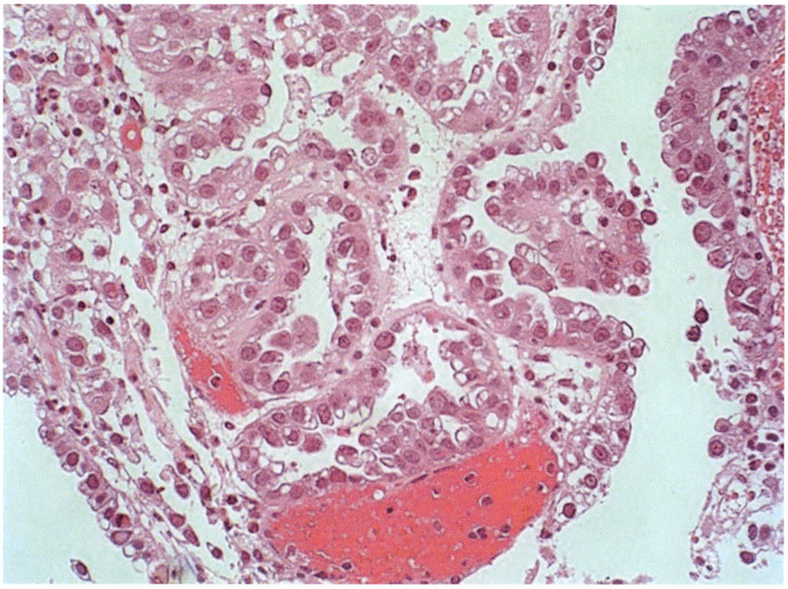

Fig. 2.85 Bladder adenocarcinoma of the clear cell type

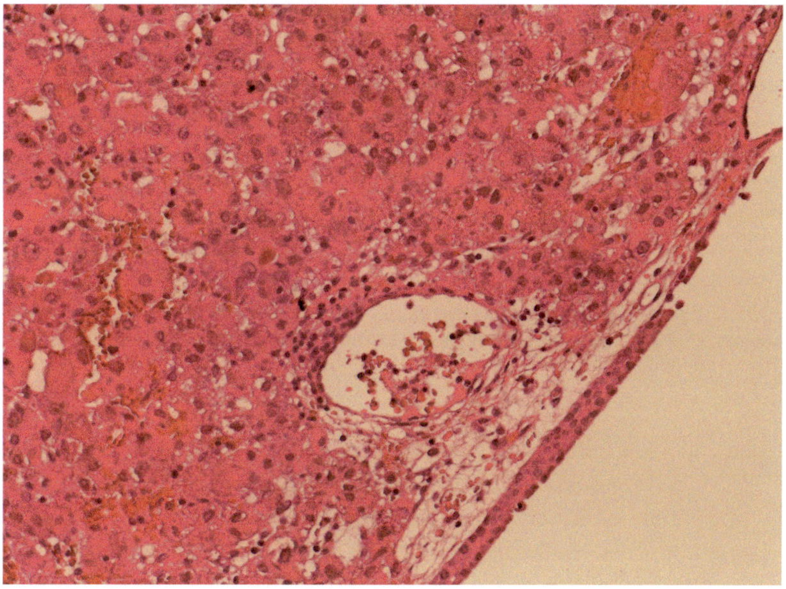

Fig. 2.86 Bladder adenocarcinoma of the hepatoid type (H&E)

this situation because primary bladder adenocarcinomas are virtually always also CDX2 positive. It is notable that CDX2 positivity has been observed in 2 % of urothelial carcinomas in a tissue microarray study; consequently, CDX2 immunostaining cannot be used to exclude a urothelial primary in cases of metastatic carcinoma of uncertain origin.

- Areas of intestinal metaplasia in the bladder also routinely stain positive for CDX2. Villin, an actin-binding protein found in epithelial cells with a brush border, is positive in colon adenocarcinoma and bladder adenocarcinomas of enteric-type, but not in urothelial carcinomas with glandular differentiation. Nuclear β-catenin staining is seen in 81 % of colorectal carcinomas involving the bladder, whereas staining restricted to the cytoplasm is typical of primary bladder adenocarcinoma.

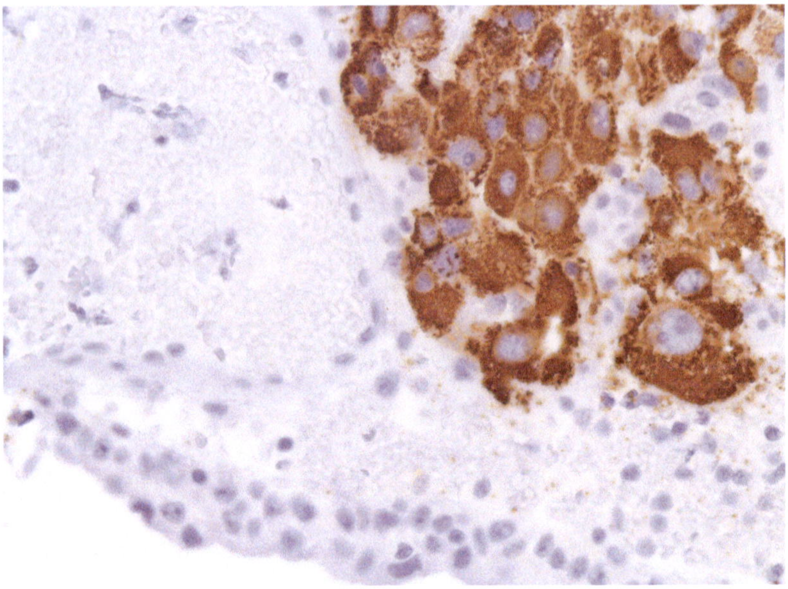

Fig. 2.87 Heppar1 is positive in hepatoid adenocarcinoma of the bladder

Table 2.16 Typical staining patterns of primary and secondary adenocarcinomas of the bladder

	34BE12	CK7	CK20	CEA	PSA	PSAP	CDX2	Villin	CA-125	Vimentin
Primary bladder adenocarcinoma	+	+/–	+/–	+	–	+/–	+	+/–	+/–	–
Clear cell carcinoma		+	+/–		–	–			+	
Prostatic adenocarcinoma	–	–	+/–	+/–	+	+	–	–	–	–
Seminal vesicle adenocarcinoma		+	–						+	
Renal cell carcinoma	–	–	–	–	–	–	–	–	–	+
Colorectal adenocarcinoma	–	–	+	+	–	–	+	+	+/–	–
Endometrial adenocarcinoma		+	–	–	–	–	+/–		+	+

34BE12 high molecular weight cytokeratin 34 E12, *CK7* cytokeratin 7, *CK20* cytokeratin 20, *CEA* carcinoembryonic antigen, *PSA* prostate specific antigen, *PSAP* prostate specific acid phosphatase, + usually positive, +/– variable staining, – usually negative

Clear cell adenocarcinoma

- Clear cell (mesonephric) adenocarcinoma is a rare variant of urinary bladder carcinoma that resembles its müllerian counterpart in the female genital tract. Patients are typically females who present with hematuria or dysuria. Occasionally clear cell adenocarcinoma has been associated with endometriosis or müllerianosis; occurrence in a bladder diverticulum has been reported.
- Tumors are typically exophytic, nodular, or sessile in appearance. Clear cell adenocarcinomas may infiltrate the bladder wall and metastasize to lymph nodes and distant organs in a pattern similar to other types of bladder cancer.
- Clear cell adenocarcinoma exhibits a distinctive histologic appearance, with a variety of architectural patterns, forming tubulocystic or papillary structures or growing in diffuse solid sheets. The tubules vary in size and may contain either basophilic or eosinophilic secretions. The papillae are generally small and their fibrovascular cores may be extensively hyalinized.
- The tumor cells range from flat to cuboidal to columnar and they may have either clear or eosinophilic cytoplasm. The cytoplasm often contains glycogen. Hobnail cells are frequently seen. Cytologic atypia is usually moderate to severe, and high mitotic counts are frequently observed. In some cases, clear cell

Table 2.17 Differential diagnosis of atypical nephrogenic metaplasia and clear cell adenocarcinoma

Characteristics	Nephrogenic adenoma	Clear cell adenocarcinoma
Sex	Male predominance (male-to-female ratio, 3:1)	Female predominance (male to female ratio, 1:2)
Mean age (years)	62	58
Clinical presentation	Hematuria and voiding symptoms	Hematuria and voiding symptoms
Biological behavior	Benign	Aggressive
Location	No apparent predilection	Prewdilection for urethra
Size	Small	Large
Microscopic findings		
Necrosis	Absent	Often present (53 %)
Mitotic figures	Absent or inconspicuous	Easily identifiable
Stromal edema	Common	Uncommon
Luminal mucin	Common	Common
Clear cell change	May be seen	Common
Hobnail cells	Common	Common
Infiltrative growth	Usually absent	Present
Psammoma bodies	Absent	May be seen
Inflammation	Invariably present	May be present
Cytologic atypia		
Nuclear enlargement	Present	Present
Nuclear hyperchromasia	Present	Present
Prominent nucleoli	Present	Present
Nuclear pleomorphism	Minimal	Present
Immunostaining		
PSA	Negative	Negative
34βE12	Positive	Positive (occasionally negative)
Cytokeratin 7	Positive	Positive
Cytokeratin 20	Negative	Positive
EMA	Positive	Positive
AMACR (P504S)	Often positive	Often positive
PAX2	Positive	Positive
PAX8	Positive	Positive
MIB labeling index	<5 %	Often >15 %
P53	Occasional focal positive	Positive
DNA ploidy	Aneuploid pattern may be seen	Unknown

Nuclear pleomorphism is more pronounced in clear cell adenocarcinoma
PSA prostate-specific antigen, *34βE12* high molecular weight cytokeratin, *EMA* epithelial membrane antigen, *AMACR* α-methylacyl CoA racemase

adenocarcinoma is associated with urothelial carcinoma, and rarely with adenocarcinoma not otherwise specified (NOS).

- Tumor cells are positive for CA-125, suggestive of Müllerian origin, but CA-125 staining may also be seen in urothelial carcinoma and carcinoma from a variety of other sites so this finding does not prove Müllerian origin.
- These tumors are typically positive for cytokeratin 7 with variable cytokeratin 20 staining. Stains for prostate specific antigen (PSA) and prostate specific acid phosphatase (PSAP) are negative. The main differential diagnostic consideration for clear cell carcinoma is nephrogenic metaplasia (Table 2.17).
- Several immunohistochemical stains have been evaluated for utility in making this distinction, but only p53 and MIB-1 appear useful, with at most focal p53 staining and MIB-1 counts of less than 14 per 200 cells in

nephrogenic adenoma and strong p53 staining and MIB-1 counts of greater than 32 per 200 cells in clear cell adenocarcinoma.

- However, p53 nuclear accumulation (up to 20 %), increased MIB-1 labeling index (up to 5 %), and aneuploid DNA patterns have been observed in atypical nephrogenic metaplasia.
- All cases of atypical nephrogenic metaplasia display positive immunoreactivity for high-molecular-weight cytokeratin (34βE12), cytokeratin 7, and EMA. In contrast to atypical nephrogenic metaplasia, clear cell carcinomas will typically display greater cytologic atypia, a significant mitotic rate, and necrosis.
- Clear cell adenocarcinoma of the urinary is positive for both cytokeratin 7 and cytokeratin 20. Positive alpha-methylacyl-CoA racemase (P504S) (AMACR) immunoreactivity for both clear cell adenocarcinoma and nephrogenic adenoma has been note. CD10 is focally positive in clear cell adenocarcinoma.
- The other differentia diagnostic considerations include clear-cell variant of urothelial carcinoma, metastatic clear cell renal carcinoma, cervical or vaginal clear cell adenocarcinoma, and in males, prostatic adenocarcinoma secondarily involving the bladder. In addition to the immunostaining characteristics noted previously, clear cell adenocarcinoma may show positive staining for carcinoembryonic antigen and LeuM-1 (CD15), but is negative for estrogen and progesterone receptors, and these stains may be helpful in the differential.

Hepatoid adenocarcinoma

- Primary hepatoid adenocarcinoma of the bladder is extremely rare, with only three well-illustrated case reports. The pathological diagnosis is based on a combination of histological features resembling hepatocellular carcinoma and positive immunostaining for alpha-fetoprotein.
- The tumor occurs in the elderly men and is biologically aggressive. Lymph node metastases are common. The histogenesis is uncertain. Tumors are composed of polygonal cells with abundant granular eosinophilic cytoplasm, vesicular nuclei and prominent nucleoli, arranged in nests and trabecular structures; the overall appearance is reminiscent of hepatocellular carcinoma.
- Occasionally, hyaline globules and bile production are seen. Immunoreactivity for alphafetoprotein (AFP), low molecular weight cytokeratin (CAM 5.2), alpha-1-antitrypsin (AAT), albumin, hepatocyte paraffin-1 (HepPar-1), epithelial membrane antigen (EMA), and a striking canalicular pattern with polyclonal anti-carcinoembryonic antigen (CEA) staining all indicate hepatocellular differentiation. The hepatic nature of the cells was further confirmed by the demonstration of albumin gene mRNA by non-isotopic in situ hybridization.

Urachal adenocarcinoma

- Urachal adenocarcinoma is far less common than non-urachal adenocarcinoma of the bladder. Urachal adenocarcinomas arise from the urachus, the fibrous remnant from the embryonic allantoic stalk connecting the umbilicus to the bladder.
- Urachal remnants are reported to occur most frequently in the bladder dome or posterior wall. Most cases of urachal adenocarcinoma occur in the fifth and sixth decades of life, which is about 10 years younger than those patients with non-urachal bladder adenocarcinoma. This tumor occurs slightly more often in men than in women. Presenting signs and symptoms may include a suprapubic mass, mucusuria or irritative symptoms.
- Urachal carcinoma usually involves the muscular wall of the bladder dome, and it may or may not destroy the overlying mucosa. The mass may be relatively small and discrete, but in some cases it forms a large mass invading the retropubic space of Retzius and may extend as far as the anterior abdominal wall.
- Mucinous lesions tend to calcify, and these calcifications on plain x-ray films of the abdomen may be the initial clinical manifestation. The mucosa of the urinary bladder remains intact in early stages of the disease, but it eventually becomes ulcerated as the tumor extends towards the bladder cavity.
- The cut surface of this tumor exhibits a glistening, light-tan appearance, reflecting its

mucinous contents. A specific staging system for this neoplasm has been proposed. Histologically, urachal adenocarcinomas are subdivided into mucinous, enteric, not otherwise specified, signet ring-cell, and mixed types; these subtypes are similar to those of adenocarcinoma of the urinary bladder.

- Specific criteria to classify a tumor as urachal in origin consisted of the following: (1) tumor in the dome of the bladder, (2) absence of cystitis cystica and cystitis glandularis, (3) invasion of muscle or deeper structures and either intact or ulcerated epithelium, (4) presence of urachal remnants, (5) presence of a suprapubic mass, (6) a sharp demarcation between the tumor and the normal surface epithelium, and (7) tumor growth in the bladder wall, extending into the space of Retzius.
- Although urachal adenocarcinoma may arise from villous adenoma of the urachus, intestinal metaplasia of the urachal epithelium is believed to be the factor predisposing to malignant transformation at this site.
- Whenever urachal adenocarcinoma or primary adenocarcinoma of the bladder is considered, direct extension or metastasis from colorectal carcinoma must be excluded. Management of urachal adenocarcinoma consists of partial or radical cystectomy, including resection of the umbilicus.
- Recurrences are common, however, especially when a partial cystectomy is done. It is important to distinguish between urachal and nonurachal adenocarcinomas for treatment purposes. Resection of urachal adenocarcinoma must include removal of the entire urachal remnant.
- Nonurachal bladder adenocarcinomas show positive immunostaining with carcinoembryonic antigen in 67 % of cases and Leu-M1 (CD15) in 73 % of cases, whereas urachal adenocarcinomas consistently stain with both.
- A recent study including 34 urachal adenocarcinoma and 6 secondary adenocarcinomas concluded that using ß-catenin (frequently membrano-cytoplasmic ß-catenin staining) and CK7 (positive in 50 % of urachal adenocarcinomas) may have value in differentiating urachal adenocarcinoma of enteric morphology from colonic adenocarcinoma.

2.2.6 Squamous Cell Neoplasms

Squamous cell carcinoma in situ

- Histologically, it is identical to squamous cell carcinoma in situ found in other organ sites. This finding is often associated with subsequent or concurrent invasive urothelial carcinoma with squamous differentiation.
- In a recent report of 11 patients, one patient had no evidence of disease at 8 months, one had residual squamous cell carcinoma-in-situ at 10 months, one had high-grade urothelial carcinoma (not otherwise specified) at rebiopsy after 6 months, 3 patients were noted to have invasive squamous cell carcinoma at intervals of 2, 3, and 4 months, respectively, and one was found to have invasive urothelial carcinoma with squamous features in the cystectomy specimen at 12 months.
- Wide-range human papillomavirus DNA signal was detected in one case. Enhanced expression of EGFR in these bladder squamous lesions suggests a possible therapeutic target in cases that are difficult to manage clinically.

Squamous cell carcinoma

- Squamous cell carcinoma is defined as a malignant neoplasm derived from the urotelium that shows a pure squamous cell phenotype. When urothelial elements (including urothelial carcinoma in situ) are present, the tumor should be classified as urothelial carcinoma with squamous differentiation.
- Risk factors associated with the development of squamous cell carcinoma include tobacco smoking, chronic non-specific urinary tract infections and schistosomiasis.
- Keratinizing squamous metaplasia may be present in the adjacent epithelium in cases of squamous cell carcinoma of the bladder, and frequently displays the full spectrum of dysplastic lesions and/or carcinoma in situ.

Table 2.18 Differential diagnosis of squamous papilloma, condyloma acuminatum, and verrucous squamous cell carcinoma of the urinary bladder

	Squamous papilloma	Condyloma acuminatum	Verrucous squamous cell carcinoma
Age (years)	62 (range, 32–82)	40 (range, 17–76)	66 (range, 43–83)
Sex (male: female)	1:6	1:1.6	1.2:1
Clinical history	Non-specific	External genitalia condyloma or history of immunosuppression	Non-specific
Clinical presentation	Irritative symptoms	Irritative symptoms	Irritative symptoms
Biological behavior	Rarely recurs	Aggressive	Aggressive
Location	No predilection	No predilection	No predilection
Extent	Small, solitary	Multiple, extensive	Diffuse, extensive
Histologic changes			
Architecture	Papillary	Papillary	Expansive and endophytic
Pushing margin	Absent	Absent	Present
Cytologic atypia	Usually not seen or mild	Usually not seen or mild	May be present
Stromal invasion	Absent	Absent	Present
P53 alteration	−/+	+	+
Human papilloma virus detection	–	+	–
DNA ploidy	Diploid	Aneuploid	Aneuploid

+ usually positive, +/– variable staining, – usually negative

Invasive squamous cell carcinoma of the bladder displays a range of differentiation, from well differentiated to poorly differentiated, with a histologic spectrum that can vary from well-defined islands of squamous cells with keratinization, prominent intercellular bridges, and minimal nuclear pleomorphism, to tumors exhibiting marked nuclear pleomorphism and only focal evidence of squamous differentiation (Table 2.18).

- Histologic grading is based on the amount of keratinization and the degree of nuclear pleomorphism using a 3-tiered system (grades 1, 2 and 3). Several morphologic variants of squamous cell carcinoma, including verrucous, basaloid, and clear cell pattern, have been recognized.

Schistosoma-associated squamous cell carcinoma

- Schistosomiasis is known to be associated with squamous cell carcinoma of the bladder (Fig. 2.88). Tumors arising in this setting are typically large, often filling the bladder lumen, and frequently polypoid or solid with visible necrosis and keratin debris; others are ulcerated infiltrating tumors.
- Histologically, the presence of keratinizing squamous metaplasia in the adjacent flat epithelium is relatively constant and may be associated with dysplasia or carcinoma in situ. The prevalence of associated squamous metaplasia in cases of squamous cell carcinoma of the bladder ranges from 17 to 60 %, and is widely variable according to geographic location of the patient population. Similar to non-schistosoma-associated squamous cell carcinoma, these tumors range from well to poorly differentiated, but most commonly are well-differentiated with prominent keratinization and intercellular bridge formation with minimal nuclear pleomorphism.
- Pathologic stage and lymph node status are significant prognostic and predictive factors, and pathologic grade according to the degree of keratinization and the degree of nuclear pleomorphism is also considered an important prognostic indicator. Radical surgical excision currently is the most widely used treatment option; neoadjuvant radiation has been reported to improve survival in aggressive tumors.

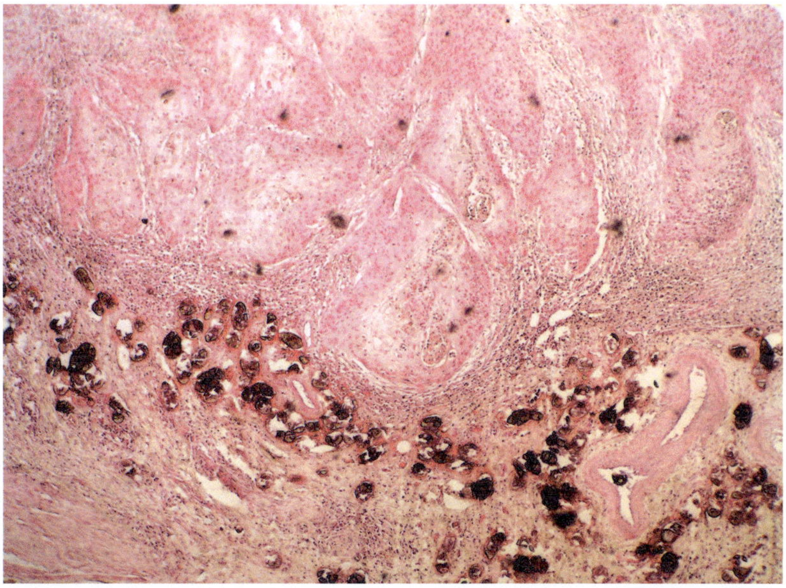

Fig. 2.88 Squamous cell carcinoma in schistosoma infection

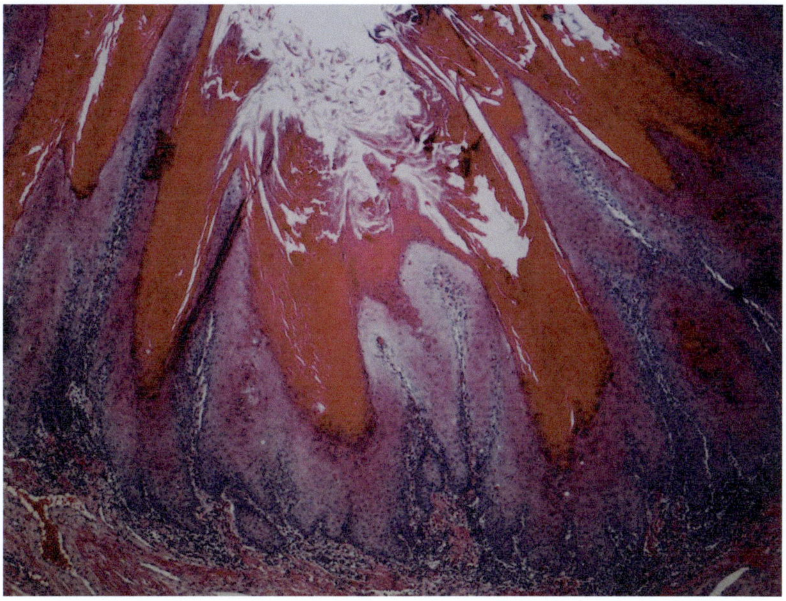

Fig. 2.89 Verrucous squamous cell carcinoma

Verrucous squamous cell carcinoma

- Verrucous carcinoma is an uncommon variant of squamous cell carcinoma that accounts for 3–5 % of squamous bladder cancers. It occurs most often in patients with schistosomiasis, but has also been reported in patients from non-endemic areas. This tumor grossly appears as a "warty" mass; histologically, it shows epithelial acanthosis and papillomatosis, minimal nuclear and architectural atypia and rounded pushing deep borders (Fig. 2.89).
- Cases of squamous carcinoma with verrucous features but which additionally have an infiltrative component have been described; it is recommended by the WHO (2004) not to diagnose such cases as verrucous carcinoma, but as regular squamous cell carcinoma. Verrucous carcinoma in the bladder is associated with minimal

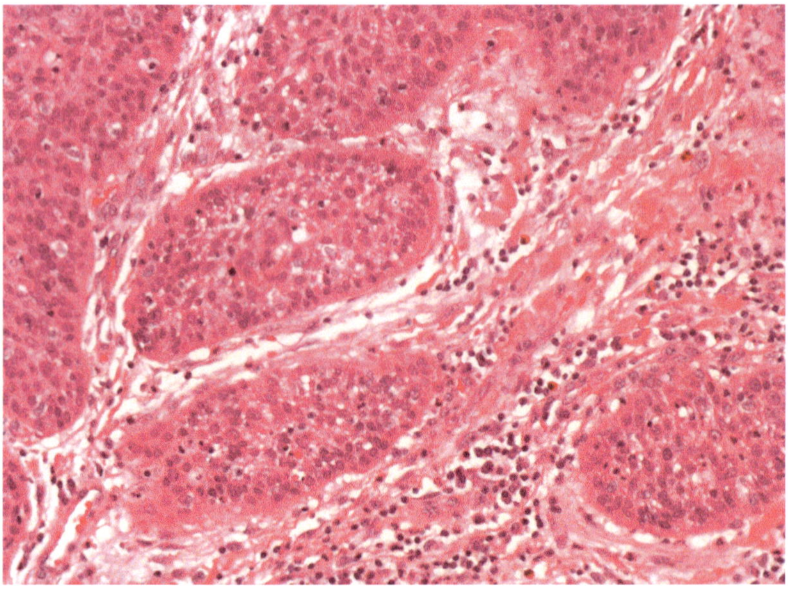

Fig. 2.90 Basaloid squamous cell carcinoma of the bladder

risk of progression whether associated with schistosomiasis or not. A link to human papilloma virus infection has not been established. P16 expression in squamous cell carcinoma is unrelated to HPV infection in these tumors.

Basaloid squamous cell carcinoma

- Basaloid squamous cell cell carcinoma has been recently recognized in the urinary bladder with one reported case. The patient had a longstanding history of recurrent urinary tract infections. Grossly, it was a sessile multilobulated tan-brown mass involving the posterior wall of the bladder. Architecturally, the tumor was characterized by small nests of basaloid cells with minimal cytoplasm arranged with peripheral palisading.
- Cytologically, the tumor cells had a high nuclear/cytoplasmic ratio with dense hyperchromatic nuclei. Central necrosis of the larger nests and pseudoglandular arrangement of the small nests was focally present. The tumor stroma was desmoplastic. Mitotic figures and apoptotic bodies were frequent. The reported case also had microscopic foci of urothelial cell carcinoma with squamous differentiation. Squamous metaplasia was present elsewhere in the bladder in addition to dysplasia and squamous cell carcinoma in situ (Figs. 2.90 and 2.91).
- The experience with basaloid squamous cell carcinoma in other organs suggests that these may have a more aggressive course than usual squamous carcinoma. This tumor is probably best categorized as urothelial carcinoma with squamous cell differentiation (basaloid type).

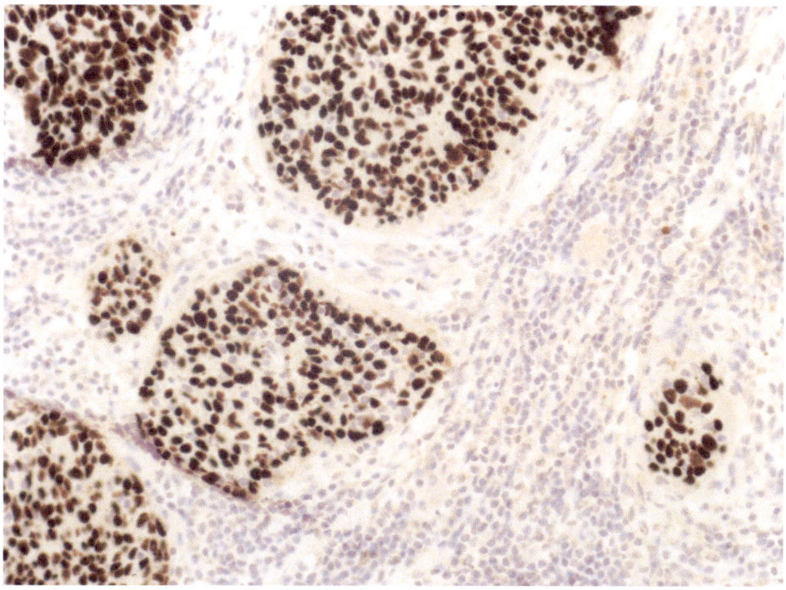

Fig. 2.91 P63 is positive in basaloid squamous cell carcinoma of the bladder

2.2.7 Neuroendocrine Tumors

Small cell carcinoma

- Small cell carcinoma is a malignant neuroendocrine neoplasm of the urothelium which histologically mimics its pulmonary counterpart. It is an extremely rare malignancy that accounts for less than 1 % of urinary bladder cancers. The demographic and clinical features of small cell carcinoma of the urinary bladder are similar to those of conventional urothelial carcinoma.
- The majority of patients are male, and most patients are in the sixth to seventh decade of life. The mean age at the time of diagnosis is 66 years, ranging from 36 to 85 years, with a male predominance (male to female ratio is 3: 1). Most patients have a history of cigarette smoking.
- There is no link between small cell carcinoma of the urinary bladder and human papilloma virus infection. Clinical presentations include site-specific and systemic symptoms. Site-specific symptoms are similar to those of urothelial carcinoma.
- Clinical presentations include hematuria, irritative symptoms such as dysuria, nocturia, frequency, urinary obstructive symptoms or localized abdominal/pelvic pain. Systemic symptoms are non-specific, and include anorexia and weight loss. Occasionally, patients have paraneoplastic syndromes with hypercalcemia, hypophosphatemia, or ectopic secretion of adrenocorticotropic hormone (ACTH) (Tables 2.19 and 2.20).

Molecular Genetics

- Recent molecular data indicate that both urothelial and small cell carcinoma originate from the same stem cell in the urothelium.
- At the molecular level, small cell carcinoma of the urinary bladder demonstrates chromosomal aberrations that are commonly seen in small cell lung cancer. Loss of 4q, 5q, 10q and 13q is common in small cell carcinoma of the urinary bladder. Allelic loss at 3p25-26, 9p21, 9q32-33, 17p13 and nonrandom inactivation of X chromosome have also been reported in a large series of small cell carcinoma of the urinary bladder. Homozygous deletion of p16 and gain or high level of amplification at 1p22-32, 3q26.3, 8q24, 12q14-21, and 5q, 6p, 8q and 20q, chromosomes 1–3, 5–7, 9, 11 and 18 have also been found.. Some of these regions contain oncogenes.
- Small cell carcinoma of the urinary bladder also shares some of the aberrant signaling pathways seen in small cell lung cancer. For instance, an autocrine loop through the c-Kit/

Table 2.19 Macroscopic and microscopic features in neuroendocrine tumors of the bladder

	SCC	LCC	Carcinoid
Gross features			
Tumor size/appearance	Variable size/polypoid	Large (2.5–6 cm)/polypoid/ ulcerated	Small (3–12 mm) ovoid or rounded sessile-polypoid masses
Growth pattern	Diffusely invasive	Invasive	Smooth surface/subepithelial/ rarely invade lamina propria
Histologic features			
Architecture	Diffuse sheets/nests	Diffuse sheets/solid nests/ trabeculae/rosette-like patterns	Anastomosing cords/glandular/ cribriform structures
Cellular shape			
Fusiform shape	Common	Rare	Absent
Poligonal shape with abundant cytoplasm	Absent	Typically present	Absent
Cuboidal/columnar	Absent	Absent	Frequent
Cell size	Small or intermediate	Large	Intermediate
Cytoplasm			
Size/quantity	Scant	Abundant	Moderate to abundant
Nucleus to cytoplasm volume ratio	High	Low	Granular eosinophilic subnuclear/ amphophilic
Nuclei			
Size	Small	Large	Small
Shape	Round to oval	Oval	Round to oval
Molding	Frequent	Absent	Absent
Nuclear rupture/crush artefact	Typical	Rare	Absent
Chromatin	Finely granular/salt and pepper	Coarse granular/vesicular	Finely stippled
Nucleolus	Inconspicuous	Prominent	Inconspicuous
Other findings			
Necrosis	Variable/frequent	Multiple large areas	Absent
Basophilic staining of vessels and stroma	Occasional	Rare	Absent
Mitotic index/activity	High	Very high	Low

Table 2.20 Immunohistochemistry patterns in neuroendocrine tumors of the bladder (summary of reported cases)

	SCC	LCC	Carcinoid
Neuroendocrine markers	Range of tumors with positive staining (%)	Range of tumors with positive staining (%)	Range of tumors with positive staining (%)
Chromogranin A	0–100	80	100
Synaptophysin	16–100	90	100
Neuron Specific Enolase (NSE)	0–100	81	100
CD56	71–83	100	100
CD57 (Leu7)	27–58		
Serotonin	77–91		
Epithelial markers			
Cytokeratin AE1/AE3	70–80	87	
CAM5.2	47–66	100	
CK 34bE12	40		
p63	0–14		
Cytokeratin 7	50–64		83
Cytokeratin 20	0		0
EMA	0–78	100	
Other markers			
TTF1	0–75	67	33
Uroplakin	0		
CD44v6	7		
S100	40	0	82
c-kit (CD117)	22–28		
EGFR	36–50		
PDGFR	100		
Ki67	15–80	67	
p16	93		
p53	54		50
c-erbB2	50		
CD45	3		

stem cell factor (SCF) pathway has been frequently identified in SCLC. It is well known that c-Kit, a transmembrane receptor tyrosine kinase involved in many physiological and pathological processes including hematopoiesis and carcinogenesis, is a target of the tyrosine kinase inhibitor imatinib. c-Kit expression can be detected in up to 40 % of small cell carcinoma of the urinary bladder.

Pathology

- Most tumors appear as a single large, solid, polypoid mass. but may also appear sessile and ulcerated, and extensively infiltrate the bladder wall. The lateral walls and dome of the bladder are the most frequent topographies but rare cases may arise in a bladder diverticulum.
- Histologically, small cell carcinoma of the urinary bladder consists of sheets or nests of small or intermediate-size cells with nuclear molding, scant cytoplasm, inconspicuous nucleoli and evenly dispersed finely stippled chromatin. Mitotic figures are readily evident and may be frequent. There may be extensive nuclear disruption, which can make diagnosis difficult in biopsy specimens (Figs. 2.92, 2.93, and 2.94).
- Punctate or geographical necrosis is common, and DNA encrustation of blood vessel walls (Azzopardi phenomenon) may be noted. Occasionally, tumor rosettes are present. Vascular invasion is invariably present. In the great majority of cases, extensive tumor infiltration of detrusor muscle is evident.

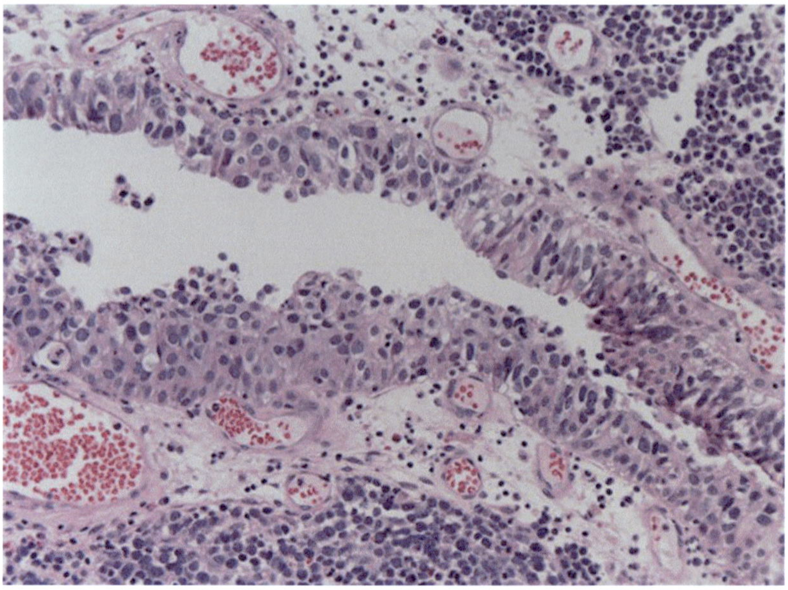

Fig. 2.92 Microscopic features of small cell carcinoma of the bladder (low power) as compared with overlying urothelium (*center*)

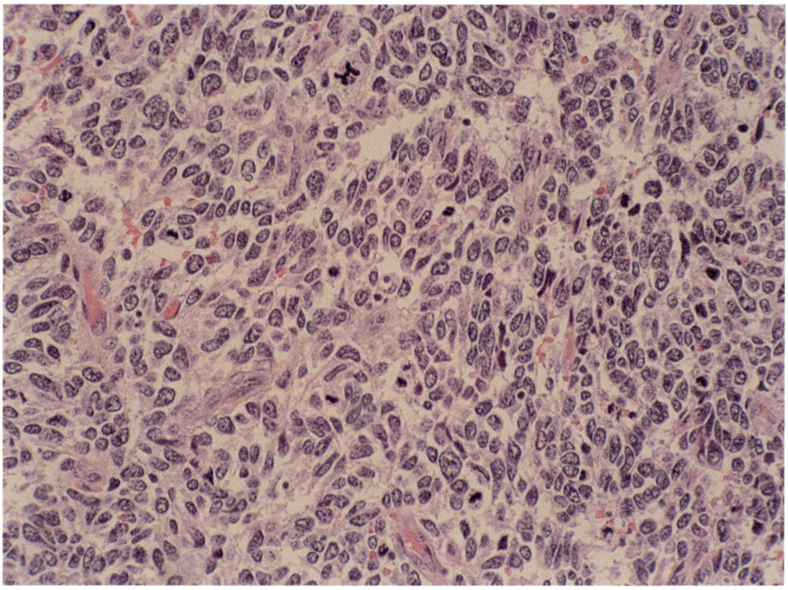

Fig. 2.93 High mitotic rate in small cell carcinoma

- Co-existing non-small cell carcinoma components, in the form of carcinoma-in-situ, conventional urothelial carcinoma, adenocarcinoma, squamous cell carcinoma, or sarcomatoid carcinoma, are present in 12–61 % of cases.

Immunohistochemistry

- The immunohistochemical profile of small cell carcinoma of the urinary bladder has been extensive investigated. It typically exhibits both epithelial and neuroendocrine differentiation.
- Likewise, the diagnosis of small cell carcinoma can be made on the typical morphologic features alone, even if neuroendocrine differentiation cannot be demonstrated. Markers that have been helpful in confirming neuroendocrine differentiation in small cell carcinoma include neuron specific enolase, chromogranin, synaptophysin, Leu 7, protein gene

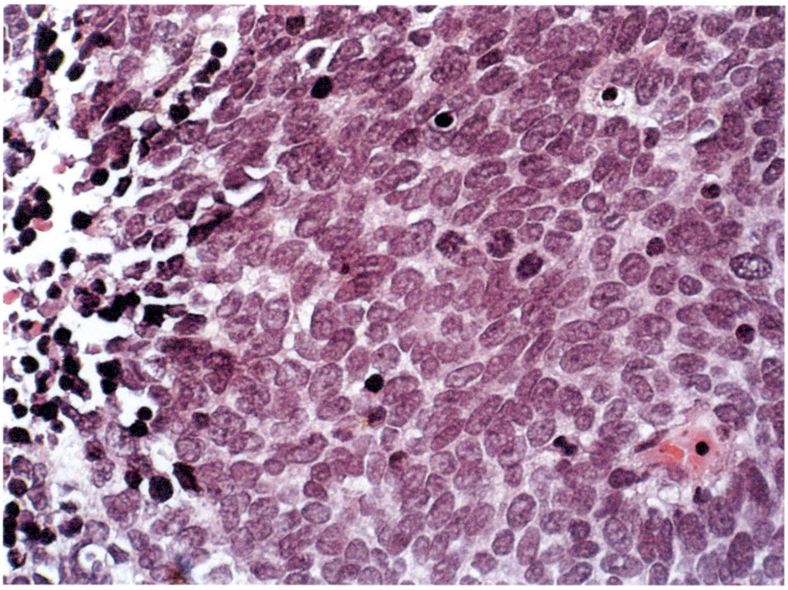

Fig. 2.94 Histologically, cells show molding of nuclei

product 9.5 (PGP9.5), serotonin, vasoactive intestinal peptide and others. Neuroendocrine differentiation has been demonstrated in 30–100 % cases of small cell carcinoma by various markers in different studies.

- Chromogranin A appears to be a relatively insensitive marker, demonstrable immunohistochemically in only a third of cases.
- Positive immunostaining for cytokeratin 7 has been observed in about 60 % of cases. Cytokeratin 20 and uroplakin III immunostains are negative in small cell carcinoma of the urinary bladder. Strong and focally intense cytoplasmic dot-like CAM5.2 reactivity is reported in about two-thirds of cases studied.
- Positive immunostaining for cytokeratin 34ßE12 has been observed in 40 % of cases, and positive EMA immunostaining in about 78 % of cases. p53 is over-expressed in 52 % of cases. Reported frequencies of Ki67 expression have varied from 15 to 80 %.
- CD44v6 may be useful in distinguishing poorly differentiated urothelial carcinoma from small cell carcinoma. CD44, a member of a family of transmembrane glycoproteins, mediates cell-cell and cell-matrix adhesion, the latter by serving as a receptor for hyaluronate binding. CD44v6 splice variant is an isoform conferring metastatic potential and has been correlated with aggressive behavior in some cancers.
- CD44v6 immunoreactivity is demonstrable in 60 % of cases of urothelial carcinoma, compared with only 7 % positivity in small cell carcinoma.
- Thyroid transcription factor 1 (TTF-1) is a nuclear transcriptional factor protein, which is expressed in thyroid and lung epithelium. TTF-1 is considered to be a reliable marker for distinguishing primary adenocarcinomas of the lung from adenocarcinomas of extrapulmonary origin, and for distinguishing pulmonary small cell carcinoma from Merkel cell carcinoma. About 40 % of cases of small cell carcinoma of the urinary bladder had positive TTF-1 staining. Therefore TTF-1 immunostaining cannot reliably distinguish between a lung or urinary bladder primary in cases of metastatic small cell carcinoma of uncertain primary location.

Differential Diagnosis

- The main differential diagnoses include metastasis of small cell carcinoma from another site, lymphoma, lymphoepithelioma-like carcinoma, plasmacytoid carcinoma and poorly differentiated urothelial carcinoma.
- Immunohistochemical studies can be quite helpful in distinguishing these entities in

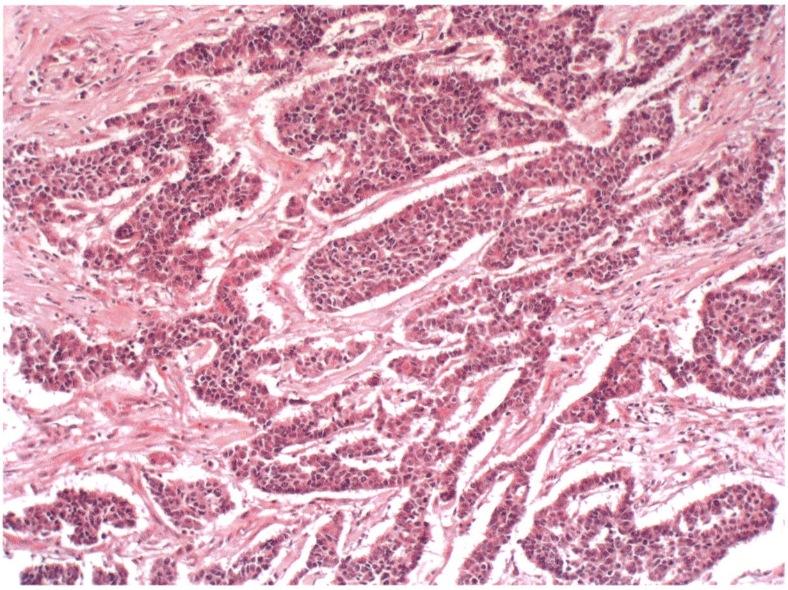

Fig. 2.95 Microscopic features of large cell neuroendocrine carcinoma of the bladder (low power)

difficult cases. Small cell carcinoma can occasionally mimic malignant lymphoma when the tumor cells of small cell carcinoma appear to grow in a discohesive pattern, a finding that may result from artifacts produced by fixation and specimen processing. Lymphoma shows positive immunostaining for leukocyte common antigen (LCA), and negative immunostaining for keratin and neuroendocrine markers that typically are positive in small cell carcinoma.

- Plasmacytoid carcinoma, poorly differentiated urothelial carcinoma, and squamous cell carcinoma do not express neuroendocrine markers such as synaptophysin or chromogranin, as does small cell carcinoma.
- Large cell neuroendocrine carcinoma is morphologically characterized by large sized tumor cells with low nuclear to cytoplasmic ratios, coarse chromatin and frequent nucleoli and high mitotic activity with areas of necrosis; confirmation of its true nature requires positive immunostaining with appropriate neuroendocrine markers.
- Small cell carcinoma metastatic to the urinary bladder can only be distinguished from a bladder primary by knowledge of the clinical setting.

Large cell neuroendocrine carcinoma

- Large cell neuroendocrine carcinoma is a poorly differentiated and high-grade neuroendocrine tumor, morphologically identical to their counterparts in the lung. Primary large cell neuroendocrine carcinomas of the urinary bladder are rare, and experience with these tumors is limited to a few anecdotal case reports.
- The age at diagnosis ranges from 32 to 82 years of age. These tumors are either pure or can be associated with other components, such as typical urothelial carcinoma, squamous cell carcinoma, adenocarcinoma or sarcomatoid carcinoma (Figs. 2.95, 2.96, and 2.97).
- Immunohistochemically, the tumor cells frequently show immunoreactivity to chromogranin A, CD56, neuron-specific enolase, and synaptophysin. In addition to neuroendocrine markers, the tumor cells typically show positive immunostaining for cytokeratins CAM 5.2 and AE1/AE3 and for epithelial membrane antigen (EMA), and may show focal positivity for vimentin.
- In situ hybridization for the detection of Epstein-Barr virus in one reported case was negative. These tumors are aggressive and tend to metastasize systemically despite aggressive adjuvant therapy. Metastasis from a lung primary should be considered before diagnosing a primary bladder large cell neuroendocrine carcinoma.

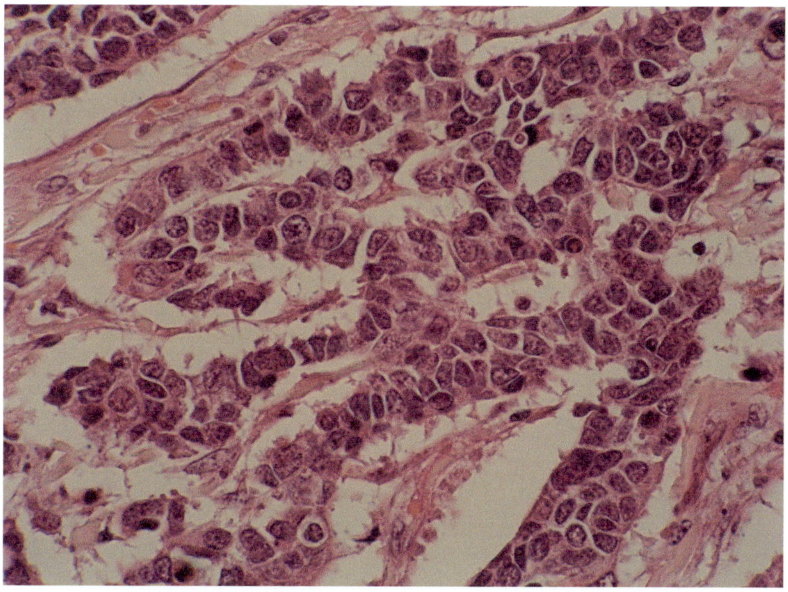

Fig. 2.96 Microscopic features of large cell neuroendocrine carcinoma of the bladder (high power)

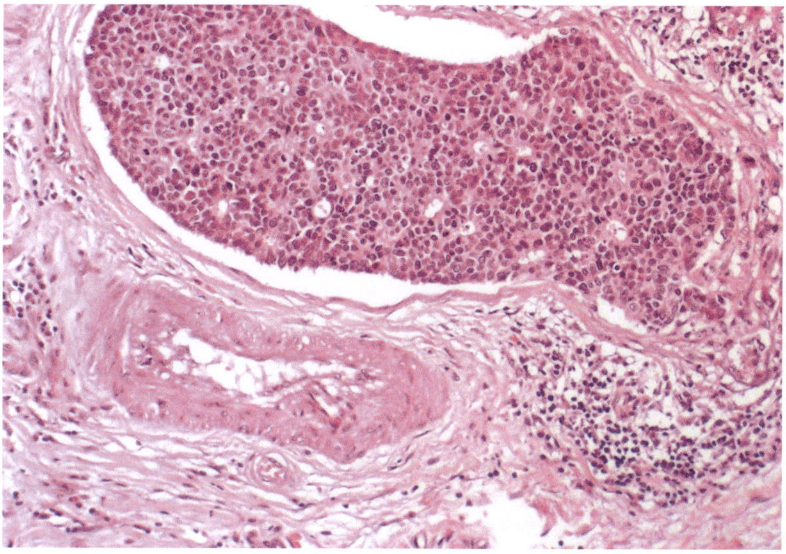

Fig. 2.97 Carcinoid tumor of the bladder trigone

Carcinoid

- Carcinoid is a potentially malignant neuroendocrine neoplasm derived from the urothelium. Less than two dozen cases of carcinoid tumours of the urinary bladder have been reported, usually occurring in elderly patients (range 29–75 years of age), with slight male predominance. Hematuria is common, but irritative voiding symptoms may be the first symptom.
- Association with carcinoid syndrome has not been reported. Most tumours are submucosal with a predilection for the trigone. They range in size from 0.3 to 3 cm. Carcinoid tumours are often polypoid at cystoscopy. Coexistence of carcinoid with other urothelial neoplasia, such as inverted papilloma and adenocarcinoma, has been reported.
- Carcinoid tumours of the bladder are histologically similar to their counterparts in other organ sites (Figs. 2.97 and 2.98). The tumor cells have abundant amphophilic cytoplasm and are arranged in an insular, acinar, trabecular,

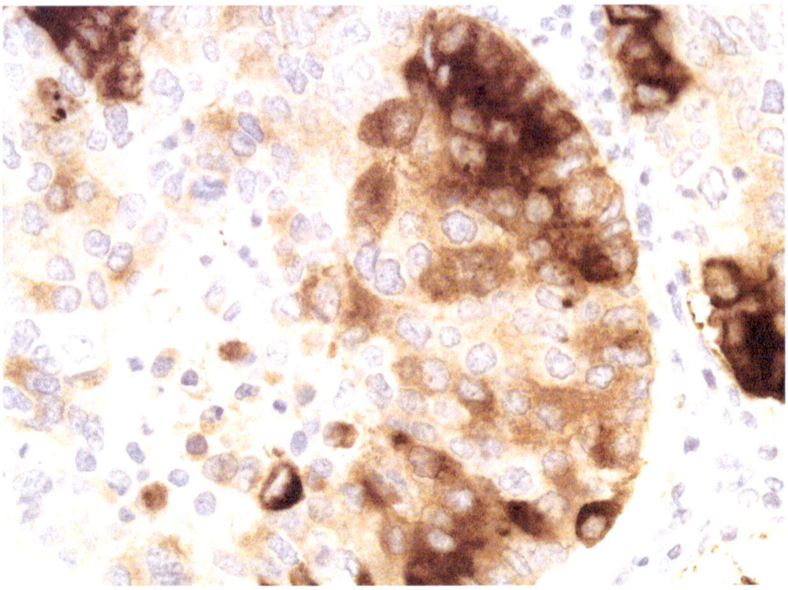

Fig. 2.98 Chromogranin is positive in carcinoid tumor

or pseudoglandular pattern with a delicate vascular stroma. An organoid growth pattern, resembling paraganglioma, is sometimes seen. Tumor cell nuclei have finely stippled chromatin and inconspicuous nucleoli. Mitotic figures are infrequent, and tumor necrosis is absent.

- Tumor cells show immunoreactivity for neuroendocrine markers (neuron-specific enolase, chromogranin, serotonin, and synaptophysin) and cytokeratin (AE1/AE3). Differential diagnostic considerations include paraganglioma, nested variant of urothelial carcinoma and metastatic prostate carcinoma. About 25 % of patients have or develop regional lymph node or distant metastasis but the majority are cured by excision.

Paraganglioma

- Primary paraganglioma of the bladder occurs infrequently. Females are more likely to develop bladder paraganglioma: the male to female ratio is 1:3. The tumor tends to occur in young patients (mean, 45 years) and symptoms are present in over 80 % of cases.
- Presenting symptoms include hematuria, hypertension which may be exacerbated during voiding, and other symptoms of catecholamine excess. At cystoscopic examination, small (<3 cm), dome-shaped nodules covered by normal mucosa are found in the trigone, dome or lateral wall (Figs. 2.99 and 2.100).
- In contrast to extra-adrenal paragangliomas at other sites, of which approximately 10 % exhibit malignant behavior, the frequency of malignancy in bladder paragangliomas is about 20 %.
- No reliable histologic criteria exist to distinguish malignant from benign neoplasms. The findings of nuclear pleomorphism, mitotic figures, and necrosis are not reliable predictor of clinical outcome in patients with paraganglioma of the urinary bladder. Malignancy in these tumors can only be confirmed by the occurrence of regional or distant metastases. No metastases or tumor recurrences have been observed in patients whose tumors were confined within the bladder wall.

Genetics

- Genomic analyses have identified germline mutations responsible for sporadic as well as familial paraganglioma syndromes. The susceptibility genes include SDHB, SDHC, and SDHD. Succinate dehydrogenase (SDH), which consists of four polypeptides, [SDHA, SDHB (1p36), SDHC (1q21), and SDHD (11q23)], is the major mitochondrial enzyme linking the aerobic respiratory chain and the Krebs cycle, which oxidizes succinate to fumarate.

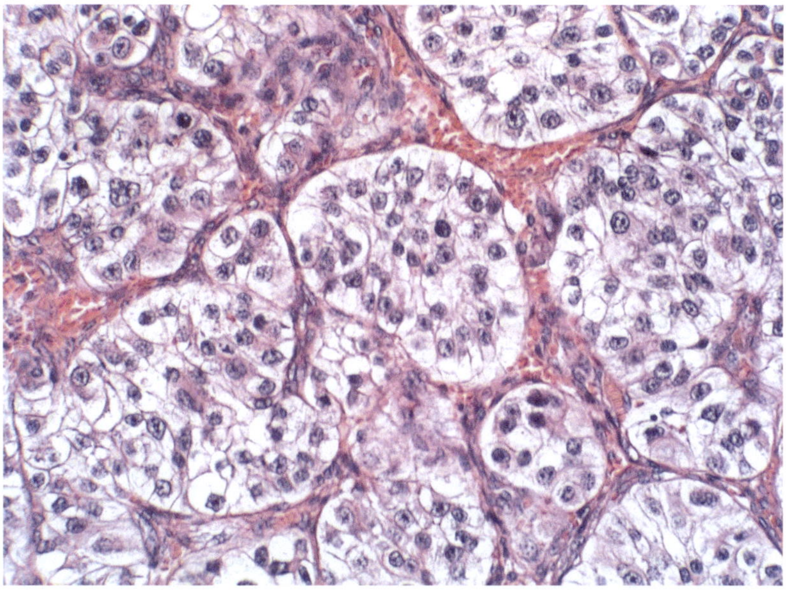

Fig. 2.99 Paraganglioma of the bladder

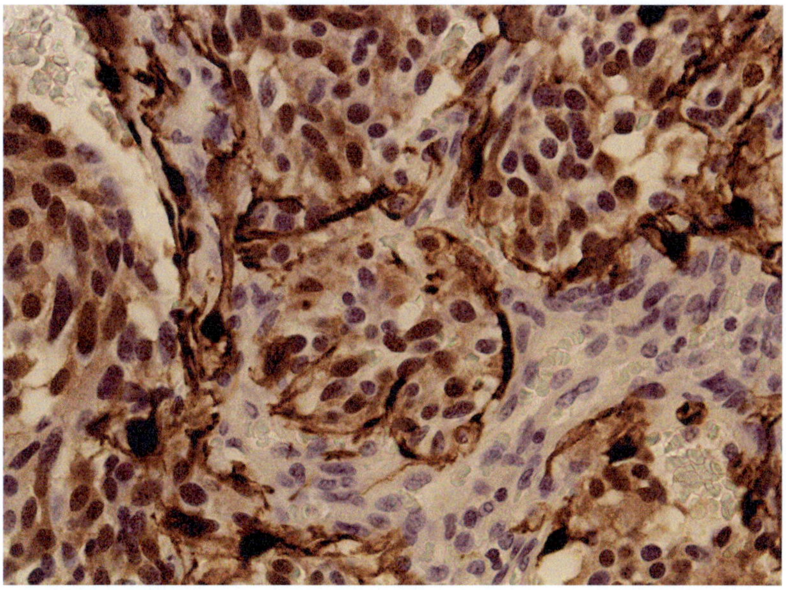

Fig. 2.100 S-100 protein immunohistochemistry highlight sustentacular cells in the periphery of paraganglioma nests

- The SDH genes are tumor suppressor genes, the inactivation of which is involved in the hypoxia-angiogenic pathway activating the transcription factor hypoxia-inducible factor (HIF). Nonsense and missense mutations, insertions, and small and large deletions have been reported in the SDH genes of patients with pheochromocytoma or paraganglioma. These mutations are generally seen in younger patients. SDHD mutations have been identified in patients with pheochromocytoma or functional paraganglioma. Patients with these mutations usually have a paternal family history of disease due to maternal imprinting.
- SDHB gene mutations are usually associated with abdominal paragangliomas and are often identified in patients with no family history of the disease. The SDHB gene mutation is associated with a high risk of malignancy.

- HIF dysregulation is also linked to inactivation of the VHL tumor suppressor gene (3p25-26), which is seen in von Hippel-Lindau disease. Pheochromocytomas or paragangliomas may be seen in this disease. Other autosomally dominant diseases associated with pheochromocytomas/paragangliomas include multiple endocrine neoplasia type 2 (due to mutation of the RET proto-oncogene) and neurofibromatosis type 1 (due to a mutation in NF-1, a tumor suppressor gene).
- Genetic aberrations at other loci (2q and 16p) have also been recently found to be associated with familial pheochromocytoma. Similarly, Lemeta et al. found abnormalities in tumor suppressor genes located at 6q23-24 which may play a role in the tumorigenesis of pheochromocytomas.

Pathology

- Histologically, bladder paraganglioma is similar to its counterparts in other body sites; most are covered by normal urothelium. The tumor consists of round or polygonal epithelioid cells with abundant eosinophilic or granular cytoplasm. Tumor cell nuclei are centrally located, and are vesicular with finely granular chromatin. The cells are arranged in discrete nests (zellballen), with intervening vascular septa. Sustentacular cells may be present. Mitotic figures, necrosis, and vascular invasion are usually absent.

Immunohistochemistry

- Paraganglioma typically demonstrates immunoreactivity with neuroendocrine markers such as chromogranin, synaptophysin, and neuron specific enolase. The sustentacular cells exhibit immunostaining for S-100 protein. Tumor cells are often immunoreactive for vimentin, but usually show no immunoreactivity for cytokeratins 7, 20, or pancytokeratin AE1/AE3.

Differential diagnosis

- The differential diagnosis for this tumor includes granular cell tumor, nested variant of urothelial carcinoma, metastatic large cell neuroendocrine carcinoma, and malignant melanoma.
- Granular cell tumor has abundant eosinophilic granular cytoplasm, shows strongly positive immunostaining for S-100 protein, and lacks the zellballen growth pattern, the fine vascular stroma, chromogranin immunoreactivity, and sustentacular cell S-100 protein immunostaining. The nested variant of urothelial carcinoma also lacks a fine vascular network and is immunohistochemically negative for S-100 protein and chromogranin.
- Metastatic large cell neuroendocrine carcinoma is characterized by necrosis, abundant mitotic activity, and cellular anaplasia. While it is immunoreactive for neuroendocrine markers similar to paraganglioma, it is also immunoreactive for cytokeratin and negative for sustentacular cell S-100 protein immunoreactivity.
- History is important in differentiating paraganglioma from metastatic carcinoid. Carcinoid tumor is negative for sustentacular cell S-100 protein immunoreactivity. Malignant melanoma must be considered in the differential diagnosis since paraganglioma may contain melanin pigment.

2.2.8 Soft Tissue Tumors

- Pure sarcomas of the urinary bladder are all rare and have been described only in small series and isolated case reports. Myofibroblastic proliferations, including pseudosarcomatous myofibroblastic tumor and postoperative spindle cell nodule still invoke a degree of uncertainty for classification and differential diagnosis.
- Other rare benign lesions of the bladder include leiomyoma, hemangioma and neurofibroma. Other examples of benign soft tissue tumors are rarely described. Malignant mesenchymal tumors of the urinary bladder include leiomyosarcoma, rhabdomyosarcoma, angiosarcoma and malignant fibrous histiocytoma (undifferentiated sarcoma) (Tables 2.21 and 2.22).
- Recognizing these spindle cell lesions and differentiating them from sarcomatoid carcinoma is important as these two diagnostic categories have differing therapeutic as well as prognostic implications.

Table 2.21 Immunohistochemistry of spindle cell lesions of the bladder

	Sarcomatoid carcinoma	IMT	LMS	Leiomyoma	MFH	Neurofibroma	PSCN	RMS
ALK-1		Pos				Rare pos	Neg	
α-1-Antichymotrypsin					Pos			
CD68					Pos			
Cytokeratin	Pos	Pos/neg	Neg/pos		Neg/pos	Neg	Neg/pos	Neg/pos
Desmin	Neg/pos	Pos/neg	Pos	Pos	Neg/pos		Pos/neg	Pos
EMA	Pos	Pos/neg	Neg			Neg	Neg	Neg
h-Caldesmon			Pos	Pos	Neg			Neg
Muscle-specific actin	Pos/neg	Pos	Pos	Pos	Neg/pos		Pos	Pos
MYOD1			Neg		Neg			Pos
Myogenin			Neg		Neg			Pos
Myoglobin		Neg						Pos/neg
NSE								Neg/pos
Smooth muscle actin	Neg/pos	Pos	Pos	Pos	Neg/pos		Pos/neg	Neg/pos
S-100 protein		Neg	Neg		Neg	Pos		Neg
Vimentin	Pos/neg	Pos	Pos	Pos	Pos		Pos	Pos
CD31					Neg			
CD34			Neg/pos		Neg			Neg

ALK anaplastic lymphoma kinase, *IMT* inflammatory myofibroblastic tumor, *PSCN* postoperative spindle cell nodule, *LMS* leiomyosarcoma, *MFH* malignant fibrous histiocytoma, *RMS* rhabdomyosarcoma, *EMA* epithelial membrane antigen, *NSE* neuron-specific enolase, *Pos* positive, *Neg* negative, *Neg/Pos* variable staining

Table 2.22 Differential features of selected soft tissue tumors of the urinary bladder

	Cytologic atypia	Mitotic figures	Atypical mitotic figures	Tumor necrosis	Inflammation	Invasion of muscle	Other features
Sarcomatoid carcinoma	Present	Present	Present	Present	Often present	May be present	Concomitant carcinoma
IMT	Minimal	Few	Absent	Surface only	Often prominent	May be present	Delicate capillaries
Leiomyoma	Minimal	Rare	Absent	Absent	Absent	Absent	Well circumscribed
Leiomyosarcoma	Present	Present	Present	Present	Sparse	Present	Uniform appearance
MFH	Present	Present	Present	Present	Present	Present	Multinucleated cells
Neurofibroma	Varies	Absent	Absent	Absent	Sparse	Absent	Strands of collagen
PSCN	Minimal	Variable	Absent	Absent	Present	Absent	Delicate capillaries
RMS	Present	Present	Present	Varies	Absent	May be present	Cambium layer in embryonal RMS, alveolar appearance
Angiosarcoma	Present	Present	Present	May be present	Present	May be present	Anastomosing vessels

ALK anaplastic lymphoma kinase, *IMT* inflammatory myofibroblastic tumor, *MFH* malignant fibrous histiocytoma, *PSCN* postoperative spindle cell nodule, *RMS* rhabdomyosarcoma

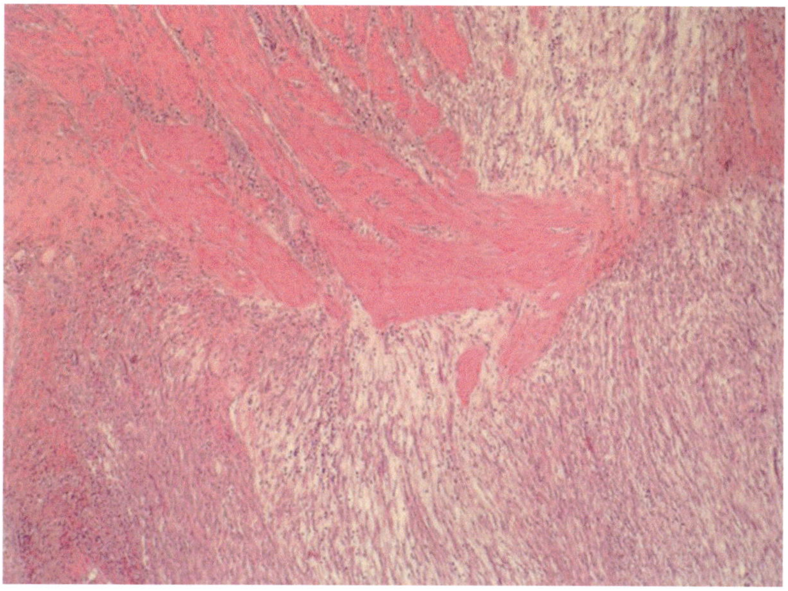

Fig. 2.101 Inflammatory myofibrobastic tumor invading the bladder wall

Inflammatory myofibroblastic tumor (IMT)

- Is a controversial entity, and has had many designations, including inflammatory pseudotumor, inflammatory pseudosarcomatous fibromyxoid tumor, nodular fasciitis, pseudosarcomatous myofibroblastic proliferation, and fibromyxoid pseudotumor. It was initially described as a lesion showing spindle cells in a myxoid stroma with scattered chronic inflammatory cells.
- The most frequent presenting symptom is hematuria; other symptoms include irritative and/or obstructive voiding symptoms, abdominal pain, or the discovery of a mass lesion. Rarely, constitutional symptoms including fever and weight loss have been reported, possibly due to the release of cytokines.
- Grossly, the lesion is either a polypoid mass or a submucosal nodule. The tumor may or may not cause surface ulceration and the cut surface is often pale, firm and glistening.

Pathology

- There is a proliferation of spindle cells with elongated eosinophilic cytoplasmic processes in a loose edematous or myxoid background (Figs. 2.101, 2.102, and 2.103).
- The nuclei may be large with occasional atypia. Single, prominent nucleoli may be present. Occasional mitotic figures are seen, none of which is atypical. The mitotic rates vary from 0 to 20 mitoses per 10 HPF (high power fields). Inflammation, usually chronic and consisting of a lymphoplasmacytic infiltrate is invariably seen. Some lesions have infiltrates of eosinophils or neutrophils, which may be focally prominent. Extravasated red blood cells may be present.
- Three histologic patterns have been recognized, the most common of which is the "nodular fasciitis-like" pattern with myxoid, vascular, and inflammatory areas.
- A second pattern, designated "fibrous histiocytoma-like", has a more compact spindle cell proliferation and scattered lymphocytes, plasma cells or eosinophils.
- The third pattern, designated "scar or desmoid-like", has dense collagen with fewer spindled and inflammatory cells.
- Infiltration into the muscularis propria or even perivesical involvement may be seen. Typically, the lesion occurs in young patients (9–42 years) with a female predominance. The tumor size ranges from 1.5 to 13 cm. Follow up data has revealed no evidence of metastases, but the lesion may recur after surgery.

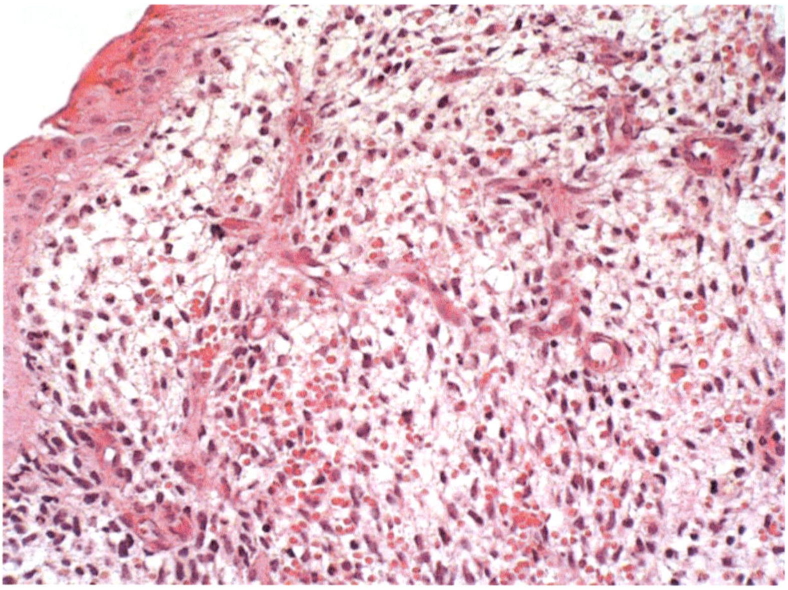

Fig. 2.102 Inflammatory myofibrobastic tumor showing myxoid appearance

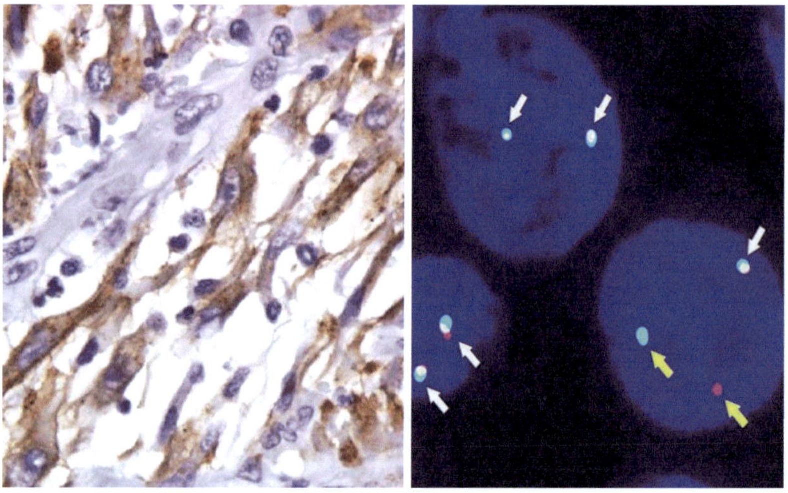

Fig. 2.103 Inflammatory myofibrobastic tumor. ALK positive immunohistochemistry (*left*) and ALK translocation by FISH (*right*) showing normal signal (*white arrow*) and split (break apart) signal (*yellow arrow*)

Immunohistochemistry

- Utility of immunostaining in separating this lesion from other spindle cell lesions of the bladder is limited. Immunoreactivity for actin and vimentin is usually present but may be focal. P53 staining is weak or absent in inflammatory myofibroblastic tumor and postoperative spindle cell nodule but strongly and diffusely positive in rhabdomyosarcoma, leiomyosarcoma or sarcomatoid carcinoma.
- Pancytokeratin reactivity, which may be patchy, is seen in many cases of inflammatory myofibroblastic tumor. Nevertheless, cytokeratin may be seen in other nonepithelial tumors such as leiomyosarcoma. Actin immunoreactivity may not help differentiate benign from malignant tumors, since α-smooth muscle actin (SMA) is positive in 43 % of sarcomas, 63 % of inflammatory myofibroblastic tumor and an intermediate percentage of postoperative spindle cell nodule. Rhabdomyosarcoma rarely expresses SMA but leiomyosarcoma often does.
- Inflammatory myofibroblastic tumor, postoperative spindle cell nodule may be reactive for desmin, but this marker may be present in

leiomyosarcoma at other sites. Inflammatory myofibroblastic tumor shows variable staining for EMA. Inflammatory myofibroblastic tumor is negative for myoglobin, whereas rhabdomyosarcoma is usually positive for skeletal muscle markers such as myogenin or MyoD1. Strong coexpression of SMA and cytokeratin is characteristic of vesical myofibroblasts, and thus should characterize inflammatory myofibroblastic tumor.

Differential diagnosis

- The main differential diagnoses include post-operative spindle cell nodule, embryonal rhabdomyosarcoma, and leiomyosarcoma.
- Post-operative spindle cell nodule reportedly is more likely to have eosinophils. Inflammatory myofibroblastic tumor may be confused with myxoid leiomyosarcoma since both may have a myxoid stroma.
- Morphologically, leiomyosarcoma is more uniform in its cellularity and exhibits more cytologic atypia. Inflammatory myofibroblastic tumor, on the other hand, has a more prominent network of small blood vessels and a more extensive inflammatory infiltrate.
- Inflammatory myofibroblastic tumor may have necrosis at the site of surface ulceration and it may infiltrate into the detrusor muscle, but it typically does not exhibit deep necrosis as may be seen in a sarcoma. Recently, positive cytoplasmic immunostaining for anaplastic lymphoma kinase (ALK-1) has been identified in 89 % of inflammatory myofibroblastic tumor in the bladder. The ALK-1 staining was confirmed by fluorescence in situ hybridization to mRNA from a fusion gene resulting from translocation of the ALK gene on chromosome 2p23 to the clathrin heavy chain region on chromosome 17q23. It has been suggested that ALK negative cases are less likely to recur. Neither ALK-1 staining nor translocation of the ALK-1 gene has been identified in any case of bladder leiomyosarcoma or rhabdomyosarcoma. However, spindle cell lesions in sites other than the urinary bladder may display ALK-1 expression, which has been reported in 40 % of inflammatory myofibroblastic tumor, 19 % of rhabdomyosarcomas and 10 % of leiomyosarcomas at other sites.

Post-operative spindle cell nodule (PSCN)

- It is characterized by nodules up to 4 cm in size occurring in the lower genital tract and lower urinary tract months after surgical instrumentation or resection. Patients range in age from 29 to 79 years, and typically present with hematuria and/or obstructive voiding symptoms. Some PSCN are found incidentally by CT scan or at cystoscopy. Microscopically the tumors are uniform, composed of intersecting fascicles of plump spindle cells with delicate vessels, focal hyalinization, and moderate collagen deposition (Fig. 2.104).
- The spindle cells have abundant, tapering, eosinophilic cytoplasm. The nuclei vary only slightly in size and there is no cytologic atypia. There are numerous mitotic figures, ranging from 1 to 25 per 10hpf, none of which is abnormal. All lesions have ulceration with acute inflammatory cells in the ulcer bed, as well as scattered chronic inflammatory cells in deeper areas.
- The tumor has infiltrating margins with smooth muscle destruction. Moderate edema and small foci of hemorrhage may be identified. No recurrences or metastases have been reported, but bladder wall eosinophilia may be prominent following resection of the lesion. The proliferating cells are immunoreactive for cytokeratin AE1/AE3, CAM5.2 and vimentin in some cases, similar to the findings in IMT. Some cases exhibit only immunoreactivity for vimentin.
- The differential diagnoses for PSCN include sarcomatoid carcinoma, myxoid leiomyosarcoma, rhabdomyosarcoma, and malignant fibrous histiocytoma (see inflammatory myofibroblastic tumor section for discussion).
- Findings that are helpful in distinguishing PSCN from sarcoma include the lack of necrosis or myxoid degeneration, lack of nuclear atypia, and predominance of chronic over acute inflammation. P53 immunostaining may be helpful in distinguishing these lesions, being noted only rarely in PSCN, but showing strong and diffuse staining in malignant lesions.

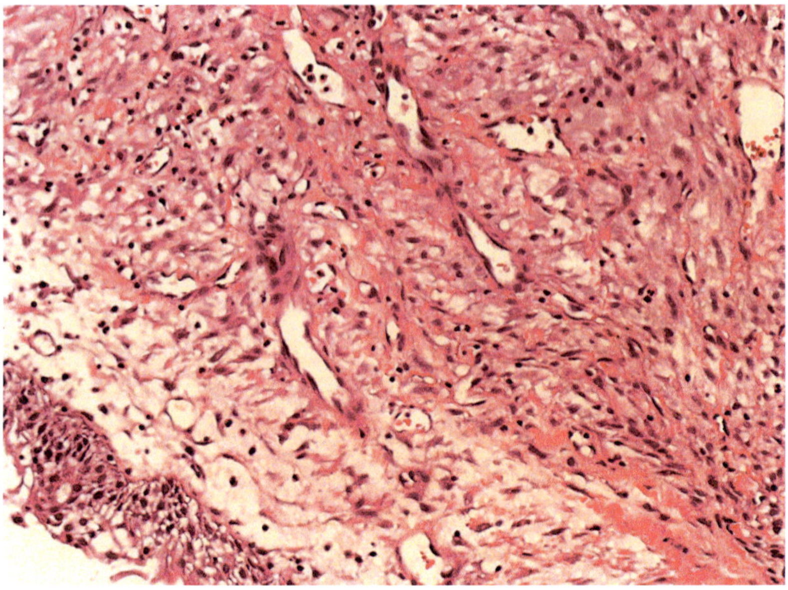

Fig. 2.104 Histologic features of postoperative spindle cell nodule

Leiomyoma

- Although rare, leiomyoma is the most common benign neoplasm of the bladder. About 60 % occurred in the third through sixth decades with an average patient age of 44 years. Leiomyoma of the bladder is more common in women, with a male: female ratio of 1:3. About 19 % of patients are asymptomatic; others present with obstructive voiding symptoms (49 %), irritative symptoms (38 %), hematuria (11 %), or flank pain (13 %).
- Leiomyomas are most often endovesical, followed be extravesical, or intramural. Grossly, the tumors are small, well circumscribed, white nodules without hemorrhage or necrosis, and a tumor size of 1.6–5.8 cm. Microscopically, leiomyoma consists of intersecting fascicles of smooth muscle cells with moderate to abundant eosinophilic cytoplasm (Figs. 2.105 and 2.106).
- Cellularity is usually limited, and myxoid change is absent in most cases. The nuclei are oval to cigar-shaped, centrally located, and blunt-ended, and lack significant nuclear atypia, mitotic activity and necrosis. Examples of angioleiomyoma have been reported. Leiomyoma is immunoreactive for smooth muscle actin (SMA), actin, desmin, and vimentin. Some may express CD34 but most are negative for cytokeratin and S-100 protein.

Hemangioma

- Mean age at diagnosis is 30–58 years. Male-to-female ratio is 3.7:1. The usual presenting symptom is gross hematuria, but other complaints may include irritative voiding symptoms and abdominal pain. Endoscopically, a sessile, blue, raised mass may be seen. The lesion is usually small (median 0.7 cm).
- Hemangiomas are most often found on the posterior and lateral walls of the bladder. The histologic findings in bladder hemangioma are the same as those noted in other sites. Cavernous hemangioma is the most common type reported in the bladder, but capillary or arteriovenous types may infrequently be seen (Fig. 2.107).
- The differential diagnosis for bladder hemangioma includes angiosarcoma and Kaposi sarcoma, both of which exhibit more cytologic atypia. Exuberant granulation tissue contains prominent inflammation, which is not a feature of hemangioma. Multiple hemangiomas may be associated with syndromes predisposing to their development, including Klippel-Trenaunay-Weber and Sturge-Weber syndromes.

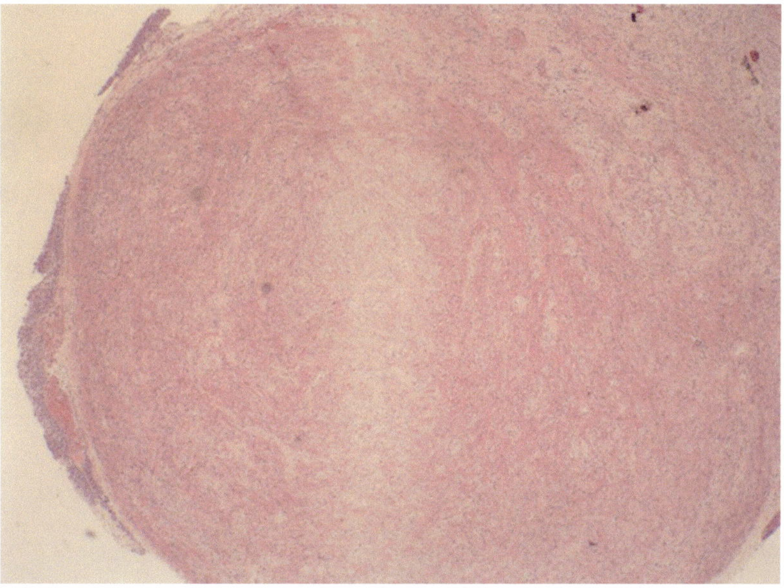

Fig. 2.105 Subepithelial leiomyoma of the bladder

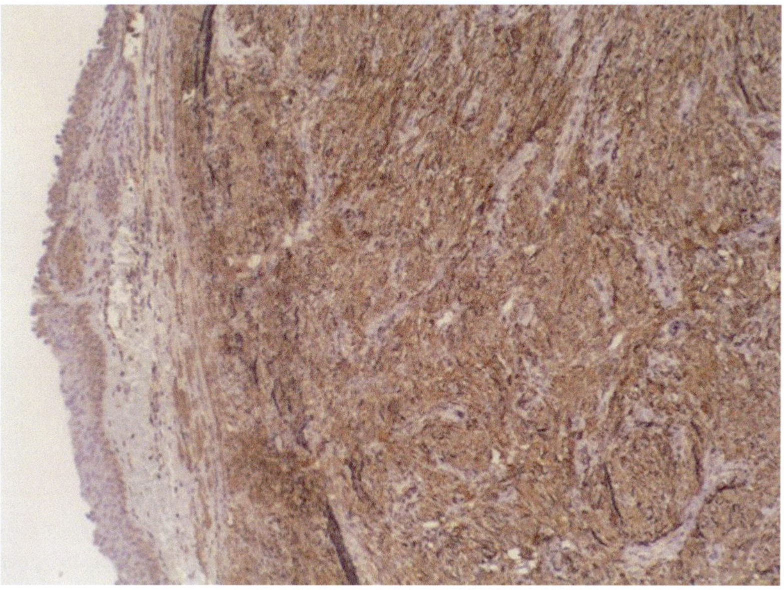

Fig. 2.106 Smooth muscle actin expression in bladder leiomyoma

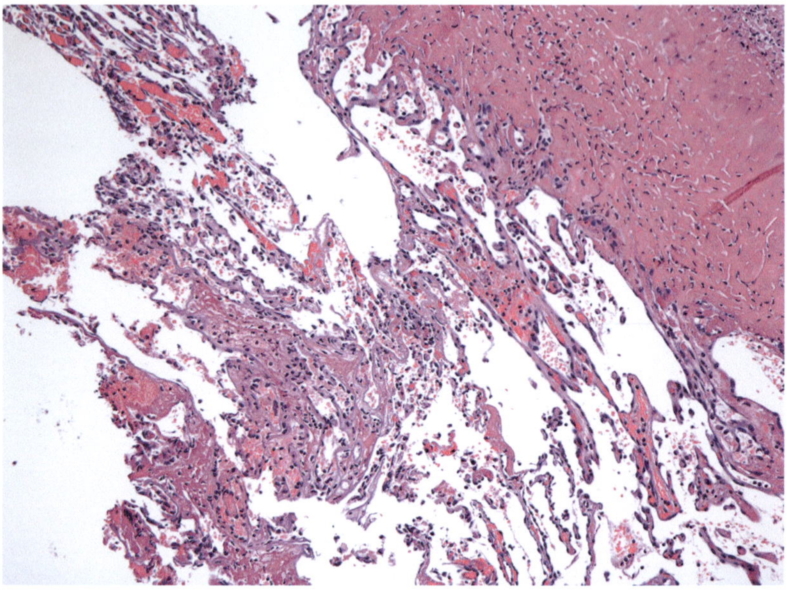

Fig. 2.107 Bladder hemangioma

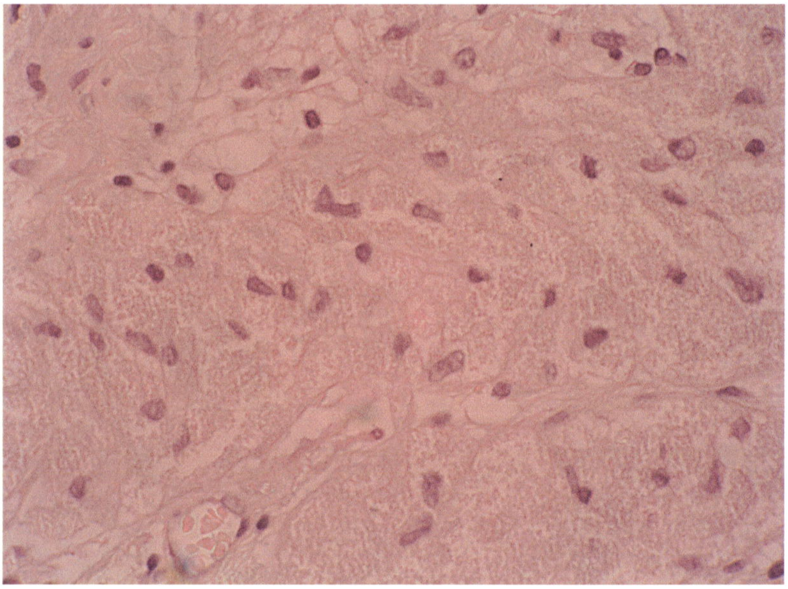

Fig. 2.108 Bladder myoblastoma showing granular cytoplasm of the cells

Granular cell tumour

- This tumor is rarely seen in the urinary bladder but reported cases have occurred in adult patients 23–70 years of age. There is no gender predilection. They are usually solitary, well circumscribed and vary in size up to 12 cm.
- Histologically, the cells have abundant granular eosinophilic cytoplasm and vesicular nuclei. S-100 protein is invariably expressed in the tumor cells (Figs. 2.108 and 2.109).
- A congenital granular cell tumor of the gingiva with systemic involvement including urinary bladder has been reported. Rare cases of malignant granular cell tumor of the bladder are on record.

Solitary fibrous tumors

- Solitary fibrous tumor of the urinary bladder has recently been recognized. It occurs in older patients who present with pain or hematuria. The tumor is typically a polypoid

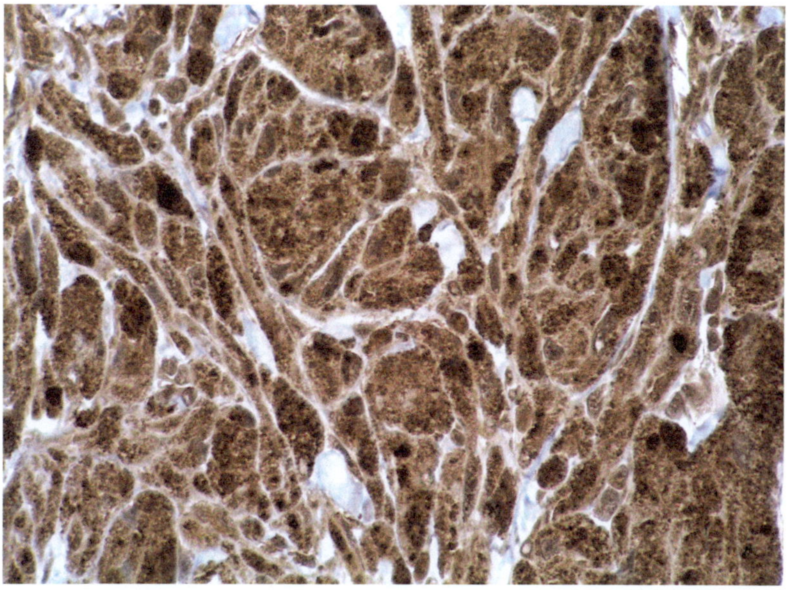

Fig. 2.109 Myoblastoma cells are positive for S-100

submucosal mass. Histopathologic features include spindle cells arranged haphazardly in a variably collagenous stroma.
- Dilated vessels reminiscent of hemangiopericytoma are present. All solitary fibrous tumours of the bladder have had a benign course, although the number of cases is small, and follow-up has been short term in several cases. The proliferating cells typically show CD34 immunoreactivity.

Perivascular epithelioid cell tumor (PEComa)
- Perivascular epithelioid cell tumor (PEComa) is a rare mesenchymal neoplasm with indolent biological behavior. All cases involving the urinary bladder have occurred in patients less than 50 years old. One of characteristic histologic features of this tumor is the delicate vascular stroma between the tumor cell nests (Figs. 2.110, 2.111, 2.112, and 2.113).
- Clear to eosinophilic, epithelioid and spindled cells are arranged in fascicles or packets. Mitotic figures are inconspicuous. Immunohistochemically the cells are positive for HMB-45 and smooth muscle actin, but negative for S-100 protein, Melan-A, desmin, and pan-cytokeratin.
- Clear cell myomelanocytic tumor, another member of the PEComa family, has also been reported in the urinary bladder. The single reported case arose from the muscularis propria in a 33-year-old woman.

Neurofibroma
- Neurofibroma of the urinary bladder is rare. Most of these lesions occur in the setting of neurofibromatosis type 1 rather than as isolated lesions. Classically, neurofibromas of the urinary bladder occur in young patients with a slight male predominance. The average age at diagnosis is 17 years.
- Presenting symptoms include hematuria, irritative symptoms, and pelvic mass. Neurofibroma is a benign tumor of various nerve sheath cells, including Schwann cells, perineurium-like cells, fibroblasts, and intermediate type cells.
- The histologic findings are the same as in neurofibromas of other organs: tumors are composed of a hypocellular proliferation of spindle cells, loosely arranged into fascicles with scattered "shredded carrot" bundles of collagen. Individual cells have wavy, bland nuclei.
- Some bladder neurofibromas were transmural with both diffuse and plexiform growth patterns with submucosal involvement and subepithelial pseudo-Meissnerian corpuscles on biopsy. A few mast cells are present.
- Immunohistochemical staining was reactive in all cases for S-100 protein as well

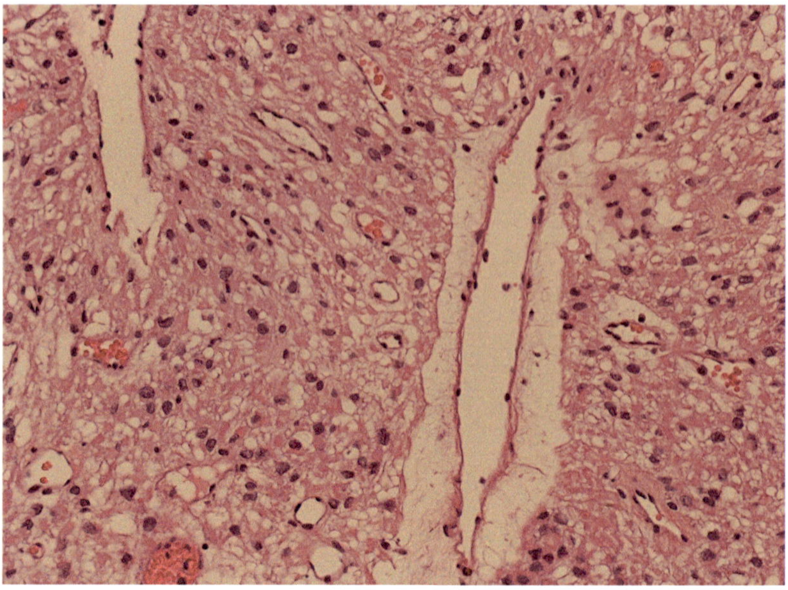

Fig. 2.110 Pecoma of the urinary bladder showing a cellular area

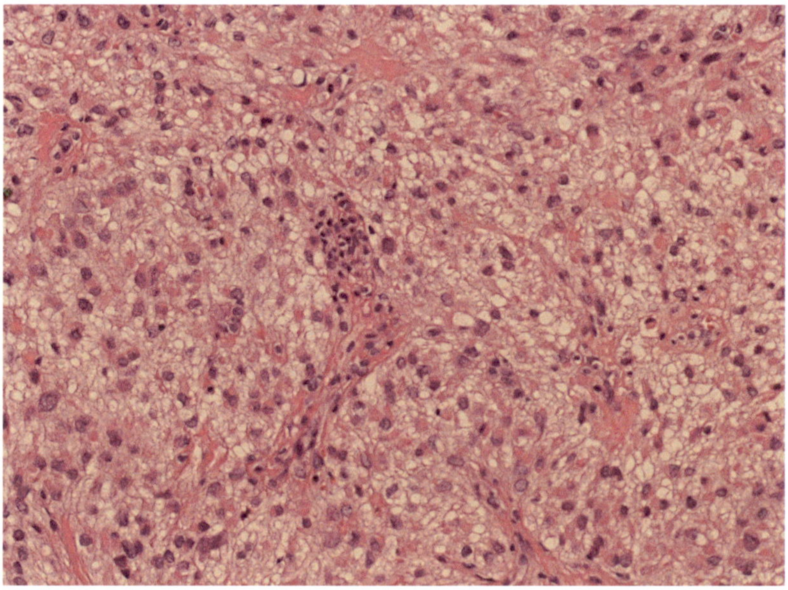

Fig. 2.111 Pecoma of the urinary bladder showing clear cells

as Type IV collagen. Three were positive for neurofilament protein in axons. A recent report indicates that bladder neurofibromas do not express ALK-1 protein. The differential diagnosis of bladder neurofibroma includes other spindle cell tumors such as leiomyoma, post-operative spindle cell nodule, myofibrobastic tumor, low grade leiomyosarcoma, other nerve sheet tumors and rarely rhabdomyosarcoma.

Schwannoma

- Schwannoma of the urinary bladder is derived from Schwann cells in nerve sheaths. It occurs in both men and women, and is often associated with von Recklinghausen's disease. The age at presentation ranges from the fourth to sixth decade.
- The presenting symptoms include bladder pressure, suprapubic pain, back pain, urgency, and frequency. No recurrences have been reported.

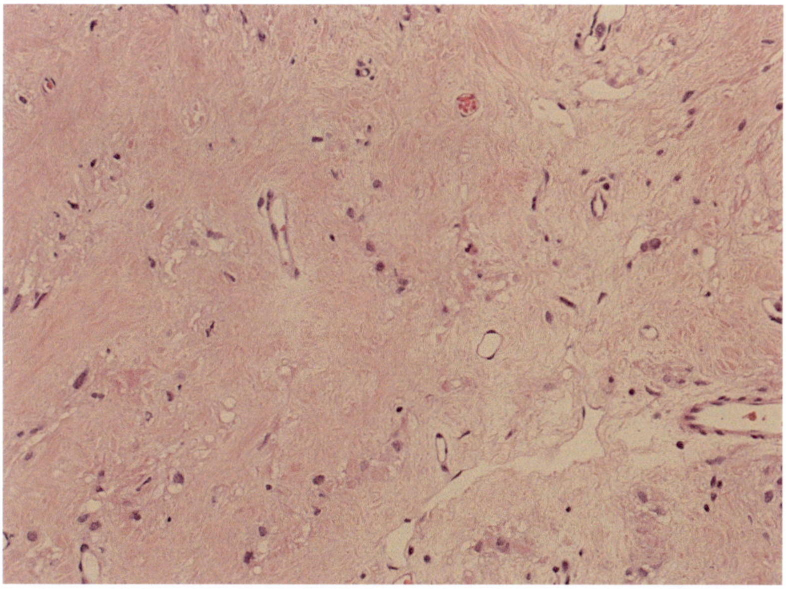

Fig. 2.112 Hypocellular area of a pecoma of the urinary bladder

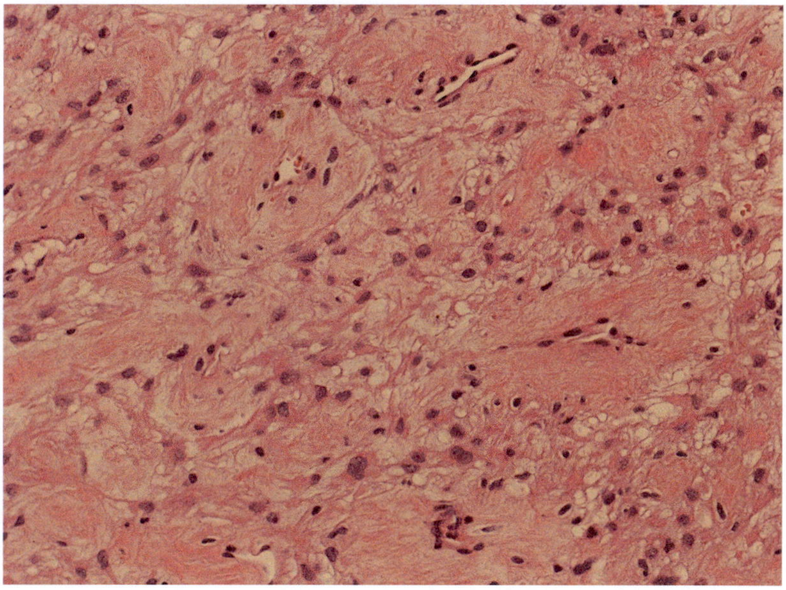

Fig. 2.113 Hypocellular area of a pecoma of the urinary bladder with hyalinized vessels wall

- The tumor appears as a circumscribed mass, often arising from the lateral wall, beneath a normal mucosa. It may or may not extend into the perivesical fat. Histologically, schwannoma consists of spindle cells with uniform round to oval nuclei arranged in a palisading or organoid pattern.
- There is no nuclear pleomorphism and mitotic figures are infrequent. Tumor cells show positive immunostaining for S-100 protein, neuron-specific enolase, and vimentin. Immunostains for myoglobin, keratins, actin (HHF-35), and desmin are negative.

Primitive neuroectodermal tumor

- Primary primitive neuroectodermal tumor (PNET) of the bladder is an extremely rare and aggressive neoplasm. It is morphologically a small round blue cell tumor without rosette formation and with extensive areas of necrosis. Tumor cells show strong expression

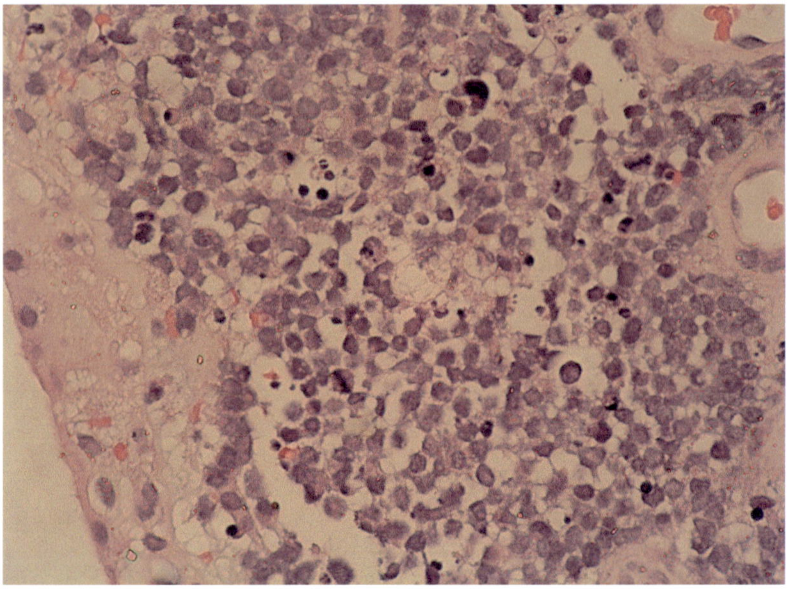

Fig. 2.114 Small cell proliferation with necrosis characteristic of peripheral neuroectodermal tumor

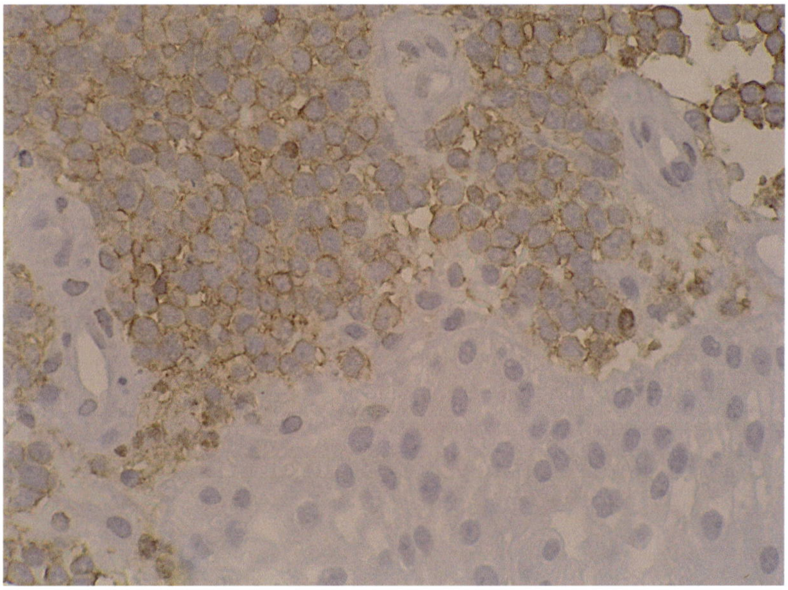

Fig. 2.115 CD99 positive peripheral neuroectodermal tumor. Overlying urothelium is negative

of CD99, vimentin, and CD117 (c-kit), and focal reactivity to cytokeratin and S-100 protein (Figs. 2.114 and 2.115).

- Ultrastructural study reveals sparse neurosecretory granules. Molecular genetic analysis supports the diagnosis of PNET by showing the EWS/FLI-1 fusion transcript type 2 by RT-PCR and EWS gene rearrangement by FISH. A patient treated with imatinib following systemic chemotherapy and radical surgery remains alive after 8 years follow-up.

Malignant peripheral nerve sheath tumor (MPNST)

- Malignant peripheral nerve sheath tumor is rare in the urinary bladder. Only a few cases have been documented, predominantly in patients less than 40 years old. Some have arisen in the setting of neurofibromatosis type 1, possibly originating in neurofibromas of autonomic nerve plexuses in the bladder wall. MPNST is typically a highly malignant and rapidly growing tumor.

- Patients present with hematuria, and a suprapubic mass is sometimes noted. The lesion has been seen arising from the trigone, as well as from the lateral and posterior walls of the bladder. It may form multiple large nodules with surface ulceration and areas of necrosis. The tumor may infiltrate the entire thickness of the bladder wall, involving perivesical soft tissues or pelvic peritoneum. Distant metastases may be present at diagnosis.
- Prognosis is generally poor with local recurrence or distant metastases often evident within 2 months of initial surgical resection.

Pathology

- MPNST is a poorly differentiated tumor that grows in sheets and nodules consisting of interlacing fascicles of malignant spindle cells. The tumor cells are pleomorphic, with variable amounts of eosinophilic cytoplasm. Most have a single nucleus, but multinucleated tumor cells may be present.
- Nuclei are round to oval with prominent irregular eosinophilic nucleoli, or elongated and tapered with marked atypia. Mitotic activity may be moderate. An extensive infiltrate of acute and chronic inflammatory cells, including eosinophils, may be present. An epithelioid variant as well as a variant with rhabdomyoblastic differentiation, (malignant triton tumor) have been described.

Immunohistochemistry

- Immunohistochemical stains can help with the identification of this tumor, which typically shows positive immunostaining for S-100 protein and vimentin, and focally positive staining for neuron-specific enolase (NSE). It usually does not stain for epithelial membrane antigen (EMA), cytokeratin AE1/AE3, muscle-specific actin, desmin, myoglobin, cytokeratin, chromogranin, or neurofilament.
- In one case, rhabdomyoblastic differentiation with focal immunostaining for myoglobin was identified in a tumor that arose in an infant with neurofibromatosis type 1.
- The differential diagnosis of this tumor includes epithelioid sarcoma, undifferentiated carcinoma, melanoma, epithelioid angiosarcoma, rhabdoid tumor, carcinosarcoma, and epithelioid leiomyosarcoma. Immunoreactivity to HMB45 or Melan-A, or strong diffuse S100 protein immunoreactivity would favor melanoma.
- Carcinosarcoma would show evidence of epithelial differentiation with immunoreactivity for cytokeratins and EMA. Unlike epithelioid sarcoma, tumor cells of MPNST are immunoreactive for S-100 protein, focally immunoreactive for NSE, and are not immunoreactive for EMA or cytokeratins. Immunohistochemistry can also be used to help rule out endothelial, muscular and neuroendocrine differentiation as well as anaplastic lymphoma.

Leiomyosarcoma

- Leiomyosarcoma is the most common malignant mesenchymal tumor of the urinary bladder in adults. It is rare but has been reported in patients ranging from 15 to 75 years of age. There is male predominance.
- Some leiomyosarcomas develop a number of years after the administration of cyclophosphamide. Acrolein, a degradation product of cyclophosphamide, is thought to be the causative agent.
- Patients present with gross hematuria, obstructive voiding symptoms, dysuria, or abdominal mass. Most often the tumor is located in the dome of the bladder, and less frequently in the lateral walls.
- Grossly, the tumor is large, unencapsulated, often polypoid with surface ulceration, and exhibits invasive growth involving all layers of the bladder. The cut surface is usually firm or fleshy with a fibrous or myxoid appearance. Some are hemorrhagic, with varying degrees of necrosis.

Pathology

- Interlacing bundles and fascicles of elongated, eosinophilic cytoplasmic processes and spindled to elongate hyperchromatic nuclei are common. High grade lesions have significant nuclear pleomorphism with hyperchromasia and irregular nuclear membranes (Fig. 2.116).

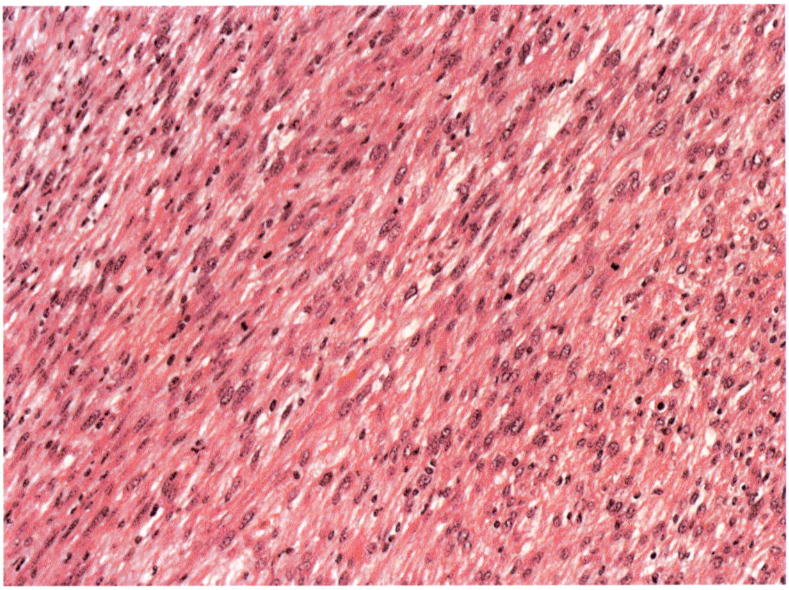

Fig. 2.116 Microscopic features of leiomyosarcoma of the bladder with high mitotic index

- Pleomorphic, vesicular nuclei with macronucleoli and frequent bizarre mitotic figures, interspersed with some multinucleate giant cells characterize high grade lesions. The pleomorphism of high grade leiomyosarcoma is usually identifiable at low power, along with tumor cell necrosis, increased mitotic activity, and infiltration of the muscularis propria.
- Grading influences prognosis, and is based on the degree of cytologic atypia and mitotic activity. Low grade leiomyosarcoma has fewer than 5 mitoses per HPF, mild to moderate cytologic atypia, minimal necrosis and an infiltrative margin.
- High grade leiomyosarcoma has more than 5 mitoses per HPF, moderate to marked cytologic atypia and may show abundant necrosis.
- Several morphologic variants including myxoid and epithelioid types have been described. Myxoid leiomyosarcoma may contain moderate numbers of thin-walled blood vessels, and epitheliod leiomyosarcoma has rounded tumor cells, which occasionally exhibit clear and vacuolated cyotoplasm.
- Immunohistochemically, leiomyosarcomas usually stain positively for vimentin, with variable staining for SMA (43–100 %), and desmin (0–60 %). Infrequently, they show positive immunostaining with epithelial markers including cytokeratins (CAM5.2, AE1/AE3) (10 %) and epithelial membrane antigen (5 %). ALK-1 immunostain is usually negative.
- Leiomyosarcoma must be differentiated from several other tumors, including leiomyoma, sarcomatoid carcinoma, rhabdomyosarcoma, postoperative spindle cell tumor and pseudosarcomatous myofibroblastic proliferations. Sarcomatoid carcinoma can be recognized if one is aware of a history of a high-grade urothelial carcinoma or of concurrent urothelial in situ or invasive carcinoma.
- Therefore, extensive tissue sampling is recommended before rendering a diagnosis of leiomyosarcoma in the bladder. Sarcomatoid carcinoma is typically immunopositive for low molecular weight cytokeratin and EMA and usually immunonegative for myogenous markers such as desmin and SMA, although in rare cases with muscle differentiation, these markers may be diffusely positive.
- While leiomyosarcomas may show cytokeratin immunoreactivity, the staining is usually focal and weak. Another differential consideration, rhabdomyosarcoma, may have a myxoid appearance but this tumor is extremely rare in adults. Features of rhabdomyosarcoma include the presence of cross-striations and/or

a cambium layer, as well as positive staining for myogenin.

Rhabdomyosarcoma

- Rhabdomyosarcoma is infrequently seen in the urinary bladder, and the great majority occurs during childhood and adolescence. Only a few cases of bladder rhabdomyosarcoma in adults have been reported. Rhabdomyosarcoma is the most frequent malignant tumor of the bladder in children. Children with neurofibromatosis type 1 have an increased prevalence of rhabdomyosarcoma with a predominance of bladder or prostate primaries.
- Patients with rhabdomyosarcoma classically present with hematuria; some have obstructive voiding symptoms, and in some cases an abdominal mass is evident. The most frequent site of involvement is adjacent to the trigone.
- Several histologic variants of rhabdomyosarcoma are seen in the bladder, with embryonal type, including the botryoid subtype, being the most common.
- Grossly, rhabdomyosarcoma, including the sarcoma botryoides variant, appears as a polypoid gelatinous and lobulated mass protruding into bladder lumen with variable hemorrhage and necrosis. The shiny, lobulated, grape-like appearance of the most common type of bladder sarcoma in children is the source of the name sarcoma botryoides.
- Most tumors have a superficial covering epithelium. The botryoid subtype of embryonal RMS demonstrates a "cambium" layer, or condensed layer of small round rhabdomyoblasts under the intact epithelium. The main tumor mass in botryoid rhabdo-myosarcoma may be a pauci-cellular myxoid tumor. These hypocellular areas may be admixed with more cellular areas, especially where the tumor infiltrates deeply into the muscle wall.
- Histologically, well differentiated tumor cells (rhabdomyoblasts) have hyperchromatic small nuclei. The cells are small and elongated with frequent cross-striations. Less differentiated rhabdomyoblasts have medium-sized or large, irregularly shaped hyperchromatic nuclei with a small rim of cytoplasm and a high mitotic rate. Often atypical mitotic figures and bizarre cells are seen.
- A rare variant reported to occur in the bladder is alveolar rhabdomyosarcoma. This sarcoma has closely packed alveolar spaces separated by thin fibrovascular septa lined by a single layer of cuboidal hyperchromatic tumor cells. The polygonal cells lining the fibrovascular septa have a hobnail appearance, with nuclei projecting away from the basement membrane. Tumor cells floating in the alveolar spaces have been described.
- The solid type of alveolar rhabdomyosarcoma grows in confluent sheets, but the cells are similar to those of the classic pattern. Mixed alveolar and embryonal types occur, and their biologic behavior is similar to that of pure alveolar RMS. The botryoid subtype, which tends not to infiltrate deeply into the muscle, are associated with an overall excellent prognosis. Deeply infiltrating embryonal RMS and alveolar RMS, on the other hand, often portend a poor prognosis even with modern multimodality therapy.
- Immunohistochemical stains of rhabdomyosarcoma usually show positivity for desmin, MyoD1 or myogenin. Also, muscle-specific actin, myoglobin, and myosin may be positive. Rhabdomyoblasts may stain for neuron-specific enolase and infrequently for cytokeratin. The alveolar variant has been reported to stain focally with S-100. The differential diagnosis of bladder rhabdomyosarcoma includes pseudosarcomatous myofibroblastic tumor, leiomyosarcoma, neurofibroma and sarcomatoid carcinoma.

Angiosarcoma

- Angiosarcoma of the bladder is exceedingly rare and carries a very poor prognosis with most patients died of disease within two years of diagnosis. Angiosarcoma can arise in any part of the bladder. The age at presentation ranges from 38 to 85 years. There is a male predominance.
- The development of angiosarcoma has been linked to certain environmental exposures including vinyl chloride, arsenic, and therapeutic irradiation. All cases have presented

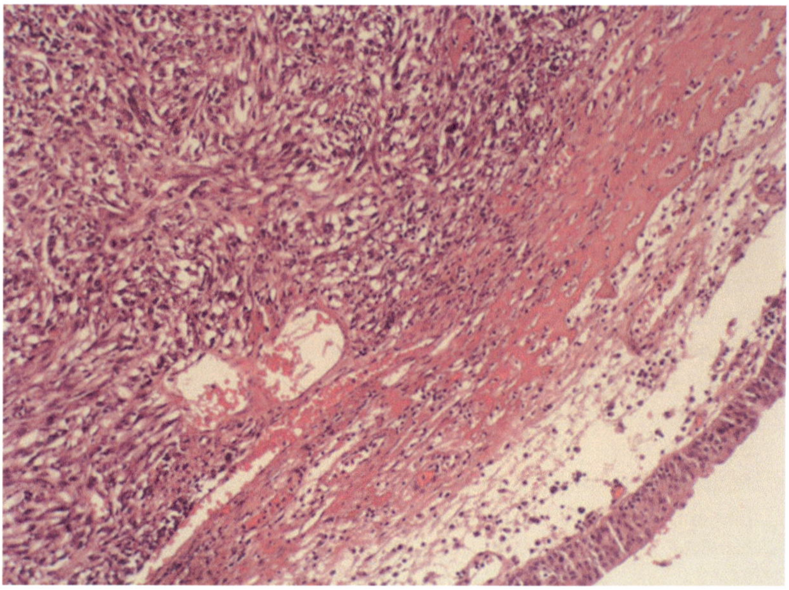

Fig. 2.117 Malignant fibrohistiocytoma of the bladder (low power)

with hematuria. Other reported symptoms include flank or groin pain and dysuria. The disease has often extended locally beyond the bladder or metastasized at time of presentation. Frequent sites of metastasis are lung and liver.

- Histologically, angiosarcoma of the bladder is composed of anastomosing vascular channels lined by atypical endothelial cells. The endothelial cells often are pleomorphic with large hyperchromatic nuclei, prominent nucleoli and abundant mitotic figures. The vascular lining cells may protrude into the lumen imparting a hobnail appearance. There may be no intervening stroma. The vascular channels range in size from small capillaries to sinusoidal spaces.
- A solid growth pattern of monomorphic epithelioid cells with vesicular chromatin and moderate eosinophilic cytoplasm arranged in sheets and nests has been described. Infiltration into the deep muscle layer may be present with either vascular or solid growth patterns.
- Immunohistochemically, angiosarcoma stains positively for vimentin, CD31, and CD34. Cytokeratins may be positive. The differential diagnosis for angiosarcoma of the bladder is hemangioma, which is usually small and lacks cytologic atypia, anastomosing channels, and solid areas. Kaposi sarcoma may be seen in the urinary bladder, especially in immunocompromised patients. The differential also includes high grade urothelial carcinoma.

Malignant fibrous histiocytoma (undifferentiated sarcoma)

- Primary malignant fibrous histiocytoma (MFH) of the bladder is rare. It occurs most commonly in men from 45 to 79 years of age, with gross hematuria at time of presentation. The tumor is often large at presentation and involves all layers of the bladder wall.
- The overlying urothelium may be either normal or ulcerated. Four morphologic variants are recognized, including myxoid, inflammatory, storiform-fascicular, and pleomorphic types. Histologically, these tumors are composed of spindled or polygonal cells with variably sized oval to round nuclei. The nuclei have coarse chromatin and prominent nucleoli. Mitotic activity is usually moderate to high. Multinucleated giant cells are scattered throughout. Inflammatory type malignant fibrous histiocytoma is characterized by an abundance of inflammatory cells, especially neutrophils infiltrating between fascicles of tumor cells (Figs. 2.117, 2.118, 2.119, and 2.120).

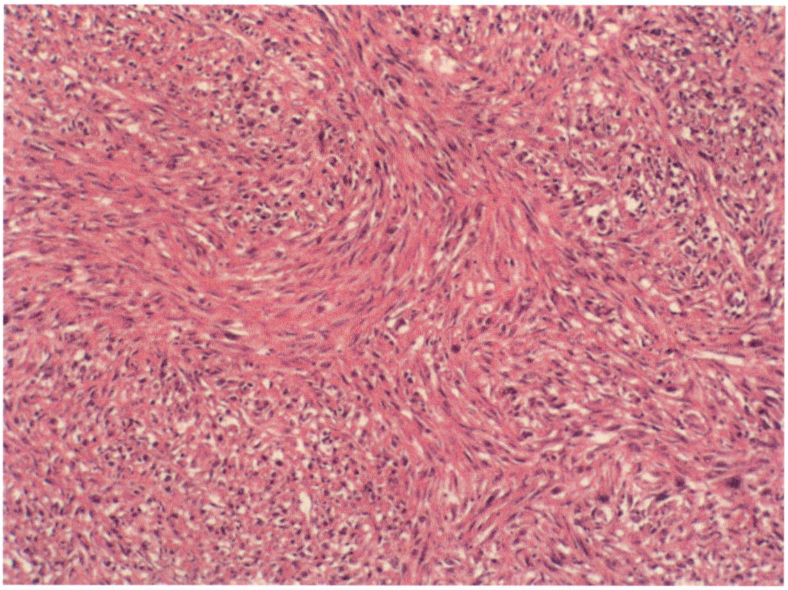

Fig. 2.118 Malignant fibrohistiocytoma of the bladder with storiform pattern

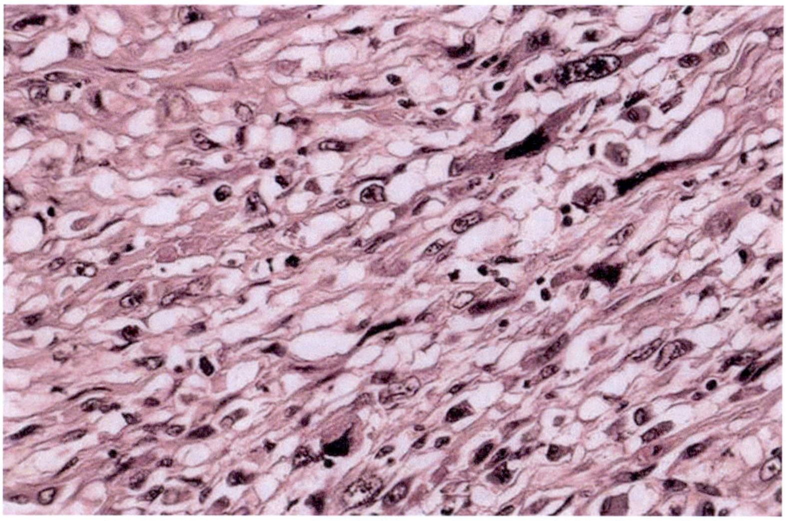

Fig. 2.119 Pleomorphic malignant fibrohistiocytoma of the bladder

- Immunohistochemical stains can help differentiate malignant fibrous histiocytoma from other spindle cell neoplasms in the bladder. Typically, malignant fibrous histiocytoma is nonreactive for cytokeratin. It is often reactive for vimentin, alpha-1-antichymotrypsin, and focally reactive for CD68.
- Several tumors enter into the differential diagnosis of malignant fibrous histiocytoma. Sarcomatoid carcinoma of the bladder may have a similar appearance, but an epithelial component immunoreactive to cytokeratin and EMA is usually identifiable in sarcomatoid carcinoma.
- Differentiating malignant fibrous histiocytoma from pseudosarcomatous myofibroblastic tumor or postoperative spindle cell nodule may be difficult. Mixed acute and chronic inflammatory cells and a history of a surgical procedure favors post-operative spindle cell nodule. Malignant fibrous histiocytoma of the bladder is a highly aggressive tumor with a high local recurrence rate and frequent metastasis.

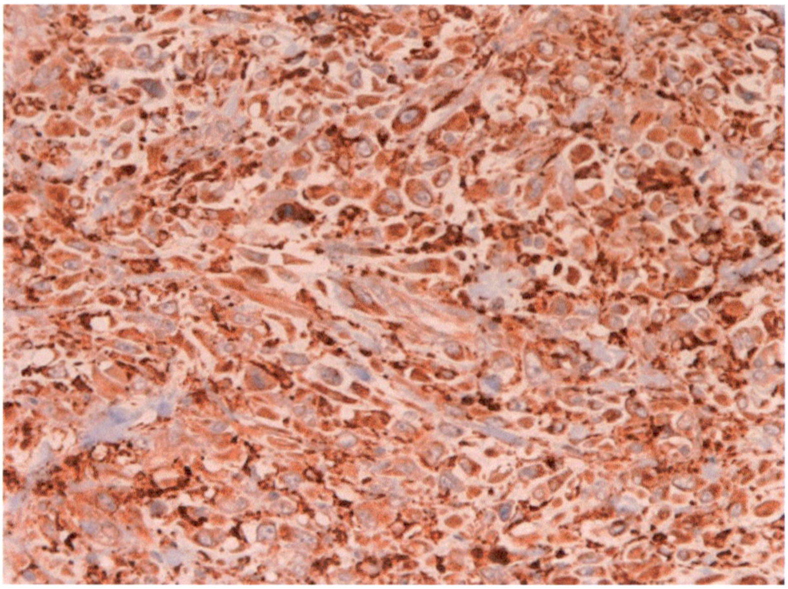

Fig. 2.120 CD68 positive expression in malignant fibrohistiocytoma of the bladder

Osteosarcoma

- Defined as a malignant tumour showing osteoid production, osteosarcoma of the urinary bladder occurs in male patients 60–65 years of age. Some have a history of radiation therapy for urothelial carcinoma. Most osteosarcomas arise in the trigone region. Hematuria, dysuria, urinary frequency, and recurrent urinary tract infections are the most common presenting symptoms.
- Osteosarcoma of the urinary bladder presents as a solitary, large, polypoid, gritty, often deeply invasive, variably hemorrhagic mass. Histologically, tumors are composed of cytologically malignant cells surrounding variably calcified, woven bone lamellae. Foci of chondrosarcomatous differentiation or spindle cell areas may also be observed. The cytologic atypia differentiates osteosarcoma from stromal osseous metaplasia occurring in some urothelial carcinomas.
- By definition, a recognizable malignant epithelial component is diagnostic of sarcomatoid carcinoma (carcinosarcoma) even when osteoid is present. Urothelial sarcomatiod carcinoma is the most important differential diagnostic consideration for osteosarcoma of the bladder.
- Osteosarcoma of the urinary tract is an aggressive tumour associated with a poor prognosis. The majority of patients have advanced stage at presentation and die of disease within 6 months, often with lung metastases. The stage of the disease at time of diagnosis is the best predictor of survival.

Other rare soft tissue tumors arising in the bladder

- Other malignant mesenchymal neoplasms such as malignant peripheral nerve sheath tumor, lipoma and liposarcoma, chondrosarcoma, hemangiopericytoma, and Kaposi sarcoma may rarely involve the bladder. The diagnosis requires that bladder involvement by direct extension from another site be excluded.
- In the case of primary chondrosarcoma of the bladder, sarcomatoid carcinoma must be excluded. Immunostaining for cytokeratin is negative.
- A single case report on alveolar soft part sarcoma arising in the bladder has been reported. The tumor showed strong nuclear immunoreactivity for TFE3.

2.2.9 Malignant Melanoma

- Malignant melanoma may occur in the urinary bladder as a primary or metastatic

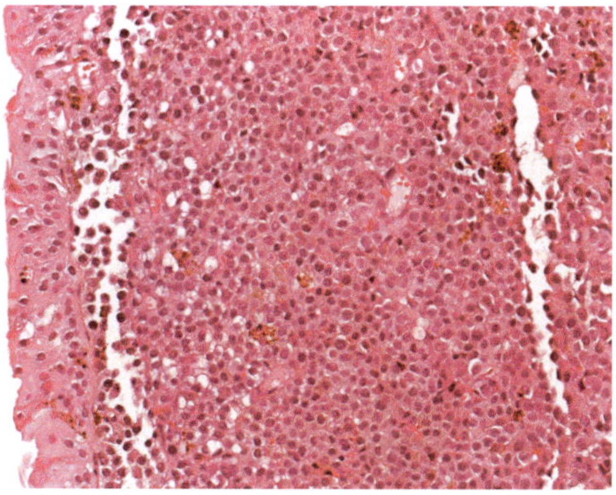

Fig. 2.121 Malignant melanoma of the urinary bladder

tumour. All patients have been adults, with men and women being equally affected. Gross hematuria is the most frequent presenting symptom but some patients with bladder melanoma have presented with symptomatic metastases.

- Metastatic melanoma in the bladder is much more common than melanoma primary in the bladder. The generally accepted criteria for determining that melanoma is primary in the bladder are: lack of a cutaneous lesion history, failure to find a regressed melanoma of the skin, failure to find a different visceral primary, and pattern of spread consistent with bladder primary.
- Almost all of the tumours have appeared darkly pigmented at cystoscopy and on gross pathologic examination. Their sizes range from less than 1 to 8 cm. Histologically, the tumours show classic features of malignant melanoma: pleomorphic nuclei, spindle and polygonal cytoplasmic contours, and intracytoplasmic melanin pigment. Pigment production is variable and may be absent (Fig. 2.121).
- One example of clear cell melanoma has been reported. A few of the tumours are associated with melanosis of the vesical epithelium. One malignant melanoma arose in a bladder diverticulum.
- Immunohistochemical procedures have shown positive reactions with antibodies to S-100 protein and with HMB-45 or Melan A.

2.2.10 Germ Cell Tumors

- A number of germ cell neoplasms may arise rarely in the bladder, including dermoid cyst, teratoma, seminoma, choriocarcinoma, and yolk sac tumor. Rare cases of teratoma arising in the bladder have been described in both adults and children. Dermoid cyst typically occurs in women between 30 and 49 years of age who present with nonspecific bladder symptoms. Typical histologic features include calcifications and structures consistent with hair and/or teeth or other differentiated elements.
- Pure choriocarcinoma of the bladder in the absence of recognizable papillary or solid urothelial carcinoma is a rare, and is associated with an aggressive clinical course. Diagnostic features include syncytiotrophoblastic giant cells and cytotrophoblast cells that display human chorionic gonadotropin (HCG) immunoreactivity.
- Chriocarcinoma should not be confused with urothelial carcinoma with syncytiotrophoblastic giant cells (see previous discussion). One reported case had isochromosome 12 by fluorescence in situ hybridization. Patients usually have symptoms typical of other bladder cancers, including hematuria, dysuria and frequency. Some male patients may have gynecomastia. Increased urinary levels of HCG may be present in some patients.

2.2.11 Hematologic Malignancies

- Malignant lymphoma may occur in the urinary bladder as a primary lesion or as part of a systemic disease. Lymphomas constitute less than 1 % of bladder neoplasms. Secondary involvement of the bladder is common (12–20 %) in advanced stage systemic lymphoma.
- Bladder lymphomas may form solitary (70 %) or multiple (20 %) masses at cystoscopy. Occasionally there may be diffuse thickening (10 %) of the bladder wall. Ulceration is rare (<20 %) in primary, but common in secondary lesions. Frankly hemorrhagic changes of the

mucosa have been observed. Schistosomiasis may be associated with a T-cell lymphoma of the bladder.

- Papillary urothelial tumors may present simultaneously with bladder lymphoma, either primary or secondary. Primary marginal zone B-cell lymphoma of mucosa-associated lymphoid tissue (MALT lymphoma) of the bladder has an excellent prognosis after therapy. Lymphoepithelial lesions may be seen and they should not confused with lymmphoepithelioma-like carcinoma or lymphoid rich variant urothelial carcinoma.
- Other types of primary bladder lymphoma, such as Burkitt lymphoma, T-cell lymphoma, Hodgkin lymphoma and plasmacytoma are very rare. Among secondary bladder lymphomas, diffuse large B-cell lymphoma is the single most frequent histological subtype, followed by follicular, small cell, low grade MALT, mantle cell, Burkitt and Hodgkin lymphoma. Involvement of the urinary bladder by acute myeloid leukemia (granulocytic sarcoma or myeloid sarcoma) is rare and relevant clinical data and high index of suspicion are critical to avoid misdiagnosis.

2.2.12 Tumor-Like Conditions

Papillary-polypoid cystitis

- May be clinically and microscopically mistaken for papillary urothelial carcinoma. The designation papillary cystitis is used when thin finger-like papillae are present, and polypoid cystitis refers to lesions with edematous and broad-based papillae. In both, there is typically abundant chronic inflammation in the stroma accompanied by prominent and often ectatic blood vessels.
- In bullous cystitis, the lesion is wider than lesions of polypoid or papillary cystitis. Long-standing cases of polypoid cystitis may have a fibrous rather than edematous stroma.
- Occasionally Papillary-Polypoid Cystitis may be associated with reactive and metaplastic changes in the overlying or adjacent urothelium with squamous metaplasia being the most common. The urothelium may be hyperplastic, but it lacks cytologic atypia. Occasionally the overlying urothelium can take the appearance of a pseudocarcinomatous epithelial hyperplasia.
- Papillary-Polypoid cystitis should be differentiated from low grade papillary urothelial carcinoma. Two clinical settings suggest that an exophytic bladder lesion is reactive or inflammatory: patients with an indwelling catheter, and those with vesical fistula (Figs. 2.122, 2.123, 2.124, 2.125, 2.126, 2.127, 2.128, 2.129, 2.130, and 2.131).

Encrusted Cystitis

- This uncommon condition occurs when urea-splitting organisms alkalinize the urine, creating superficial deposits of inorganic salts. In rare instances, encrusted cystitis may mimic a neoplasm. Microscopically, calcified deposits are mixed with fibrin and necrotic debris on the mucosal surface or submucosa; muscle involvement is uncommon

Xanthogranulomatous cystitis

- Sheets of foamy histiocytes, often admixed with other inflammatory cells, without well formed granulomas that lack Michaelis-Gutman bodies.

Malakoplaquia

- Inflammatory lesion that is caused by impaired intraphagosomal digestion resulting in histiocytis accumulation. In the bladder is typically associated with a bacterial infection related to E Coli.
- On gross examination, are typically soft yellow plaques. Histologically, it consist of sheets of histiocytes with granular eosinophilic cytoplasm called von Hanseman cells. These cells have small basophilic intracytoplasmic inclusions (Michaelis-Gutmann bodies).

BCG granuloma

- BCG induces a marked inflammatory response with denudation of the urothelium. The lamina propria typically shows a mixed inflammatory infiltrate and small epithelioid granulomas showing multinucleated giant cells.

Squamous metaplasia

- Squamous metaplasia is a frequent finding in patients with *Schistosomia haematobium*

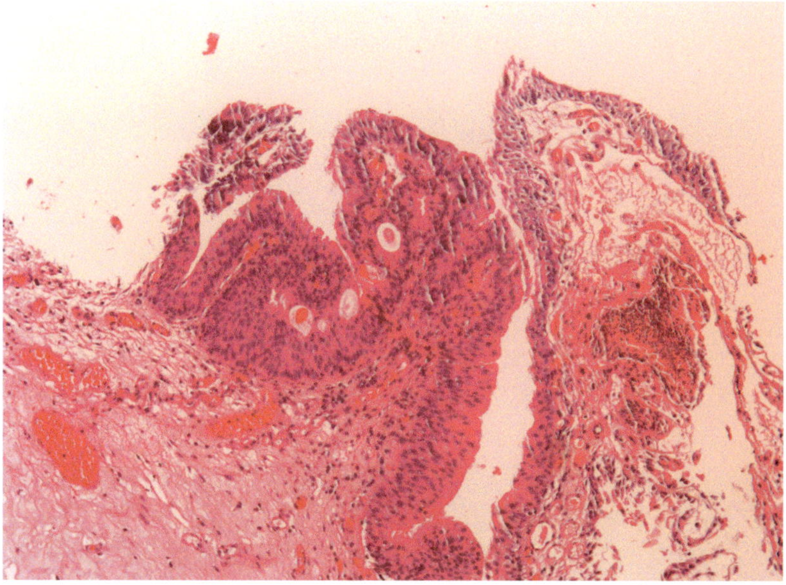

Fig. 2.122 Cystitis papillary-polypoid

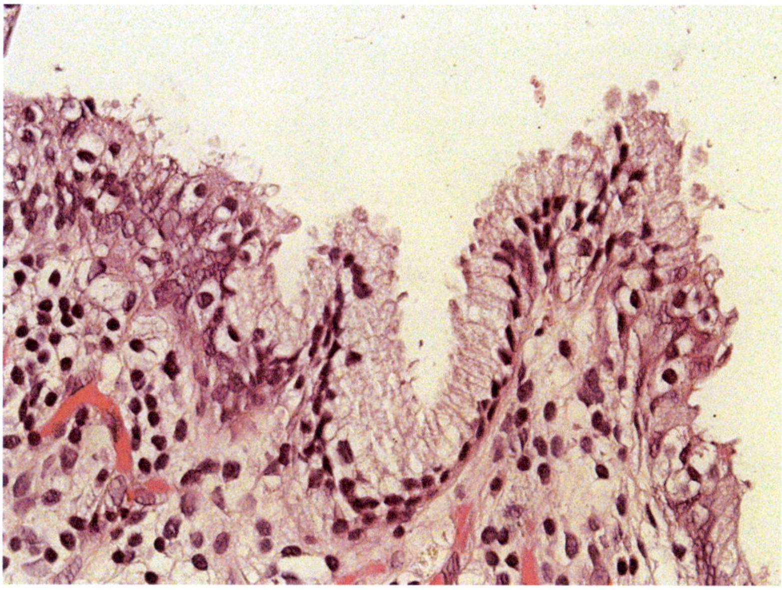

Fig. 2.123 Bladder endocervicosis

infection, nonfunctioning bladder, exstrophy, or severe chronic cystitis. It is more common in women than men, and often occurs on the anterior wall.

- At cystoscopy, the mucosa is thickened and typically white or gray-white. Microscopically, there is squamous mucosa of variable thickness that is often covered by a layer of keratin. Cytologic atypia is uncommon, but may include dysplasia or carcinoma in situ, raising the possibility of invasive carcinoma elsewhere in the specimen.
- Squamous metaplasia should be distinguished from nonkeratinizing glycogenated squamous epithelium, similar to that of the vaginal type, which is a normal finding in the trigone and bladder neck in up to 86 % of women.

Cistitis glandularis et cystica

- Cystitis glandularis is thought to arise from Brunn's nests, similar to cystitis cystica and is

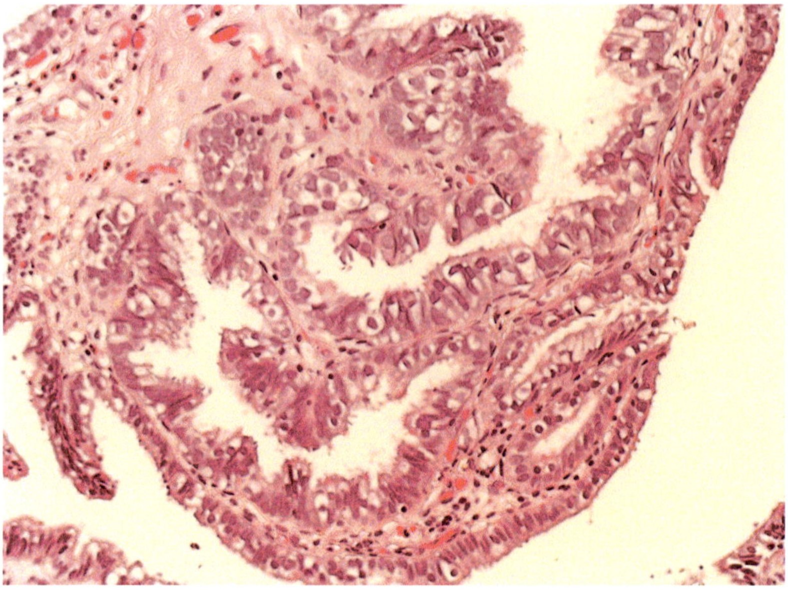

Fig. 2.124 Bladder endosalpingiosis

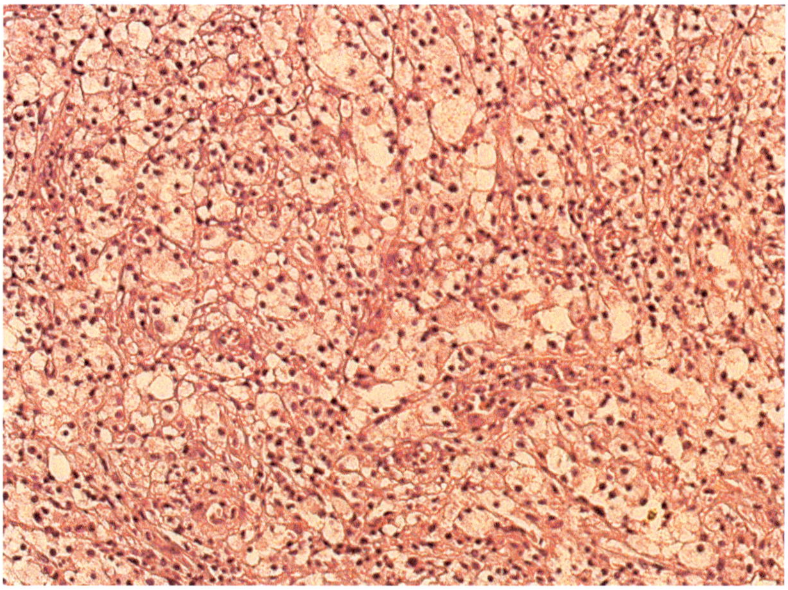

Fig. 2.125 Cystitis xanthogranulomatosa

frequently associated with voiding symptoms. Cystitis glandularis is characterized by a central lining of cuboidal or columnar cells surrounded by layers of urothelial cells and some authors believe to be a metaplastic change of the urothelial lining in response to chronic inflammation or irritation.

- It is present in 71 % of serially sectioned bladders, and, like von Brunn's nests, is most common in the trigone. It may be responsible for unusual bladder masses in children, and rare cases are associated with pelvic lipomatosis. Cystitis glandularis is present in some patients with neuropathic bladder and chronic indwelling urinary catheter.
- These lesions have characteristic immunostaining with CK7, similar to normal urothelium, and lack of expression for CDX2 and CK20, markers associated with intestinal differentiation.

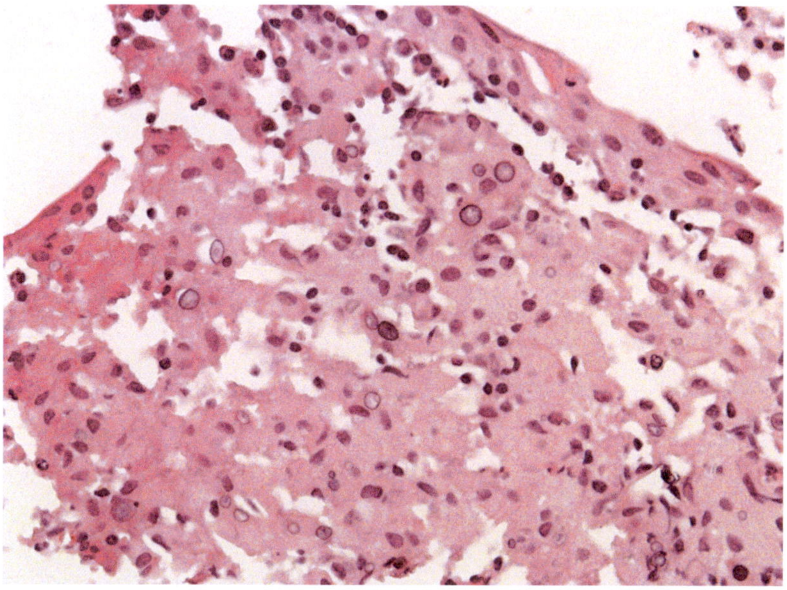

Fig. 2.126 Malakoplaquia

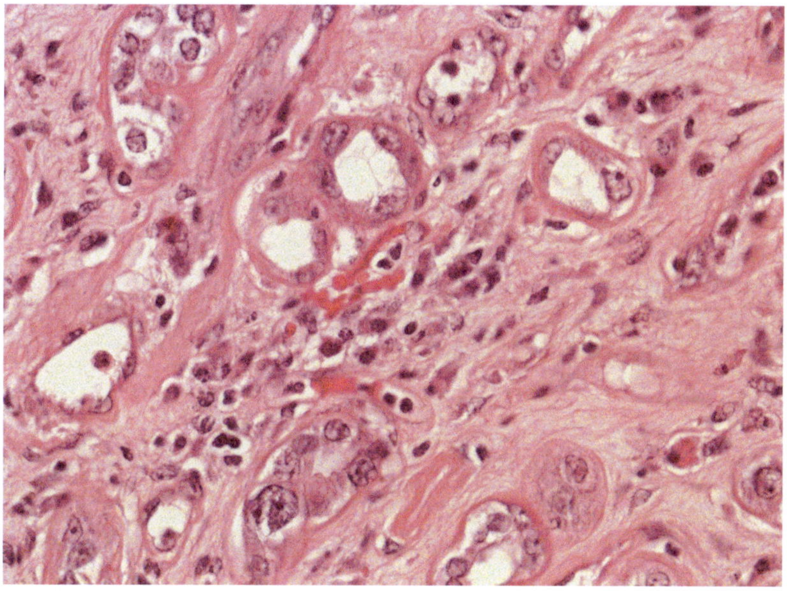

Fig. 2.127 Nephrogenic adenoma with nuclear atypia

Intestinal metaplasia

- Consists of tall columnar and goblet cells with prominent mucin production resembling colonic epithelium. Paneth and neuroendocrine cells are present. Atypia and mitosis are not a common feature of intestinal metaplasia of the bladder.
- A form off intestinal metaplasia with polypoid appearance has been described as lorid cystitis glandularis, is usually an incidental finding, and is distinguished from adenocarcinoma by the lack of stromal infiltration and absence of marked cytologic abnormalities.

Nephrogenic adenoma

- Nephrogenic metaplasia (adenoma) is most common in the bladder (55 % of cases) but may also involve the urethra (41 %) and ureter (4 %). It usually occurs in adults men. Most patients have a history of an operative procedure or one or more irritants including calculi,

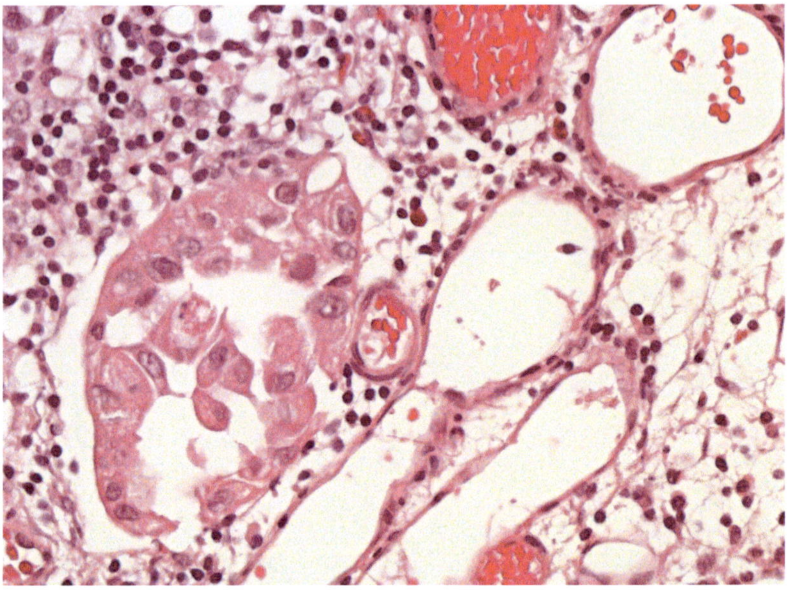

Fig. 2.128 Nephrogenic adenoma with nuclear atypia

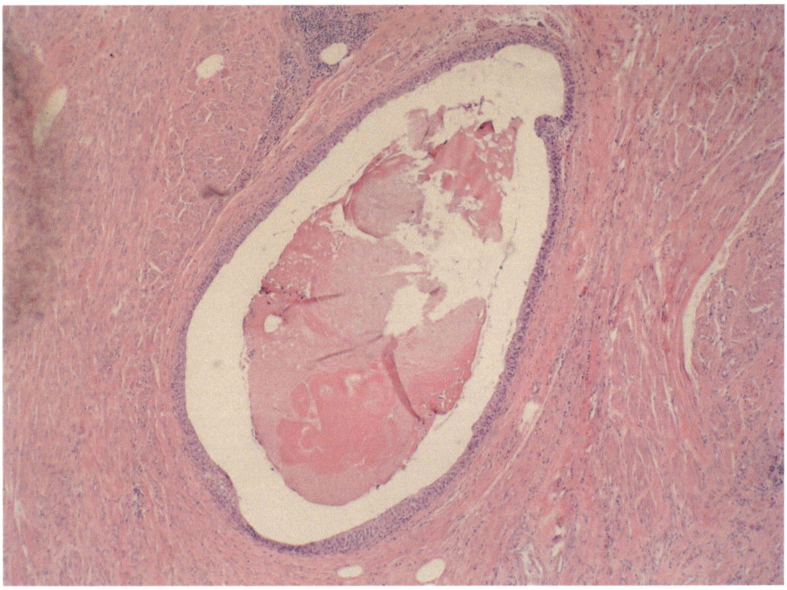

Fig. 2.129 Urachal cyst

trauma, cystitis, and tuberculosis. About 8 % of patients have undergone kidney transplantation; in these patients, cells of nephrogenic adenoma derive from tubular cells of the renal transplant, and are not metaplastic proliferations of the recipient's bladder urothelium.

- Microscopically, tubules are the most common histologic finding, but the proliferation may also be cystic, polypoid, papillary, and, rarely, diffuse. The tubules appear as small, round, hollow acini reminiscent of renal tubules. They are occasionally solid and surrounded by a prominent basement membrane that is highlighted by periodic acid-Schiff stain. The tubules frequently become dilated and cystic, but may also appear as near-solid nests.
- The lumens often contain eosinophilic or basophilic secretions that are weakly mucicarminophilic. Most of the cells lining the

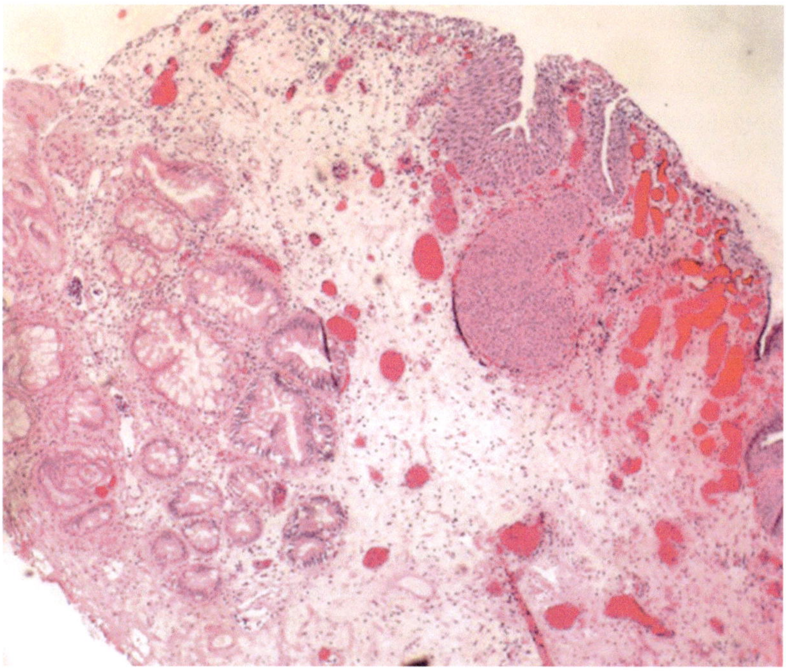

Fig. 2.130 Intestinal metaplasia

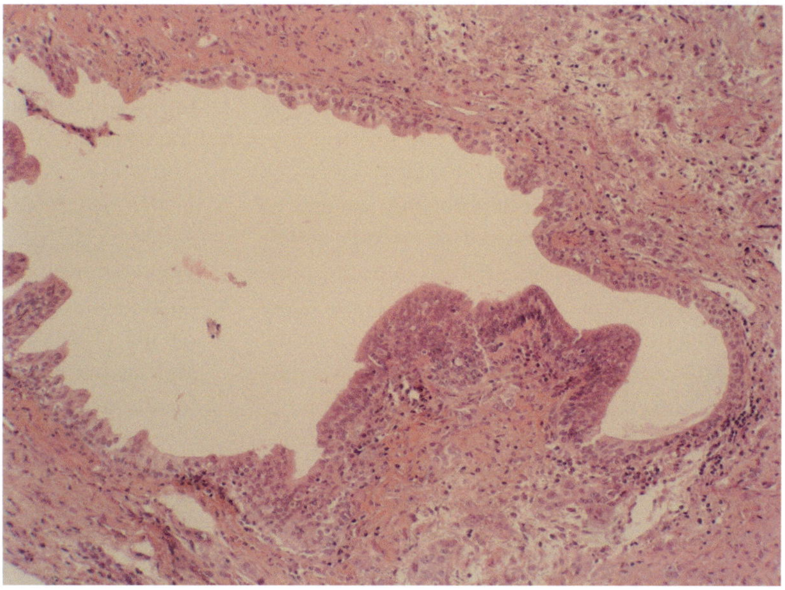

Fig. 2.131 Mullerian cyst

tubules, cysts, and papillae are cuboidal or low columnar with scant cytoplasm; occasionally, the cells have abundant clear cytoplasm. Hobnail cells line the tubules and cysts in up to 70 % of cases, and large cysts may be lined by flattened cells. Small amounts of mucin may be present in the cells of nephrogenic metaplasia, but glycogen is usually scant or absent. Nuclear abnormalities are uncommon and, when present, appear reactive or degenerative.

- Mitotic figures are rare or absent. The stroma is typically described as edematous with a variable infiltrate of inflammatory cells, sometimes prominent. Other stromal features sometimes include dilated vessels, calcification, amyloid-like plaque, or multinucleate giant cells. There is often marked chronic cystitis which may partially obscure nephrogenic metaplasia; squamous and glandular metaplasia may coexist with nephrogenic metaplasia.

- Rare cases of nephrogenic metaplasia are associated with prominent stromal calcification, malacoplakia, or cytomegalovirus infection.
- The most common differential diagnostic considerations of nephrogenic metaplasia are adenocarcinoma, and urothelial carcinoma with pseudoglandular differentiation.
- In some cases, the metaplasia is composed of minute mucin-containing tubules lined by single cells with compressed nuclei that simulates signet-ring cell carcinoma. Hobnail cells suggest the possibility of clear cell carcinoma of the bladder, but such cells are focally present in 70 % of cases of nephrogenic metaplasia. Solid tubules with cells containing clear cytoplasm also suggest clear cell carcinoma, but this is an uncommon and focal finding in nephrogenic metaplasia.
- Histopathologic features that favor clear cell adenocarcinoma over nephrogenic metaplasia include a predominance of clear cells, severe cytologic atypia, high mitotic rate, the presence of tumor necrosis, high MIB-1 count, and strong staining for p53. When present in the prostatic urethra, nephrogenic metaplasia may be mistaken for prostatic adenocarcinoma.
- In the differential diagnosis of adenocarcinoma, nephrogenic adenoma may be positive for alpha-methylacyl-CoA racemase (AMACR or P504S) it might be confused with prostatic adenocarcinoma, particularly when involving the prostatic urethra.
- Similarly, lesions frequently show absence of high molecular weight cytokeratin and p63, which may falsely confirm this impression.
- Nephrogenic adenoma is positive for PAX-2 and PAX-8.
- Nephrogenic adenoma with cytologic atypia, defined as the presence of nuclear enlargement, hyperchromasia, and prominent nucleoli, these lesions may be highly concerning for malignancy; however, none of reported cases developed bladder carcinoma.
- A rare variant of nephrogenic adenoma admixed with fibromyxoid areas composed of spindled cells resembling fibroblasts or small vessels and a fibromyxoid extracellular matrix, has been reported as fibromyxoid nephrogenic adenoma.
- Nephrogenic adenoma should be differentiated from urothelial carcinoma with small tubules, a rare variant of urothelial carcinoma that demonstrate a marked predominance of small tubules and acini. In differentiation of this lesion from nephrogenic adenoma, morphologic evaluation for the characteristic tubular and papillary components, cuboidal to low-columnar epithelium, and occasional hobnail appearance of nephrogenic adenoma may be helpful.
- Urothelial carcinoma with small tubules may show extensive invasion of the bladder wall in opposition to its bland histology. Urothelial carcinoma with small tubules shows immunoprofile similar to urothelial carcinoma.

Endometriosis

- The bladder is the most common organ (80 %) in the urinary tract to harbor foci of ectopic endometrial tissue. Most cases occur in women during the reproductive years
- Histopathologic diagnosis is typically based on the presence of both endometrial glands and stroma. In some cases these features may be obscured, leading to significant differential diagnostic difficulties.
- The glands observed in these lesions typically resemble those of an inactive or proliferative pattern endometrium, although occasionally a secretory pattern is seen. The stromal component at least focally resembles normal endometrial stroma, although it may be quite inconspicuous or may be obscured by infiltrating histiocytes, either with foamy or hemosiderin-laden cytoplasm
- Awareness of a variety of histologic findings in cases of endometriosis is also important to avoid misdiagnosis. Although overall the process is uncommon in the urinary tract,

endometriosis in general sometimes demonstrates abundant extracellular mucin, postmenopausal changes, or treatment-related changes. Features, that may cause confusion with a glandular malignancy.
- Immunohistochemistry may be helpful in demonstrating endometrial components. Positivity with CD10, similar to normal or neoplastic endometrium may be a useful diagnostic feature, although nonspecific to endometrial tissue. In cases of ureteral endometriosis, it was observed significant positivity for ER, PR, CK7, and CA125 in the epithelial component, with CD10 expression in the stromal component.

Endocervicosis
- The term "endocervicosis" refers to an uncommon glandular tumor-like condition occurring in the bladder of women between 31 and 44 years of age. All reported lesions were diagnostically challenging, and some were misinterpreted as adenocarcinoma. Symptoms include suprapubic pain, dysuria, frequency, or hematuria. Typically arises in the posterior wall and posterior dome of the bladder.
- Microscopically, there is variable extensive involvement of the wall by irregular benign-appearing or mildly atypical endocervical-type glands, some of that are typically cystically dilated. Although the stroma surrounding the glands may demonstrate a constellation of patterns including normal smooth muscle, an acutely and chronically inflamed fibrous cuff, endometrial-type stroma, or elastosis; a desmoplastic response is not present and may help in the discrimination from adenocarcinoma.
- Differentiation from intestinal metaplasia (cystitis glandularis of the intestinal type) may be challenging; however, the architectural pattern of deep muscular involvement in endocervicosis is a contrasting feature to the superficial location of cystitis glandularis. Intestinal metaplasia appears to be composed more uniformly of goblet-type cells with genuine intestinal differentiation, as evidenced by intestinal markers immunohistochemistry.
- Immunohistochemical markers appear likewise to confirm the benign and endocervical origin of these lesions, as at least in the setting of individual cases. In a case report, HBME-1+, estrogen receptor and progesterone receptor exhibited a similar strong pattern of staining in the bladder lesion as compared to control endocervix (heterogeneous staining). DF3, a marker of apomucin MUC1, was strongly positive in both lesional tissue and controls, and low proliferative index with MIB-1 (Ki67), supports the lesion's benign nature.

Endosalpingiosis
- In such cases, the epithelium of a tubal-type component may be lined by low cuboidal, partially ciliated cells, intermingled with intercalated cells and peg cells, similar to endosalpingiosis seen elsewhere.
- Differentiation from atrophic endometriosis (without significant endometrial stroma) may be achieved frequently based on relative abundance or lack of a ciliated cell component.

Mullerianosis
- Collectively referred to as Müllerianosis, sometimes components of endometriosis, endocervicosis, and endosalpingiosis may be seen in varying combination in the bladder

Mullerian cyst
- Cysts observed in men that lie between the bladder and rectum

Amyloidosis
- Primary localized amyloid typically present in lamina propria with vascular involvement. Congo red or thioflavin T stain bladder amyloid which most frequently is AL type (immunoglobulin light chain).

Fallopian tube prolapse
- Fragments of fallopian tube prolapsed into the bladder after fistula secondary to surgery

Hamartoma
- Polypoid lesion composed of foci resembling von Brunn nests, cystitis glandularis, or cystitis cystica dispersed irregularly in a fibrous, muscular or myxoid stroma, that can be focally cellular.

Proteinoma
- Tamm-Horsfall protein may accumulate in the bladder where it produces a tumor-like proteinoma with waxy eosinophilic extracellular material or homogeneous eosinophilic flecks

in areas of fibrinous exudate. It has no clinical significance.

Suture Granuloma

- Granuloma occasionally arises in response to silk sutures introduced at the time of herniorrhaphy, diverticulectomy or other surgical procedure, producing a mass in or adjacent to the bladder. The process primarily involves the bladder wall and perivesical tissue, producing an intraluminal mass visible at cystoscopy. Microscopically, there is a histiocytic reaction to suture with foreign body-giant cells and varying degrees of fibrosis and chronic inflammation.

Collagenoma

- Submucosal accumulation of collagen that is comprised of a dense homogeneous, eosinophilic and acellular material. This occurs as a result of local collagen injections to treat urinary incontinence.

Ectopic prostate

- Also known as prostate-type polyp seen rarely in the bladder trigone that include histologically benign prostatic glands that react with PSA and PAP.

Fibroepithelial polyp

- Rare polypoid lesion that may be seen in the bladder of any age showing edematous stroma with scattered blood vessels and may rarely have atypical stromal cells.

Patent urachus and urachal cyst

- Patent urachus is lined by urothelium or metaplastic epithelium without atypia. Urachal cysts may vary in size. Most are covered by urothelium, flattened attenuated epithelium, or cuboidal/columnar epithelium.

Other tumor-like conditions

- Polyomavirus infection (nuclear inclusion atypia), schistosoma, HPV condyloma, tuberculosis, diverticula (lack of muscle fibers in the wall), paraganglia, postsurgical necrobiotic granuloma, sarcoidosis, giant cell cystitis, follicular cystitis, submucosal ossification and calcification, bladder melanosis, or subepithelial hemorrhage may rarely present as tumor-like condition or being the subject of differential diagnosis with a neoplastic disease.

2.2.13 Metastatic Tumors and Secondary Extension

- The urinary bladder is secondarily involved by a wide spectrum of malignancies. The most common primary sites with direct extension to the bladder and their relative frequencies include colon. (21 %), prostate (19 %), rectum (12 %), and cervix (11 %).
- The most common distant sites of origin of tumors metastatic to the bladder and their relative frequencies are stomach (4 %), skin (4 %), lung (3 %), and breast (2.5 %). Secondary tumor deposits are almost always solitary (97 %), and 54 % of these are located in the bladder neck or trigone. Over half of secondary tumors are adenocarcinomas.
- In terms of differential diagnosis, few secondary tumors have distinctive histological features, making it difficult to make the appropriate diagnosis. Hence knowledge of the history and clinical setting are particularly important in these cases. Immunohistochemistry is useful for distinguishing primary tumors of the urinary bladder from metastases or direct extension from other sites.
- Urothelial carcinoma involving gynecologic organs can be challenging. Immunohistochemistry shows strong CK7 and focal to diffuse strong CK20 positivity in all cases, as well as at least focal p16 positivity in many cases. HPV in situ hybridization was negative in all cases, therefore can be used in differential diagnosis.

2.2.14 Metastatic Urothelial Carcinoma

- When urothelial carcinoma presents at other sites, recognition of urothelial origin may be difficult, particularly since squamous and glandular differentiation are common in high-grade urothelial carcinoma. Differential cytokeratin expression may be of value in the confirmation of metastatic urothelial carcinoma. Expression of the combination of

GATA 3, Uroplakin III, thrombomodulin, high molecular weight cytokeratin (34βE12), and cytokeratin 20 is strongly suggestive of urothelial origin in the setting of metastatic carcinoma of unknown primary while the expression of two of these three is still suggestive, albeit more weakly. Expression of uroplakin III is highly specific for tumors of urothelial origin.

- Ovarian Brenner tumors, which histologically resemble urothelial neoplasms, may stain with uroplakin III and, therefore, may be included as a possible alternate primary site for uroplakin III positive metastatic carcinomas in female patients.
- Some immunophenotypic differences between Brenner tumors and urothelial carcinomas of the bladder do exist. Urothelial carcinomas are frequently positive for thrombomodulin and cytokeratin 20 while Brenner tumors typically do not stain with these antibodies.
- Ovarian transitional cell carcinomas rarely (6 %) express uroplakin III and typically have a uroplakin III -/cytokeratin 20-/WT1+ phenotype in contrast to the uroplakin III positive phenotype observed in 82 % of Brenner tumors.
- In fact, the differences in staining with uroplakin III and other markers suggests that Brenner tumors are the only true urothelial neoplasms of the ovary, with ovarian transitional cell carcinomas representing a pattern of poorly differentiated adenocarcinoma.

2.3 The Renal Pelvis and Ureter

- Tumors arising in the renal pelvis, the ureter and the urethra are morphologically similar to those in the bladder (Table 2.23) The incidence of these tumors ranges 0.7–1.1 per 100,000 and there is a male to female ratio of 1.7–1 with an increasing incidence in females.
- Tumors of the ureter and renal pelvis account for 8 % of all urinary tract neoplasms and are more common in older patients (mean 70

Table 2.23 WHO histological classification of tumors of renal pelvis and ureter

Epithelial tumors
Benign
Urothelial papilloma
Inverted papilloma
Squamous cell papilloma
Villous adenoma
Malignant
Urothelial carcinoma
Nested
Microcystic
Inverted
Micropapillary
Clear cell
With squamous differentiation
With glandular differentiation
Lymphoepithelioma-like
Sarcomatoid
Giant cell
Squamous cell carcinoma
Adenocarcinoma
Small cell carcinoma
Undifferentiated carcinoma
Non-epithelial tumors
Benign
Fibroepithelial polyp
Leiomyoma
Fibrous-histiocytoma
Neurofibroma
Haemangioma
Lipoma
Hibernoma
Malignant
Leiomyosarcoma
Rhabdomyosarcoma
Fibrosarcoma
Angiosarcoma
Osteosarcoma
Malignant schwannoma
Miscellaneous
Pheochromocytoma
Carcinoid
Lymphoma
Plasmacytoma
Wilms' tumour
Choriocarcinoma
Malignant melanoma

years). More than 90 % are urothelial carcinomas. Hematuria and flank pain are the chief presenting symptoms.

Benign epithelial tumors

- In this location, most benign epithelial tumors are urothelial papilloma, inverted papilloma, villous adenoma and squamous papilloma. Most lesions are incidental findings and show similar histology to bladder cases. Synchronous inverted papilloma of the urinary bladder and the renal pelvis may occur. Benign epithelial tumors are rare in the upper urinary tract.

Urothelial carcinoma

- Carcinoma arising in the renal pelvis and calyces are twice as common as those of the ureter. Multifocality is frequent as it is the association with a bladder neoplasm.
- Bilateral synchronous or metachronous ureteral and renal pelvic carcinomas may occur. Etiologic and predisposing factors additional to those for bladder malignancy include phenacetin abuse, papillary necrosis, Balkan nephropathy, thorium containing radiologic contrast material, urinary tract infections or nephrolithisis.
- Some tumors of the ureter are associated with hereditary non-polyposis colon cancer syndrome (Lynch syndrome).
- Grossly, tumors may be papillary, polypoid, nodular, ulcerative or infiltrative. Some tumors distend the entire pelvis while others ulcerate and infiltrate, causing thickening of the wall (Figs. 2.132, 2.133, and 2.134).
- A high grade tumor may appear as an ill-defined mass that involves the renal parenchyma, mimicking a primary renal cell carcinoma. Hydronephrosis and stones may be present in renal pelvic tumors while hydroureter and/or stricture may accompany ureteral neoplasms.
- Microscopically, renal pelvis and bladder urothelial malignancies mirrors bladder urothelial neoplasia and therefore, occur with similar histology including papillary non-invasive or invasive tumors, carcinoma-in-situ and solid invasive carcinoma.
- The entire morphologic spectrum of urothelial carcinoma and its variants may be seen and tumor types include those showing squamous and glandular differentiation, inverted growth, or different morphologic variants (nested, microcystic, micropapillary, clear cell and plasmacytoid) and poorly differentiated or undifferentiated carcinoma (lymphoepithelioma-like, sarcomatoid and giant cell) (Fig. 2.3).
- Sarcomatoid carcinoma is rare in the pelvis and ureter, have a poor prognosis and shows either homologous or heterologous stromal elements (Fig. 2.4). Rare cases of choriocarcinoma reported in this location are viewed at this time as high grade urothelial carcinoma with trophoblastic differentiation.
- Some urothelial carcinomas in this location display alpha-fetoprotein expression at immunohistochemistry. Synchronous renal cell carcinoma and urothelial cell carcinoma may coexist.
- Urothelial tumors should be graded following the proposal for the bladder urothelial tumors made by the World Health Organization (WHO) in 2004 or until validated, both the WHO, 1973 and WHO, 2004 can be stated in the final pathology report.
- There is a separate Tumor Node and Metastases (TNM) staging system for tumors of the renal pelvis and ureter according to the AJCC/TNM,

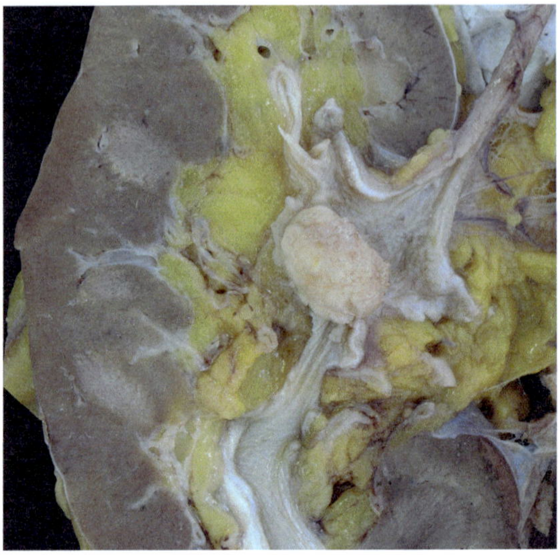

Fig. 2.132 Gross features of a carcinoma of the renal pelvis

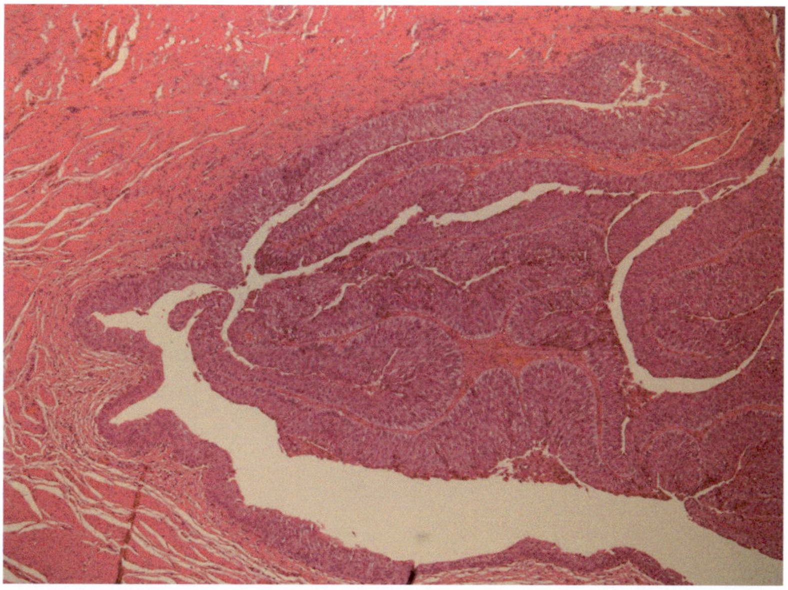

Fig. 2.133 Microscopic features of a low grade papillary urothelial carcinoma of the renal pelvis

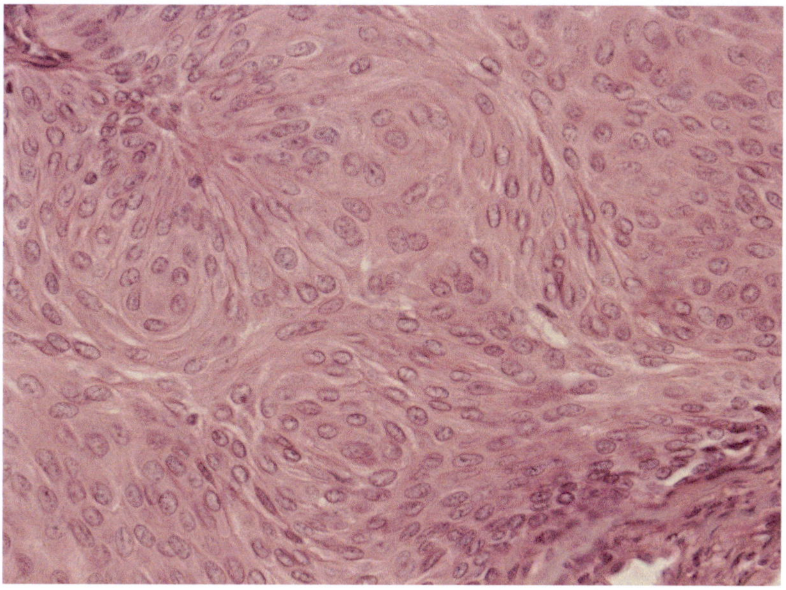

Fig. 2.134 Microscopic features of a low grade papillary urothelial carcinoma of the renal pelvis with inverted growth and squamoid eddies (whorled distribution of urothelial cells)

2010 revision (Table 2.24) The most important prognostic factor is tumor stage.

- In evaluating these specimens, it is important to avoid over-staging as pT3 tumors that invade the muscularis (pT2) but shows extension into renal tubules in a pagetoid or intramucosal pattern with no stromal infiltration. Survival for patients with pTa/pTis lesions is essentially 100 % but declines up to 75 % in patients with pT2. Survival for patients with pT3 and pT4 tumors, tumors with nodal involvement and patients with residual tumor after surgery is poor.
- It has been suggested that Ki-67 overexpression might be of prognostic value and that ErbB2 expression could be a predictor of

Table 2.24 TNM classification of tumors of the renal pelvis and ureter

T – primary tumour	
TX	Primary tumour cannot be assessed
T0	No evidence of primary tumour
Ta	Papillary noninvasive carcinoma
Tis	Carcinoma in situ
T1	Tumour invades subepithelial connective tissue
T2	Tumour invades muscularis
T3	(Renal pelvis) Tumour invades beyond muscularis into peripelvic fat or renal parenchyma
	(Ureter) Tumour invades beyond muscularis into periureteric fat
T4	Tumour invades adjacent organs or through the kidney into perinephric fat
N – regional lymph nodes	
NX	Regional lymph nodes cannot be assessed
N0	No regional lymph node metastasis
N1	Metastasis in a single lymph node 2 cm or less in greatest dimension
N2	Metastasis in a single lymph node more than 2 cm but not more than 5 cm in greatest dimension, or multiple lymph nodes, none more than 5 cm in greatest dimension
N3	Metastasis in a lymph node more than 5 cm in greatest dimension
M – distant metastasis	
MX	Distant metastasis cannot be assessed
M0	No distant metastasis
M1	Distant metastasis

disease progression and disease-related survival in upper urothelial carcinoma

Squamous cell carcinoma

- Squamous cell carcinoma is very rare but may occur in the renal pelvis were it follows in frequency to urothelial carcinoma. Squamous differentiation in an otherwise urothelial carcinoma is seen in about 40 % cases of the renal pelvis.
- Pure squamous cell carcinomas are usually high grade and stage tumors and frequently invade the kidney; usually occur in the background of nephrolithiasis, chronic inflammation or being associated with squamous metaplasia. Some squamous cell carcinoma may present with hypercalcemia; but are unrelated to Epstein-Barr virus infection. Survival at 5 years follow up is poor.

Adenocarcinoma

- Pure adenocarcinoma of the renal pelvis and ureters are rare showing similar morphologic types as in the bladder (enteric, mucinous or signet-ring cell). Glandular (intestinal) metaplasia, nephrolithiasis and repeated infections are predisposing factors.
- Most adenocarcinomas are high grade and are widely invasive at presentation.

Soft tissue tumors of renal pelvis and ureter

- Rare examples of non-epithelial tumors and tumor-like conditions arising in the renal pelvis and/or ureter have been described including leiomyoma, neurofibroma, fibroushistiocytoma, hemangioma, lipoma, hibernoma glomus tumor (Figs. 2.135 and 2.136).
- Fibroepithelial polyp is a tumor-like condition growing as an exophytic intraluminal mass of vascular connective and inflammatory cells covered by normal urothelium; rare cases may have a prominent peudosarcomatous stroma.
- Malignant soft tissue tumors include leiomyosarcoma and less frequently rhabdomyosarcoma, osteosarcoma, fibrosarcoma, angiosarcoma, malignant schwannoma, and Ewing sarcoma; gastrointestinal stromal tumor-like lesions as well as myofibroblastic proliferations may occur.

Other tumors

- Few cases of ureteric pheochromocytoma have been reported. Pelvic and ureteric carcinoid is similarly rare and must be differentiated from metastatic disease. Small cell carcinoma of the renal pelvis is a rarity observed in elderly patients.
- These aggressive tumors usually contain foci of urothelial carcinoma and have a typical neuroendocrine immunohistochemical profile. Renal pelvic and ureteric lymphomas are usually associated with systemic disease, while localized pelvic plasmacytoma has been reported.
- Wilms tumor confined to the renal pelvis or extending into the ureter and cases of malignant melanoma of the renal pelvis may be seen rarely in the literature. A curious case of tumor-like lesion of the renal pelvis composed of Liesegang rings has been reported.

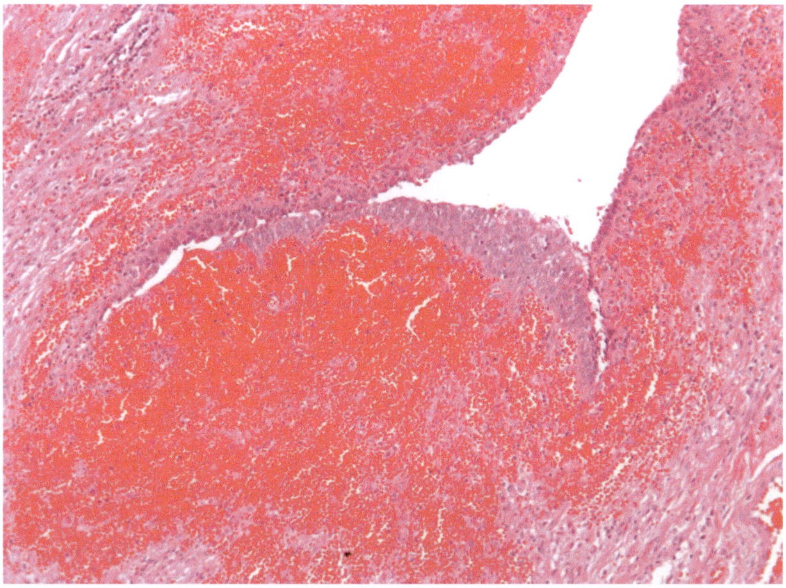

Fig. 2.135 Subepithelial hemorrhage (Antopol-Goldman lesion) seen in the renal pelvis

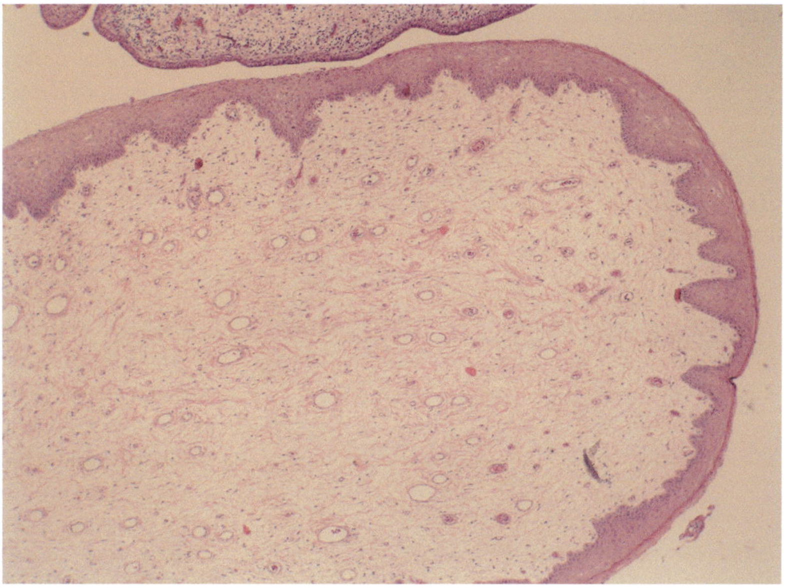

Fig. 2.136 Fibroepithelial polyp

2.4 The Urethra

- This category includes epithelial and non-epithelial neoplasms of the male and female urethra, from urinary bladder to the urethral meatus, and tumors arising in the accessory glands (Cowper and Littre glands as well as Skene glands in the female (Table 2.25).
- Epithelial tumors of the urethra are rare and three to four times more common in women than in men. Urethral carcinomas occurring in men are strikingly different in clinical and pathologic features when compared to tumors in women. This difference seems to be attributable to the distinct differences in the anatomy and histology of the urethra in the two sexes.
- Benign epithelial tumors are exquisitely rare in the urethra of either sex. Congenital diverticulum as well as acquired strictures of the

Table 2.25 Histological classification of the tumors of the urethra

Epithelial tumors
Benign
Squamous papilloma
Villous adenoma
Urothelial papilloma including inverted papilloma
Malignant
Primary
Sqamous cell carcinoma
Urothelial carcinoma
Adenocarcinoma
Clear cell carcinoma
Non-clear cell carcinoma
Enteric
Colloid (mucinous) carcinoma
Signet-ring cell carcinoma
Adenocarcinoma, not otherwise specified (NOS)
Adenosquamous carcinoma
Neuroendocrine carcinoma
Undifferentiated carcinoma
Secondary
Non-epithelial tumors
Benign
Leiomyoma
Hemangioma
Glomangiomyoma
Malignant
Malignant melanoma
Non-Hodgkin-lymphoma
Plasmocytoma
Tumour-like lesions
Fibroepithelial polyp
Prostatic polyp
Carcuncle
Condyloma accuminatum
Nephrogenic adenoma (metaplasia)
Tumors of accessory glands
Malignant
Carcinoma of skenes, littres and cowpers glands

female urethra, contribute to female preponderance of carcinomas. Columnar and mucinous adenocarcinomas and are thought to arise from glandular metaplasia, whereas cribriform adenocarcinoma that shows PSA staining seems to originate from Skene glands.

Benign epithelial tumors of the urethra

- Tumors occurring in males are similar to those in the female urethra. Some reports on squamous papilloma, villous adenoma and urothelial papilloma of the urethra are available but overall are rare. Inverted papilloma has also being reported in the urethra.
- The histological features are identical to neoplasms described in the urinary bladder and other sites. Villous adenoma of the urethra has been shown to occur associated with tubulovillous adenoma and adenocarcinoma of the rectum.
- Rare cases of adenoma nephrogenico (nephrogenic metaplasia) may be seen in the ureter or renal pelvis. Some may invade and reach perirenal fat tissue that should not be misdiagnosed as malignant.

Carcinoma of the urethra

- Tumors involving the distal urethra and meatus are most common and appear as exophytic nodular, infiltrative or papillary lesions with frequent ulceration. Tumors involving the proximal urethra that are urothelial exhibit macroscopic diversity with cases showing papillary growth, carcinoma in situ (erythematous or white plaque-like) or the nodular/infiltrative growth of invasive carcinoma (Figs. 2.137, 2.138, 2.139, 2.140, and 2.141).
- Adenocarcinomas are often large infiltrative or expansile neoplasms which may have an exophytic surface. They can be mucinous, gelatinous or cystic. These tumors may occur within urethral diverticulum (Fig. 2.6). Other tumors may occur in the penile urethra, bulbomembranous urethra or the prostatic urethra, which often determines the gross and histological appearance. These tumors may grow as ulcerative, nodular, papillary, cauliflower-like or ill-defined lesions.
- Microscopically, there are some differences between female and male urethral carcinomas, mainly because of its different anatomic location. Distal urethral and meatus tumors are squamous cell carcinomas (70 %), and tumors of the proximal urethra are urothelial carcinomas (20 %) or adenocarcinomas (10 %).

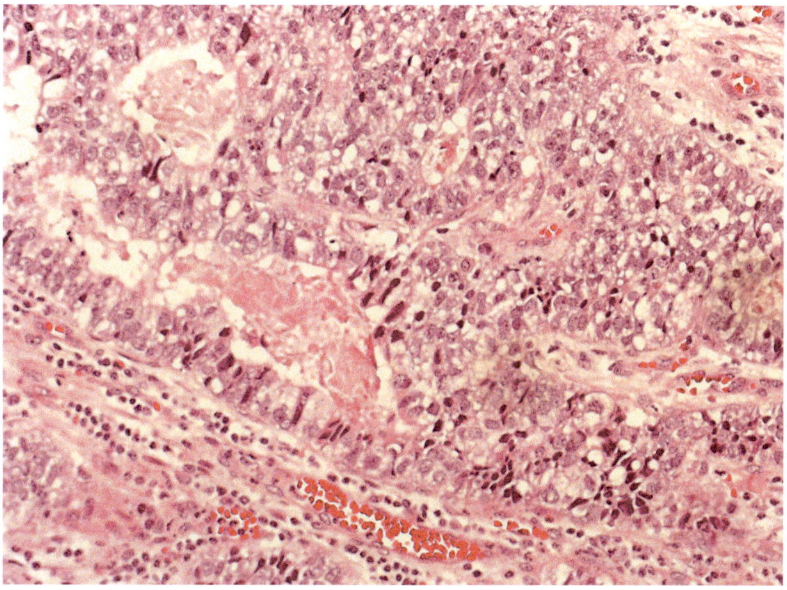

Fig. 2.137 Adenocarcinoma urethral with features suggesting of embryonal type

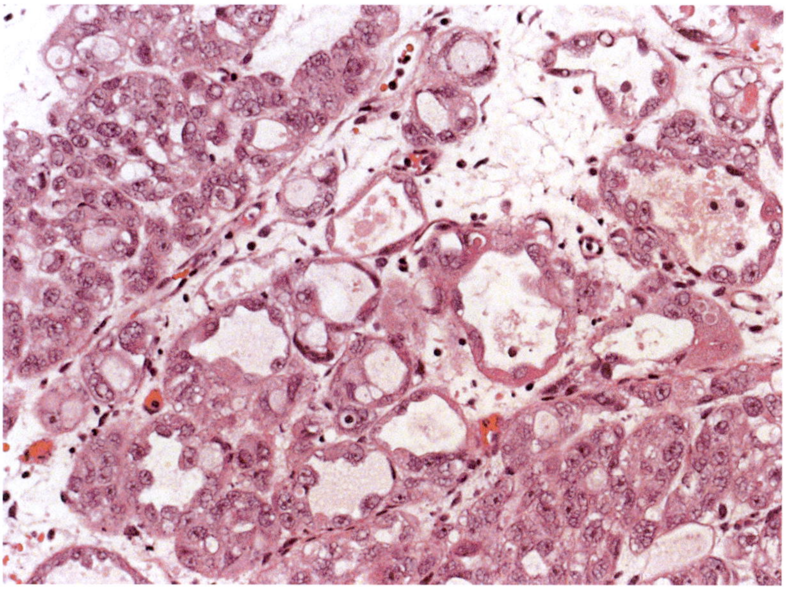

Fig. 2.138 Clear cell type adenocarcinoma of the urethra

- Squamous cell carcinomas of the urethra span the range from well differentiated (including the rare verrucous carcinoma) to moderately differentiated (most common) to poorly differentiated.
- Urothelial neoplasms may be non-invasive, papillary low-grade or high-grade carcinomas, carcinoma in situ (CIS) or invasive urothelial carcinoma. CIS may involve suburethral glands, focally or extensively, a fact that should not be mistake as invasion.
- Deeply invasive carcinomas are high grade, with or without papillary component, and characterized by irregular nests, sheets or cords of cells accompanied by a desmoplastic and/or inflammatory response.

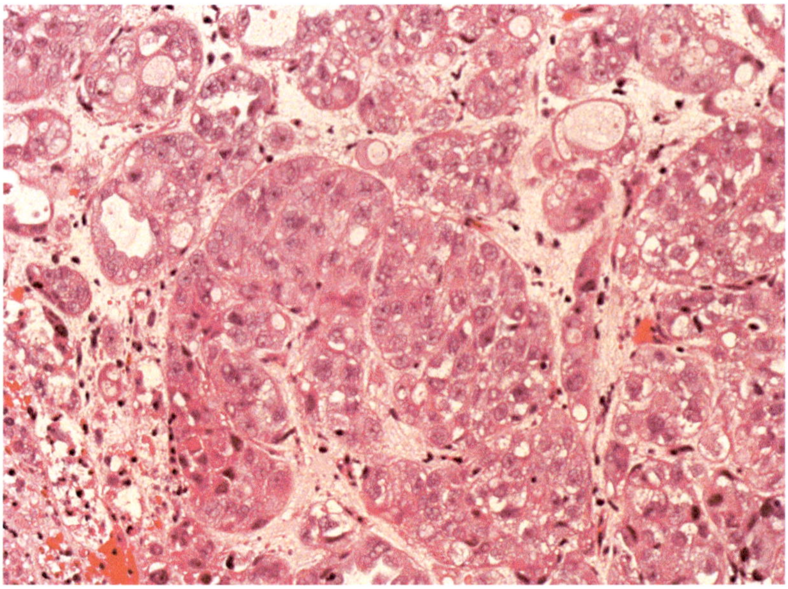

Fig. 2.139 Clear cell type adenocarcinoma of the urethra. Different area of the case depicted in Fig. 2.138

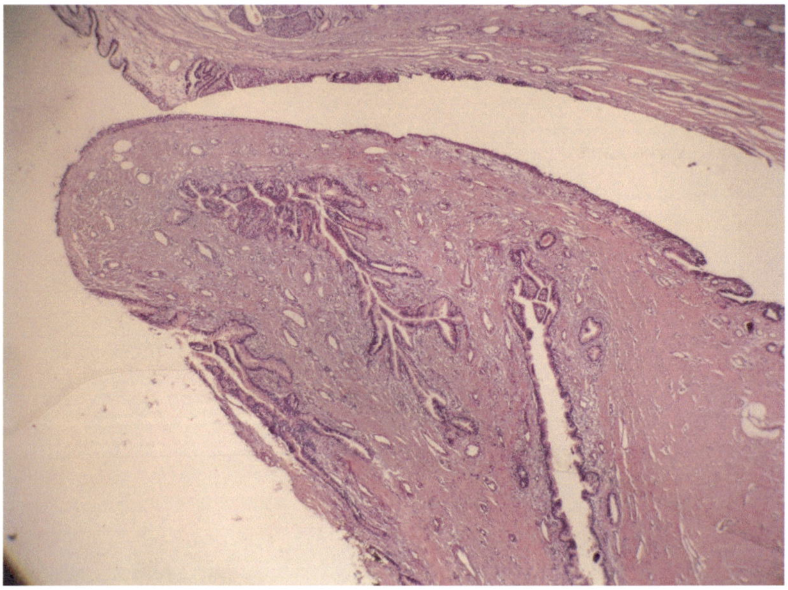

Fig. 2.140 Urethal polyp

- Tumors may exhibit squamous or glandular differentiation or unusual morphologic variations (nested, microcystic, micropapillary, clear cell or plasmacytoid). A small cell or sarcomatoid carcinoma component is rarely seen. In the penile and bulbomembranous urethra about 75 % of carcinomas are squamous cell carcinoma followed by urothelial carcinomas (usually prostatic urethra and less commonly bulbomembranous and penile urethra), adenocarcinomas (usually bulbomembranous urethra) or undifferentiated carcinoma.
- Squamous cell carcinomas are similar in histology to invasive squamous cell carcinomas at other sites.
- Urothelial carcinoma may involve the prostatic urethra, exhibiting the same grade and histological spectrum described in the female urethra. It may be synchronous or metachronous to bladder neoplasia. Features unique to

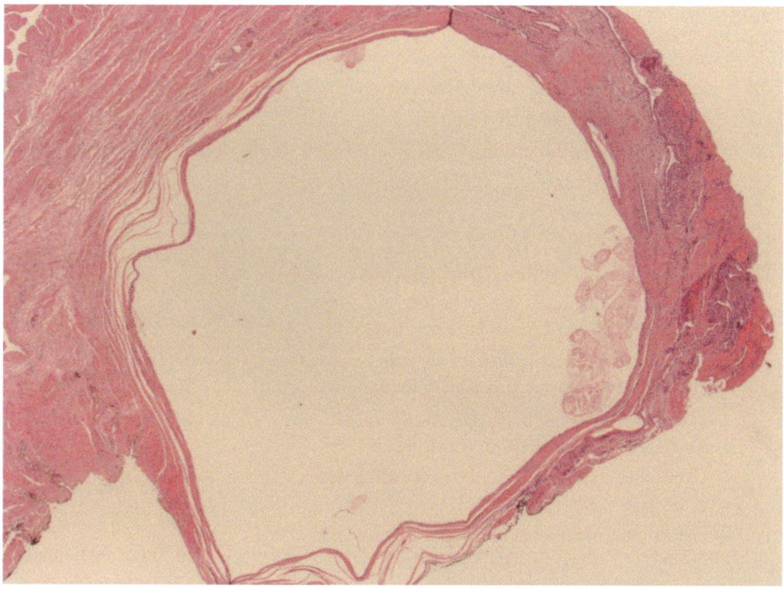

Fig. 2.141 Paraurethral cyst

prostatic urethral urothelial cancers are the frequent proclivity of high-grade tumors to extend into the prostatic ducts and acini in a pagetoid fashion.

- Adenocarcinoma of the female urethra may be seen in the form of two patterns, clear cell adenocarcinoma (approximately 40 %) and non-clear cell adenocarcinoma (approximately 60 %), the later frequently exhibiting similar patterns as in other portions of the urinary tract (enteric, mucinous, signet-ring cell or adenocarcinoma not otherwise specified). Clear cell adenocarcinoma are usually characterized by pattern heterogeneity within the same neoplasm and show solid, tubular, tubulocystic or papillary patterns.
- The cytologic features vary from low grade (resembling nephrogenic adenoma focally) to high grade (more frequently). Necrosis, mitotic activity and extensive infiltrative growth are commonly observed. Relationship to nephrogenic adenoma remains uncertain.
- Urothelial neoplasms are graded as outlined in the urinary bladder. Adenocarcinomas and squamous cell carcinomas are usually graded following similar carcinomas in other organs – well, moderately, and poorly differentiated carcinomas using the classic criteria of degree of differentiation.
- Bulbourethral gland carcinomas may show a mucinous, papillary, adenoid cystic, acinar or tubular architecture. Female periurethral gland adenocarcinomas are clear cell or mucinous and often show prostatic specific antigen immunoexpression.
- There is a separate Tumor Node and Metastases (TNM) staging system for tumors of the urethra. The overall prognosis is relatively poor. Tumor stage and location are important prognostic factors. In females and males, proximal tumors have better overall survival than distal tumors with 5-year survival of 51 % for proximal versus 6 % for distal in female, and 50 % for proximal and 20 % for distal tumors in males (Table 2.26).
- In both sexes, high pT tumor stage and the presence of lymph node metastasis are adverse prognostic parameters. A number of tumor-like conditions entering the differential diagnosis of urethral carcinoma include nephrogenic metaplasia (adenoma), fibroepithelial and prostatic polyps, condyloma acuminatum and caruncle.

Non-epithelial tumors of the urethra

- Rare examples of non-epithelial tumors arising in the urethra have been described. Benign tumors include leiomyoma with similar morphology and immunoprofile as in other organs;

Table 2.26 TNM classification of tumors of the urethra

T – primary tumour	
TX	Primary tumour cannot be assessed
T0	No evidence of primary tumour
	Urethra (male and female)
Ta	Noninvasive papillary, polypoid, or verrucous carcinoma
Tis	Carcinoma in situ
T1	Tumour invades subepithelial connective tissue
T2	Tumour invades any of the following: corpus spongiosum, prostate, periurethral muscle
T3	Tumour invades any of the following: corpus cavernosum, beyond prostatic capsule, anterior vagina, bladder neck
T4	Tumour invades other adjacent organs
	Urothelial (transitional cell) carcinoma of prostate (prostatic urethra)
Tis pu	Carcinoma in situ, involvement of prostatic urethra
Tis pd	Carcinoma in situ, involvement of prostatic ducts
T1	Tumour invades subepithelial connective tissue
T2	Tumour invades any of the following: prostatic stroma, corpus spongiosum, periurethral muscle
T3	Tumour invades any of the following: corpus cavernosum, beyond prostatic capsule, bladder neck (extra- prostatic extension)
T4	Tumour invades other adjacent organs (invasion of bladder)
N – regional lymph nodes	
NX	Regional lymph nodes cannot be assessed
N0	No regional lymph node metastasis
N1	Metastasis in a single lymph node 2 cm or less in greatest dimension
N2	Metastasis in a single lymph node more than 2 cm in greatest dimension, or multiple lymph nodes
M – distant metastasis	
MX	Distant metastasis cannot be assessed
M0	No distant metastasis
M1	Distant metastasis

in female patients leiomyoma may show expression of estrogen receptors.

- Leiomyoma may occur as a part of diffuse leiomyomatosis syndrome (esophageal and rectal leiomyoma). Hemangioma and plasmacytoma have also being described.
- Malignant melanoma has also been described in the male and female urethra with some cases of amelanotic melanoma mimicking urethral carcinoma.
- Primary non-Hodgkin lymphoma has also being described.

Molecular pathology

- Urothelial carcinomas of the renal pelvis, ureter and urinary bladder show molecular similarities to bladder carcinoma, but microsatellite instability (MSI) is more common in upper urinary tract cancers.
- Deletions on chromosome 9p and 9q occur in 50–75 % of all patients and frequent deletions at 17p in addition to p53 mutations are seen in advanced invasive tumors. 20–30 % of all upper urinary tract cancers demonstrate MSI and loss of the mismatch repair proteins MSH2, MLH1 or MSH6.
- Mutations in the sequences of TGFß-RII, Bax, MSH3, and MSH6 genes are found in 20–33 % of cases with MSI, indicating a molecular pathway of carcinogenesis that is similar to some mismatch repair-deficient colorectal cancers.
- Tumors with MSI have different clinical and histological features including low tumor stage and grade, papillary growth and a higher prevalence in female patients; some of these tumors exhibit and inverted growth pattern.
- Squamous cell carcinoma of the urethra is associated with HPV infection in female and male patients. High risk human papillomaviruses (HPV) 16 or 18 may be detected in up to 60 % of urethral carcinomas in women. In men, about 30 % of squamous cell carcinomas tested positive for HPV16; tumors in the bulbar urethra are usually negative. Some HPV16 positive tumors might have a more favorable prognosis.
- Low risk HPV infection plays a crucial role in the etiology of condyloma acuminatum of the urethra. The association of urothelial carcinoma with HPV, both in the urethra and the urinary bladder remains controversial, but the variable reported incidence might be related to geographical or demographic issues.

Suggested Reading

Achiche MA, Bouhaoula MH, Madani M, Azaiez M, Chebil M, Ayed M. Primary transitional cell carcinoma of the bulbar urethra. Prog Urol. 2005;15(6):1145–8.

Al Bashir S, Yilmaz A, Gotto G, Trpkov K. Long term outcome of primary urothelial papilloma: a single institution cohort. Pathology. 2014;46:37–40.

Alexander RE, Lopez-Beltran A, Montironi R, Maclennan GT, Post KM, Bilbo SA, Jones TD, Huang W, Rao Q, Sen JD, Meehan K, Cornwell A, Miravalle L, Cheng L. KRAS mutation is present in a small subset of primary urinary bladder adenocarcinomas. Histopathology. 2012a. doi:10.1111/j.1365-2559.2012.04309.x.

Alexander RE, Hu Y, Kum JB, Montironi R, Lopez-Beltran A, Maclennan GT, Idrees MT, Emerson RE, Ulbright TM, Grignon DG, Eble JN, Cheng L. p16 expression is not associated with human papillomavirus in urinary bladder squamous cell carcinoma. Mod Pathol. 2012b;25(11):1526–33. doi:10.1038/modpathol.2012.103.

Algaba F, Arce Y, Lopez-Beltran A, et al. Intraoperative frozen section diagnosis in urological oncology. Eur Urol. 2005;47:129–36.

Al-Quran SZ, Olivares A, Lin P, et al. Myeloid sarcoma of the urinary bladder and epididymis as a primary manifestation of acute myeloid leukemia with inv(16). Arch Pathol Lab Med. 2006;130:862–6.

Alvarez KJ, Lopez-Beltran A, Anglada CF, et al. Clinicopathologic differences between bladder neoplasm with low malignant potential and low-grade carcinoma. Actas Urol Esp. 2001;25:645–50.

Amin MB, Ro JY, Lee KM, et al. Lymphoepithelioma-like carcinoma of the urinary bladder. Am J Surg Pathol. 1994;18:466–73.

Amin MB, Patel RM, Oliveira P, et al. Alveolar soft-part sarcoma of the urinary bladder with urethral recurrence: a unique case with emphasis on differential diagnoses and diagnostic utility of an immunohistochemical panel including TFE3. Am J Surg Pathol. 2006;30:1322–5.

Amin MB, Trpkov K, Lopez-Beltran A, et al. Best practices recommendations in the application of immunohistochemistry in the bladder lesions – report from the International Society of Urologic Pathology Consensus Conference. Am J Surg Pathol. 2014;38(8):e20–34.

Baldwin L, Lee AH, Al-Talib RK, et al. Transitional cell carcinoma of the bladder mimicking lobular carcinoma of the breast: a discohesive variant of urothelial carcinoma. Histopathology. 2005;46:50–6.

Bannach G, Grignon D, Shum D. Sarcomatoid transitional cell carcinoma vs pseudosarcomatous stromal reaction in bladder carcinoma: an immunohistochemical study. J Urol Pathol. 1993;1:105–13.

Bates AW, Baithun SI. The significance of secondary neoplasms of the urinary and male genital tract. Virchows Arch. 2002;440:640–7.

Baud E, Catilina P, Boiteux J-P, et al. Human bladder cancers and normal bladder mucosa present the same hot spot of heterozygous chromosome-9 deletion. Int J Cancer. 1998;77:821–4.

Baydar D, Amin MB, Epstein JI. Osteoclast-rich undifferentiated carcinomas of the urinary tract. Mod Pathol. 2006;19:161–71.

Bayley JP, van Minderhout I, Weiss MM, et al. Mutation analysis of SDHB and SDHC: novel germline mutations in sporadic head and neck paraganglioma and familial paraganglioma and/or pheochromocytoma. BMC Med Genet. 2006;7:1.

Beltran AL, Cheng L, Montironi R, et al. Clinicopathological characteristics and outcome of nested carcinoma of the urinary bladder. Virchows Arch. 2014;465(2):199–205.

Bolkier M, Ginesin Y, Lichtig C, et al. Lymphangioma of bladder. J Urol. 1983;129:1049–50.

Bollito ER, Pacchioni D, Lopez-Beltran A, et al. Immunohistochemical study of neuroendocrine differentiation in primary glandular lesions and tumors of the urinary bladder. Anal Quant Cytol Histol. 2005;27:218–24.

Bostwick DG, Lopez-Beltran A. Bladder biopsy interpretation. Washington, DC: United Pathologists Press; 1999.

Bozas G, Tassidou A, Moulopoulos LA, Constandinidis C, Bamias A, Dimopoulos MA. Non-Hodgkin's lymphoma of the renal pelvis. Clin Lymphoma Myeloma. 2006;6(5):404–6.

Chan TY, Epstein JI. Radiation or chemotherapy cystitis with "pseudocarcinomatous" features. Am J Surg Pathol. 2004;28:909–13.

Cheng L, Darson M, Cheville JC, et al. Urothelial papilloma of the bladder: clinical and biologic implications. Cancer. 1999a;86:2098–101.

Cheng L, Cheville JC, Neumann RM, et al. Natural history of urothelial dysplasia of the bladder. Am J Surg Pathol. 1999b;23:443–7.

Cheng L, Cheville JC, Neumann RM, et al. Survival of patients with carcinoma in situ of the urinary bladder. Cancer. 1999c;85:2469–74.

Cheng L, Neumann RM, Bostwick DG. Papillary urothelial neoplasms of low malignant potential. Clinical and biologic implications. Cancer. 1999d;86:2102–8.

Cheng L, Weaver AL, Neumann RM, et al. Substaging of T1 bladder carcinoma based on the depth of invasion as measured by micrometer. A new proposal. Cancer. 1999e;86:1035–43.

Cheng L, Neumann RM, Weaver AL, et al. Predicting cancer progression in patients with stage T1 bladder carcinoma. J Clin Oncol. 1999f;17:3182–7.

Cheng L, Montironi R, Bostwick DG. Villous adenoma of the urinary tract: a report of 23 cases, including 8 with coexistent adenocarcinoma. Am J Surg Pathol. 1999g;23:764–71.

Cheng L, Scheithauer BW, Leibovich BC, et al. Neurofibroma of the urinary bladder. Cancer. 1999h;86:505–13.

Cheng L, Nascimento AG, Neumann RM, et al. Hemangioma of the urinary bladder. Cancer. 1999i;86:498–504.
Cheng L, Leibovich BC, Cheville JC, et al. Squamous papilloma of the urinary tract is unrelated to condyloma acuminata. Cancer. 2000a;88:1679–86.
Cheng L, Cheville JC, Neumann RM, et al. Flat intraepithelial lesions of the urinary bladder. Cancer. 2000b;88:625–31.
Cheng L, Cheville JC, Sebo TJ, et al. Atypical nephrogenic metaplasia of the urinary tract: a precursor lesion? Cancer. 2000c;88:853–61.
Cheng L, Leibovich B, Cheville J, et al. Paraganglioma of the urinary bladder: can biologic potential be predicted? Cancer. 2000d;88:844–52.
Cheng L, MacLennan GT, Zhang S, et al. Laser capture microdissection analysis reveals frequent allelic losses in papillary urothelial neoplasm of low malignant potential of the urinary bladder. Cancer. 2004a;101:183–8.
Cheng L, Pan CX, Yang XJ, et al. Small cell carcinoma of the urinary bladder: a clinicopathologic analysis of 64 patients. Cancer. 2004b;101:957–62.
Cheng CW, Chan LW, Chan CK, et al. Is surveillance necessary for inverted papilloma in the urinary bladder and urethra? ANZ J Surg. 2005a;75:213–7.
Cheng L, Jones TD, McCarthy RP, et al. Molecular genetic evidence for a common clonal origin of urinary bladder small cell carcinoma and coexisting urothelial carcinoma. Am J Pathol. 2005b;166:1533–9.
Cheng L, Montironi R, Davidson DD, Lopez-Beltran A. Staging and reporting of urothelial carcinoma of the urinary bladder. Mod Pathol. 2009;22 Suppl 2:S70–95. Review.
Cheng L, Davidson DD, Maclennan GT, Williamson SR, Zhang S, Koch MO, Montironi R, Lopez-Beltran A. The origins of urothelial carcinoma. Expert Rev Anticancer Ther. 2010;10(6):865–80. Review.
Cheng L, Zhang S, MacLennan GT, Williamson SR, Lopez-Beltran A, Montironi R. Bladder cancer: translating molecular genetic insights into clinical practice. Hum Pathol. 2011a;42(4):455–81.
Cheng L, Zhang S, Alexander R, Maclennan GT, Hodges KB, Harrison BT, Lopez-Beltran A, Montironi R. Sarcomatoid carcinoma of the urinary bladder: the final common pathway of urothelial carcinoma dedifferentiation. Am J Surg Pathol. 2011b;35(5):e34–46. Review.
Cheng L, Maclennan GT, Lopez-Beltran A. Histologic grading of urothelial carcinoma: a reappraisal. Hum Pathol. 2012;43(12):2097–108.
Chow N, Cairns P, Eisenberger CF, et al. Papillary urothelial hyperplasia is a clonal precursor to papillary transitional cell bladder cancer. Int J Cancer. 2000;89:514–8.
Cummings JM, Wehry MA, Parra RO, et al. Schwannoma of the urinary bladder: a case report. Int J Urol. 1998;5:496–7.
Dalbagni G, Herr HW, Reuter VE. Impact of a second transurethral resection on the staging of T1 bladder cancer. Urology. 2002;60:822–4.
Dell'Atti C, Missere M, Restaino G, Carlino S, Cucci E, Ciuffreda M, Sallustio G. Primary lymphoma of the female urethra. Rays. 2005;30(3):269–72.
Drew PA, Furman J, Civantos F, et al. The nested variant of transitional cell carcinoma: an aggressive neoplasm with innocuous histology. Mod Pathol. 1996;9:989–94.
Eble JN, Young RH. Stromal osseous metaplasia in carcinoma of the bladder. J Urol. 1991;145:823–5.
Eble JN, Sauter G, Epstein JI, et al. World Health Organization classification of tumours: pathology and genetics of tumours of the urinary system and male genital organs. Lyon: IARC Press; 2004.
Edge SB, Byrd DR, Compton CC, et al. Cancer staging handbook from the AJCC Cancer Staging Manual. 7th ed. New York: Springer; 2010.
Egawa S, Uchida T, Koshiba K, et al. Malignant fibrous histiocytoma of the bladder with focal rhabdoid tumor differentiation. J Urol. 1994;151:154–6.
Eltoum IA, Moore 3rd RJ, Cook W, et al. Epithelioid variant of malignant peripheral nerve sheath tumor (malignant schwannoma) of the urinary bladder. Ann Diagn Pathol. 1999;3:304–8.
Engel JD, Kuzel TM, Moceanu MC, et al. Angiosarcoma of the bladder: a review. Urology. 1998;52:778–84.
Epstein JL, Amin MB, Reuter VR, et al. The Bladder Consensus Conference Committee. The World Health Organization/International Society of Urologic Pathology consensus classification of urothelial (transitional cell) neoplasms of the urinary bladder. Am J Surg Pathol. 1998;22:1435–8.
Farrow GM, Utz DC. Observation on microinvasive transitional cell carcinoma of the urinary bladder. Clin Oncol. 1982;1:609–15.
Farrow G, Utz D, Rife C, et al. Clinical observations on sixty-nine cases of in situ carcinoma of the urinary bladder. Cancer Res. 1977;37:2794–8.
Ferrero Doria R, Garcia Victor F, Moreno Perez F, Gasso Matoses M, Diaz Calleja E. Cavernous haemangioma as the cause of ureteral pyelic junction obstruction. Arch Esp Urol. 2005;58(9):960–3.
Fine SW, Chan TY, Epstein JI. Inverted papillomas of the prostatic urethra. Am J Surg Pathol. 2006;30(8):975–9.
Fletcher MS, Aker M, Hill JT, et al. Granular cell myoblastoma of the bladder. Br J Urol. 1985;57:109–10.
Fossa S. Rare and unusual tumors of the genitourinary tract. Curr Opin Oncol. 1992;4:463–8.
Freeman A, Geddes N, Munson P, et al. Anaplastic lymphoma kinase (ALK 1) staining and molecular analysis in inflammatory myofibroblastic tumours of the bladder: a preliminary clinicopathological study of nine cases and review of the literature. Mod Pathol. 2004;17:765–71.
Fujii Y, Kawakami S, Koga F, et al. Long-term outcome of bladder papillary urothelial neoplasms of low malignant potential. BJU Int. 2003;92:559–62.
Goluboff ET, O'Toole K, Sawczuk IS. Leiomyoma of bladder: report of case and review of literature. Urology. 1994;43:238–41.

Grignon D, Ro J, Ayala A, et al. Primary adenocarcinoma of the urinary bladder: a clinicopathologic analysis of 72 cases. Cancer. 1990;67:2165–72.

Grignon DJ, Ro JY, Mackay B, et al. Paraganglioma of the urinary bladder: immunohistochemical, ultrastructural, and DNA flow cytometric studies. Hum Pathol. 1991;22:1162–9.

Gulley ML, Amin MB, Nicholls JM, et al. Epstein-Barr virus is detected in undifferentiated nasopharyngeal carcinoma but not in lymphoepithelioma-like carcinoma of the urinary bladder. Hum Pathol. 1995;26:1207–14.

Gulmann C, Paner GP, Parakh RS, Hansel DE, Shen SS, Ro JY, Annaiah C, Lopez-Beltran A, Rao P, Arora K, Cho Y, Herrera-Hernandez L, Alsabeh R, Amin MB. Immunohistochemical profile to distinguish urothelial from squamous differentiation in carcinomas of urothelial tract. Hum Pathol. 2013;44(2):164–72. doi:10.1016/j.humpath.2012.05.018. pii: S0046-8177(12)00194-3.

Guo CC, Fine SW, Epstein JI. Noninvasive squamous lesions in the urinary bladder: a clinicopathologic analysis of 29 cases. Am J Surg Pathol. 2006;30:883–91.

Gupta A, Wang HL, Policarpio-Nicolas ML, et al. Expression of alpha-methylacyl-coenzyme A racemase in nephrogenic adenoma. Am J Surg Pathol. 2004;28:1224–9.

Halat S, Eble JN, Grignon DJ, Lacy S, Montironi R, MacLennan GT, Lopez-Beltran A, Tan PH, Baldridge LA, Cheng L. Ectopic prostatic tissue: histogenesis and histopathological characteristics. Histopathology. 2011;58(5):750–8. doi:10.1111/j.1365-2559.2011.03799.x. Epub 2011 Mar 25.

Hanna NH, Ulbright TM, Einhorn LH. Primary choriocarcinoma of the bladder with the detection of isochromosome 12p. J Urol. 2002;167:1781.

Harik LR, Merino C, Coindre JM, et al. Pseudosarcomatous myofibroblastic proliferations of the bladder: a clinicopathologic study of 42 cases. Am J Surg Pathol. 2006;30:787–94.

Harnden P, Mahmood N, Southgate J. Expression of cytokeratin 20 redefines urothelial papillomas of the bladder. Lancet. 1999;353:974–7.

Hartmann A, Moser K, Kriegmair M, et al. Frequent genetic alterations in simple urothelial hyperplasias of the bladder in patients with papillary urothelial carcinoma. Am J Pathol. 1999;154:721–7.

Hartmann A, Rosner U, Schlake G, et al. Clonality and genetic divergence in multifocal low-grade superficial urothelial carcinoma as determined by chromosome 9 and p53 deletion analysis. Lab Invest. 2000;80:709–18.

Hasegeli UA, Altundag K, Saglam A, et al. Granulocytic sarcoma of the urinary bladder. Am J Hematol. 2004;75:262–3.

Herawi M, Parwani AV, Edlow D, Smolev JK, Epstein JI. Glomus tumor of renal pelvis: a case report and review of the literature. Hum Pathol. 2005;36(3):299–302.

Herr HW. Staging invasive bladder tumors. J Surg Oncol. 1992;51:217–20.

Hes O, Curik R, Mainer K, Michal M. Urothelial signet-ring cell carcinoma of the renal pelvis with collagenous spherulosis: a case report. Int J Surg Pathol. 2005;13(4):375–8.

Hodges KB, Lopez-Beltran A, Emerson RE, et al. Clinical utility of immunohistochemistry in the diagnoses of urinary bladder neoplasia. Appl Immunohistochem Mol Morphol. 2010;18:401–10.

Hodges KB, Lopez-Beltran A, Maclennan GT, Montironi R, Cheng L. Urothelial lesions with inverted growth patterns: histogenesis, molecular genetic findings, differential diagnosis and clinical management. BJU Int. 2011;107(4):532–7.

Holmang S, Johansson SL. Bilateral metachronous ureteral and renal pelvic carcinomas: incidence, clinical presentation, histopathology, treatment and outcome. J Urol. 2006;175(1):69–72.

Holmang S, Hedelin H, Anderstrom C, et al. The relationship among multiple recurrences, progression and prognosis of patients with stages Ta and T1 transitional cell cancer of the bladder followed for at least 20 years. J Urol. 1995;153:1823–7.

Hruby G, Choo R, Lehman M, Herschorn S, Kapusta L. Female clear cell adenocarcinoma arising within a urethral diverticulum. Can J Urol. 2000;7(6):1160–3.

Huang HY, Ko SF, Chuang JH, et al. Primary yolk sac tumor of the urachus. Arch Pathol Lab Med. 2002;126:1106–9.

Huang Q, Chu PG, Lau SK, et al. Urothelial carcinoma of the urinary bladder with a component of acinar/tubular type differentiation simulating prostatic adenocarcinoma. Hum Pathol. 2004;35:769–73.

Iczkowski KA, Shanks JH, Allsbrook WC, et al. Small cell carcinoma of urinary bladder is differentiated from urothelial carcinoma by chromogranin expression, absence of CD44 variant 6 expression, a unique pattern of cytokeratin expression, and more intense gamma-enolase expression. Histopathology. 1999;35:150–6.

Jacobs MA, Bavendam T, Leach GE. Bladder leiomyoma. Urology. 1989;34:56–7.

Jewett HJ. Carcinoma of the bladder: influence of depth of infiltration on the 5-year results following complete extirpation of the primary growth. J Urol. 1952;67:672–80.

Jimenez RE, Gheiler E, Oskanian P, et al. Grading the invasive component of urothelial carcinoma of the bladder and its relationship with progression-free survival. Am J Surg Pathol. 2000;24:980–7.

Jones TD, Cheng L. Papillary urothelial neoplasm of low malignant potential: evolving terminology and concepts. J Urol. 2006;175:1995–2003.

Jones EC, Young RH. Myxoid and sclerosing sarcomatoid transitional cell carcinoma of the urinary bladder: a clinicopathologic and immunohistochemical study of 25 cases. Mod Pathol. 1997;10:908–16.

Jones EC, Clement PB, Young RH. Inflammatory pseudotumor of the urinary bladder: a clinicopathological, immunohistochemical, ultrastructural, and flow cytometric study of 13 cases. Am J Surg Pathol. 1993;17:264–74.

Jones TD, Wang M, Eble JN, et al. Molecular evidence supporting field effect in urothelial carcinogenesis. Clin Cancer Res. 2005a;11:6512–9.

Jones TD, Kernek KM, Yang XJ, et al. Thyroid transcription factor 1 expression in small cell carcinoma of the urinary bladder: an immunohistochemical profile of 44 cases. Hum Pathol. 2005b;36:718–23.

Jones TD, Zhang S, Lopez-Beltran A, et al. Urothelial carcinoma with an inverted growth pattern can be distinguished from inverted papilloma by fluorescence in-situ hybridization, immunohistochemistry, and morphologic analysis. Am J Surg Pathol. 2007;31(12):1861–7.

Kakizoe T, Matumoto K, Nishio Y, et al. Significance of carcinoma in situ and dysplasia association with bladder cancer. J Urol. 1985;133:395–8.

Kapusta L, Weiss MA, Lopez-Beltran A, Srigley JR. Inflammatory myofibroblastic tumors of the kidney. Am J Surg Pathol. 2003;27:658–66.

Kato T, Kubota Y, Saitou M, et al. Osteosarcoma of the bladder successfully treated with partial cystectomy. J Urol. 2000;163:548–9.

Kato H, Kobayashi S, Islam AM, Nishizawa O. Female para-urethral adenocarcinoma: histological and immunohistochemical study. Int J Urol. 2005;12(1):117–9.

Kaufmann O, Volmerig J, Dietel M. Uroplakin III is a highly specific and moderately sensitive immunohistochemical marker for primary and metastatic urothelial carcinomas. Am J Clin Pathol. 2000;113:683–7.

Kawachi Y, Ishi K. Inverted transitional cell carcinoma of the ureter. Int J Urol. 1996;3:313–5.

Keck B, Stoehr R, Wach S, Rogler A, Hofstaedter F, Lehmann J, Montironi R, Sibonye M, Fritsche HM, Lopez-Beltran A, Epstein JI, Wullich B, Hartmann A. The plasmacytoid carcinoma of the bladder – rare variant of aggressive urothelial carcinoma. Int J Cancer. 2011;129(2):346–54.

Kiemeney L, Witjes J, Heibroek R, et al. Dysplasia in normal-looking urothelium increases the risk of tumour progression in primary superficial bladder cancer. Eur J Cancer. 1994;30A:1621–5.

Kirkali Z, Tuzel E. Transitional cell carcinoma of the ureter and renal pelvis. Crit Rev Oncol Hematol. 2003;47(2):155–69.

Kirkali Z, Chan T, Manoharan M, et al. Bladder cancer: epidemiology, staging and grading, and diagnosis. Urology. 2005;66:4–34.

Koss LG, Tiamson EM, Robbins MA. Mapping cancerous and precancerous bladder changes. A study of the urothelium in ten surgically removed bladders. JAMA. 1974;227:281–6.

Krober SM, Aepinus C, Ruck P, et al. Extranodal marginal zone B cell lymphoma of MALT type involving the mucosa of both the urinary bladder and stomach. J Clin Pathol. 2002;55:554–7.

Kunze E, Francksen B, Schulz H. Expression of MUC5AC apomucin in transitional cell carcinomas of the urinary bladder and its possible role in the development of mucus-secreting adenocarcinomas. Virchows Arch. 2001;439:609–15.

Kuroda N, Shiotsu T, Ohara M, Hirouchi T, Mizuno K, Miyazaki E. Female urethral adenocarcinoma with a heterogeneous phenotype. APMIS. 2006;114(4):314–8.

Lahoti C, Schinella R, Rangwala AF, et al. Carcinosarcoma of urinary bladder: report of 5 cases with immunohistologic study. Urology. 1994;43:389–93.

Lambert I, Debiec-Rychter M, Dubin M, et al. Solid alveolar rhabdomyosarcoma originating from the urinary bladder in an adult. Diagnostic value of molecular genetics. Histopathology. 2004;44:508–10.

Lamm K. Chondroid and osseous metaplasia in carcinoma of the bladder. J Urol Pathol. 1995;3:255–62.

Langner C, Hutterer G, Chromecki T, Winkelmayer I, Rehak P, Zigeuner R. pT classification, grade, and vascular invasion as prognostic indicators in urothelial carcinoma of the upper urinary tract. Mod Pathol. 2006a;19(2):272–9.

Langner C, Hutterer G, Chromecki T, Leibl S, Rehak P, Zigeuner R. Tumor necrosis as prognostic indicator in transitional cell carcinoma of the upper urinary tract. J Urol. 2006b;176(3):910–3.

Langner C, Hutterer G, Chromecki T, Rehak P, Zigeuner R. Patterns of invasion and histological growth as prognostic indicators in urothelial carcinoma of the upper urinary tract. Virchows Arch. 2006c;448(5):604–11.

Leblanc B, Duclos AJ, Benard F, et al. Long-term followup of initial Ta grade 1 transitional cell carcinoma of the bladder. J Urol. 1999;162:1946–60.

Lee KH, Ryu SB, Lee MC, et al. Primary large cell neuroendocrine carcinoma of the urinary bladder. Pathol Int. 2006;56:688–93.

Lemos N, Melo CR, Soares IC, et al. Plasmacytoma of the urethra treated by excisional biopsy. Scand J Urol Nephrol. 2000;34:75–6.

Lopez-Beltran A. Bladder cancer: clinical and pathological profile. Scand J Urol Nephrol Suppl. 2008; 42(Suppl 218):95–109. Review.

Lopez-Beltran A. Rare lesions and tumors of the urinary bladder. Selected issues. Tumori. 2012;98(2):274–7. doi:10.1700/1088.11943.

Lopez-Beltran A, Cheng L. Stage pT1 bladder carcinoma: diagnostic criteria, pitfalls and prognostic significance. Pathology. 2003;35:484–91.

Lopez-Beltran A, Cheng L. Histologic variants of urothelial carcinoma: differential diagnosis and clinical implications. Hum Pathol. 2006;37:1371–88.

Lopez-Beltran A, Montironi R. Non-invasive urothelial neoplasms: according to the most recent WHO classification. Eur Urol. 2004;46:170–6.

Lopez-Beltran A, Martin J, Garcia J, et al. Squamous and glandular differentiation in urothelial bladder carcinomas. Histopathology, histochemistry and immunohistochemical expression of carcinoembryonic antigen. Histol Histopathol. 1988;3:63–8.

Lopez-Beltran A, Nogales F, Donne CH, et al. Adenocarcinoma of the urachus showing extensive calcification and stromal osseous metaplasia. Urol Int. 1994;53:110–3.

Lopez-Beltran A, Lopez-Ruiz J, Vicioso L. Inflammatory pseudotumor of the urinary bladder. A clinicopathological analysis of two cases. Urol Int. 1995;55:173–6.

Lopez-Beltran A, Escudero AL, Cavazzana AO, et al. Sarcomatoid transitional cell carcinoma of the renal pelvis. A report of five cases with clinical, pathological, immunohistochemical and DNA ploidy analysis. Pathol Res Pract. 1996;192:1218–24.

Lopez-Beltran A, Pacelli A, Rothenberg HJ, et al. Carcinosarcoma and sarcomatoid carcinoma of the bladder: clinicopathological study of 41 cases. J Urol. 1998;159:1497–503.

Lopez-Beltran A, Cheng L, Andersson L, et al. Preneoplastic non-papillary lesions and conditions of the urinary bladder: an update based on the Ancona International Consultation. Virchows Arch. 2002a;440:3–11.

Lopez-Beltran A, Luque RJ, Mazzuchelli R, et al. Changes produced in the urothelium by traditional and newer therapeutic procedures for bladder cancer. J Clin Pathol. 2002b;55:641–7.

Lopez-Beltran A, Luque RJ, Oliveira PS, et al. Urothelial carcinoma of the bladder, lipid cell variant (UCBLCV). Immunohistochemical and clinico-pathologic findings in seven cases (Abstract). Mod Pathol. 2002c;15:171A.

Lopez-Beltran A, Luque RJ, Quintero A, et al. Hepatoid adenocarcinoma of the urinary bladder. Virchows Arch. 2003;442:381–7.

Lopez-Beltran A, Sauter G, Gasser T, et al. Urothelial tumors: infiltrating urothelial carcinoma. In: Eble JN, Sauter G, Epstein JI, Sesterhenn I, editors. World Health Organization classification of tumors. Pathology and genetics of tumors of the urinary system and male genital organs. Lyon: IARC Press; 2004a.

Lopez-Beltran A, Bassi P, Pavone-Macaluso M, et al. Handling and pathology reporting of specimens with carcinoma of the urinary bladder, ureter, and renal pelvis. Eur Urol. 2004b;45:257–66.

Lopez-Beltran A, Requena MJ, Luque RJ, et al. Cyclin D3 expression in primary Ta/T1 bladder cancer. J Pathol. 2006a;209:106–13.

Lopez-Beltran A, Perez-Seoane C, Montironi R, et al. Primary primitive neuroectodermal tumour of the urinary bladder: a clinico-pathological study emphasising immunohistochemical, ultrastructural and molecular analyses. J Clin Pathol. 2006b;59:775–8.

Lopez-Beltran A, Requena MJ, Alvarez-Kindelan J, et al. Squamous differentiation in primary urothelial carcinoma of the urinary tract as seen by MAC387 immunohistochemistry. J Clin Pathol. 2007;60:332–5.

Lopez-Beltran A, Blanca A, Montironi R, Cheng L, Regueiro JC. Pleomorphic giant cell carcinoma of the urinary bladder. Hum Pathol. 2009a;40(10):1461–6. Epub 2009 May 20.

Lopez-Beltran A, Requena MJ, Montironi R, Blanca A, Cheng L. Plasmacytoid urothelial carcinoma of the bladder. Hum Pathol. 2009b;40(7):1023–8. Epub 2009 Mar 17.

Lopez-Beltran A, Cheng L, Comperat E, Rouprêt M, Blanca A, Menendez CL, Montironi R. Large cell undifferentiated carcinoma of the urinary bladder. Pathology. 2010a;42(4):364–8.

Lopez-Beltran A, Montironi R, Blanca A, Cheng L. Invasive micropapillary urothelial carcinoma of the bladder. Hum Pathol. 2010b;41(8):1159–64. Epub 2010 Apr 8.

Lopez-Beltran A, Jimenez RE, Montironi R, Patriarca C, Blanca A, Menendez CL, Algaba F, Cheng L. Flat urothelial carcinoma in situ of the bladder with glandular differentiation. Hum Pathol. 2011;42(11):1653–9. Epub 2011 Apr 29.

Lopez Beltran A, Montironi R, Cheng L. Microcystic urothelial carcinoma: morphology, immunohistochemistry and clinical behaviour. Histopathology. 2014;64:872–9.

Lott S, Lopez-Beltran A, MacLennan GT, et al. Soft tissue tumors of the urinary bladder, part I: myofibroblastic proliferationas, benign neoplasms, and tumors of uncertain malignant potential. Hum Pathol. 2007a;38(6):807–23.

Lott S, Lopez-Beltran A, Montironi R, et al. Soft tissue tumors of the urinary bladder: part II: malignant neoplasms. Hum Pathol. 2007b;38(7):963–77.

Mahadevia PS, Koss LG, Tar IJ. Prostatic involvement in bladder cancer. Prostate mapping in 20 cystoprostatectomy specimens. Cancer. 1986;58:2096–102.

Malmstrom PU, Bush C, Norlen BJ. Recurrence, progression, and survival in bladder cancer. A retrospective analysis of 232 patients with greater than or equal to 5-year follow-up. Scand J Urol Nephrol. 1987;21:185–95.

Martignoni G, Eble JN. Carcinoid tumors of the urinary bladder. Immunohistochemical study of 2 cases and review of the literature. Arch Pathol Lab Med. 2003;127:e22–4.

Martin JE, Jenkins BJ, Zuk RJ, et al. Human chorionic gonadotrophin expression and histological findings as predictors of response to radiotherapy in carcinoma of the bladder. Virchows Arch A Pathol Anat Histopathol. 1989;414:273–7.

Martin SA, Sears DL, Sebo TJ, et al. Smooth muscle neoplasms of the urinary bladder: a clinicopathologic comparison of leiomyoma and leiomyosarcoma. Am J Surg Pathol. 2002;26:292–300.

Mazzucchelli R, Cheng L, Lopez-Beltran A, Scarpelli M, Montironi R. Clinicopathological significance of lymphovascular invasion in urothelial carcinoma. Anal Quant Cytol Histol. 2012a;34(4):173–9.

Mazzucchelli R, Cheng L, Lopez-Beltran A, Scarpelli M, Montironi R. Classification and grading of noninvasive and invasive neoplasms of the urothelium. Anal Quant Cytol Histol. 2012b;34(3):111–9.

McKenney JK, Desai S, Cohen C, et al. Discriminatory immunohistochemical staining of urothelial carcinoma in situ and non-neoplastic urothelium: an analysis of cytokeratin 20, p53, and CD44 antigens. Am J Surg Pathol. 2001a;25:1074–8.

McKenney JK, Gomez JA, Desai S, et al. Morphologic expressions of urothelial carcinoma in situ: a detailed evaluation of its histologic patterns with emphasis

on carcinoma in situ with microinvasion. Am J Surg Pathol. 2001b;25:356–62.
Mearini E, Zucchi A, Costantini E, et al. Primary Burkitt's lymphoma of bladder in patient with AIDS. J Urol. 2002;167:1397–8.
Melamed M, Voutsa N, Grabstald H. Natural history and clinical behavior of in situ carcinoma of the human urinary bladder. Cancer. 1964;17:1533–45.
Mills SE, Bova GS, Wick MR, et al. Leiomyosarcoma of the urinary bladder. A clinicopathologic and immunohistochemical study of 15 cases. Am J Surg Pathol. 1989;13:480–9.
Montironi R, Lopez-Beltran A. The 2004 WHO classification of bladder tumors: a summary and commentary. Int J Surg Pathol. 2005;13:143–53.
Montironi R, Scarpelli M, Mazzucchelli R, et al. Subvisual changes in chromatin organization state are detected by karyometry in the histologically normal urothelium in patients with synchronous papillary carcinoma. Hum Pathol. 2003a;34:893–901.
Montironi R, Lopez-Beltran A, Mazzuchelli R, et al. Classification and grading of the non-invasive neoplasms: recent advances and controversies. J Clin Pathol. 2003b;56:91–5.
Montironi R, Cheng L, Lopez-Beltran A, Scarpelli M, Mazzucchelli R, Mikuz G, Kirkali Z, Montorsi F. Inverted (endophytic) noninvasive lesions and neoplasms of the urothelium: the Cinderella group has yet to be fully exploited. Eur Urol. 2011;59(2):225–30.
Morton MJ, Zhang S, Lopez-Beltran S, et al. Telomere shortening and chromosomal abnormalities in intestinal metaplasia of the urinary bladder. Clin Cancer Res. 2007;13(20):6232–6.
Mostofi FK, Sobin LH, Torloni H. Histological typing of urinary bladder tumours. Geneva: World Health Organization; 1973.
Murphy WM, Deanna DG. The nested variant of transitional cell carcinoma: a neoplasm resembling proliferation of Brunn's nests. Mod Pathol. 1992;5:240–3.
Noel JC, Fayt I, Aguilar SF. Adenosquamous carcinoma arising in villous adenoma from female vulvar urethra. Acta Obstet Gynecol Scand. 2006;85(3):373–6.
Nogales FF, Andujar M, Lopez-Beltran A, Martinez JL, Zuluaga A. Adenocarcinoma of the renal pelvis. Urol Int. 1994;52:172–5.
Offersen BV, Knap MM, Marcussen N, et al. Intense inflammation in bladder carcinoma is associated with angiogenesis and indicates good prognosis. Br J Cancer. 2002;87:1422–30.
Ogishima T, Kawachi Y, Saito A, et al. Sarcomatoid carcinoma and carcinosarcoma of the urinary bladder. Int J Urol. 2002;9:354–8.
Ohsawa M, Aozasa K, Horiuchi K, et al. Malignant lymphoma of bladder. Report of three cases and review of the literature. Cancer. 1993;72:1969–74.
Olgac S, Mazumdar M, Dalbagni G, Reuter VE. Urothelial carcinoma of the renal pelvis: a clinicopathologic study of 130 cases. Am J Surg Pathol. 2004;28(12):1545–52.
Oliva E, Amin MB, Jimenez R, et al. Clear cell carcinoma of the urinary bladder: a report and comparison of four tumors of mullerian origin and nine of probable urothelial origin with discussion of histogenesis and diagnostic problems. Am J Surg Pathol. 2002;26:190–7.
Omeroglu A, Paner GP, Wojcik EM, et al. A carcinosarcoma/sarcomatoid carcinoma arising in a urinary bladder diverticulum. Arch Pathol Lab Med. 2002;126:853–5.
Orozco R, Martin A, Murphy W. Carcinoma in situ of the urinary bladder: clues to host involvement in human carcinogenesis. Cancer. 1994;74:115–22.
Owens CL, Epstein JI. Significance of denuded urothelium in papillary urothelial lesions. Am J Surg Pathol. 2007;31:298–303.
Pan CX, Zhang H, Lara PNJ, et al. Small-cell carcinoma of the urinary bladder: diagnosis and management. Expert Rev Anticancer Ther. 2000;6:1707–13.
Pan C-C, Yu I-T, Yang A-H, et al. Clear cell myomelanocytic tumor of the urinary bladder. Am J Surg Pathol. 2003;27:689–92.
Pan CX, Yang XJ, Lopez-Beltran A, et al. c-kit Expression in small cell carcinoma of the urinary bladder: prognostic and therapeutic implications. Mod Pathol. 2005;18:320–3.
Paner GP, McKenney JK, Barkan GA, et al. Immunohistochemical analysis in a morphologic spectrum of urachal epithelial neoplasms: diagnostic implications and pitfalls. Am J Surg Pathol. 2011;35:787–98.
Paner GP, Cox RM, Richards K, Akki A, Gokden N, Lopez-Beltran A, Krausz T, McKenney JK, Steinberg GD. Pseudoangiosarcomatous urothelial carcinoma of the urinary bladder. Am J Surg Pathol. 2014;38(9):1251–9.
Pant-Purohit M, Lopez-Beltran A, Montironi R, MacLennan GT, Cheng L. Small cell carcinoma of the urinary bladder. Histol Histopathol. 2010;25(2):217–21. Review.
Parfitt JR, Bella AJ, Wehrli BM, et al. Primary PEComa of the bladder treated with primary excision and adjuvant interferon-alpha immunotherapy: a case report. BMC Urol. 2006;6:20.
Parwani AV, Herawi M, Volmar K, et al. Urothelial carcinoma with rhabdoid features: report of 6 cases. Hum Pathol. 2006;37:168–72.
Patriarca C, Colecchia M, Lopez Beltran A, Sirugo G, Bollito E, di Pasquale M. Nest-like features in bladder, simulating the nested variant of urothelial carcinoma. Int J Surg Pathol. 2011;19(1):11–9.
Perez-Montiel D, Wakely PE, Hes O, Michal M, Suster S. High-grade urothelial carcinoma of the renal pelvis: clinicopathologic study of 108 cases with emphasis on unusual morphologic variants. Mod Pathol. 2006;19(4):494–503.
Pich A, Chiusa L, Formiconi A, et al. Biologic differences between noninvasive papillary urothelial neoplasms of low malignant potential and low-grade (grade 1) papillary carcinomas of the bladder. Am J Surg Pathol. 2001;25:1528–33.
Proppe KH, Scully RE, Rosai J. Postoperative spindle cell nodules of genitourinary tract resembling sarcomas. A report of eight cases. Am J Surg Pathol. 1984;8:101–8.

Prout MN, Davis Jr HL. Hemangiopericytoma of the bladder after polyvinyl alcohol exposure. Cancer. 1977;39:1328–30.
Rao Q, Williamson SR, Lopez-Beltran A, Montironi R, Huang W, Eble JN, Grignon DJ, Koch MO, Idrees MT, Emerson RE, Zhou XJ, Zhang S, Baldridge LA, Cheng L. Distinguishing primary adenocarcinoma of the urinary bladder from secondary involvement by colorectal adenocarcinoma: extended immunohistochemical profiles emphasizing novel markers. Mod Pathol. 2013;26(5):725–32. doi:10.1038/modpathol.2012.229. Epub 2013 Jan.
Ro JY, Ayala AG, el-Naggar A. Muscularis mucosa of urinary bladder. Importance for staging and treatment. Am J Surg Pathol. 1987;11:668–73.
Ro JY, el-Naggar AK, Amin MB, et al. Inflammatory pseudotumor of the urinary bladder. Am J Surg Pathol. 1993;17:1193–4.
Samaratunga H, Khoo K. Micropapillary variant of urothelial carcinoma of the urinary bladder; a clinicopathological and immunohistochemical study. Histopathology. 2004;45:55–64.
Samaratunga H, Makarov DV, Epstein JN. Comparison of WHO/IUP and WHO classification of non-invasive papillary urothelial neoplasms for risk of progression. Urology. 2002;15:315–9.
Sangoi AR, Beck AH, Amin MB, Cheng L, Epstein JI, Hansel DE, Iczkowski KA, Lopez-Beltran A, Oliva E, Paner GP, Reuter VE, Ro JY, Shah RB, Shen SS, Tamboli P, McKenney JK. Interobserver reproducibility in the diagnosis of invasive micropapillary carcinoma of the urinary tract among urologic pathologists. Am J Surg Pathol. 2010;34(9):1367–76.
Schmitz-Drager BJ, van Roeyen CR, Grimm MO, et al. P53 accumulation in precursor lesions and early stages of bladder cancer. World J Urol. 1994;12:79–83.
Shalev M, Mistry S, Kernen K, Miles BJ. Squamous cell carcinoma in a female urethral diverticulum. Urology. 2002;59(5):773.
Shimasaki N, Inoue K, Nishigawa H, Kuroda N, Shuin T. Combined small cell carcinoma and sarcomatoid squamous cell carcinoma in the renal pelvis. Int J Urol. 2005;12(7):686–9.
Shirai T, Fukushima S, Hirose M, et al. Epithelial lesions of the urinary bladder in 313 autopsy cases. Jpn J Cancer Res. 1987;78:1073–80.
Sidransky EA, Frost P, von Eschenbach A, et al. Clonal origin of bladder cancer. N Engl J Med. 1992;326:737–40.
Spruck 3rd CH, Ohneseit PF, Gonzalez-Zulueta M, et al. Two molecular pathways to transitional cell carcinoma of the bladder. Cancer Res. 1994;54:784–8.
Sung L, Anderson JR, Arndt C, et al. Neurofibromatosis in children with rhabdomyosarcoma: a report from the Intergroup Rhabdomyosarcoma study IV. J Pediatr. 2004;144:666–8.
Sung MT, Maclennan GT, Lopez-Beltran A, et al. Natural history of urothelial inverted papilloma. Cancer. 2006a;107:2622–7.
Sung MT, Eble JN, Wang M, et al. Inverted papilloma of the urinary bladder: a molecular genetic appraisal. Mod Pathol. 2006b;19:1289–94.
Sung MT, Lopez-Beltran A, Eble JN, et al. Divergent pathway of intestinal metaplasia and cystitis glandularis of the urinary bladder. Mod Pathol. 2006c;19:1395–401.
Sung MT, Wang M, Maclennan G, et al. Histogenesis of sarcomatoid urothelial carcinoma of the urinary bladder: evidence for a common clonal origin with divergent differentiation. J Pathol. 2007;211:420–30.
Sung MT, Zhang S, MacLennan GT, et al. Histogenesis of clear cell adenocarcinoma in the urinary tract: evidence of urothelial origin by histology, immunohistochemistry and fluorescence in situ hybridization analysis. Clin Cancer Res. 2008;14(7):1947–55.
Tajima Y, Aizawa M. Unusual renal pelvic tumor containing transitional cell carcinoma, adenocarcinoma and sarcomatoid elements (so-called sarcomatoid carcinoma of the renal pelvis). A case report and review of the literature. Acta Pathol Jpn. 1988;38:805–14.
Talbert ML, Young RH. Carcinomas of the urinary bladder with deceptively benign-appearing foci. A report of three cases. Am J Surg Pathol. 1989;13:374–81.
Talwar N, Dargan P, Arora MP, Sharma A, Sen AK. Primary squamous cell carcinoma of the renal pelvis masquerading as pyonephrosis: a case report. Indian J Pathol Microbiol. 2006;49(3):418–20.
Tamas EF, Epstein JI. Detection of residual tumor cells in bladder biopsy specimens: pitfalls in the interpretation of cytokeratin stains. Am J Surg Pathol. 2007;31:390–7.
Tamas EF, Nielsen ME, Schoenberg MP, et al. Lymphoepithelioma-like carcinoma of the urinary tract: a clinicopathological study of 30 pure and mixed cases. Mod Pathol. 2007;20:828–34.
Taylor G, Jordan M, Churchill B, et al. Yolk sac tumor of the bladder. J Urol. 1983;129:591–4.
Vakar-López F, Abrams J. Basaloid squamous cell carcinoma occurring in the urinary bladder. Arch Pathol Lab Med. 2000;124:455–9.
van Rhijn BW, Lurkin I, Radvanyi F, et al. The fibroblast growth factor receptor 3 (FGFR3) mutation is a strong indicator of superficial bladder cancer with low recurrence rate. Cancer Res. 2001;61:1265–8.
van Rhijn BW, Montironi R, Zwarthoff EC, et al. Frequent FGFR3 mutations in urothelial papilloma. J Pathol. 2002;198:245–51.
van Rhijn BW, van der Kwast TH, Vis AN, et al. FGFR3 and P53 characterize alternative genetic pathways in the pathogenesis of urothelial cell carcinoma. Cancer Res. 2004;64:1911–4.
Velazquez EF, Soskin A, Bock A, Codas R, Cai G, Barreto JE, Cubilla AL. Epithelial abnormalities and precancerous lesions of anterior urethra in patients with penile carcinoma: a report of 89 cases. Mod Pathol. 2005;18(7):917–23.
Vizcaino JR, Macedo-Dias JA, Teixeira-de-Sousa JM, Silva RM, Carpenter S. Pseudotumour of renal pelvis: Liesegang rings mimicking a solid neoplasm of the renal pelvis. Histopathology. 2005;47(1):115–7.

Volmar KE, Chan TY, De Marzo AM, et al. Florid von Brunn nests mimicking urothelial carcinoma: a morphologic and immunohistochemical comparison to the nested variant of urothelial carcinoma. Am J Surg Pathol. 2003;27:1243–52.

Wagner U, Sauter G, Moch H, et al. Patterns of p53, erbB-2, and EGF-r expression in premalignant lesions of the urinary bladder. Hum Pathol. 1995;26:970–8.

Wang X, Jones TD, MacLennan GT, et al. P53 expression in small cell carcinoma of the urinary bladder: biological and prognostic implications. Anticancer Res. 2005;25:2001–4.

Wang X, MacLennan GT, Lopez-Beltran A, et al. Small cell carcinoma of the urinary bladder: histogenesis, genetics, diagnosis, biomarkers, treatment, and prognosis. Appl Immunohistochem Mol Morphol. 2007a;15:8–18.

Wang X, Zhang S, MacLennan GT, et al. Epidermal growth factor receptor protein expression and gene amplification in small cell carcinoma of the urinary bladder. Clin Cancer Res. 2007b;13:953–7.

Wasco MJ, Daignault S, Zhang Y, et al. Urothelial carcinoma with divergent histologic differentiation (mixed histologic features) predicts the presence of locally advanced bladder cancer when detected at transurethral resection. Urology. 2007;70:69–74.

Westra WH, Grenko RT, Epstein J. Solitary fibrous tumor of the lower urogenital tract: a report of five cases involving the seminal vesicles, urinary bladder, and prostate. Hum Pathol. 2000;31:63–8.

Wiedemann A, Muller H, Jaussi J, Rabs U. Mesonephric carcinoma of the urethra. A case report. Urol A. 2005;44(4):396–400.

Williamson SR, Lopez-Beltran A, Montironi R, Cheng L. Glandular lesions of the urinary bladder: clinical significance and differential diagnosis. Histopathology. 2010. doi:10.1111/j.1365-2559.2010.03651.x.

Williamson SR, Zhang S, Yao JL, Huang J, Lopez-Beltran A, Shen S, Osunkoya AO, MacLennan GT, Montironi R, Cheng L. ERG-TMPRSS2 rearrangement is shared by concurrent prostatic adenocarcinoma and prostatic small cell carcinoma and absent in small cell carcinoma of the urinary bladder: evidence supporting monoclonal origin. Mod Pathol. 2011a;24(8):1120–7. doi:10.1038/modpathol.2011.56.

Williamson SR, Zhang S, Lopez-Beltran A, Shah RB, Montironi R, Tan PH, Wang M, Baldridge LA, MacLennan GT, Cheng L. Lymphoepithelioma-like carcinoma of the urinary bladder: clinicopathologic, immunohistochemical, and molecular features. Am J Surg Pathol. 2011b;35(4):474–83.

Williamson SR, Zhang S, Lopez-Beltran A, Montironi R, Wang M, Cheng L. Telomere shortening distinguishes inverted urothelial neoplasms. Histopathology. 2013a;62(4):595–601. doi:10.1111/his.12030. Epub 2013 Feb 5.

Williamson SR, Scarpelli M, Lopez-Beltran A, Montironi R, Conces MR, Cheng L. Urethral caruncle: a lesion related to IgG4-associated sclerosing disease? J Clin Pathol. 2013b;66(7):559–62.

Williamson SR, Lopez-Beltran A, Maclennan GT, Montironi R, Cheng L. Unique clinicopathologic and molecular characteristics of urinary bladder tumors in children and young adults. Urol Oncol. 2013c;31(4):414–26.

Yoshimura I, Kudoh J, Saito S, et al. p53 gene mutation in recurrent superficial bladder cancer. J Urol. 1995;153:1711–5.

Younes M, Sussman J, True LD. The usefulness of the level of the muscularis mucosae in the staging of invasive transitional cell carcinoma of the urinary bladder. Cancer. 1990;66:543–8.

Young RH, Oliva E. Transitional cell carcinomas of the urinary bladder that may be underdiagnosed. A report of four invasive cases exemplifying the homology between neoplastic and non-neoplastic transitional cell lesions. Am J Surg Pathol. 1996;20:1448–54.

The Prostate and Seminal Vesicles

3

Contents

3.1 **Basic Anatomy and Histology** 196
3.1.1 The Prostate 196
3.1.2 The Seminal Vesicles and Ejaculatory Ducts 201

3.2 **Adenocarcinoma of the Prostate** 202
3.2.1 Preneoplastic Lesions and Conditions 202

3.3 **Diagnostic Criteria for Prostate Adenocarcinoma** 214
3.3.1 Histologic Features of Prostate Cancer 215

3.4 **Rare Histologic Subtypes of Prostatic Carcinoma** 224
3.4.1 Pseudohyperplastic Adenocarcinoma 224
3.4.2 Foamy Gland Adenocarcinoma 225
3.4.3 Atrophic Adenocarcinoma 226
3.4.4 Adenocarcinoma with Glomeruloid Features 228
3.4.5 Mucinous and Signet Ring Cell Adenocarcinoma 228
3.4.6 Oncocytic Adenocarcinoma 229
3.4.7 Lymphoepithelioma-Like Carcinoma of the Prostate 230
3.4.8 Prostatic Ductal Adenocarcinoma 232
3.4.9 Intraductal Carcinoma 237
3.4.10 Small Cell Carcinoma 239
3.4.11 Sarcomatoid Carcinoma (Carcinosarcoma) 241
3.4.12 PIN-Like Carcinoma 243
3.4.13 Pleomorphic Giant Cell Carcinoma 244

3.5 **Gleason Grading of Prostate Cancer** 247
3.5.1 Gleason Patterns 248
3.5.2 Reporting Gleason Scores in Prostate Needle Biopsies 250
3.5.3 Reporting Gleason Scores in Radical Prostatectomies 251
3.5.4 Grading Variants and Variations of Adenocarcinoma of the Prostate 252
3.5.5 Correlation Between Needle Biopsy and RP Gleason Scores 252
3.5.6 Pathology of the Prostate After Treatment 254

3.6 **Pathologic Prognosis of Prostate Cancer** 261
3.6.1 Prostate Biopsy 261
3.6.2 Prognostic Factors After Radical Prostatectomy 266

3.7 **Basic Molecular Pathology of Prostate Cancer** 271

3.8 **Rare Forms of Prostatic Tumours** 274

3.9 **Tumors and Tumor-Like Conditions of the Prostate Stroma** 288

3.10 **Miscellaneous Primary Tumours of the Prostate** 298

3.11 **Secondary Tumours Involving the Prostate** 298

3.12 **Seminal Vesicles** 302

Suggested Reading 306

A. Lopez-Beltran et al., *Rare Tumors and Tumor-like Conditions in Urological Pathology*,
DOI 10.1007/978-3-319-10253-5_3,

3.1 Basic Anatomy and Histology

3.1.1 The Prostate

- The adult prostate surrounds the urethra and is located posterior to the inferior symphysis pubis, superior to the urogenital diaphragm, and anterior to the rectum. It measure 5 cm × 4 cm × 3 cm and weighs 20 g from ages 20 to 50, with an increase to 30 g from ages 60 to 80.
- The three-zone model defines the central zone, the transition zone, and the peripheral zone.
- Cancer tends to arise in the peripheral zone (20 % do arise in the transition zone), and BPH typically arise in the transition zone (Figs. 3.1, 3.2, 3.3, 3.4, 3.5 and 3.6). The central zone is more resistant to disease. The prostatic urethra exits the prostate at the apex where it is continuous con the membranous urethra.
- The paired ejaculatory ducts run through the central zone from the seminal vesicles to their exit at the posterior urethral protuberance, known as the verumontanum (Fig. 3.7). Within the verumontanum is the prostatic utricle, located between the ejaculatory ducts (Fig. 3.8).
- The anterior fibromuscular stroma is present anteriorly over the prostate and extends from the bladder neck to the apex of the prostate.
- Adult prostate gland is a branching duct-acinar embedded in a fibromuscular stroma. The epithelium has two cell layers: the luminal/secretory and the basal layer with some neuroendocrine cells in the epithelium (Figs. 3.3 and 3.4). The cytoplasm of secretory cell is cleared with yellow-brown pigment (lipofuscin) but not mucin.
- Secretory cells are positive for CKAE1/AE3, CK 8–18, PSA, PAP, PSMA, p501S and NKX3-1. P504S (racemase) may show a focal non-circumferential positivity in secretory cells.
- Lipofuscin can also be found in the cytoplasm of seminal vesicle and ejaculatory duct epithelium (Fig. 3.9).
- Basal cells have a dense cytoplasm, and small hyperchromatic nuclei. They react with p63, CK5/6 and high molecular weight CK clone 34βE12 (CK903).
- Neuroendocrine cells are less frequent and show an immunohistochemical profile more similar to secretory cells with variable androgen receptor and PSA/PAP expression. They express a number of immunohistochemical markers including chromogranin, synaptophisin, neuron-specific enolase, and many others.
- Urothelium is also normally present in the prostate sometimes showing a cleared cytoplasm. It is PSA negative and p63 positive.
- Intraluminal contents of normal prostate glands include degenerated epithelial cells, corpora amylacea and calculi. Rarely, it may contain focal blue-tinged mucin, pink amorphous acellular secretions, and crystalloids.
- The prostatic stroma, including fibroblasts, smooth muscle, vasculature and nerves, and rarely adipocytes (carcinoma in fat should be viewed as extraprostatic extension). There are zonal differences in prostatic fibromuscular stroma density.
- The prostate does not have a true capsule. The so called outer prostatic "capsule" is a band of concentrically placed fibromuscular and vascular tissue that is inseparable from prostatic stroma and surrounding fascia. This is absent in the apex.
- Histologically, nerves are seen in the periprostatic neurovascular bundle, in the outer fibromuscular band, and in the prostate itself. Paraganglia (cleared cells that should not be mistaken as carcinoma) are usually adjacent to neurovascular bundles but may be seen deeper. Posterolateral prostate shows abundant adipose tissue together with neurovascular bundles.
- Bulbourethral Cowper glands are extrinsic to the prostate but eventually may be seen in prostate biopsies. Histologically they are tubuloalveolar glands with lobules of acini, admixed with excretory ducts and ductuli. Frequently they are associated with skeletal muscle fibers. The cells are cuboidal to columnar, pale-staining mucinous cytoplasm and small, bland, basally located nuclei. A basal cell layer is not readily apparent

with H&E. Immunohistochemistry remains unsettled with studies suggesting PSA or PSAP positive or negative. It is unclear if 34βE12 highlights basal cells but acinar cells are 34βE12 negative.

- Distorted colorectal epithelium can potentially be confused with prostatic adenocarcinoma since it is negative for basal cell markers 34βE12 and p63.

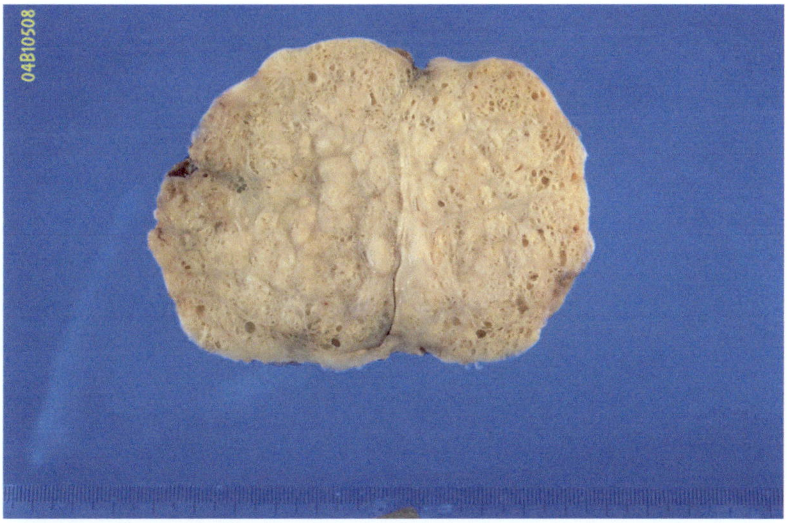

Fig. 3.1 Simple retropubic prostatectomy showing benign hyperplasia of the transition zone

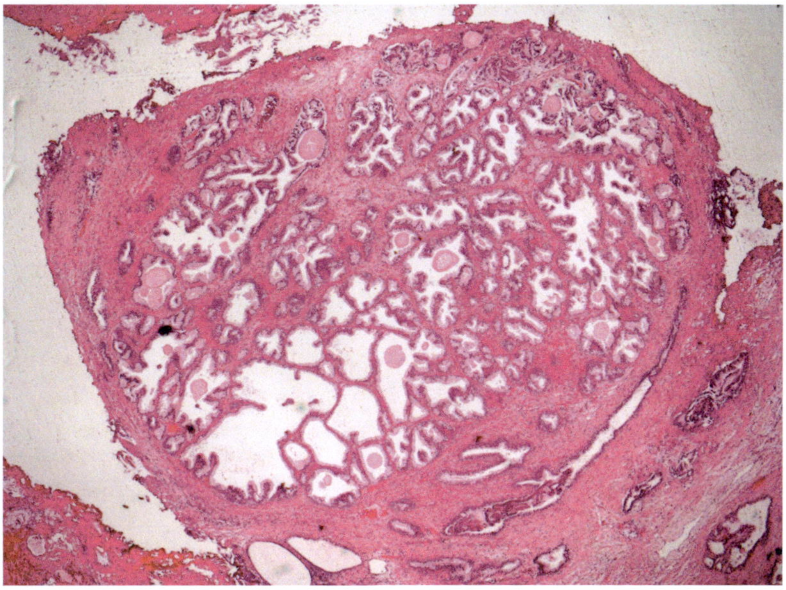

Fig. 3.2 Low power histology of a nodule of benign hyperplasia of the prostate

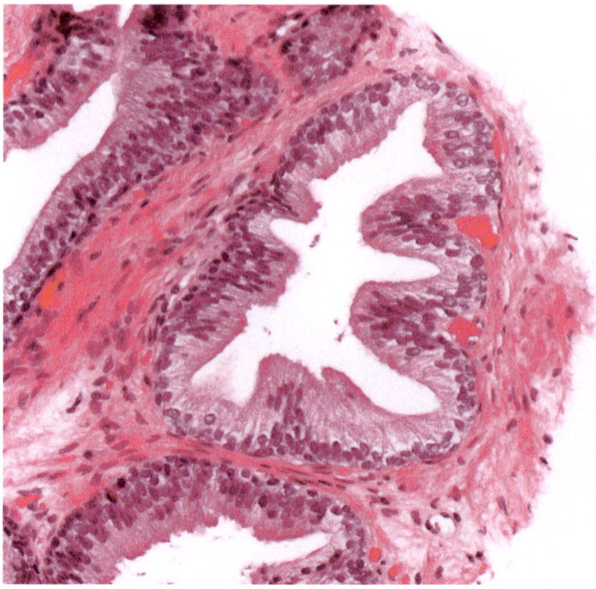

Fig. 3.3 Microscopically, prostate glands show basal cell layer and the secretory cells towards the lumen

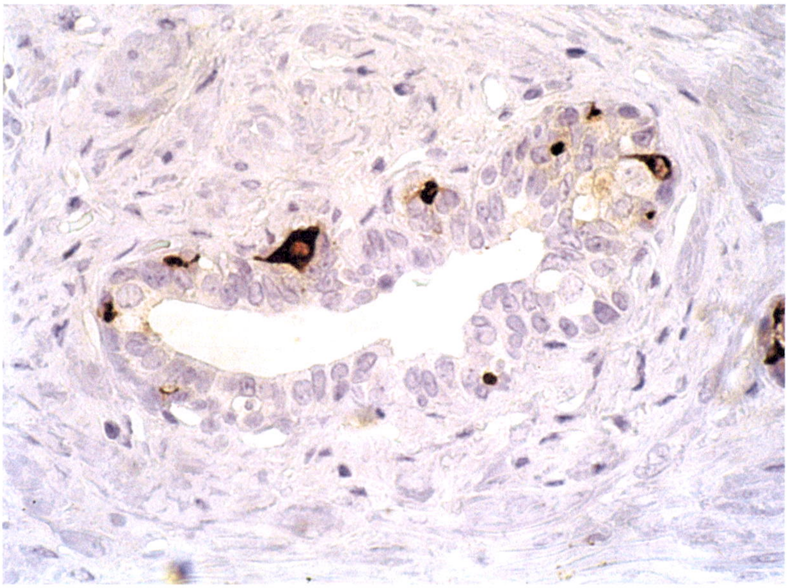

Fig. 3.4 Neuroendocrine cells are present within the basal cells but may extend to luminal surface

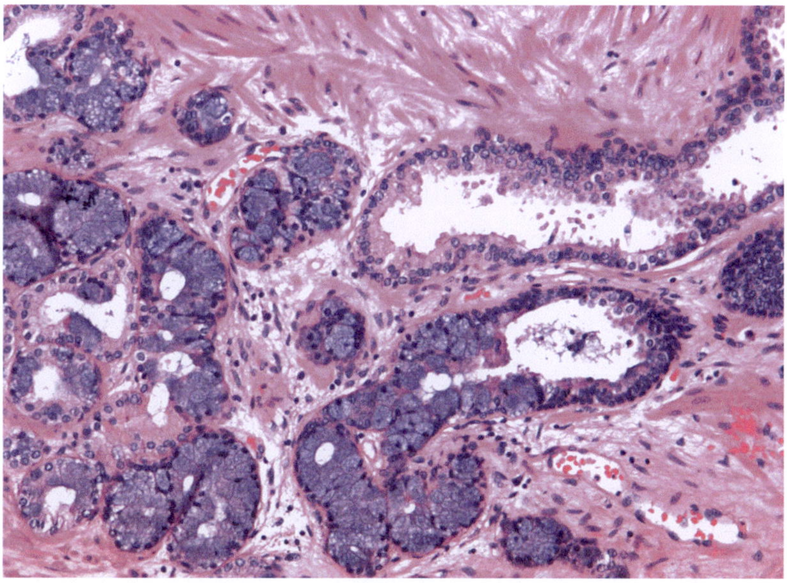

Fig. 3.5 Mucinous metaplasia may be occasionally seen in some prostate glands

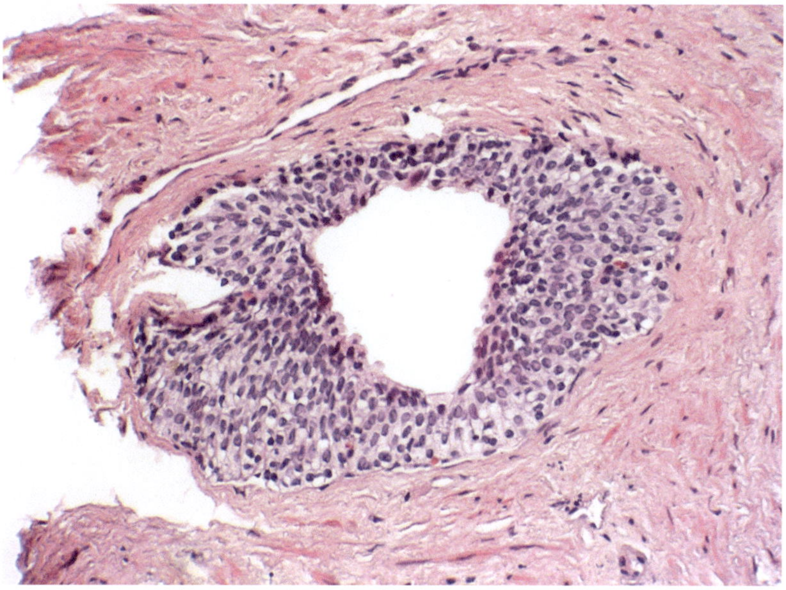

Fig. 3.6 Urothelial metaplasia is focally seen in some prostate glands

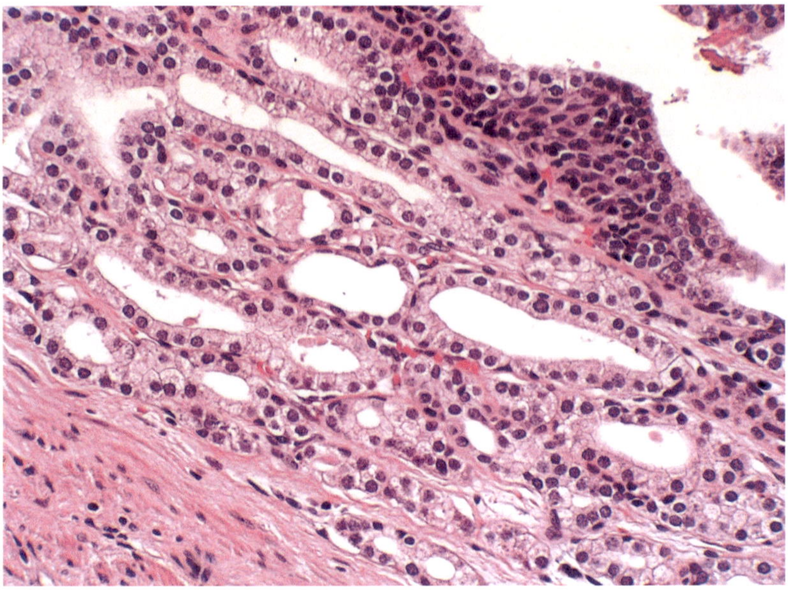

Fig. 3.7 Histology of the verumontanum glands

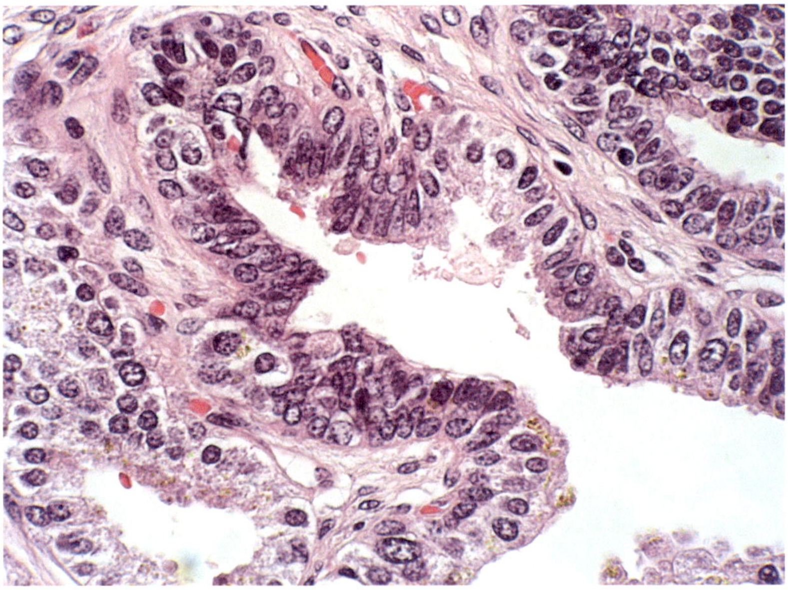

Fig. 3.8 Microscopic appearance of ejaculatory ducts

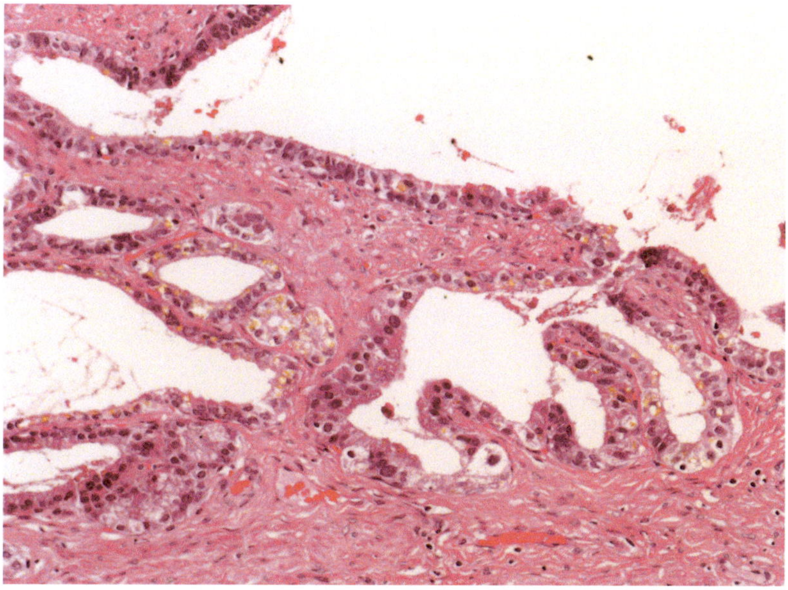

Fig. 3.9 Lipofucsin in seminal vesicle epithelium

3.1.2 The Seminal Vesicles and Ejaculatory Ducts

- Seminal vesicles lie posterolateral to the base of the urinary bladder and anterior to Denonvilliers fascia. Seminal vesicle wall consists of a thick circumferential coat of smooth muscle and the ejaculatory ducts are surrounded by a collagenous stroma. Uncommonly, one may see small hyaline globules in the SVs wall (Fig. 3.10).
- Seminal vesicle and ejaculatory ducts share histogenesis from the wolffian system with the prostatic central zone.
- The SVs epithelium is composed of ducts and acini with a two-cell lining layer of secretory cells and basal cells. Lipofuscin (yellow-brown pigment) can be found in the cytoplasm of secretory cells in SVs and ejaculatory duct epithelium, and rarely in stromal cells. It is characteristic to see scattered nuclei exhibiting enlargement and degenerative-type hyperchromasia. This is a helpful feature to separate SVs/ejaculatory ducts epithelium from prostate epithelium.
- The immunoprofile of secretory cells of SVs/ejaculatory ducts is CKAE1/AE3+, CAM5.2+, PAX-2+, MUC 6+, PSA-, PAP- and P504S (racemase) -. Basal cells are p63+.

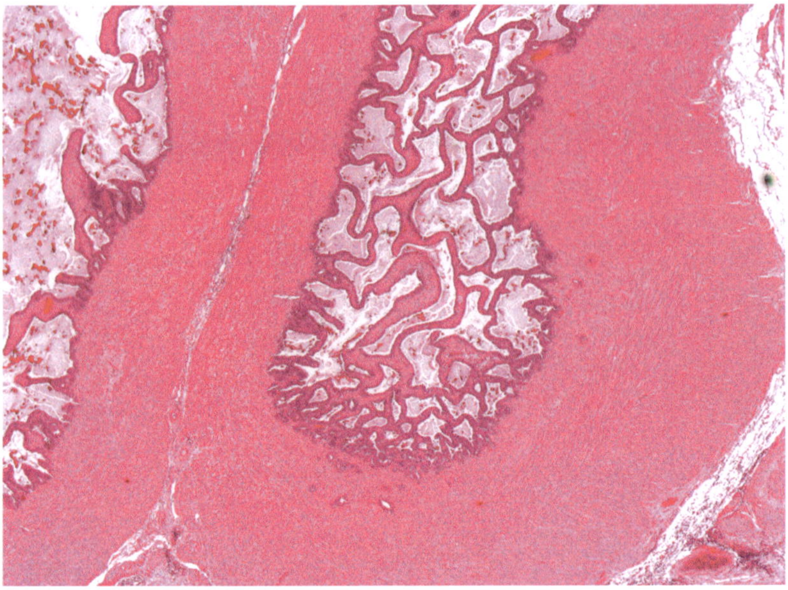

Fig. 3.10 Seminal vesicle wall consists of a thick circumferential coat of smooth muscle

3.2 Adenocarcinoma of the Prostate

- The incidence of prostate cancer (PCa) has raised dramatically in the past 25 years owing to early detection programs that employ serum prostate-specific antigen (PSA). In developed countries, PCa is the most commonly diagnosed non-skin malignancy in men.
- Multiple factors contribute to the development of PCa as well as to its progression to an androgen-independent state: dietary factors, inherited susceptibility factors, gene defects, and androgens and their receptors.
- Most prostate cancer patients are asymptomatic nowadays, detected by digital rectal examination and imaging methods in the setting of high serum PSA level. Most cancers arise in the peripheral zone, so that transition zone enlargement sufficient to cause bladder outlet obstruction usually indicates hyperplasia.
- The test most used is serum PSA and its derivatives. PSA is elevated beyond the arbitrary cut-off point of 4.0 ng/ml in the majority of patients with prostate cancer (sensitivity of 20 % and specificity of 60–70 %). It may also be greater than 4.0 ng/ml in benign conditions including benign prostatic hyperplasia (BPH).
- After therapy of localized PCa, PSA is expected to decline to a nadir of <0.2 ng/mL. PSA elevation afterward (≥0.2 ng/mL) on two occasions is considered biochemical recurrence.

3.2.1 Preneoplastic Lesions and Conditions

3.2.1.1 Prostatic Intraepithelial Neoplasia

- Prostatic intraepithelial neoplasia (PIN) refers to the preinvasive end of the continuum of cellular proliferations within the lining of prostatic ducts, ductuli, and acini (Figs. 3.11, 3.12, 3.13 and 3.14).
- It is currently recommended compression of the PIN classification into two grades: low-grade (formerly PIN grade 1) or high-grade PIN (formerly PIN grades 2 and 3) (HGPIN) (Table 3.1).

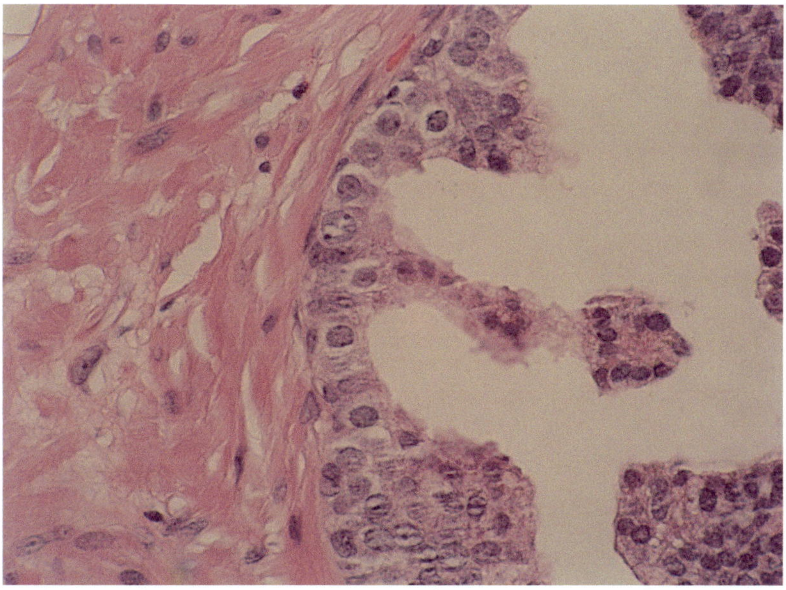

Fig. 3.11 Microscopic aspect of prostate intraepithelial neoplasia

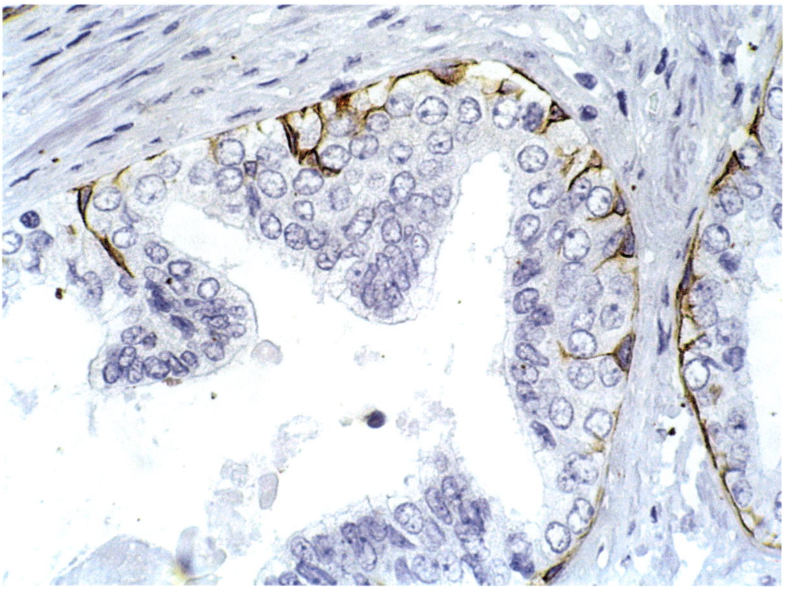

Fig. 3.12 Discontinuous basal cell layer seen with basal cell cytokeratin in prostate intraepithelial neoplasia

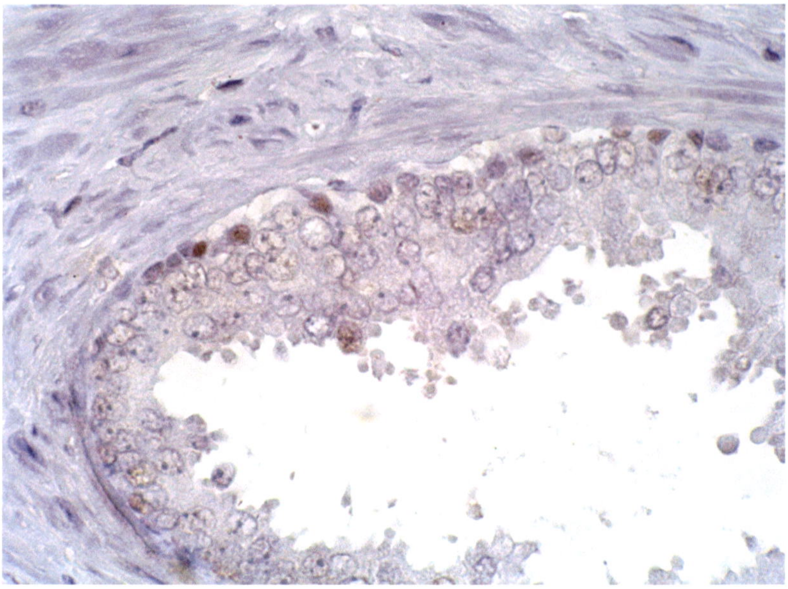

Fig. 3.13 Discontinuous basal cell layer seen with p63 in prostate intraepithelial neoplasia

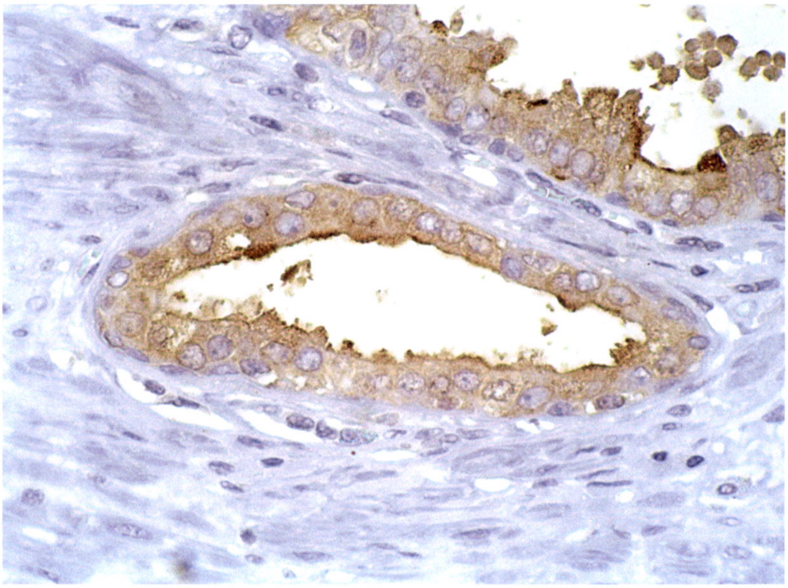

Fig. 3.14 PSA cytoplasmic expression in prostate intraepithelial neoplasia

Table 3.1 Differential diagnoses of prostate adenocarcinoma

Common:
Atrophy
Post-atrophic hyperplasia
Partial atrophy
Basal cell hyperplasia
Atypical adenomatous hyperplasia (adenosis)
Inflammatory-associated atypia
High-grade PIN
Less common:
Cowper's gland
Nephrogenic metaplasia
Clear cell cribriform hyperplasia
Seminal vesicle/ejaculatory ducts
Paraganglia
Xanthoma

3.2.1.2 Diagnostic Criteria for HGPIN

- The classification of PIN into low-grade and high-grade is chiefly based on the cytological characteristics of the cells. The nuclei of cells composing low-grade PIN are enlarged, vary in size, have slightly increased chromatin content, and possess small or inconspicuous nucleoli.
- HGPIN is characterised by cells with large nuclei of relatively uniform size, an increased chromatin content, which may be irregularly distributed, and prominent nucleoli that are similar to those of carcinoma cells. The basal cell layer is intact or rarely interrupted in low-grade PIN, but may have frequent disruptions in high-grade lesions.
- There are four main patterns of HGPIN: tufting, micropapillary, cribriform, and flat. The tufting pattern is the most common, present in 97 % of cases, although most cases have admixed patterns. There are no known clinically important differences between the architectural patterns of HGPIN, and their recognition appears to be only of diagnostic utility. Other unusual patterns of HGPIN include the signet ring-cell pattern, small cell neuroendocrine pattern, mucinous pattern, inverted-type, squamous-type and foamy pattern (Figs. 3.15, 3.16, 3.17, 3.18, 3.19, 3.20, 3.21 and 3.22).
- HGPIN is multicentric in 70 % of radical prostatectomies with cancer, including 65 % of those involving the non-transition zone and 7 % of those involving the transition zone; 2 % of cases have concomitant single foci in all zones.
- The peripheral zone of the prostate, the area in which the majority of prostatic carcinomas occur (70 %), is also the most common location for HGPIN where frequently is multicentric.
- Early stromal invasion (PIN with microinvasion), the earliest evidence of carcinoma, occurs at sites of acinar out pouching and basal cell disruption in acini with HGPIN. Such microinvasion is present in about 2 % of high power microscopic fields of HGPIN, and is seen with equal frequency with all architectural patterns.
- Evidence linking HGPIN and prostate cancer has been found in morphological, immunohistochemical, morphometric, molecular and genetic studies. Virtually all such studies have indicated that HGPIN is related more closely to prostate cancer than to benign epithelium. HGPIN was more extensive in small cancers than in larger cancers, presumably due to "overgrowth" or obliteration of HGPIN by larger cancers.
- Discrepancies in the diagnosis of HGPIN were greatest between HGPIN with cribriform proliferations.
- When the small atypical acini are too numerous and too crowded to be outpouchings or simply tangential sections, then cancer can be diagnosed. Immunohistochemical stains for the basal cell markers are of value in selected cases.
- HGPIN shows a discontinuous basal cell layer when labelled with the antibody to high-molecular-weight keratin or p63. HGPIN is considered nowadays the most frequent cause of misdiagnosis of PCa in needle prostate biopsies.
- HGPIN has a limited predictive value as a marker of adenocarcinoma in subsequent biopsy when single and unilateral. Bilateral and multifocal HGPIN increases likelihood of PCa being diagnosed in up to 10 %.
- Cancer detection rate in patients with low-grade PIN is identical to that in patients who underwent repeat biopsy for persistent elevated serum PSA or because of an abnormal digital rectal examination.

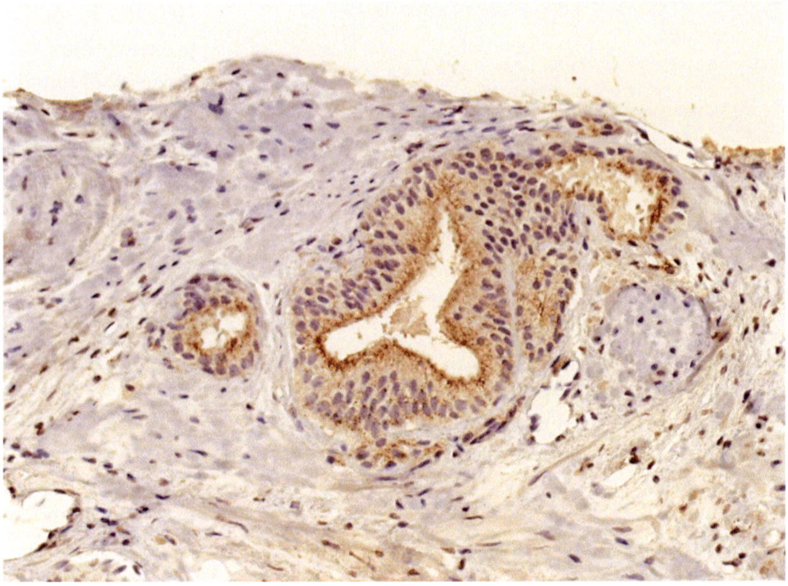

Fig. 3.15 Racemase cytoplasmic expression in prostate intraepithelial neoplasia

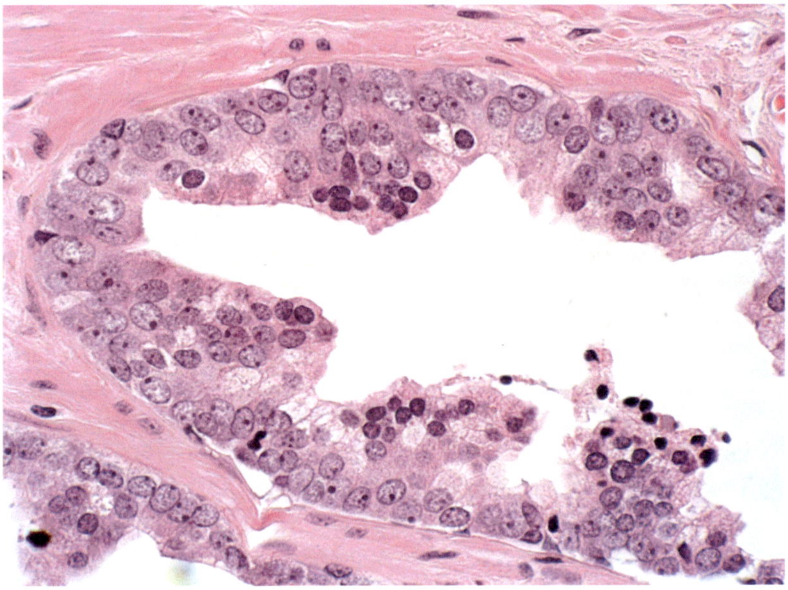

Fig. 3.16 Prostate intraepithelial neoplasia with tufting histologic pattern

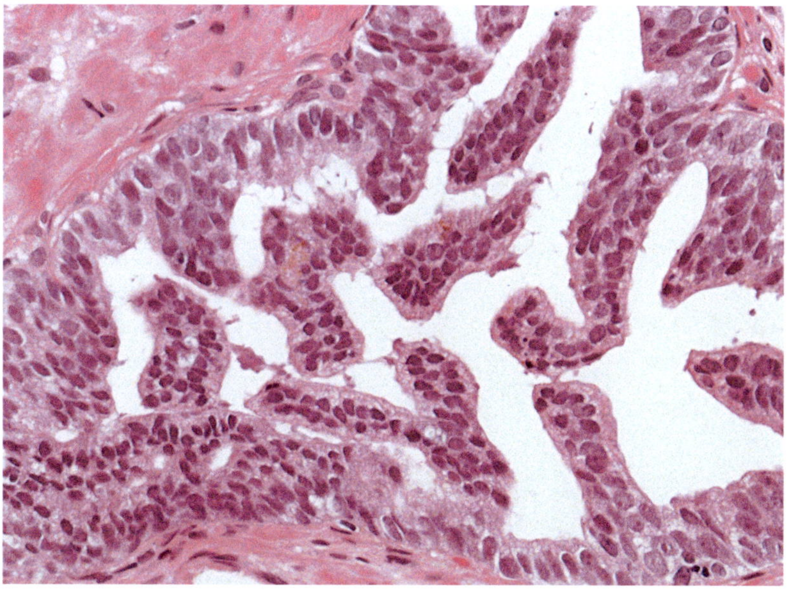

Fig. 3.17 Prostate intraepithelial neoplasia with micropapillary histologic pattern

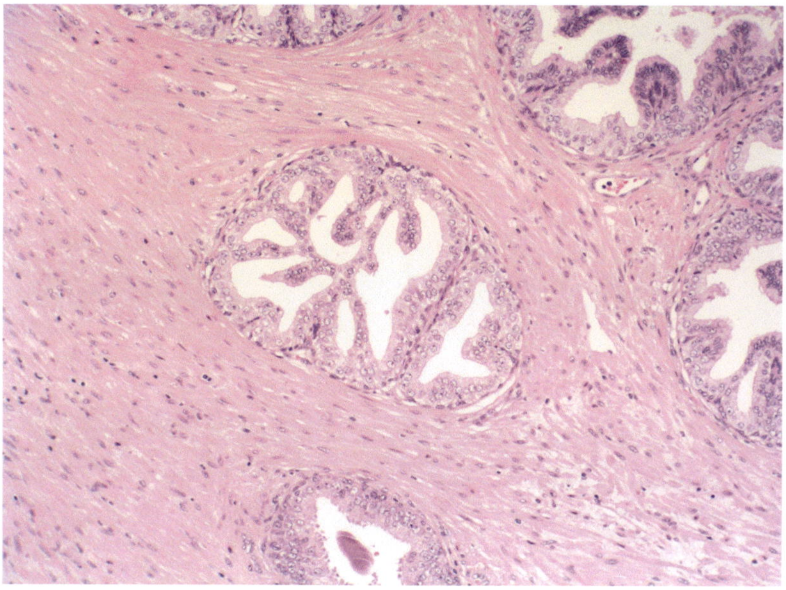

Fig. 3.18 Prostate intraepithelial neoplasia with cribriform histologic pattern

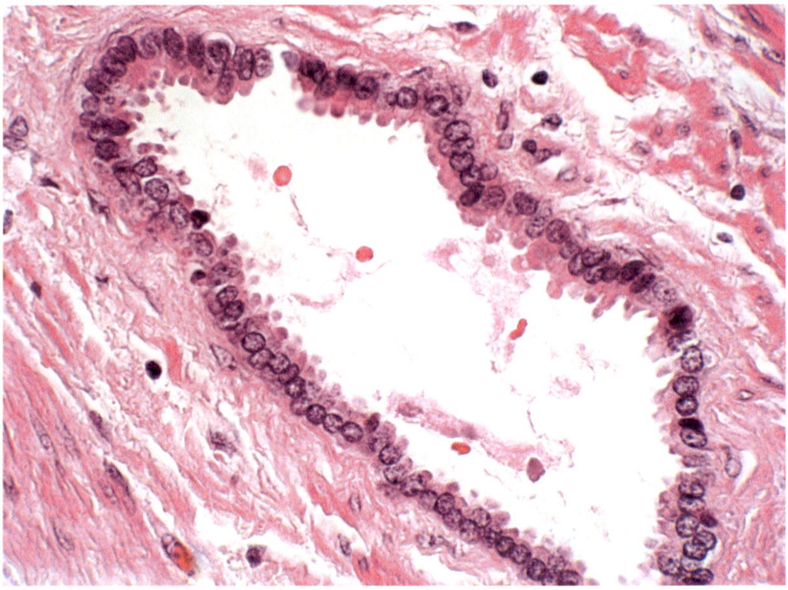

Fig. 3.19 Prostate intraepithelial neoplasia with flat histologic pattern

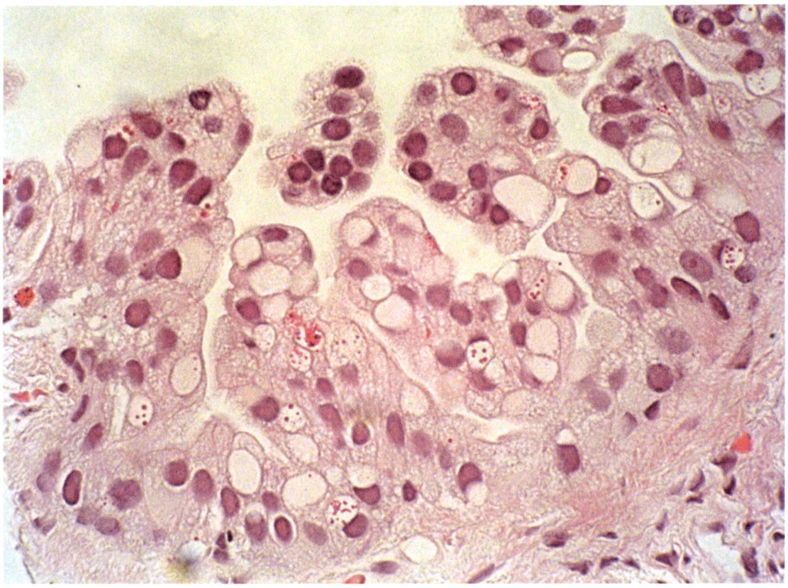

Fig. 3.20 Prostate intraepithelial neoplasia with cytoplasmic vacuoles (signet-ring) histologic pattern

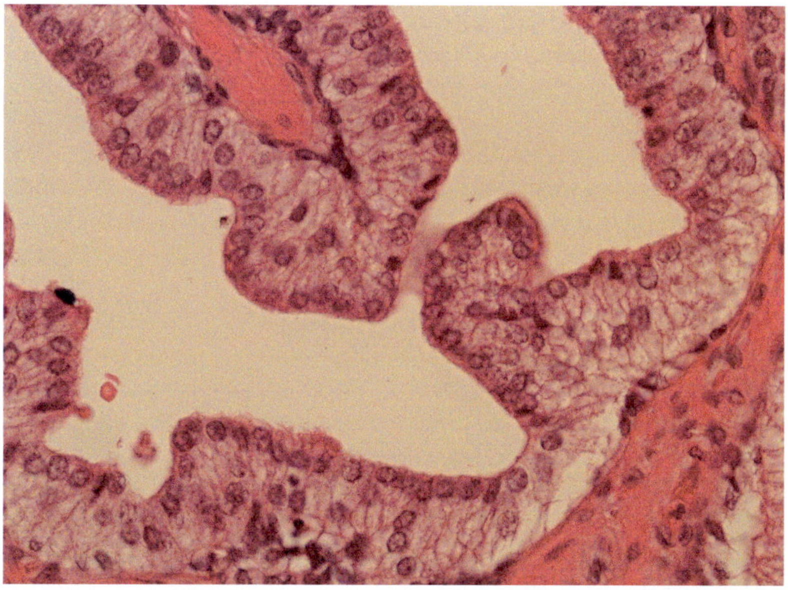

Fig. 3.21 Prostate intraepithelial neoplasia with inverted histologic pattern

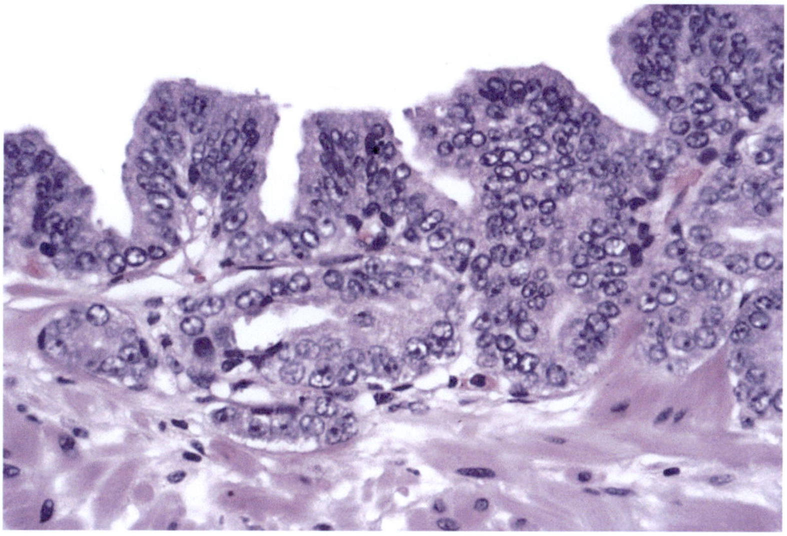

Fig. 3.22 Prostate intraepithelial neoplasia with microinvasive histologic pattern

3.2.1.3 Atypical Adenomatous Hyperplasia

- Atypical adenomatous hyperplasia (AAH, adenosis) is characterized by a circumscribed proliferation of closely packed small glands that, rather than appearing invasive, tends to merge with the surrounding, histologically benign glands.
- AAH frequently demonstrates budding acini from adjacent foci of benign hyperplastic glands, and the cells have clear cytoplasm with variable intraluminal secretions. Architecturally, AAH resembles well-differentiated adenocarcinoma of low Gleason score, and most cases of Gleason primary pattern 1 cancer are now considered within the spectrum of AAH. Recognition of the basal cell layer excludes the diagnosis of carcinoma.
- Unfortunately, identification of the basal epithelium is often difficult, as it is usually attenuated and may be discontinuous in AAH, and this may be the rule in needle biopsy specimens.
- Recognition of the basal cell layer may be facilitated by use of an antibody to p63 or to high-molecular-weight cytokeratin. An additional compelling feature is the observed positive immunoreactivity of AAH foci with Racemase (P504S). AAH lacks TMPRSS2-ERG Gene fusion as recently demonstrated.
- Nuclear and nucleolar morphology is the key differentiating feature between AAH and carcinoma, but this has less power than the presence of basal cells after immunohistochemistry. About 85 % of cases of AAH are located in the transition zone. The incidence of AAH in prostate specimens is largely variable in reported series (2–23 %) (Figs. 3.23, 3.24, 3.25 and 3.26).

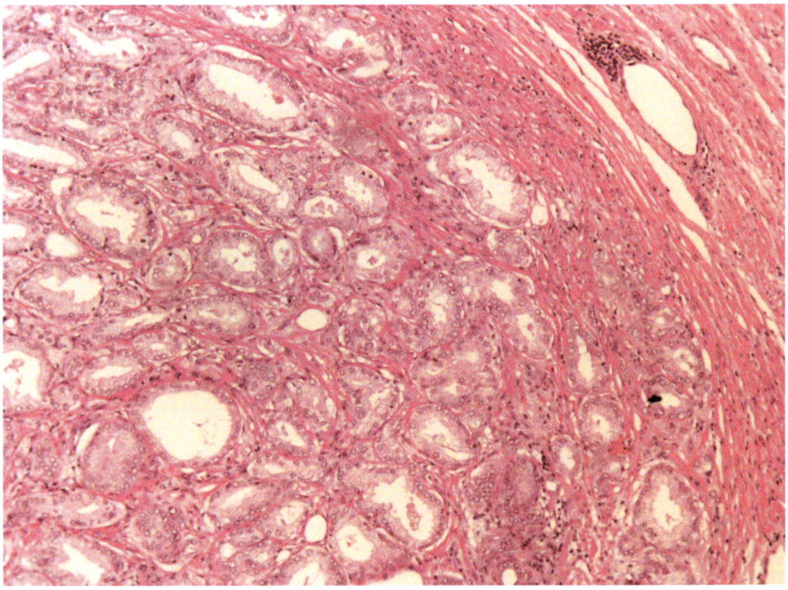

Fig. 3.23 Microscopic features of atypical adenomatous hyperplasia (adenosis) of the prostate (low power view)

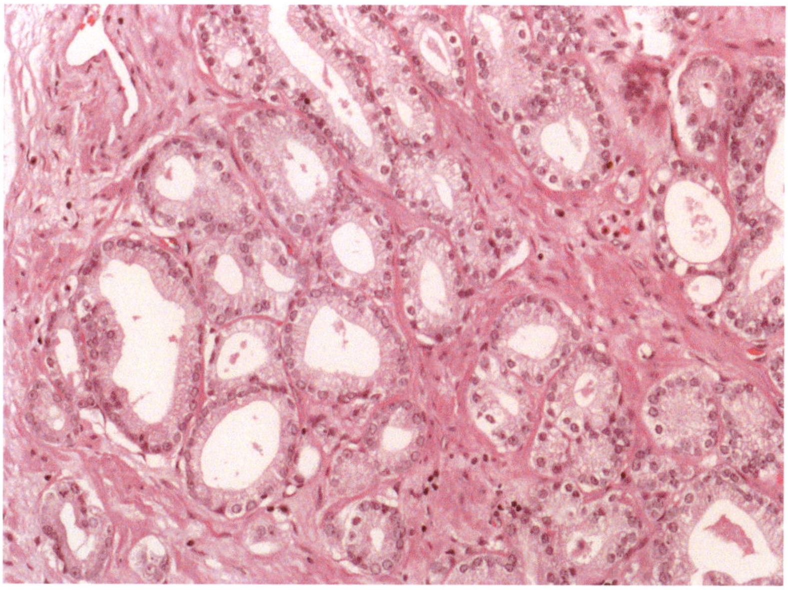

Fig. 3.24 Microscopic features of atypical adenomatous hyperplasia (adenosis) of the prostate (high power view)

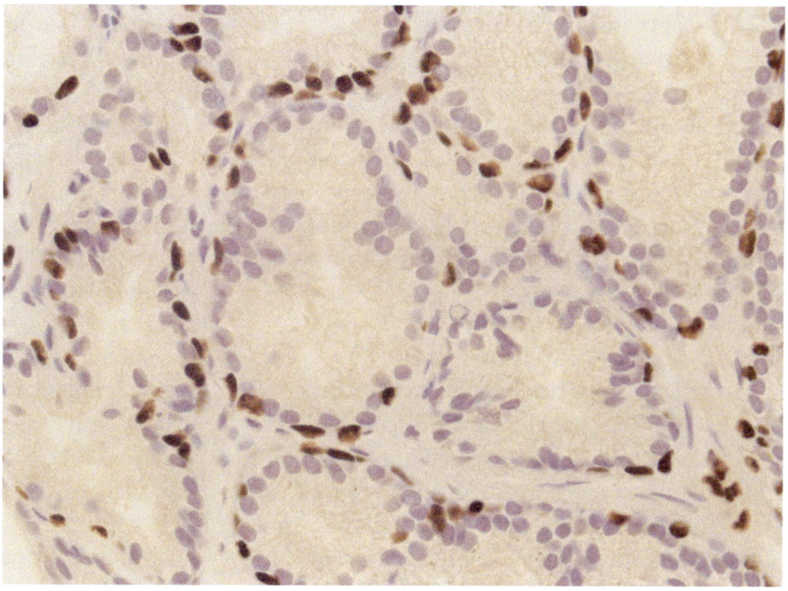

Fig. 3.25 Discontinuous p63 expression in basal cells of atypical adenomatous hyperplasia (adenosis) of the prostate

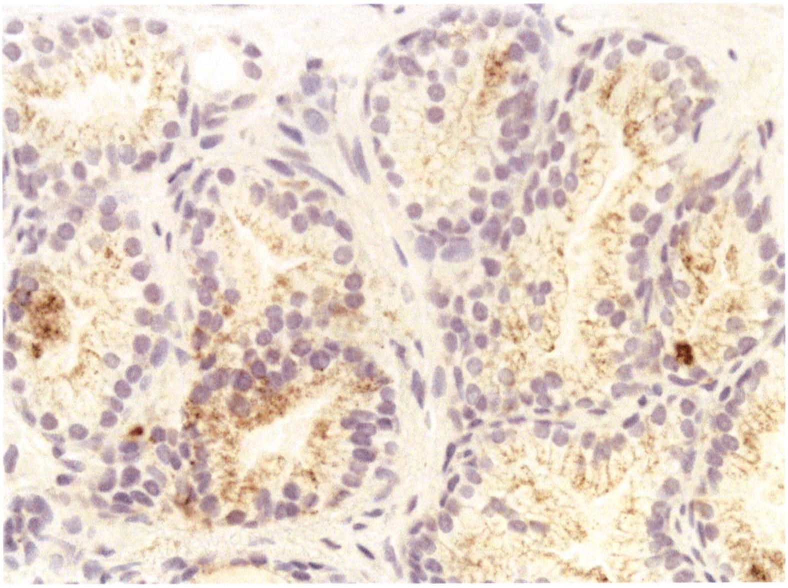

Fig. 3.26 Weak racemase expression in secretory cells of atypical adenomatous hyperplasia (adenosis) of the prostate

3.2.1.4 Post-inflammatory Atrophy (PIA)

- Recent reports suggest that post-inflammatory atrophy, may be causally linked to PIN and therefore to prostate adenocarcinoma. This hypothesis is based upon recognition of increased proliferative activity, albeit low, in the secretory cells that persist within atrophic acini.

3.2.1.5 Atypical Small Acinar Proliferation Suspicious for But Not Diagnostic of Malignancy

- Atypical focus suspicious but not diagnostic of malignancy (ASAP), also referred to as atypical small acinar proliferation suspicious for but not diagnostic of malignancy or just atypical prostate glands (ATYP), is not a preneoplastic lesion. It is descriptive diagnostic terminology used in the pathology report of a needle biopsy containing a small group of glands suspicious for adenocarcinoma, however with insufficient cytological and/or architectural atypia to establish a definitive diagnosis. In some cases (16–31 %) the lesion is associated with PIN (PIN ASAP or PIN ATYP).
- It is a broad diagnostic category that encompasses benign lesions mimicking malignant glandular proliferations and under sampled, small foci of carcinoma that harbour some but not all of the features needed for a definitive diagnosis of malignancy. It is not a diagnostic entity and is not synonymous with high-grade prostatic intraepithelial neoplasia (HGPIN).
- The widespread use of basal cell immunohistochemistry using antibodies against p63 or 34βE12 or the use of racemase (P504S) turned the use of the diagnostic term ASAP uncommon nowadays (Figs. 3.27 and 3.28; Table 3.2).

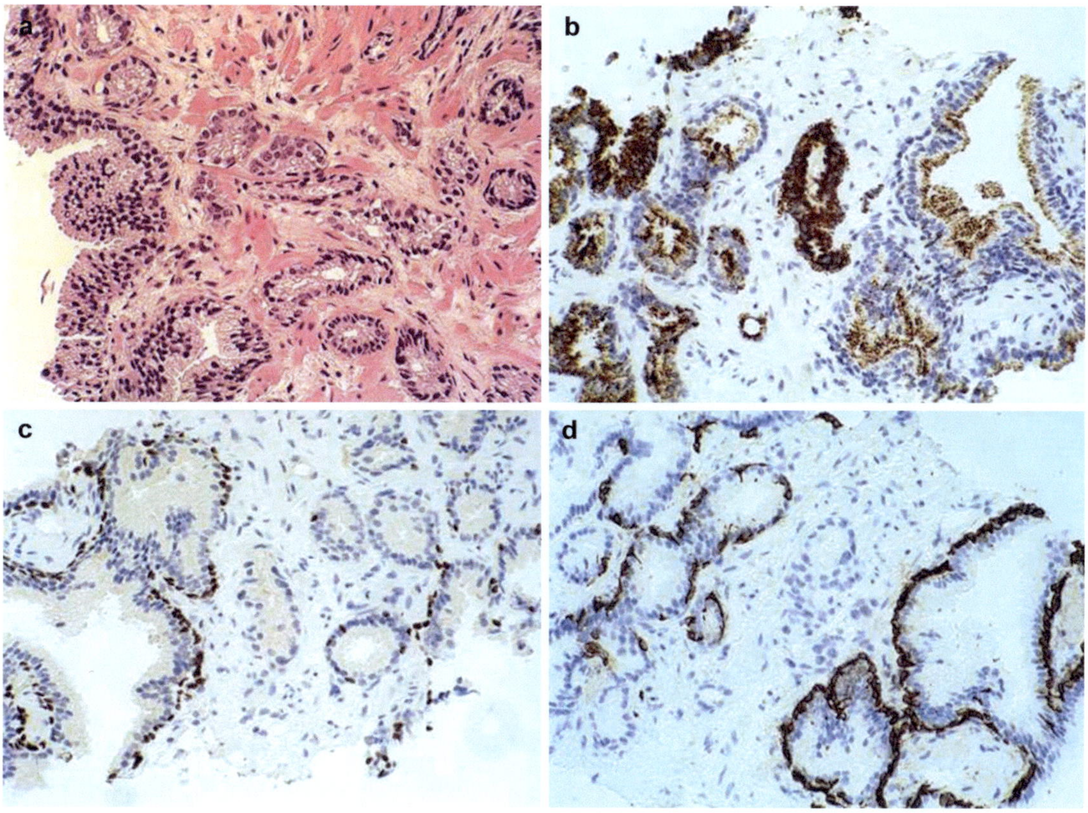

Fig. 3.27 Histologic features of atypical small acinar proliferation. (**a**) H&E; (**b**) Racemase positive; (**c**) p63 positive in a few basal cells; (**d**) Negative basal cell cytokeratin. In this scenario, the presence of p63 positive basal cells suggest that the lesion might be related to a PIN with invasion more than a carcinoma

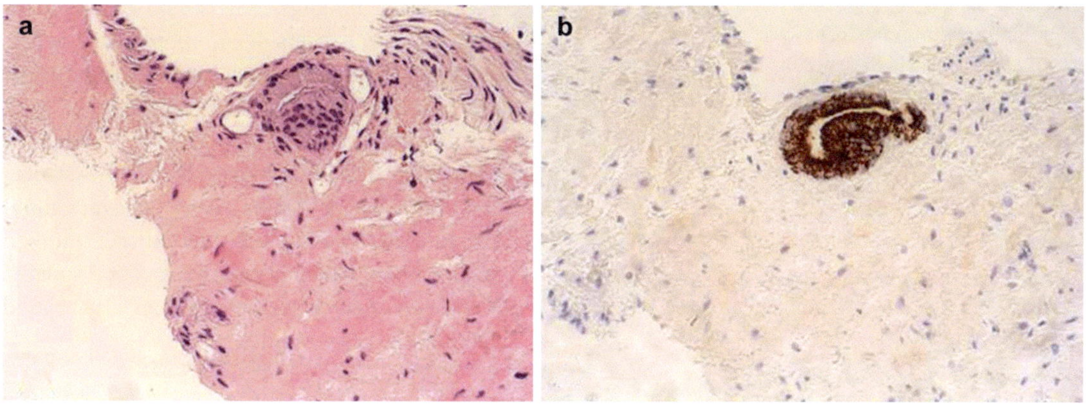

Fig. 3.28 Histologic features of atypical small acinar proliferation. (**a**) H&E; (**b**) Racemase positive; (**c**) Negative basal cell cytokeratin; (**d**) Negative p63. In this scenario, the absence of basal cells and the strong positive for racemase support malignancy even in a limited specimen

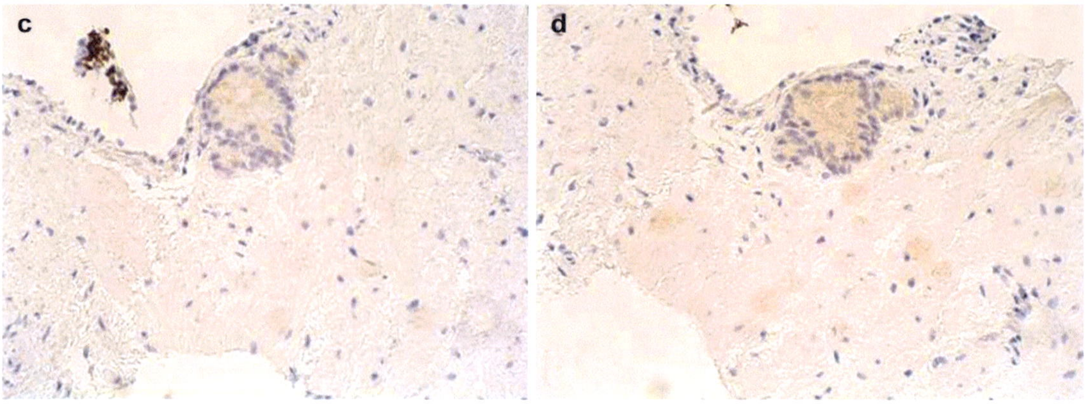

Fig. 3.28 (continued)

Table 3.2 Factors resulting in the diagnosis of atypical small acinar proliferations suspicious for malignancy

Small size of focus
Small number of acini in the focus of concern (invariably fewer than two dozen acini)
Small focus size, average 0.4 mm in diameter
Focus at core tip or biopsy edge, indicating that the focus is incompletely sampled
Loss of focus of concern in deeper levels
Conflicting morphologic findings
Distortion of acini raising concern for atrophy
Lack of convincing features of cancer (insufficient nucleomegaly or nucleolomegaly)
Clustered growth pattern mimicking a benign process such as atypical adenomatous hyperplasia
Foamy cytoplasm raising concern for foamy gland carcinoma
Conflicting immunohistochemical findings
Focally positive high molecular weight cytokeratin
Focally positive p63 staining
Negative racemase immunostain
Confounding findings
Histologic artifacts such as thick sections or overstained nuclei
Tangential cutting of adjacent high-grade PIN
Architectural or cytologic changes (nuclomegaly and nucleolomegaly) owing to inflammation or other lesions

3.3 Diagnostic Criteria for Prostate Adenocarcinoma

- Most clinically palpable prostate cancers diagnosed on needle biopsy are predominantly located posterolateral. Large transition zone tumours may extend into the peripheral zone and become palpable.
- Cancers detected on TURP are predominantly within the transition zone. Non-palpable cancers detected on needle biopsy are predominantly located peripherally, although 20 % have tumour predominantly within the transition zone. Large tumours may extend into the central zone, yet cancers uncommonly arise in this zone. Multifocal adenocarcinoma of the prostate is seen in about 85 % of prostates.
- Grossly evident cancers are firm, solid, and range in colour from white-grey to yellow-orange, the latter having increased cytoplasmic lipid; the tumours contrast with the adjacent benign parenchyma, which is typically tan and spongy. Tumours usually extend microscopically beyond their macroscopic border.

- Gross haemorrhage and necrosis are rare. Subtle tumours may be grossly recognized by structural asymmetry; for example, peripheral zone tumours may deform the periurethral fibromuscular concentric band demarcating the periurethral and peripheral prostate centrally, and peripherally may expand or obscure the out of boundaries of the prostate. Anterior and apical tumours are difficult to grossly identify because of admixed stromal and nodular hyperplasia.
- Grossly recognizable tumours tend to be larger, of higher grade and stage, and are frequently palpable, compared with grossly unapparent tumours (usually <5 mm) which are often non-palpable, small, low grade and low stage. Some large tumours are diffusely infiltrative, and may not be evident grossly.
- In countries with widespread PSA testing, grossly evident prostate cancer has become relatively uncommon (Table 3.3).

Table 3.3 Diagnostic criteria for prostatic carcinoma

Architectural features
Infiltrative pattern of malignant acini, e.g.:
Arrangement: irregular and haphazard
Spacing between acini varies widely
Variation in size
Irregular contour
Basal cell layer
Absent
Cytological features (secretory cells in single layer)
Nuclear hyperchromasia
Nuclear enlargement
Nucleolar enlargement or prominence
Mitotic figures
Amphophilic cytoplasm
Luminal findings
Crystalloids
Intraluminal blue mucin and/or pink amorphous secretions
Stromal findings
Collagenous micronodules
Immunohistochemical findings
Prostate-specific antigen
Prostatic acid phosphatase
34βE12
p63
Racemase
Additional feature
Adjacent prostatic intraepithelial neoplasia

3.3.1 Histologic Features of Prostate Cancer

- The diagnosis of carcinoma relies on a combination of architectural and cytological findings. Greater than 95 % of all carcinomas of the prostate seen in needle biopsy specimens are referred to as acinar or conventional type.

3.3.1.1 Architectural Features

- Architectural features are usually assessed at low to medium power magnification, with emphasis on spacing, size, and shape of acini. The arrangement of the acini is diagnostically useful and is the basis of the Gleason grade.
- Malignant acini usually have an irregular, haphazard arrangement, randomly scattered in the stroma in clusters or singly. The spacing between malignant acini often varies widely. Variation in acinar size is a useful criterion for cancer, particularly when small, irregular, abortive acini with primitive lumens are seen at the periphery of a focus of well-differentiated carcinoma (Fig. 3.29)
- The acini in suspicious foci are usually small or medium sized, with irregular contours that contrast with the typical smooth, round to elongated contours of benign and hyperplastic acini. Comparison with the adjacent benign prostatic acini is always of value in the diagnosis of cancer (Fig. 3.30)
- Well-differentiated carcinoma and the large acinar variant of Gleason 3 carcinoma are particularly difficult to separate from benign acini in needle biopsies because of the uniform size and spacing of acini; in such cases, greater emphasis is placed on cytologic features, immunohistochemical findings, and the presence of smaller diagnostic acini at the edge of the focus (Figs. 3.31, 3.32, 3.33 and 3.34).
- The basal cell layer is absent in prostate cancer, whereas an intact basal cell layer is present with benign acini. This is an important diagnostic feature that is not always easy to evaluate in routine tissue sections owing to false negative findings with atrophy and other mimics of cancer. Compressed stromal fibroblasts may mimic basal cells but are usually seen only focally at the periphery of acini.

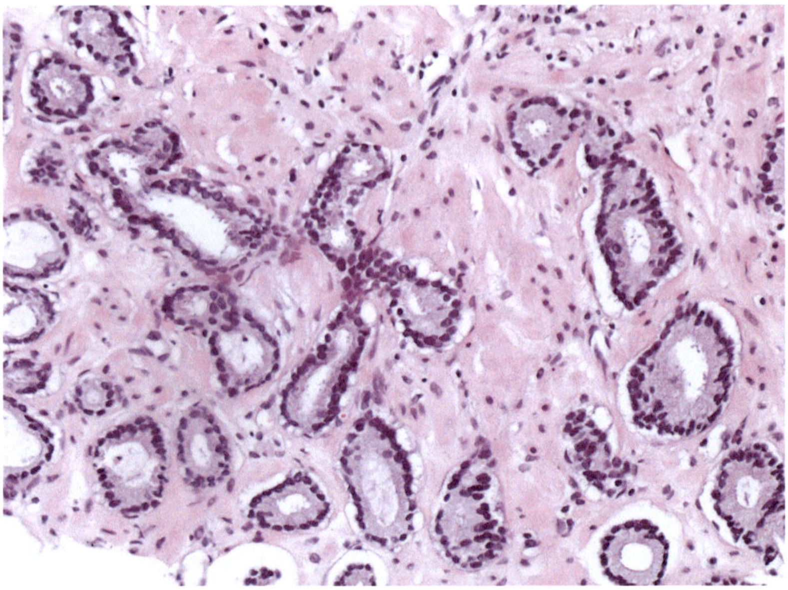

Fig. 3.29 Microscopic appearance of acinar (conventional) prostate cancer showing infiltrating acini, amphophilic cytoplasm, retraction artefact of the glands, and minimal nuclear atypia

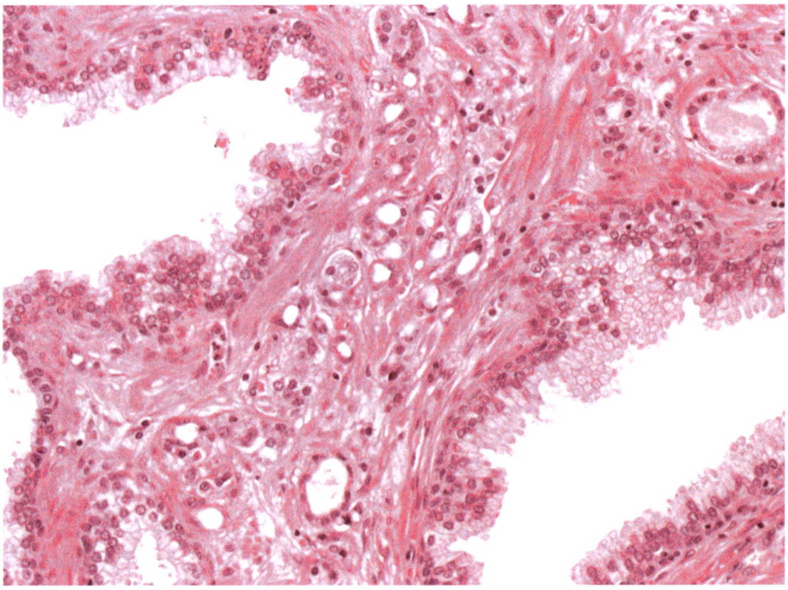

Fig. 3.30 Infiltrating acini between non-malignant ducts. Comparison with the adjacent benign prostatic acini is of value in the diagnosis of cancer

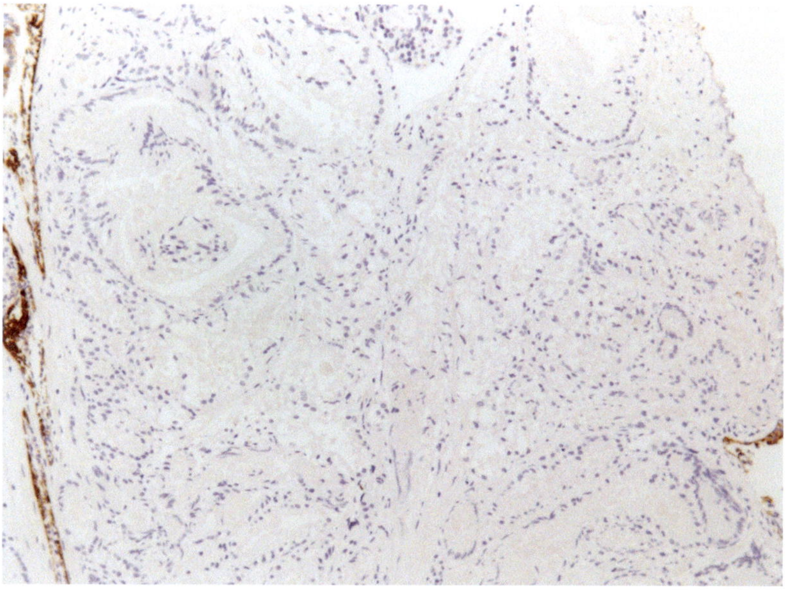

Fig. 3.31 Basal cells are typically lost in prostate carcinoma. Anti-34BE12 immunohistochemistry

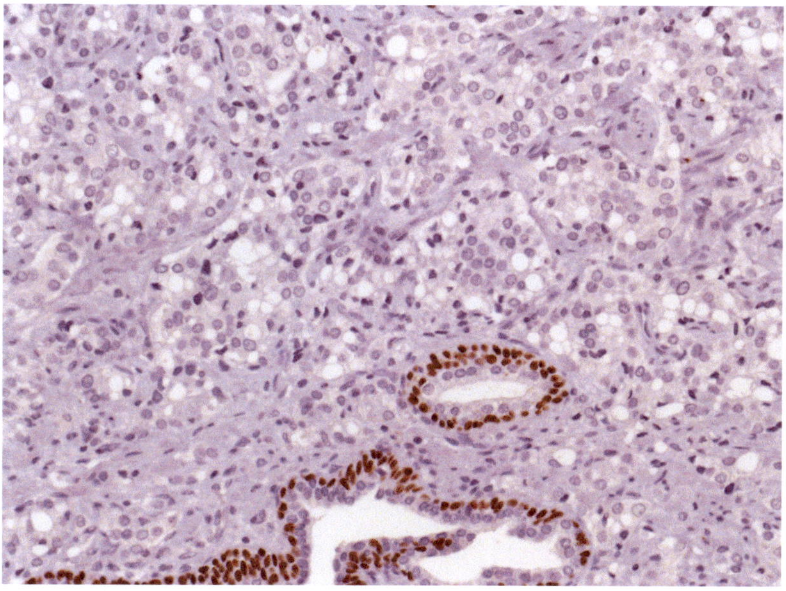

Fig. 3.32 Basal cells are typically lost in prostate carcinoma. Anti-p63 immunohistochemistry

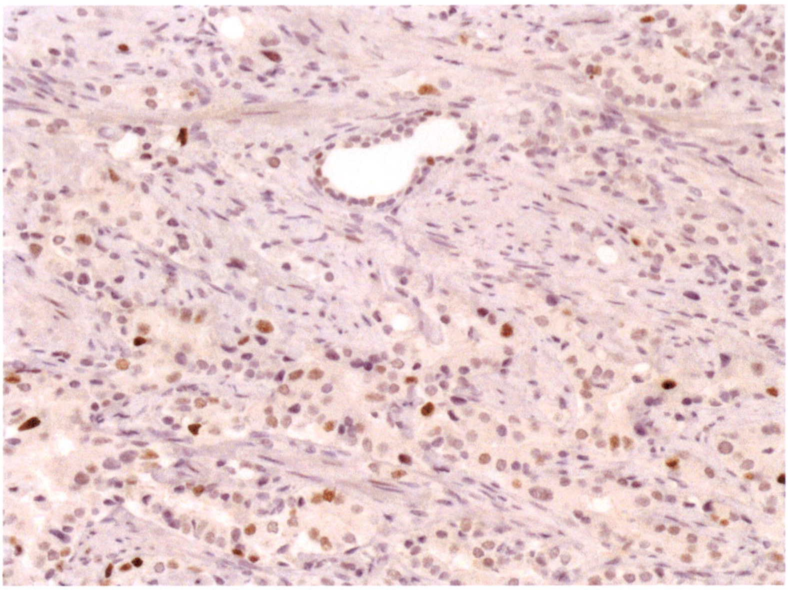

Fig. 3.33 Rare cases of prostate carcinoma may be positive with current anti-p63 antobodies, a challenging diagnostic factor

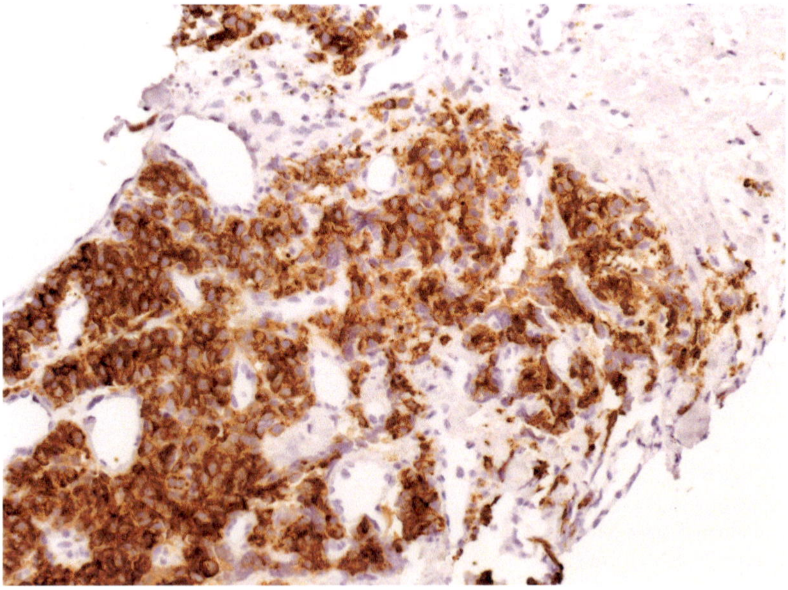

Fig. 3.34 Strong cytoplasmic expression of racemase is a characteristic of acinar prostate carcinoma

3.3.1.2 Cytological Features

- The cytological features of adenocarcinoma include nuclear and nucleolar enlargement, which occurs in most malignant cells. Every cell has a nucleolus at least 1.50 μm in diameter or larger. Artifacts such overstaining and differences in fixation often obscure the nuclei and nucleoli, so comparison with non-neoplastic cells (internal control) from the same specimen is a useful diagnostic clue (Figs. 3.35 and 3.36).

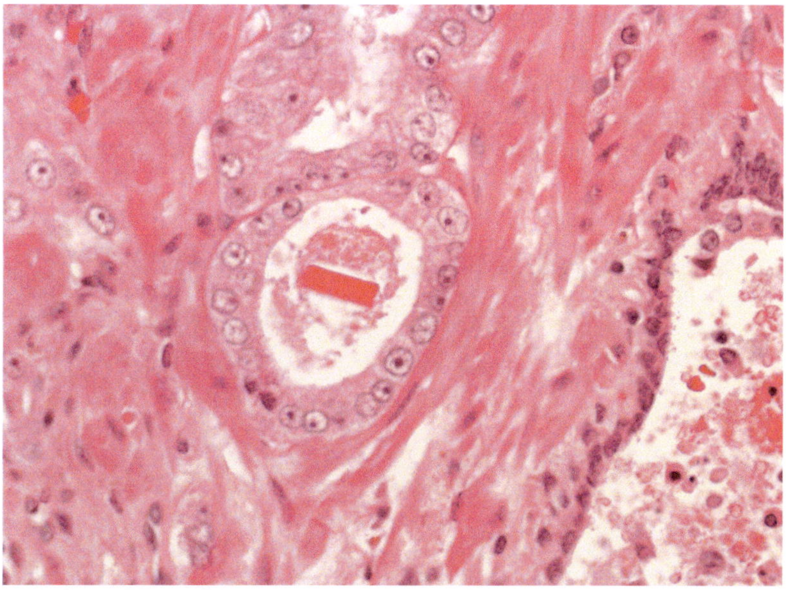

Fig. 3.35 Prominent nucleolus is characteristic of many prostate carcinomas. In this case, luminal crystals are also present

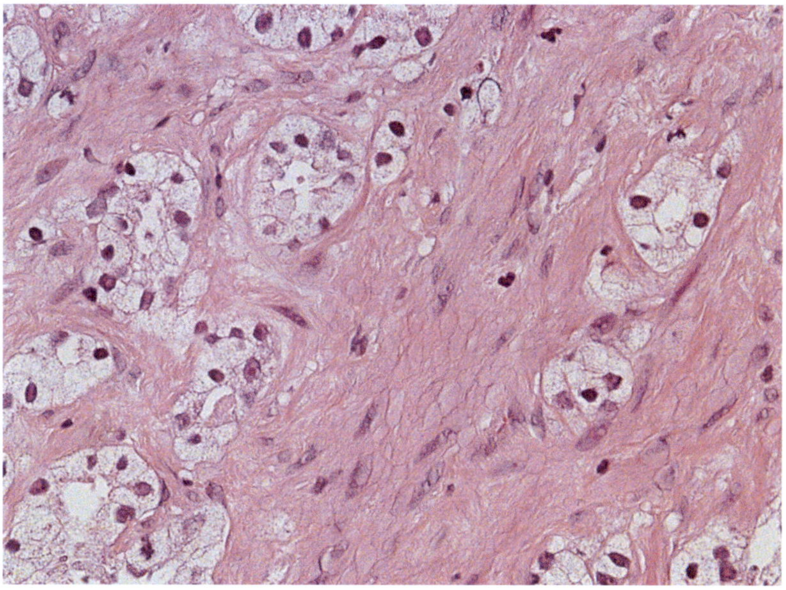

Fig. 3.36 Prominent nucleolus may not be present in some cases. This case shows clear-type cytoplasm and nucleolus-poor features

3.3.1.3 Luminal Findings

- Crystalloids are sharp, needle-like eosinophilic structures that are often present in the lumens of well-differentiated and moderately differentiated carcinoma. They are not specific for carcinoma and can be found in other conditions. The presence of crystalloids in metastatic adenocarcinoma of unknown site of origin is strong presumptive evidence of prostatic origin, although it is an uncommon finding (Fig. 3.37).
- Luminal acidic sulfated and nonsulfated mucin is often seen in acini of adenocarcinoma, appearing as amorphous, faintly basophilic secretions in routine sections. This mucin stains with Alcian blue at pH2.5, whereas normal prostatic epithelium contains periodic acid Schiff-reactive mucin that is neutral (Fig. 3.38).
- Acidic mucin is not specific for carcinoma. It may be found in prostatic intraepithelial neoplasia (PIN), atypical adenomatous hyperplasia, sclerosing adenosis, and, rarely, nodular hyperplasia.
- Intraluminal corpora amylacea may be seen occasionally in prostate cancer.

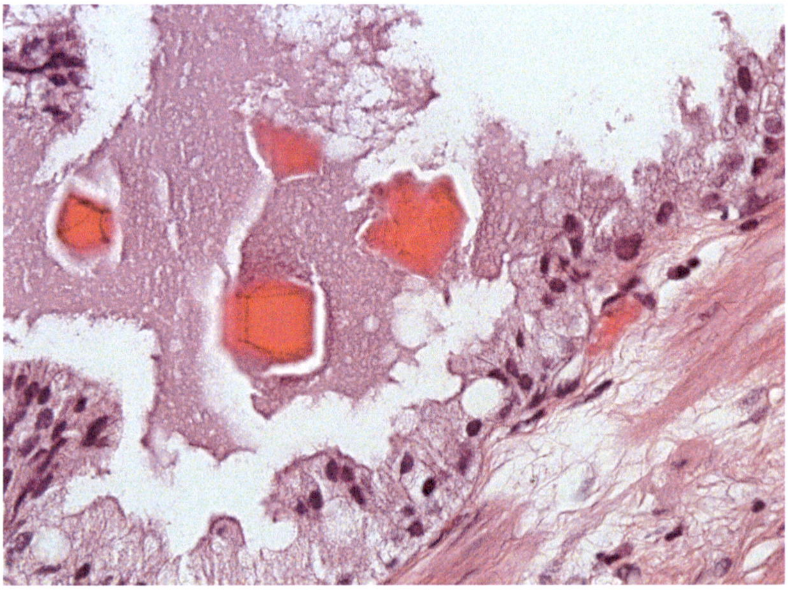

Fig. 3.37 Some prostate carcinoma may present luminal basophilic material and crystals

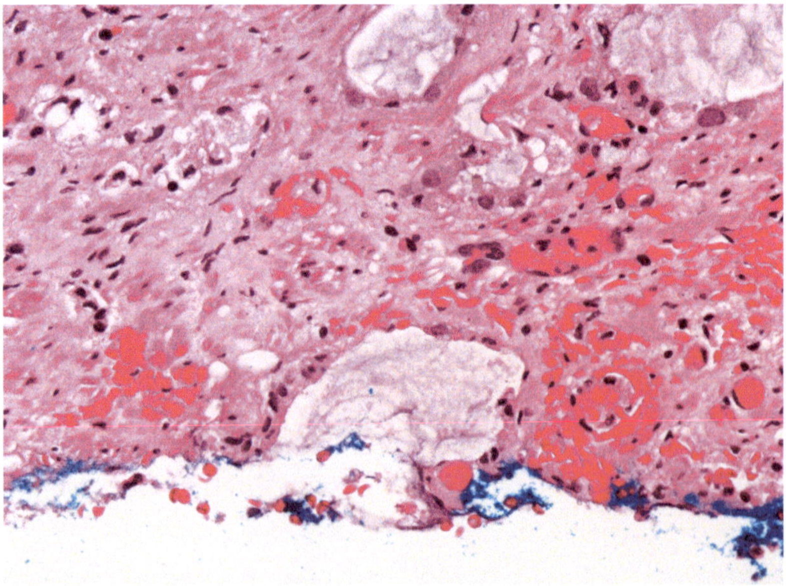

Fig. 3.38 Mucin is also present in some prostate carcinoma glands

3.3.1.4 Stromal Findings

- The stroma in cancer frequently contains young collagen, which appears lightly eosinophilic, although desmoplasia may be prominent. Muscle fibers in the stroma are sometimes split or distorted. But most frequently resembles the stroma associated with benign prostate (Fig. 3.39).
- Collagenous micronodules (mucinous fibroplasia) are a specific but infrequent and incidental finding in prostatic adenocarcinoma. They consist of microscopic nodular masses of paucicellular eosinophilic fibrilar stroma that impinge on acinar lumens. They are usually present in mucin-producing adenocarcinoma and result from extravasation of acidic mucin into the stroma (Fig. 3.40).
- Collagenous micronodules are present in about 14 % of cases of adenocarcinoma. Collagenous micronodules may be particularly valuable in challenging needle biopsy specimens. They are not observed in PIN, nodular hyperplasia, or benign epithelium.

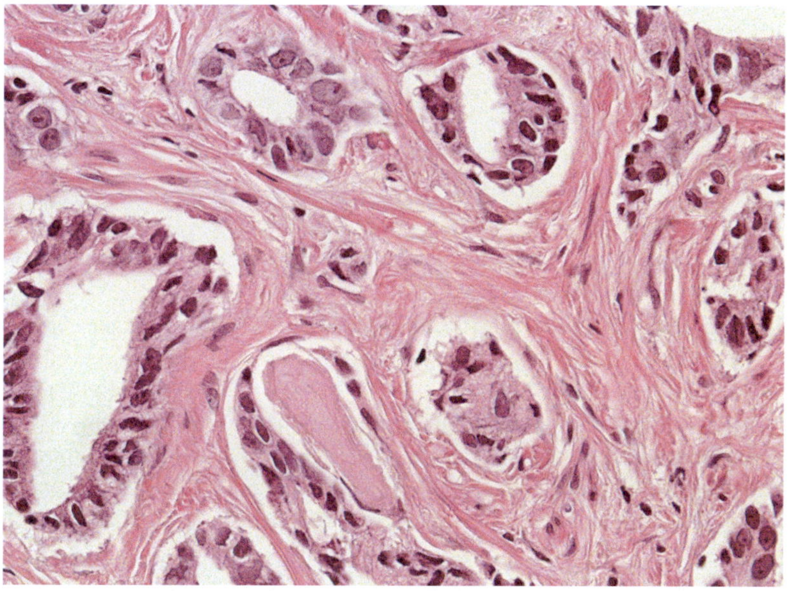

Fig. 3.39 Prostate carcinoma with prominent fibroblastic stroma

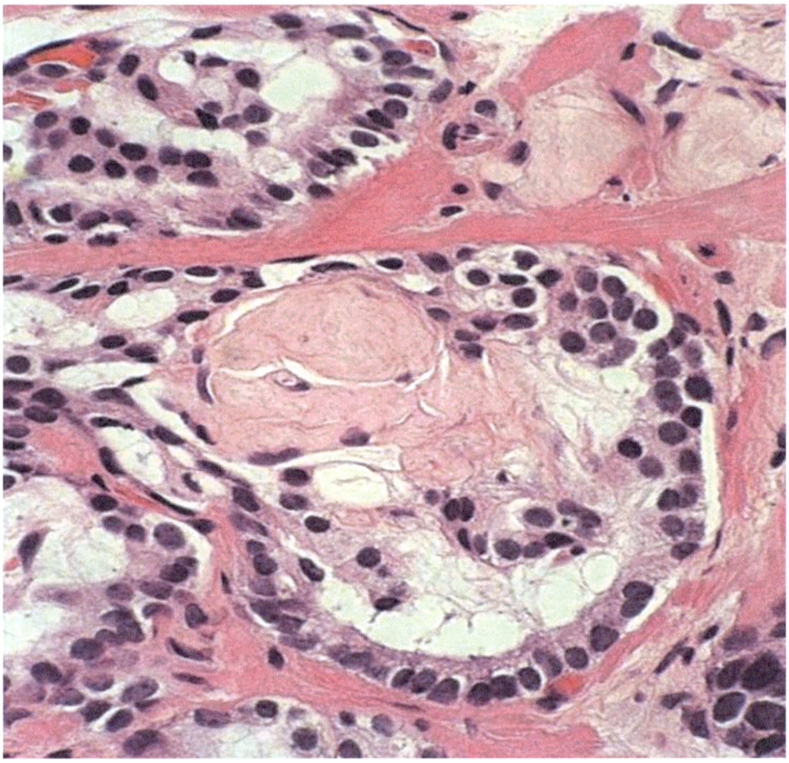

Fig. 3.40 Collagenous micronodules are a an uncommon feature of prostate carcinoma

3.3.1.5 Immunohistochemical Findings

- Important immunohistochemical markers in prostate pathology are PSA, PAP, PSMA, high-molecular-weight keratin clone 34βE12, CK 5/6, p63 and AMACR.
- Immunohistochemical expression of Prostate-Specific Antigen (PSA) is useful for distinguishing high-grade prostate cancer from urothelial carcinoma, colonic carcinoma, granulomatous prostatitis, and lymphoma. PSA also facilitates identification of the site of tumour origin in metastatic adenocarcinoma. PSA can be detected in frozen and paraffin-embedded sections and is preserved in decalcified specimens. Staining is invariably heterogeneous.
- The use of PSMA adds specificity over PSA according to some authors. Prostatic Acid Phosphatase (PAP) is a valuable immunohistochemical marker for identifying prostate cancer when used in combination with PSA.

High-molecular-weight cytokeratin (clone 34βE12) and CK5/6

- May be useful for evaluation of the basal cell layer. It is most useful in confirming the benignancy of a suggestive focus by showing an immunoreactive basal cell layer. Anti-keratin 34βE12 stains nearly all of the normal basal cells of the prostate; no staining occurs in the secretory and stromal cells.
- Uniform absence of a basal cell layer is one important diagnostic feature of invasive carcinoma and basal cells may be inapparent by Hematoxilin-Eosin (H&E) stain, basal cell specific immunostains may help to distinguish invasive prostatic adenocarcinoma from benign small acinar cancer mimics which retain their basal cell layer, e.g. glandular atrophy, post-atrophic hyperplasia, atypical adenomatous hyperplasia, sclerosing adenosis and radiation induced atypia.
- Because the basal cell layer may be interrupted or not demonstrable in small numbers of benign glands, the complete absence of a basal cell layer in a small focus of acini cannot be used alone as a definitive criterion for malignancy; rather, absence of a basal cell layer is supportive of invasive carcinoma only in acinar proliferations which exhibit suspicious cytological and/or architectural features on H&E stain.
- Conversely, some early invasive prostatic carcinomas, e.g. microinvasive carcinomas arising

in association with or independent of high grade prostatic intraepithelial neoplasia, may have residual basal cells (transitive glands). Intraductal spread of invasive carcinoma and entrapped benign glands are other proposed explanations for residual basal cells. Rare prostatic adenocarcinomas contain sparse neoplastic glandular cells which are immunoreactive for 34βE12, yet these are not in a basal cell distribution. The use of antibodies for 34βE12 is especially helpful for the diagnosis for of deceptively being appearing variants of prostate cancer.

- Immunohistochemistry for cytokeratins 7 and 20 have a limited diagnostic use in prostate pathology with the exception that negative staining for both markers, which can occur in prostate adenocarcinoma, would be unusual for transitional cell carcinoma.

p63

A nuclear protein encoded by a gene on chromosome 3q27-29 with homology to p53 (a tumour suppressor gene), has been shown to regulate growth and development in epithelium of the skin, cervix, breast and urogenital tract.

- Specific isotypes are expressed in basal cells of stratified and pseudostratified epithelia (prostate, bronchial), reserve cells of simple columnar epithelia (endocervical, pancreatic ductal), myoepithelial cells (breast, salivary glands, cutaneous apocrine/eccrine glands), urothelium and squamous epithelium. p63 has similar applications to those of high molecular weight cytokeratins in the diagnosis of prostatic adenocarcinoma, but with the advantages that p63 is less susceptible to the staining variability of 34βE12 (particularly in TURP specimens with cautery artefact), stains a subset of 34βE12 negative basal cells, and is easier to interpret because of its strong nuclear staining intensity.
- Interpretative limitations related to presence or absence of basal cells in small numbers of glands for 34βE12 apply to p63, requiring correlation with morphology. Prostatic adenocarcinomas have occasional p63 immunoreactive cells, most representing entrapped benign glands or intraductal spread of carcinoma with residual basal cells, but some true p63 positive carcinomas have been reported.
- An immunohistochemical cocktail containing monoclonal antibodies to cytokeratin 34betaE12 and p63 is in use by some authorities.

AMACR (α-Methyl-CoA Racemase, P504S)

- This mRNA was found to encode a racemase protein, for which polyclonal and monoclonal antibodies have been produced which are active in formalin-fixed, paraffin- embedded tissue. Over 80 % of prostatic adenocarcinomas are labelled with racemase.
- Certain subtypes of prostate cancer, such as foamy gland carcinoma, atrophic carcinoma, pseudohyperplastic, and treated carcinoma show lower AMACR expression. However, AMACR is not specific for prostate cancer and is present in nodular hyperplasia (12 %), atrophic glands (35 %), HGPIN (90 %) and atypical adenomatous hyperplasia (18 %).
- AMACR may be used as a confirmatory stain for prostatic adenocarcinoma, in conjunction with histology and basal cell specific markers. AMACR is expressed in other non-prostatic neoplasms including urothelial, renal and colon cancer.
- A cocktail containing 34betaE12, p63 and racemase is used by some authors.

3.3.1.6 Focal Neuroendocrine Differentiation

- About 10 % of prostatic carcinomas have zones with a large number of single or clustered neuroendocrine cells detected by chromogranin A immunohistochemistry, some cells may also be serotonin positive. Immunostaining for neuron-specific enolase, synaptophysin, bombesin/gastrin-releasing peptide and a variety of other neuroendocrine peptides may also occur in individual neoplastic neuroendocrine cells, or in a more diffuse pattern and receptors for serotonin may also be present (Fig. 3.41).
- There are conflicting studies as to whether advanced androgen independent and androgen deprived carcinomas show increased neuroendocrine differentiation. The prognostic significance of focal neuroendocrine differentiation in primary untreated prostatic carcinoma is controversial.
- In advanced prostate cancer, especially androgen independent cancer, focal neuroendocrine differentiation portends a poor prognosis.

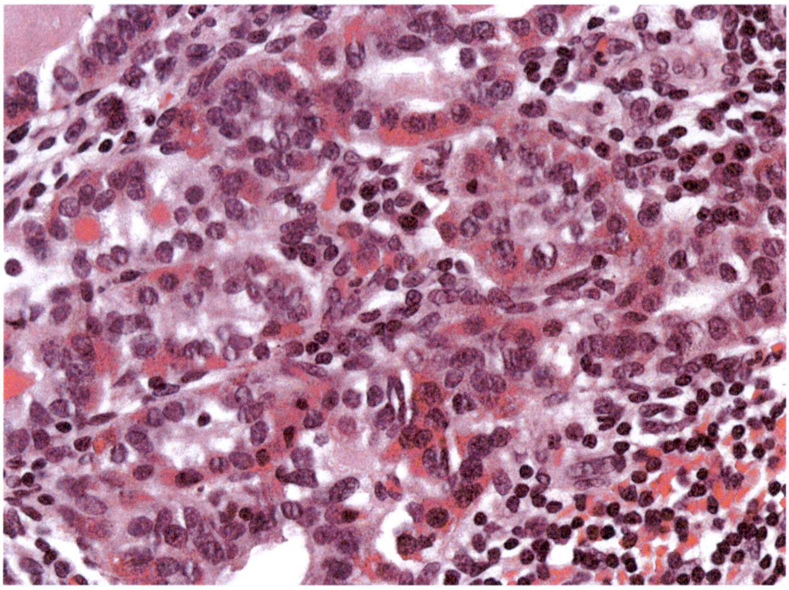

Fig. 3.41 Focally prominent of neuroendocrine cells (Paneth cell-like change) is an uncommon finding in prostate cancer

3.4 Rare Histologic Subtypes of Prostatic Carcinoma

- A wide variety of histologic subtypes and variants of adenocarcinoma may be seen in the prostate (Table 3.4).

Table 3.4 Histological classification of carcinoma of the prostate

1. Adenocarcinoma (acinar, conventional, usual type)
2. Variants of adenocarcinoma and other carcinomas
Pseudohyperplastic adenocarcinoma
Foamy gland adenocarcinoma
Atrophic adenocarcinoma
Adenocarcinoma with glomeruloid features
Mucinous (colloid) adenocarcinoma
Signet ring cell carcinoma
Oncocytic adenocarcinoma
Lymphoepithelioma-like carcinoma
PIN-like
Pleomorphic giant cell carcinoma
Prostatic duct adenocarcinoma
Small cell carcinoma and other neuroendocrine tumours
Sarcomatoid carcinoma
Basal cell carcinoma
Urothelial carcinoma
Adenosquamous carcinoma
Squamous cell carcinoma

3.4.1 Pseudohyperplastic Adenocarcinoma

- Pseudohyperplastic prostate cancer resembles benign prostate glands in that the neoplastic glands are large with branching and papillary infolding. Most occur in the transition zone which is the usual site for benign prostatic hyperplasia (Fig. 3.42).
- The recognition of cancer with this pattern is based on the architectural pattern of numerous closely packed glands as well as nuclear features more typical of carcinoma. Pseudohyperplastic cancer, it is considered Gleason score 3+3=6.
- One pattern of pseudohyperplastic adenocarcinoma consists of numerous large glands that are almost back-to-back with straight even luminal borders, and abundant cytoplasm. Comparably sized benign glands either have papillary infolding or are atrophic.
- The presence of cytological atypia in some of these glands further distinguishes them from benign glands. It is helpful to verify the absence of basal cells by immunohistochemistry.
- HOXB13 G84E variant-related prostate cancers show frequent pseudohyperplastic-type features and markedly low prevalence of ERG.
- A cystic variant of pseudohyperplastic carcinoma (microcystic carcinoma) has been recognized.

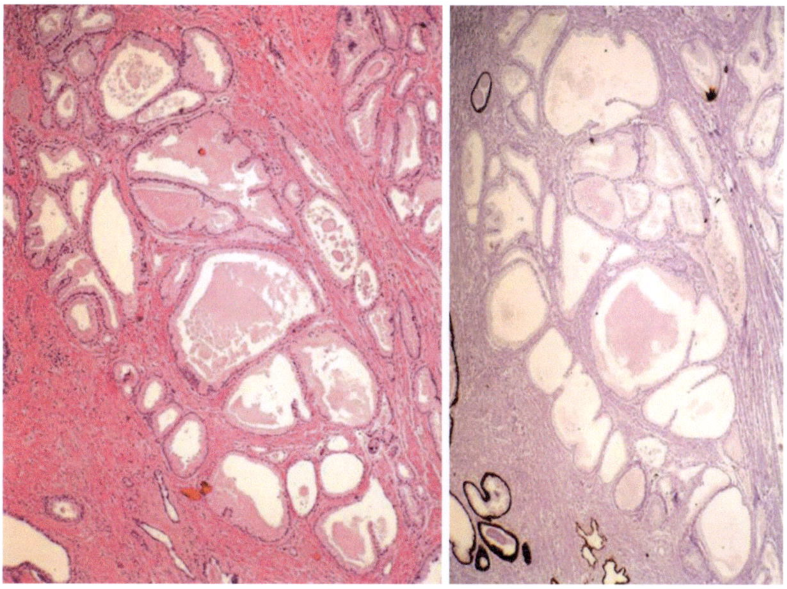

Fig. 3.42 Pseudohyperplastic carcinoma may simulate benign hyperplasia of the prostate (*left*) but lack basal cell layer (*right*)

3.4.2 Foamy Gland Adenocarcinoma

- Foamy gland (also known as xanthomatous) cancer is a variant of acinar adenocarcinoma of the prostate that is characterized by having abundant foamy appearing cytoplasm. Although the cytoplasm has a xanthomatous appearance, it does not contain lipid, but rather empty microvacuoles (Figs. 3.43 and 3.44).
- Typical features of adenocarcinoma such as nuclear enlargement and prominent nucleoli are frequently rare to absent, which makes this lesion difficult to recognize as carcinoma especially on biopsy material.
- Whereas most cases of foamy gland carcinoma would be grade as Gleason 3+3, higher grade foamy gland carcinoma exists and should be graded accordingly based on the pattern; most frequently Gleason pattern 4.
- Characteristically, the nuclei in foamy gland carcinoma are small and densely hyperchromatic. Nuclei in foamy gland cancer are round, more so than those of benign prostatic secretory cells. It is recognized as carcinoma by its architectural pattern of crowded and/or infiltrative glands, and frequently present dense pink acellular secretions.
- In most cases, foamy gland cancer is seen in association with ordinary adenocarcinoma of the prostate.

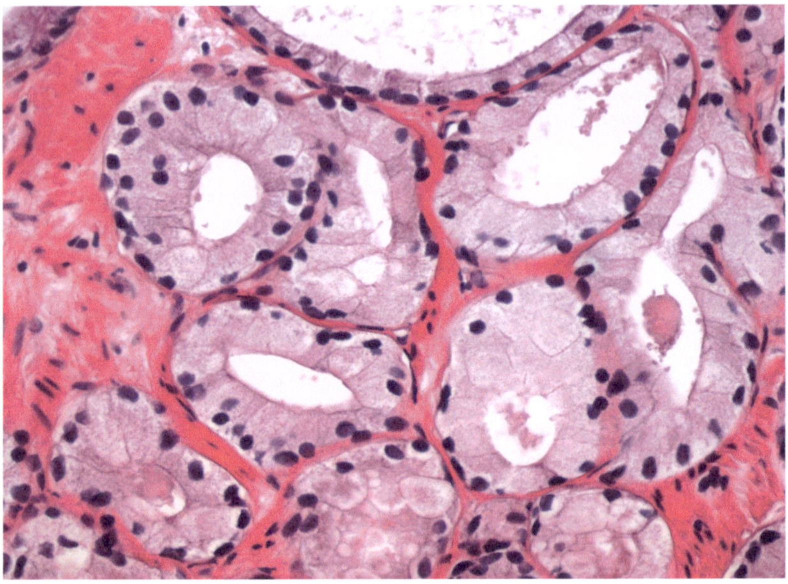

Fig. 3.43 Foamy gland adenocarcinoma showing xanthomatous cytoplasm of the cells

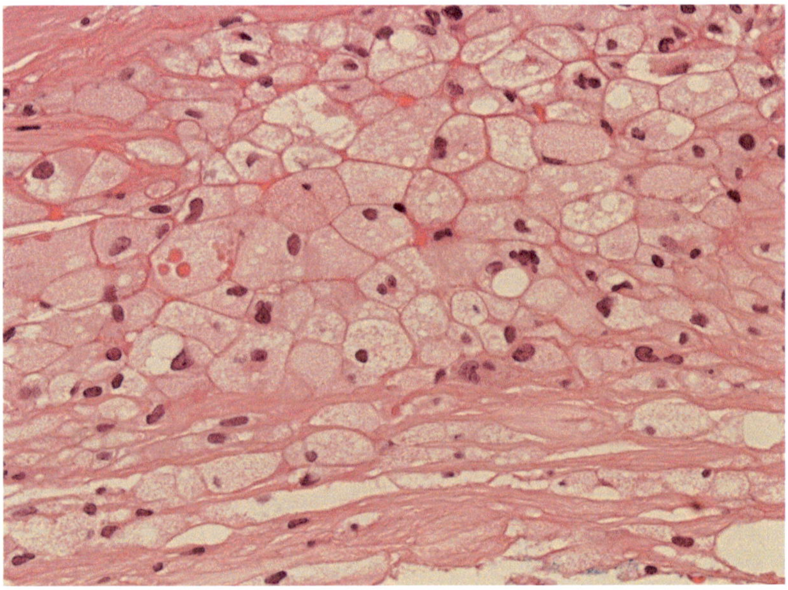

Fig. 3.44 Prostate xanthoma (this case) to be compared with foamy gland adenocarcinoma

3.4.3 Atrophic Adenocarcinoma

- An unusual variant of prostate cancer resembles benign atrophy owing to its scant cytoplasm. Atrophic prostate cancers are unrelated with a prior history of treatment (Fig. 3.45).
- The diagnosis is based on several features. First, atrophic prostate cancer may demonstrate a truly infiltrative process with individual small atrophic glands situated between larger benign glands. In contrast, benign atrophy has a lobular configuration with a centrally dilated atrophic gland surrounding by clustered smaller glands that are not truly infiltrative (Fig. 3.46).
- Whereas some forms of atrophy, are associated with fibrosis, atrophic prostate cancer

lack fibrotic stroma. Atrophic prostate cancer may also be differentiated from benign atrophy by the presence of marked cytological atypia. Atrophy may show enlarged nuclei and prominent nucleoli, although not the huge eosinophilic nucleoli seen in some atrophic prostate cancers.

- Ordinary type carcinoma is usually present. The absence of basal cell layer at immunohistochemistry is of help. AMACR is expressed in 70 % of atrophic carcinomas, which is lower compared to acinar adenocarcinoma.
- Most glands are well formed with lumina (Gleason 3), and less often exhibit fusion (Gleason 4).
- Main differential diagnosis is simple atrophy which shows a lobular growth and does not exhibit gland infiltration. Benign atrophic glands retain basal cell layer that may be discontinuous and atrophic cancer has a complete loss of basal cell layer.

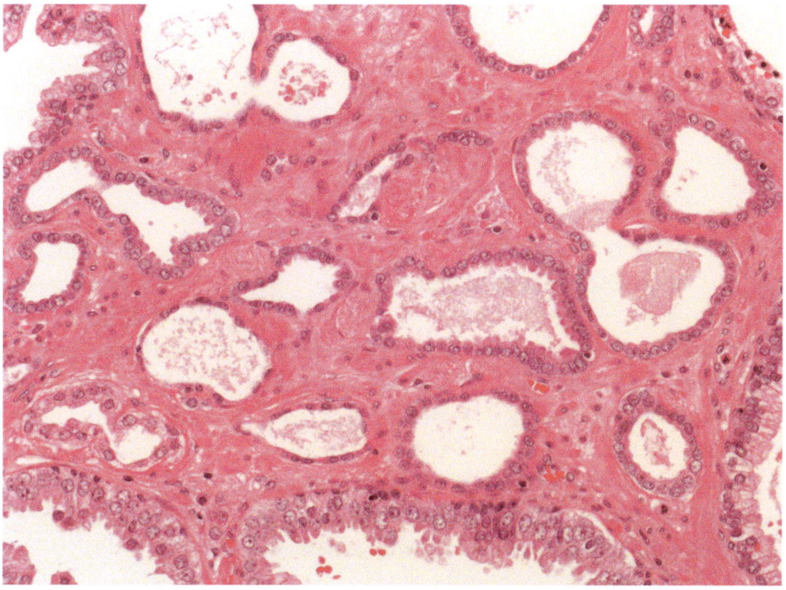

Fig. 3.45 Microscopic appearance of atrophic prostate carcinoma

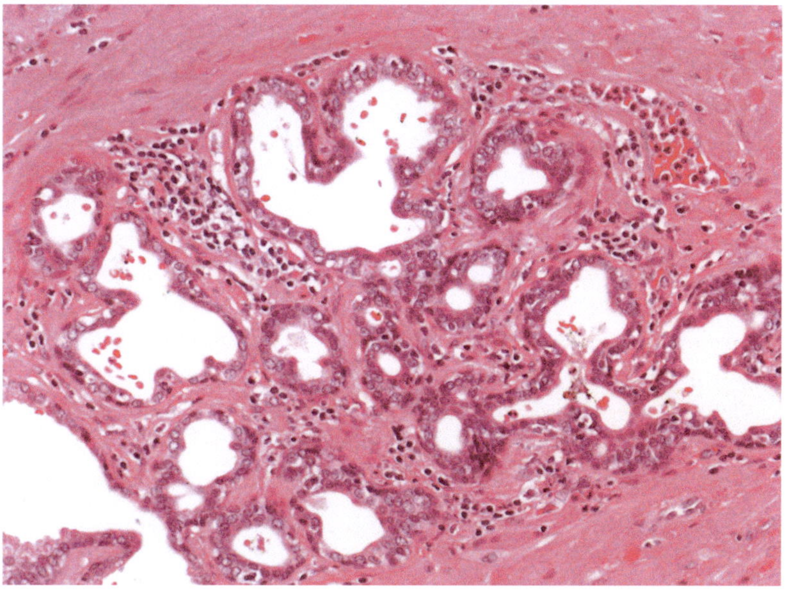

Fig. 3.46 Atrophic cancer needs to be differentiated from non-neoplastic atrophic glands. In this case lobular atrophy

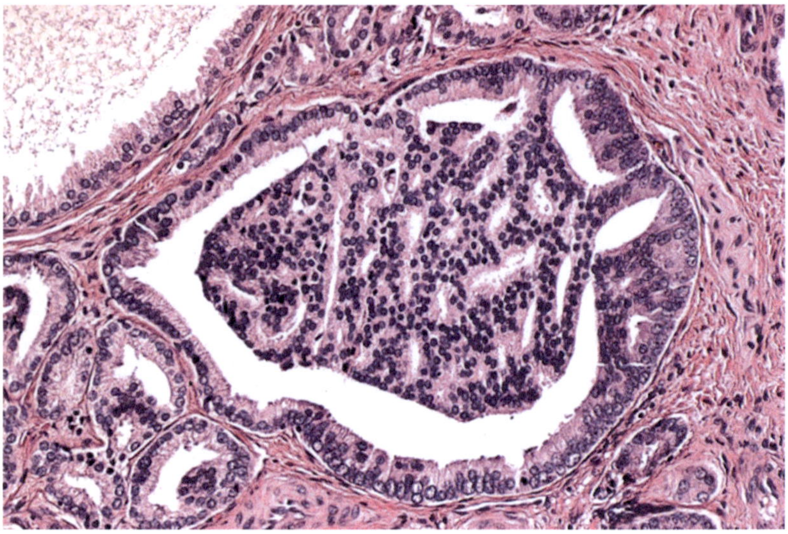

Fig. 3.47 Microscopic appearance of glomeruloid prostate cancer

3.4.4 Adenocarcinoma with Glomeruloid Features

- Prostatic adenocarcinoma with glomeruloid features is characterized by intraluminal ball-like clusters of cancer cells reminiscent of renal glomeruli. Glomeruloid structures in the prostate represent an uncommon but distinctive pattern of growth that is specific for malignancy (glomeruloid-like structures in non-malignant glands are extremely rare) (Fig. 3.47).
- Glomeruloid features may be a useful diagnostic clue for malignancy, particularly in some challenging needle biopsy specimens. This pattern of growth is usually seen in high-grade adenocarcinoma, often with extraprostatic extension. A Gleason score of 4 has been suggested for this variant of prostate cancer.

3.4.5 Mucinous and Signet Ring Cell Adenocarcinoma

- Mucinous adenocarcinoma is one of the least common morphologic variants of prostatic carcinoma. The diagnosis of mucinous (colloid) adenocarcinoma of the prostate gland should be made when at least 25 % of the tumour resected contains lakes of extracellular mucin.
- Mucinous prostate adenocarcinomas behave aggressively with most patients died or were alive with disease 5 years after therapy. Mucinous prostate adenocarcinomas have a propensity to develop bone metastases. These cases should be graded as Gleason score 4+4 (Fig. 3.48).
- Mucinous adenocarcinoma shows higher (83 %) incidence of TMPRSS2-ERG fusion that usual acinar carcinoma (about 50 %).
- Some carcinomas of the prostate may have a signet-ring-cell appearance, yet the vacuoles do not contain mucin (prostatic carcinoma with cytoplasmic vacuoles) (Fig. 3.49). These vacuolated cells may be present as singly invasive cells, in single glands, and in sheets of cells. These tumors should be graded as if the vacuoles were not present.
- Only a few cases of prostate cancer have been reported with mucin positive signet cells (signet ring mucinous adenocarcinoma). These tumors seem to be very aggressive., and should be distinguished from adenocarcinoma with cytoplasmic vacuoles (see above).

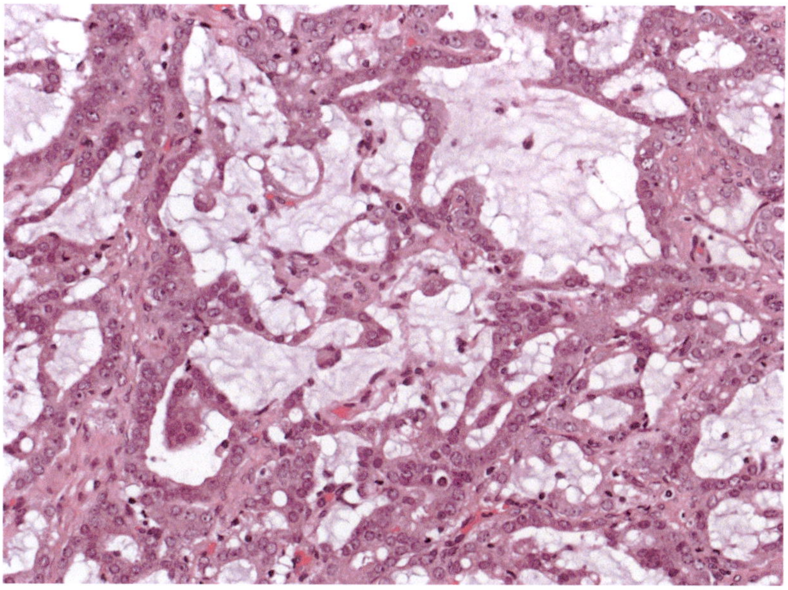

Fig. 3.48 Microscopic appearance of mucinous (colloid) adenocarcinoma

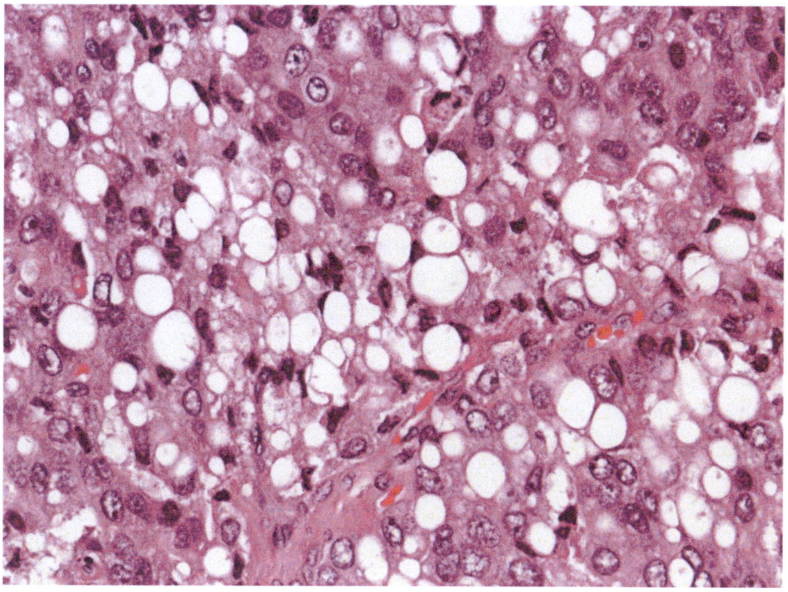

Fig. 3.49 Microscopic appearance of prostate carcinoma with cytoplasmic vacuoles (signet ring-like). This need to be separated from mucinous signet-ring carcinoma

3.4.6 Oncocytic Adenocarcinoma

- This is an exceptionally rare variant of PCa with unclear clinical significance (Fig. 3.50).
- Tumour cells have round to ovoid hyperchromatic nuclei, and have granular cytoplasm with numerous mitochondria on ultrastructural or immunohistochemical examination and are strongly positive for PSA. A high Gleason grade, elevated serum PSA and metastasis of similar morphology have been documented.

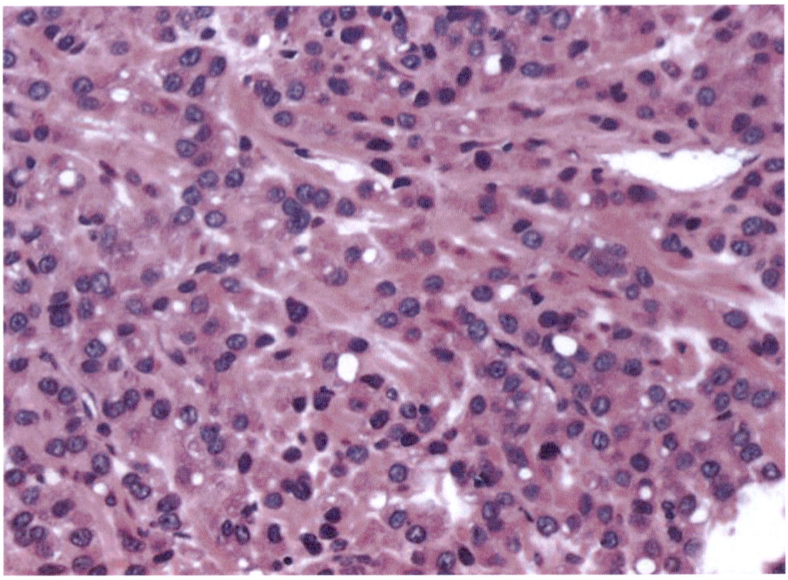

Fig. 3.50 Microscopic appearance of oncocytic prostate carcinoma

3.4.7 Lymphoepithelioma-Like Carcinoma of the Prostate

- This undifferentiated carcinoma is characterised by indistinct cytoplasmic borders with syncytial arrangement of malignant cells associated with a heavy lymphocytic infiltrate including some plasma cells and neutrophils; one case had a prominent infiltration of eosinophils. Associated ordinary adenocarcinoma is always present and may be of acinar, adenosquamous or ductal type (Figs. 3.51, 3.52 and 3.53).
- Immunohistochemical staining demonstrated that lymphoepithelioma-like carcinoma was positive for prostate-specific antigen, prostate acid phosphatase, alpha-methylacyl coenzyme A racemase, and epithelial membrane antigen; several cytokeratins (AE1/AE3, 7, 8, and 20 [rare cells]) were also immunoreactive. The mean Ki-67 labeling index was 53 % (range, 40–0 %), and the p53 expression in all cases was low (10–20 %).
- The lymphoid component was mainly composed of T with a minor subset of B cells, admixed with some dendritic cells and histiocytes as seen by S100 and CD68 immunoreactivity. Latent membrane protein 1 immunostaining and in situ hybridization for Epstein-Barr virus were negative in all 5 lymphoepithelioma-like carcinoma cases.
- DNA ploidy of lymphoepithelioma-like carcinoma tumors gave DNA histograms with aneuploid peaks. DNA ploidy of the concurrent adenocarcinoma gave DNA aneuploid peaks except in one DNA diploid case.
- The largest series included 5 patients at a mean age of 76 years with obstructive symptoms and high PSA. Most presented at advanced clinical stage. Four patients died of disease from 8 to 26 months.

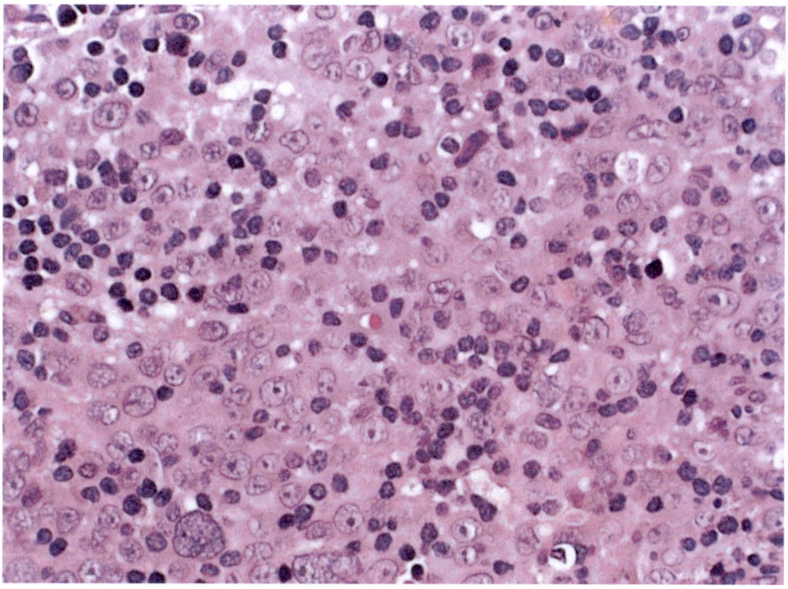

Fig. 3.51 Microscopic appearance of lymphoepithelioma-like carcinoma of the prostate

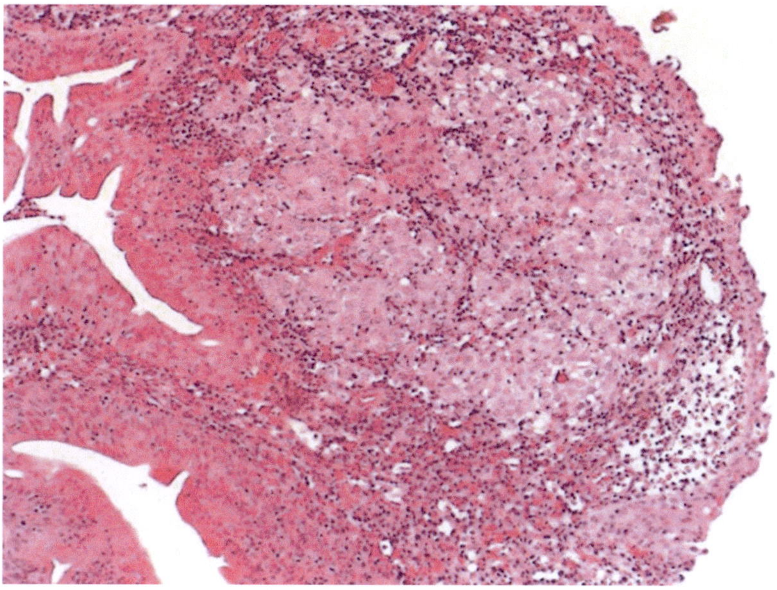

Fig. 3.52 Lymphoepithelioma-like carcinoma may also occur in the prostatic urethra

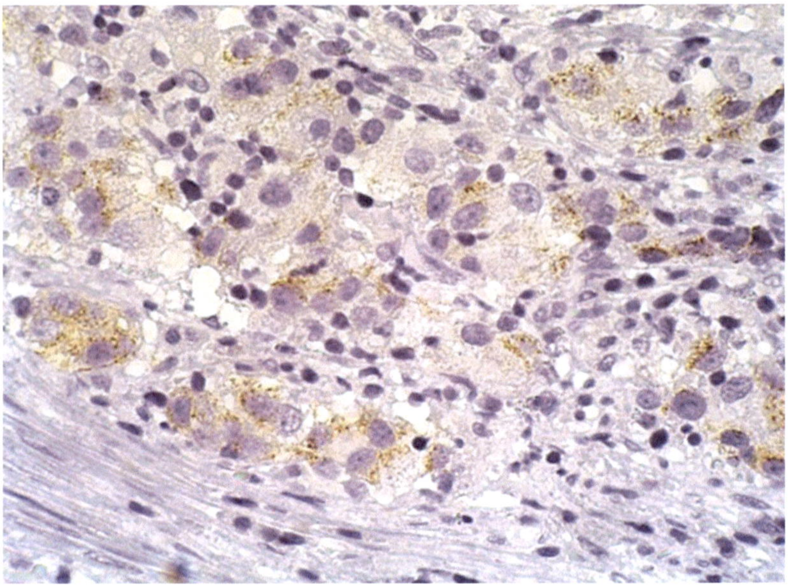

Fig. 3.53 Weak racemase positive expression in lymphoepithelioma-like carcinoma of the prostate

3.4.8 Prostatic Ductal Adenocarcinoma

- Subtype of adenocarcinoma (also known as endometrioid carcinoma) composed of larger glands lined by tall pseudostratified columnar cells. It was originally thought to originate from prostate utricle. In pure form, ductal adenocarcinoma accounts for 0.2–0.8 % of prostate cancers. It is assumed that almost all cases have an acinar component (Figs. 3.54, 3.55, 3.56, 3.57, 3.58, 3.59 and 3.60).
- Ductal adenocarcinoma may be located centrally around the prostatic urethra or more frequently located peripherally admixed with typical acinar adenocarcinoma. A centrally located adenocarcinoma may also be associated with a peripherally located acinar adenocarcinoma. Peripherally occurring ductal carcinomas typically show a white-gray firm appearance similar to acinar adenocarcinoma. These tumors may lead to enlargement or induration of the prostate.
- Centrally occurring tumours appear as exophytic polypoid or papillary masses protruding into the urethra around the verumontanum and may cause hematuria, urinary urgency and eventually urinary retention. In these cases, there may be no abnormalities on rectal examination. Because of the papillary growth, some of these cases may be misdiagnosed as papillary urothelial carcinoma of high grade arising in the urethra.
- Of importance is that serum PSA levels may be normal particularly in patients with only centrally located tumors. In most cases, transurethral resections performed for diagnosis or relief of the urinary obstruction will provide an accurate diagnostic. Transrectal needle core biopsies may also obtain diagnostic tissue when the tumour is more peripherally located. In addition, areas of ductal adenocarcinoma may be incidentally identified in prostatectomy specimens. And in those cases there is a tendency to find more advanced disease.
- A Gleason score of 4+4 (or 9 if comedonecrosis is present) applies to ductal prostatic adenocarcinoma. The recent described PIN-like ductal carcinoma should be graded as Gleason pattern 3 (Fig. 3.61).

Histology and Immunohistochemistry

- Ductal adenocarcinoma is characterized by tall columnar cells with abundant usually amphophilic cytoplasm, which form a single or pseudostratified layer. The cytoplasm of is often amphophilic and may occasionally appear clear. In some cases, there are numerous mitoses and marked cytological atypia. In other cases, the cytological atypia is minimal, which makes a diagnosis difficult particularly on needle biopsy. Peripherally located tumours are often admixed with cribriform, glandular or solid patterns as seen in acinar adenocarcinoma.

- Ductal adenocarcinomas are mostly equivalent to Gleason patterns 4. In some cases comedotype of necrosis is present and therefore considered equivalent to Gleason pattern 5.
- Ductal adenocarcinoma displays a variety of architectural patterns which are often intermingled: cribriform, papillary, individual gland or solid pattern. Immunohistochemically ductal adenocarcinoma is strongly positive for PSA and PAP and racemase (Fig. 3.60). Tumour cells are typically negative for basal cell specific markers; however, a frequently incomplete basal cell layer may be present in pre-existing ducts with cancer.
- Ductal adenocarcinoma usually spread along the urethra or into the prostatic ducts with or without stromal invasion, or may spread similar to that of acinar carcinoma with invasion to extraprostatic tissues and metastasis to pelvic lymph nodes or distal organs. Ductal adenocarcinomas appear to have a tendency to metastasize to lung and penis, but also may metastasize to bones.

Differential diagnosis and prognosis

- Ductal adenocarcinoma must be distinguished from urothelial carcinoma, ectopic prostatic tissue, benign prostatic polyps, and papillary-polypoid urethritis.
- Ductal adenocarcinoma is aggressive with 27–39 % of cases showing metastases at the time of diagnosis. Five-year survival rate is poor ranging 14–40 % of patients.

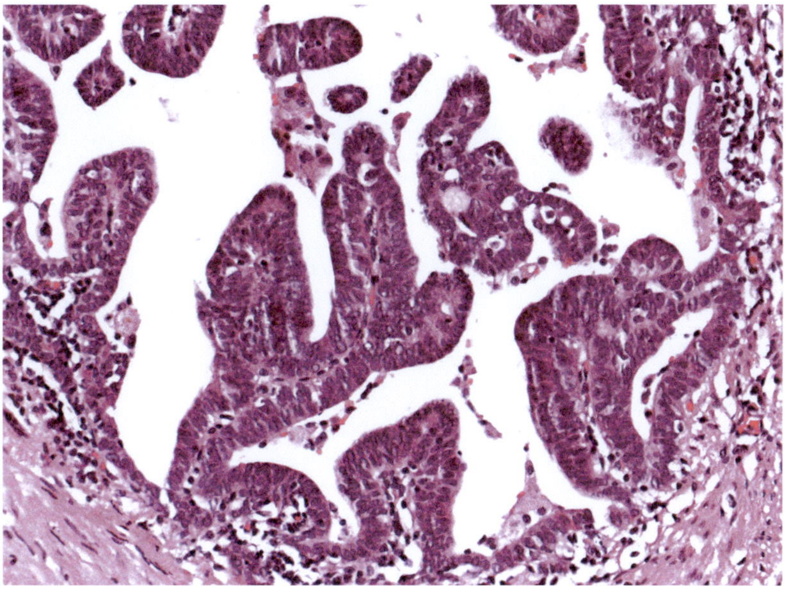

Fig. 3.54 Microscopic appearance of ductal carcinoma of the prostate with endometrioid features

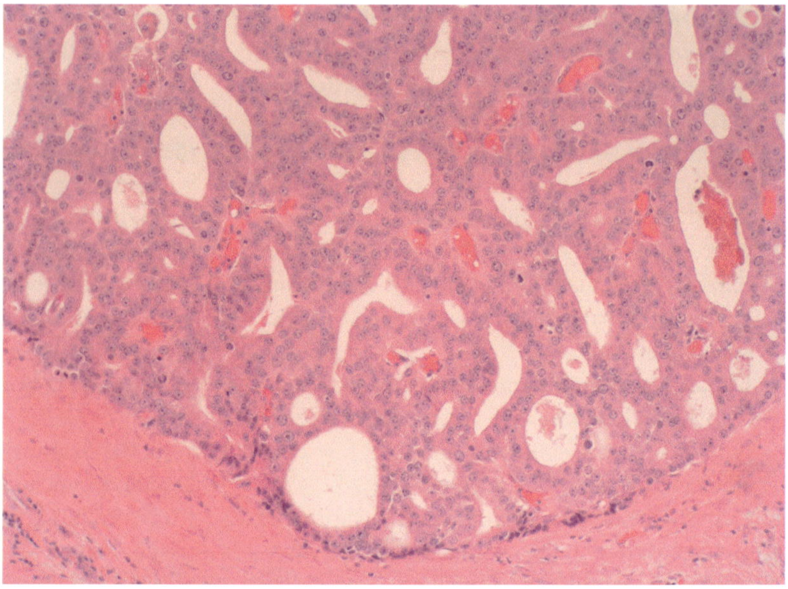

Fig. 3.55 Microscopic appearance of ductal carcinoma of the prostate with cribriform features

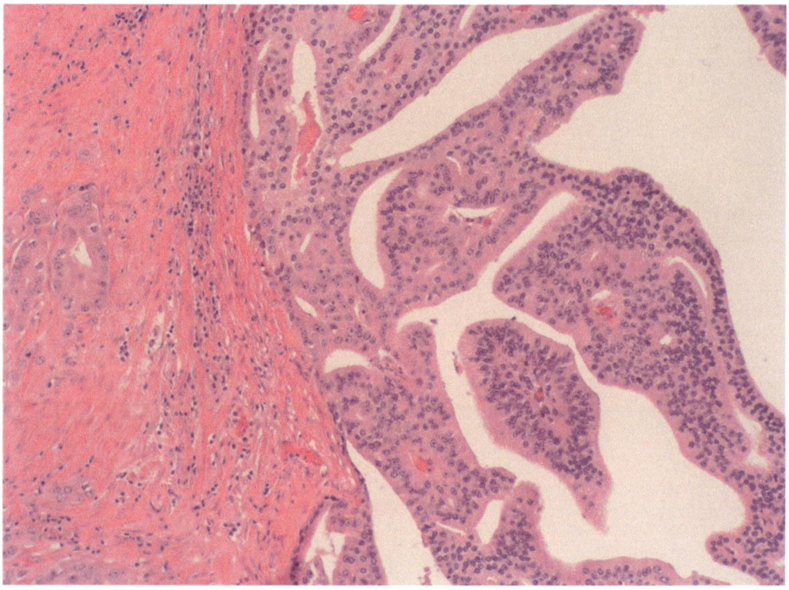

Fig. 3.56 Microscopic appearance of ductal carcinoma of the prostate with papillary features

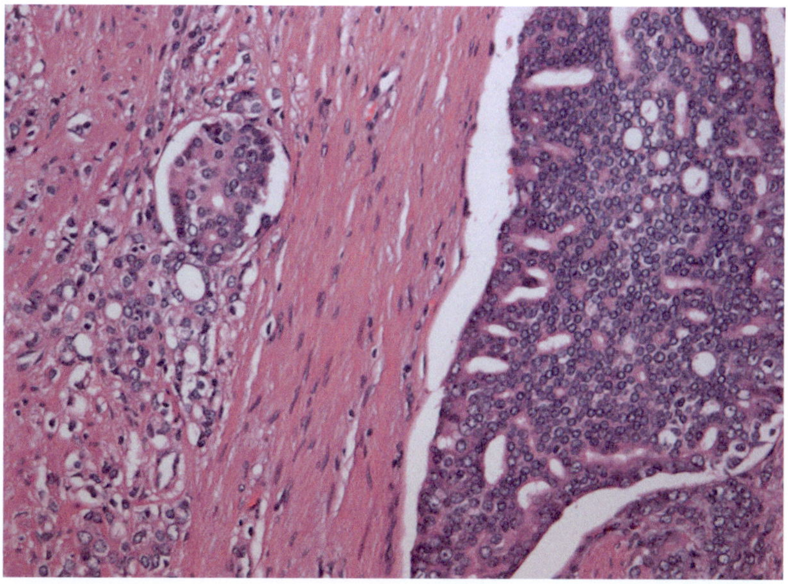

Fig. 3.57 Microscopic appearance of ductal carcinoma of the prostate with cribriform features (*right*) and associated acinar carcinoma (*left*)

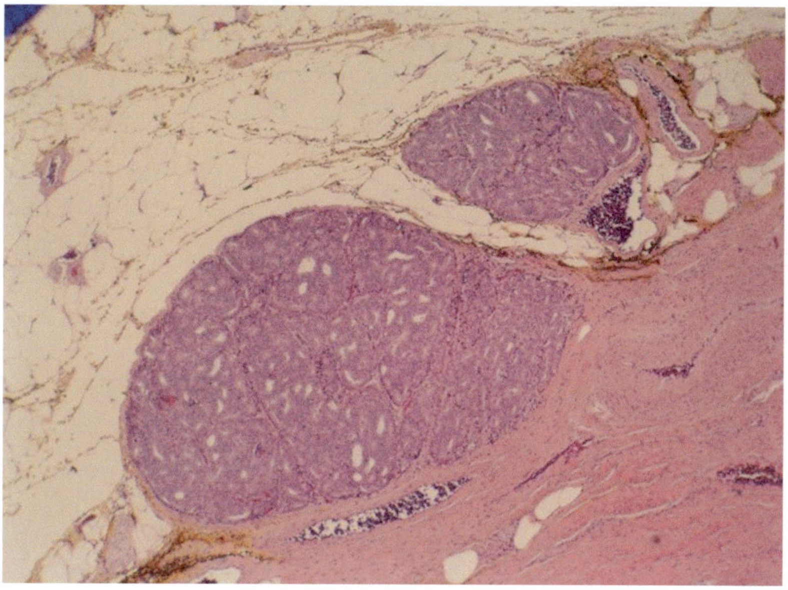

Fig. 3.58 Ductal carcinoma with extraprostatic extension

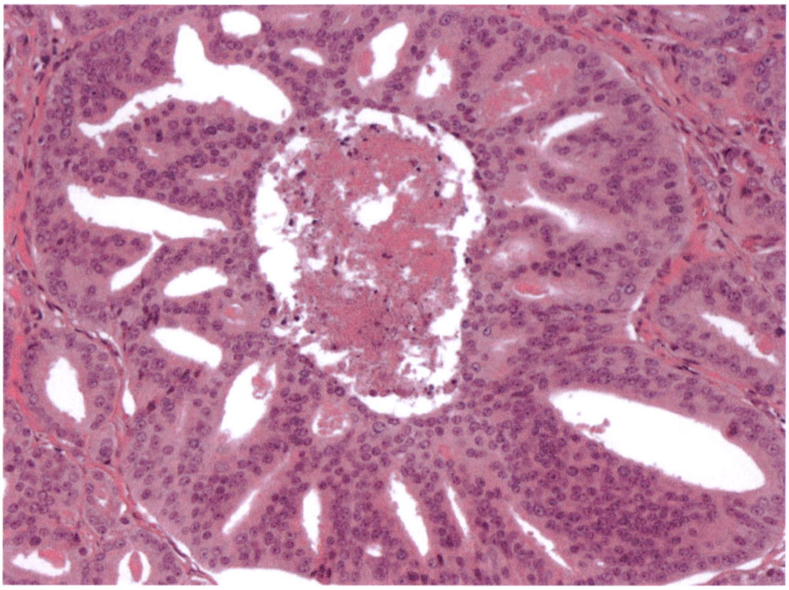

Fig. 3.59 Ductal carcinoma with comedo-type necrosis

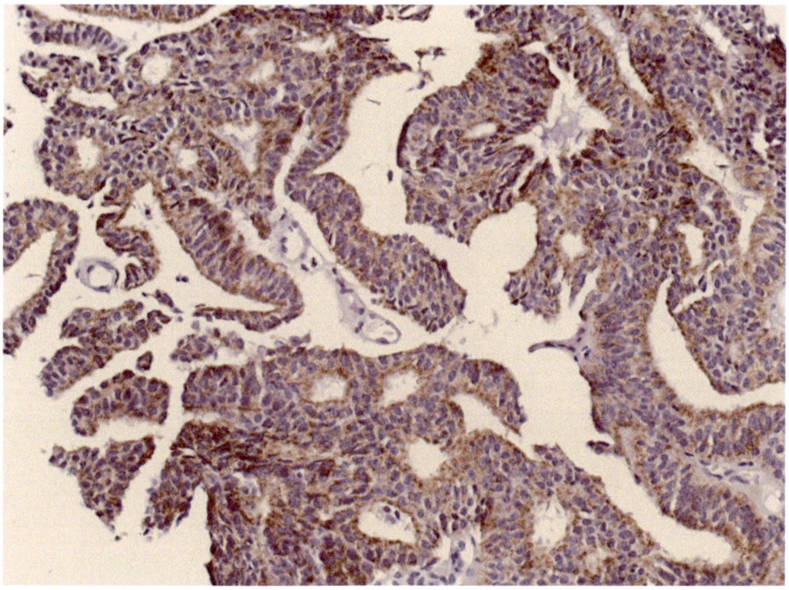

Fig. 3.60 Racemase expression in ductal carcinoma of the prostate

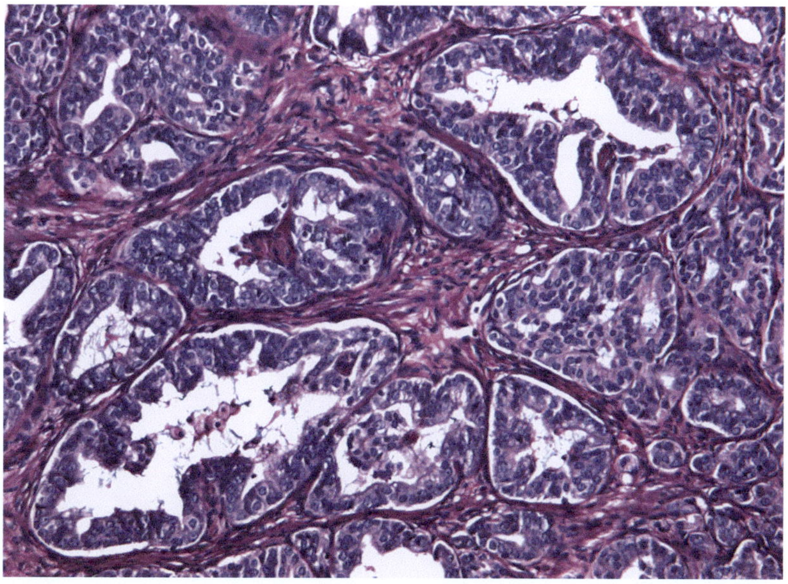

Fig. 3.61 Histologic features of PIN-like ductal carcinoma of the prostate

3.4.9 Intraductal Carcinoma

- Intraepithelial spread of prostatic carcinoma within pre-existing non-neoplastic ducts or acini is known as intraductal carcinoma (IDC). It is characterized by the preservation of basal cells and is now regarded as tumor progression prior to cancer invasion. Other suggests that is a carcinomatous evolution of high grade PIN preceding invasion (Figs. 3.62, 3.63 and 3.64).
- Diagnosis of IDC in practice is limited by its problematic distinction from PIN; both lesions retain basal cell as seen by immunohistochemistry. Most cases are seen in association with high grade PCa. IDC has been reported to occur in 18 % of radical prostatectomy samples. The incidence is higher in specimens with higher stage. In needle biopsies might be present in about 3 % of cases. Basal cell immunohistochemistry may show complete or partial basal cell layer.
- IDC as an isolated finding is rare (<1 % of biopsies) and its clinical significance remains a matter of discussion. An alternative term of atypical cribriform lesion has been suggested to report needle biopsy cases with borderline features between IDC and high grade PIN.
- Current approach to IDC is by identifying large acini and ducts containing basal cells filled with malignant epithelial cells that show solid or dense cribriform patterns. In cases with luminal pattern of loose cribriform or micropapillary, marked nuclear atypia (≥6×) or non-focal comedonecrosis is required. Other authors suggest to combine a set of major and minor criteria, as follows:

  Major criteria for diagnosis of IDC are:

1. Large glands (>2× normal)
2. Presence of basal cells (confirmed by immunohistochemistry)
3. Cytologically malignant cells with frequent mitosis
4. Cells spanning gland lumen
5. Comedonecrosis

  Minor criteria for diagnosis of IDC are:

1. Right-angle branching
2. Round smooth gland contour
3. Frequently 2 population of cells

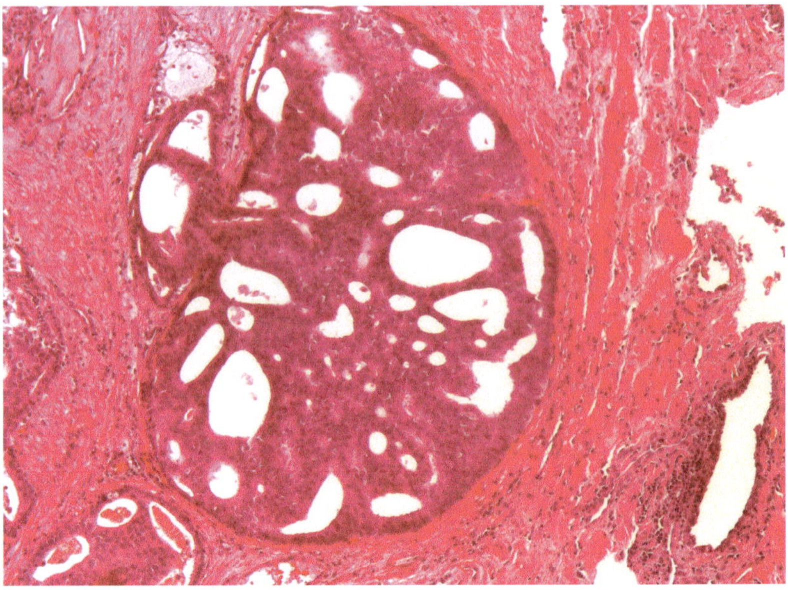

Fig. 3.62 Intraductal carcinoma of the prostate. Microscopic features

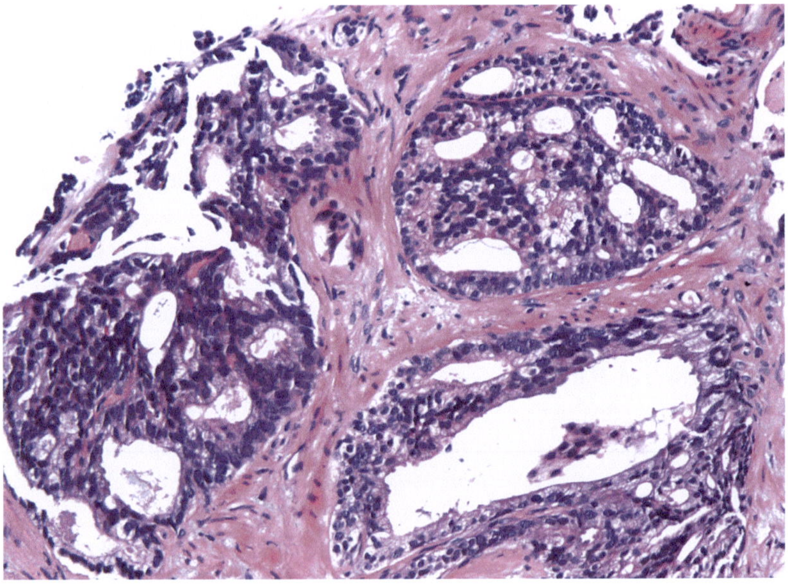

Fig. 3.63 Intraductal carcinoma of the prostate as seen in needle biopsy

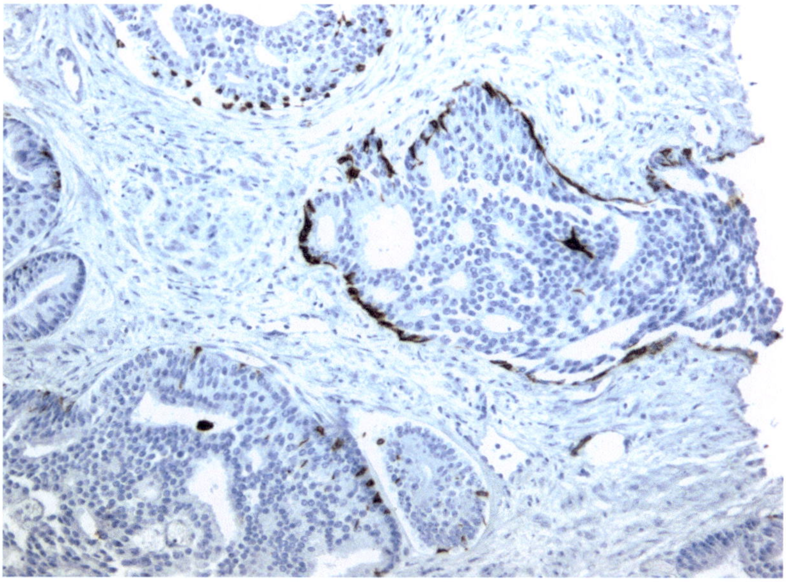

Fig. 3.64 Basal cells are still present in intraductal carcinoma as seen with antibodies against basal cell cytokeratins

3.4.10 Small Cell Carcinoma

- Small-cell carcinomas of the prostate histologically are identical to small-cell carcinomas of the lung and similar diagnostic criteria apply. About 50 % of the patients have mixed small-cell carcinoma and adenocarcinoma of the prostate.
- The average survival of patients with small-cell carcinoma of the prostate is less than a year. There is no difference in prognosis between patients with pure small-cell carcinomas and those with mixed glandular and small-cell carcinomas. The appearance of a small-cell component within the course of adenocarcinoma of the prostate indicates a terminal phase of the disease.
- Using immunohistochemistry small-cell components are negative for PSA and PAP but positive for neuroendocrine markers and ERG. By FISH analysis, small cell carcinoma from prostate may be differentiated from small cell carcinoma of the bladder since the former retains *ERG-TMPRSS2* molecular alterations.
- There are conflicting studies as to whether small cell carcinoma of the prostates is positive for thyroid transcription factor-1 (TTF-1), in order to distinguish them from a metastasis from the lung.
- Small cell carcinoma of the prostate needs to be differentiated from Gleason pattern 5 which is negative for neuroendocrine markers. No Gleason grade applies to small cell carcinoma (Figs. 3.65, 3.66 and 3.67).

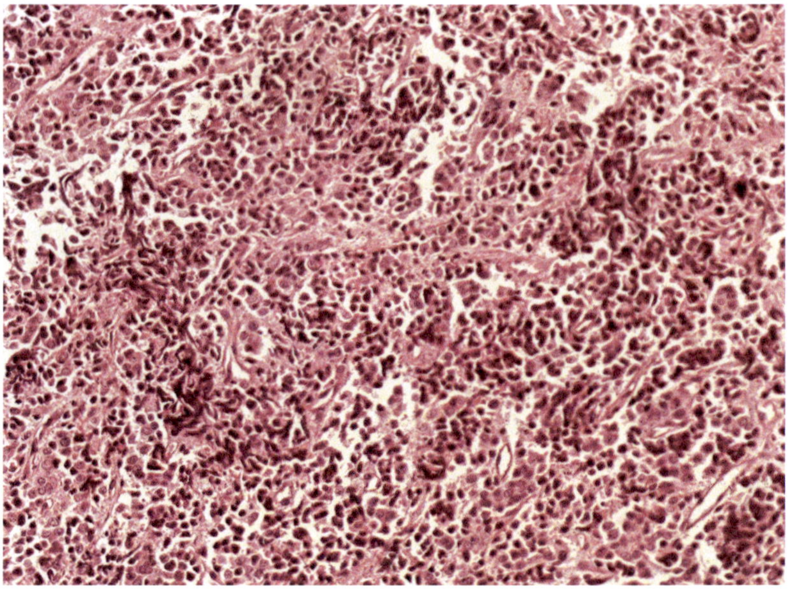

Fig. 3.65 Microscopic appearance of small cell carcinoma of the prostate

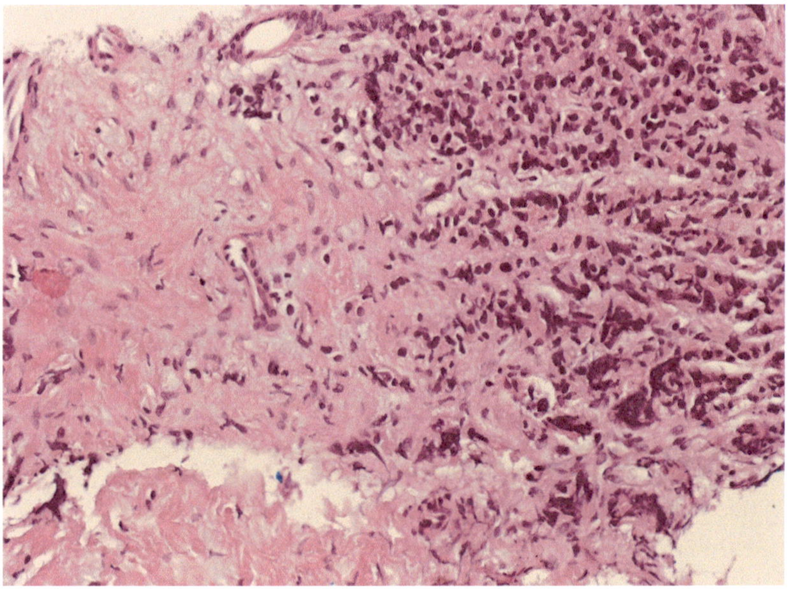

Fig. 3.66 Small cell carcinoma needs to be differentiated from small cell pattern of Gleason 5 prostate adenocarcinoma depicted in this figure

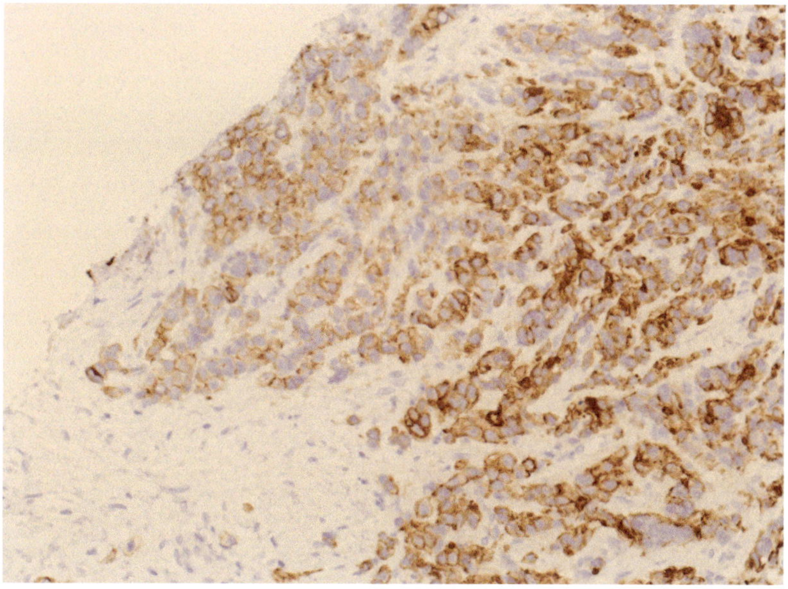

Fig. 3.67 Racemase expression in small cell pattern of Gleason 5 prostate adenocarcinoma

3.4.11 Sarcomatoid Carcinoma (Carcinosarcoma)

- In some series, carcinosarcoma and sarcomatoid carcinoma are considered as separate entities based on the presence of specific mesenchymal elements in the former. However, given their otherwise similar clinico-pathologic features and identically poor prognosis, these two lesions are best considered as one entity.
- Sarcomatoid carcinoma of the prostate is a rare neoplasm composed of both malignant epithelial and malignant spindle-cell and/or mesenchymal elements. Sarcomatoid carcinoma may be present in the initial pathologic material (synchronous presentation) or there may be a previous history of adenocarcinoma treated by radiation and/or hormonal therapy (metachronous). The gross appearance may resemble sarcoma.
- Serum PSA is within normal limits in most cases. Nodal and distant organ metastases at diagnosis are common with less than a 35 % 5-year survival.

Histology

- Microscopically, sarcomatoid carcinoma is composed of a glandular component showing variable Gleason score. The sarcomatoid component often consists of a non-specific malignant spindle-cell proliferation (Figs. 3.68 and 3.69).
- Amongst the specific mesenchymal elements is osteosarcoma, chondrosarcoma, rhabdomyosarcoma, leiomyosarcoma, liposarcoma, angiosarcoma or multiple types of heterologous differentiation. Sarcomatoid carcinoma should be distinguished from the rare carcinoma with metaplastic, benign-appearing bone or cartilage in the stroma.
- Epithelial elements react with antibodies against PSA and/or pan-cytokeratins, whereas spindle-cell elements react with markers of soft tissue tumours and variably express cytokeratins or CD10.

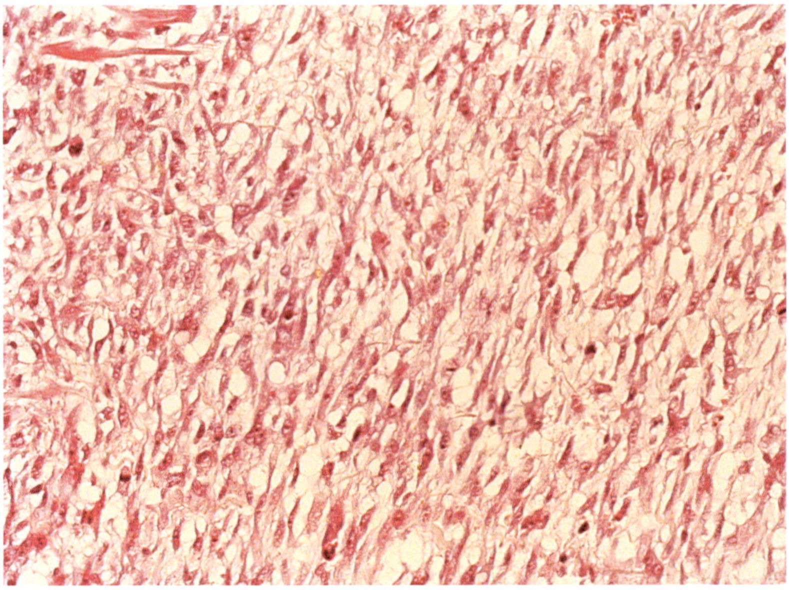

Fig. 3.68 Sarcomatoid carcinoma (carcinosarcoma) of the prostate showing myxoid spindle cell proliferation with high mitotic index

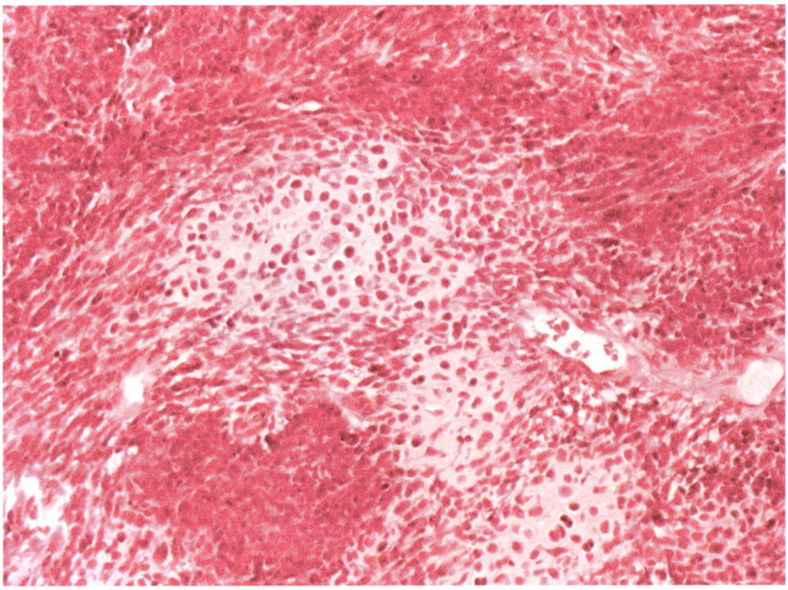

Fig. 3.69 Sarcomatoid carcinoma (carcinosarcoma) of the prostate showing chondrosarcoma and undifferentiated sarcoma

3.4.12 PIN-Like Carcinoma

- The malignant glands exhibit cellular stratification and thus morphologically resemble PIN. Patients mean age is 68 years. The malignant glands have lumina that may be tufted, micropapillary, flat or a mixture of patterns.
- Predominance of stratified tall columnar is similar to ductal carcinoma and therefore it is referred to as PIN-like ductal carcinoma. It is suggested that may behave similar to Gleason score 3 + 3 = 6 cancers.
- This unusual form of prostatic carcinoma needs to be distinguished from high grade PIN. Lack of staining for basal cell markers is a diagnostic clue (Figs. 3.70 and 3.71).

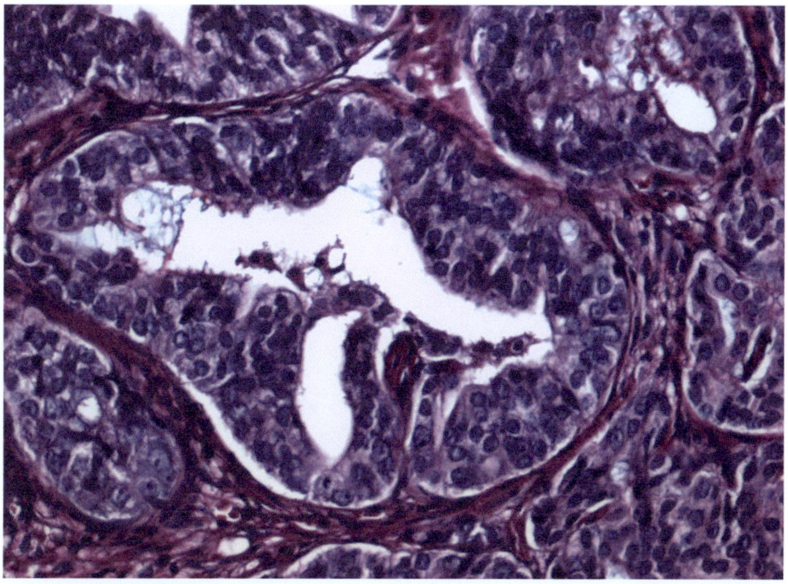

Fig. 3.70 PIN-like subtype of prostate adenocarcinoma

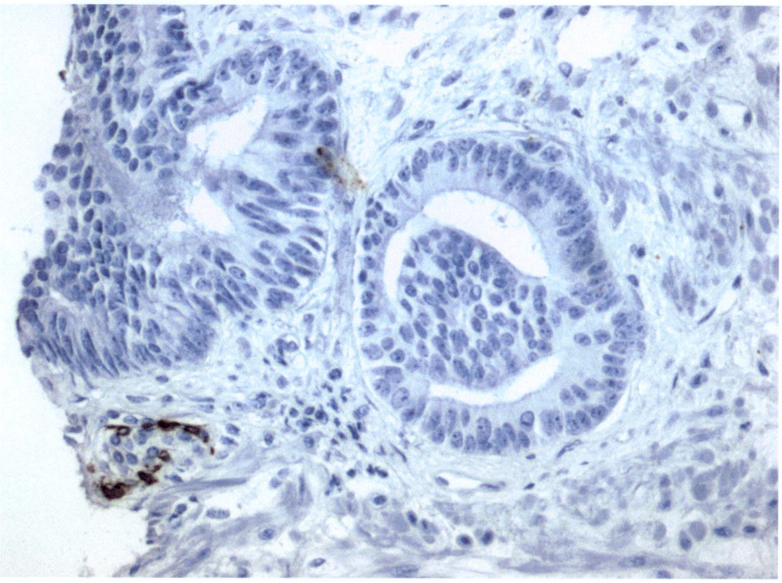

Fig. 3.71 PIN-like subtype of prostate adenocarcinoma. Lack of basal cells as seen by immunohistochemistry with anti-basal cell cytokeratin

3.4.13 Pleomorphic Giant Cell Carcinoma

- Extremely rare and aggressive variant of prostate cancer with large bizarre anaplastic giant cells. Mean age at diagnosis is 66 years. Occurs admixed with high grade prostate carcinoma Gleason score 9. Pleomorphic giant cells are DNA aneuploidy and immunoreactive for epithelial markers and focally with PSA and PAP (Figs. 3.72 and 3.73; Tables 3.5 and 3.6).

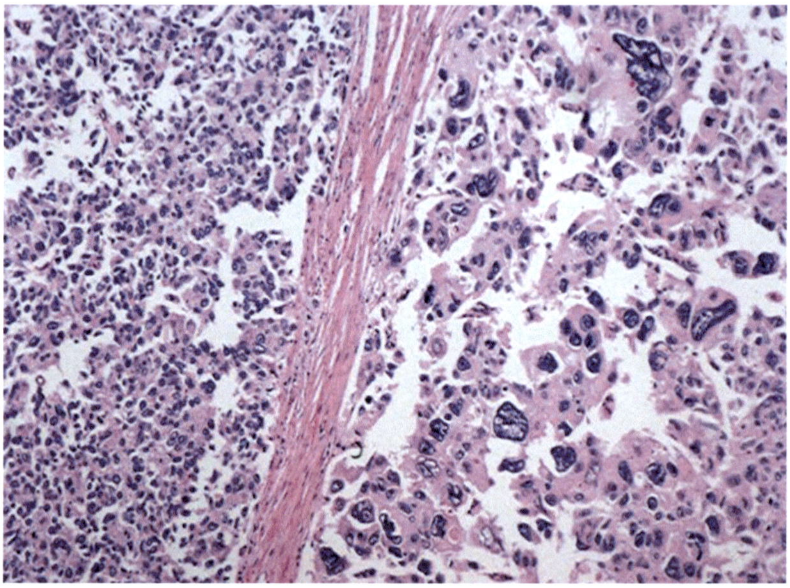

Fig. 3.72 Pleomorphic giant cell carcinoma of the prostate (*right*) as compared with high grade acinar carcinoma (*left*)

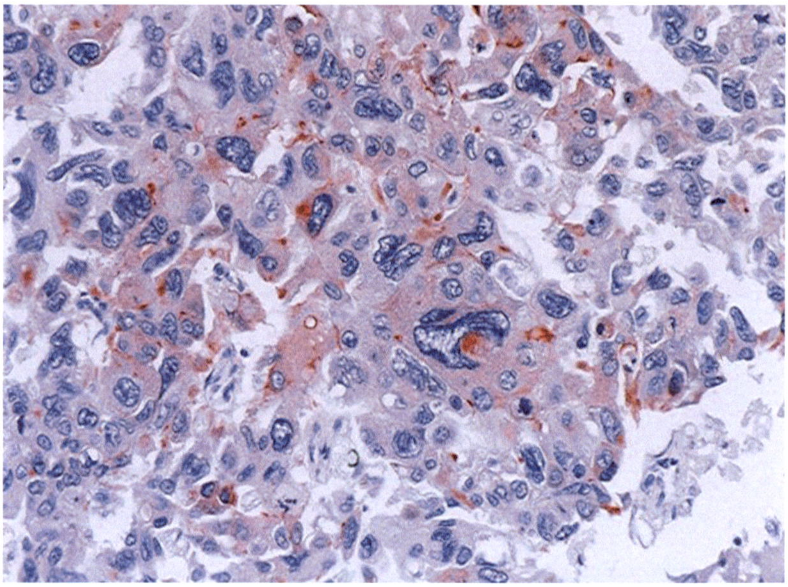

Fig. 3.73 PSA staining of pleomorphic giant cell carcinoma cells

Table 3.5 Gleason grades in histological variants and variations of prostate cancer

Variants
Ductal carcinoma [pattern 4]
Small cell carcinoma [no grade applies]
Mucinous (colloid) carcinoma [pattern 4 (some pattern 3) vs. grade according to underlying pattern]
Mucinous signet ring cell carcinoma [no grade applies]
Sarcomatoid carcinoma [no grade applies]
Pleomorphic giant cell [pattern 5]
Adenosquamous carcinoma [no grade applies]
Lymphoepithelioma-like [no grade applies]
Basal cell/adenoid cystic carcinoma [no grade applies]
Urothelial carcinoma (involving prostatic ducts and acini with or without stromal invasion) [no grade applies]
Squamous cell carcinoma [no grade applies]
Variations
Atrophic features[underlying glandular pattern]
Pseudohyperplastic [pattern 3]
Glomeruloid [pattern 3 or pattern 4]
Collagenous micronodules (mucinous fibroplasia) [underlying glandular pattern (most pattern 3)]
Focal acellular mucin extravasation [ignore mucin and use underlying glandular pattern]
Foamy gland carcinoma [underlying glandular pattern (most pattern 3)]
Non-mucinous signet ring cell features (cytoplasmic vacuoles) [underlying glandular pattern (most pattern 4 or 5)]
Hypernephroid [pattern 4]

Table 3.6 Main clinico-pathological findings in unusual variants of prostate cancer

	Clinical features	PSA	IHC	Age at	Incidence	Treatment
Small cell carcinoma[a]	Bladder outlet obstruction; disseminated disease; paraneoplastic syndrome	Usually elevated	Cells are positive for at least one of the neuroendocrine marker, i.e. chromogranin A, synaptophysin, neuron specific enolase, CD56 or TTF-1	65–72 years (range 24–89)	0.3–1 %	Chemotherapy
Ductal adenocarcinoma	Obstruction and hematuria are common; some with metastases and advanced clinical stage at diagnosis	Most above 4 ng/ml	PSA and PSAP are almost always positive; Alpha-methylacyl CoA racemase can be detected at a reduced level	63–72 years (range of 41–89 years)	1.3 %[b]	Androgen deprivation therapy may provide palliative relief, even though this cancer is less hormonally responsive than acinar adenocarcinoma
Sarcomatoid carcinoma (carcinosarcoma)	Urinary tract obstruction and symptoms of frequency, urgency and nocturia	Variable normal or elevated	Epithelial markers (cytokeratins, PSA, PSAP) and muscle markers can be detected Vimentin immunostains are uniformly positive, and S-100 protein is consistently found in chondrosarcomatous regions, others +	70 years of age (range 50–89)	Rare	Surgery followed by Chemotherapy
Basal cell carcinoma	Urinary obstruction	Variable	stained with 34betaE12 and p63 and negative for PSA, PSAP and alpha-methylacyl-coenzyme racemase; others+	Elderly	Rare	Surgery
Squamous cell carcinoma	Some arise in prostate cancer patients following endocrine therapy or radiotherapy or schistosomiasis	Most with normal serum PSA and PSAP	negative for PSA and PSAP immunostains	Average age of 68	Less than 0.6 %	Surgery
Adenosquamous carcinoma	50 % may arise in prostate cancer patients following endocrine therapy or radiotherapy	Most with Most with normal serum PSA and PSAP	Negative for PSA and PSAP immunostains	Average age of 68	Rare	Surgery
Primary urothelial carcinoma	Urinary obstruction and hematuria	Variable (limited information)	They are PSA and PSAP negative, and are frequently positive for the cytokeratins CK20, CK7, high molecular weight cytokeratins bound by antibody 34betaE12, p63, thrombomodulin, and uroplakins	(Range 45–90 years)	0.7–2.8 %	Surgery
Pleomorphic giant cell carcinoma	Urinary obstruction; metastases	Variable (limited information)	PSA, PSAP, Cytokeratins	45–77 years	Very rare	Surgery, androgen blockade, radiation therapy
LELC	Urinary obstruction	5.5 ng/ml	Cytockeratins,PSA and PSAP	66 years	Vary rare	Surgery

[a]In about one-half of cases it is pure small cell carcinoma, while in the other half there is a mixture with prostatic acinar adenocarcinoma
[b]The incidence of mixed ductal-acinar adenocarcinoma is 4.8 %

3.5 Gleason Grading of Prostate Cancer

- The Gleason grading system for prostate cancer is the predominant grading system for prostate cancer around the world. The Gleason grading system is based on glandular architecture which can be divided into five patterns of growth (also known as grades) with decreasing differentiation (Table 3.7).
- The primary and secondary pattern or grade, i.e. the most prevalent and the second most prevalent pattern or grade are added to obtain a Gleason score or sum that is to be reported. Nuclear atypia or cytoplasmic features are not evaluated. An important issue is that the initial grading of prostate carcinoma should be performed at low magnification. Then one may proceed with high power objectives to look for rare fused glands or a few individual cells.
- Gleason grading remains as one of the most significant factors in the clinical decision making activity both in needle biopsy specimens and after radical prostatectomy is performed; i.e. it predicts pathologic stage, margin status, biochemical failure, local recurrences, lymph node, disease progression or distant metastasis after prostatectomy. Radiation therapy, radical prostatectomy and other therapies are initially based on the Gleason score
- In practice Gleason scores of 7 is considered on intermediate risk, Gleason score 8 is a high risk and Geason score 9–10 are associated with worse prognosis meanwhile Gleason scores 5–6 are associated with lower progression rates after therapy. Gleason score has been included in clinical nomograms which are used with increasing frequency to predict disease progression.

Table 3.7 Diagnostic reporting of Gleason score

General features
Perform Gleason grading at low magnification using a 4× or 10× lens
Report primary pattern and secondary pattern and assign Gleason score
If only one pattern is present, double it to yield Gleason score. A Gleason score is usually assignable even if the cancer is extremely small
In a needle biopsy with more than 2 patterns (tertiary pattern), the worst pattern must be reflected in the Gleason score even if it is not the predominant or secondary pattern, use the rule "the most and the worst" (see text)
In a radical prostatectomy with more than 2 patterns, the primary and secondary patterns must be reflected in the Gleason score. Add tertiary pattern as a note in the report
Provide Gleason score for each separately involved core when identified and give overall Gleason score when mixed in one container
In general a diagnosis of Gleason score 2–4 should not be made
Do not report Gleason score after hormonal or radiation therapy except if cancer shows no treatment effect
Optional features
Provide percent of tumour with Gleason pattern 4 in Gleason score 7
Provide percent of tumour with Gleason patterns 4 and 5 in tumours with Gleason score 8–10

3.5.1 Gleason Patterns

- Pattern 1: Very well circumscribed nodule of separate, closely packed glands which do not infiltrate into adjacent benign prostatic tissue. The glands are of intermediate size and approximately equal in size and shape. The nucleus is typically small and cytoplasm frequently is abundant and pale-staining. Nuclear and cytoplasm appearance are not taken into account in diagnosis. This pattern is exceedingly rare and usually seen in transition zone cancers (Fig. 3.74).
- Pattern 2: Round to oval glands with smooth ends. The glands are more loosely arranged and not quite as uniform in size and shape as those of Gleason pattern 1. There may be minimal invasion by neoplastic glands into the surrounding non-neoplastic prostatic tissue. The glands are of intermediate size and larger than in Gleason pattern 1. The variation in glandular size and separation between glands is less than that seen in pattern 3. Although not evaluated in Gleason grading, the cytoplasm of Gleason pattern 2 cancers is abundant and pale-staining. Gleason pattern 2 is usually seen in transition zone cancers but may occasionally be found in the peripheral zone.
- Pattern 3: Is the most common pattern but is morphologically heterogeneous. The glands are infiltrative and the distance between them is more variable than in patterns 1 and 2. Malignant glands often infiltrate between adjacent non-neoplastic glands. The glands of pattern 3 vary in size and shape and are often angular. Small glands are typical for pattern 3, but there may also be large and irregular. Each gland has an open lumen and is circumscribed by stroma. This heterogeneous expression of Gleason grade 3 raised an initial subdivision in patters known as A, B, and C, respectively.
- Pattern 4: Glands appear fused, cribriform or they may be poorly defined and small. Fused glands are composed of a group of glands that are no longer completely separated by stroma. The edge of a group of fused glands is scalloped and there are occasional thin strands of connective tissue within this group. The hypernephroid pattern described by Gleason is a rare variant of fused glands with clear or very pale-staining cytoplasm. Cribriform pattern 4 glands (currently all cribriform patterns are Gleason 4 except those with necrosis) are large or they may be irregular with jagged edges. As opposed to fused glands, there are no strands of stroma within a cribriform gland. Poorly defined glands do not have a lumen that is completely encircled by epithelium.
- Pattern 5: Almost complete loss of glandular lumina which are only occasionally present. The epithelium forms solid sheets, solid strands or single cells invading the stroma; comedonecrosis may be present. Care must be applied when assigning a Gleason pattern 4 or 5 to limited cancer on needle biopsy to exclude an artifact of tangential sectioning of lower grade cancer.

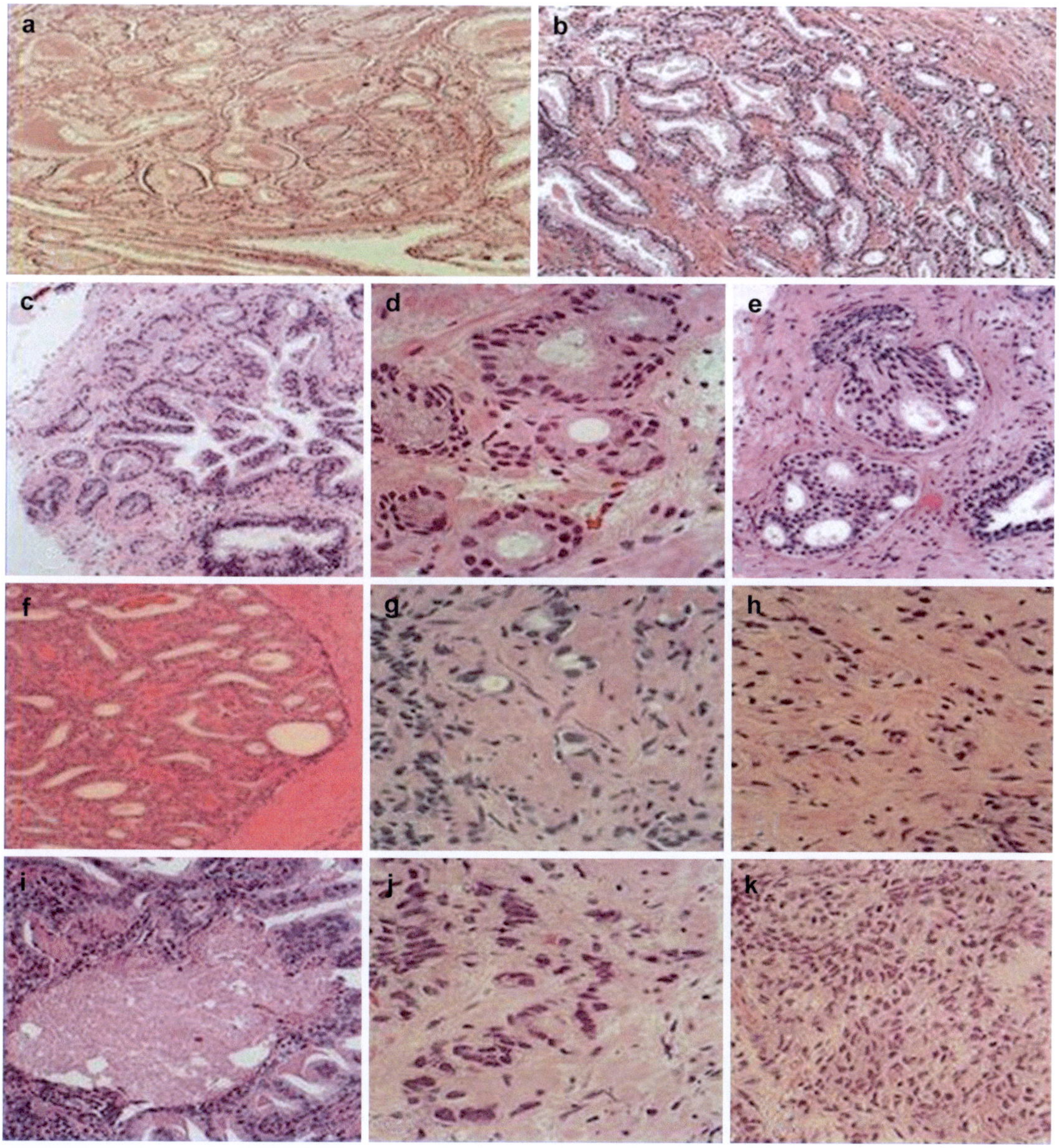

Fig. 3.74 Gleason grading of prostate cancer. (**a**) Gleason 1; (**b**) Gleason 2; (**c–e**) Gleason 3; (**f–h**) Gleason 4; (**i–k**) Gleason 5 patterns

3.5.2 Reporting Gleason Scores in Prostate Needle Biopsies

Gleason score 2–4

- The diagnosis of Gleason score 2–4 on needle biopsies should be made "rarely, if ever", and the reasons are compelling: (1) Gleason score 2–4 cancer is extraordinarily rare in needle biopsies as compared to transurethral resection specimens; (2) poor reproducibility among experts; (3) the correlation with the prostatectomy score is poor; and (4) a "low" score of Gleason 2–4 may misguide clinicians into believing that there is an indolent tumour.
- Gleason score of 1 + 1 = 2 is a grade that should not be diagnosed regardless of the type of specimen, since most of these cases in the era of Gleason, would today be referred to as atypical adenomatous hyperplasia (adenosis). Cribriform morphology is not allowed within Gleason pattern 2.

Gleason Pattern 3

- Cribriform morphology is not allowed within Gleason pattern 3. Therefore the majority of cribriform patterns should be diagnosed as Gleason pattern 4. "Individual cells" would not be allowed within Gleason pattern 3.

Gleason pattern 4

- The importance of the percentage of Gleason 4 pattern in Gleason score 7 tumours accumulates rapidly. In recently generated nomograms, patients with Gleason score 4+3 vs. 3+4 are stratified differently. Whether or not the percentage of pattern 4 tumour should be included in the report remains optional at present time. Small, ill-defined glands with poorly formed glandular lumina also warrant the diagnosis of Gleason pattern 4.

Gleason Pattern 5

- Comedonecrosis when seen in solid nests or cribriform masses should be regarded as Gleason pattern 5. However, the definition of comedonecrosis requires intraluminal necrotic cells and/or nuclear debris (karyorrhexis).

Tertiary pattern

- Another important issue in current practice is the recognition and reporting of the tertiary pattern in needle biopsies.
- This includes tumours with patterns 3, 4, and 5 in various proportions on a biopsy. Tertiary patterns are uncommon but when the worst Gleason grade is the tertiary pattern, it should influence the final Gleason score, and therefore the primary pattern and the highest grade should be recorded following the rule of "the most and the worst". A case with primary Gleason pattern 3, secondary pattern 4, and tertiary pattern 5 should be assigned a Gleason score of 8.

Needle biopsy with different cores showing different grades

- This is related to when one or more of the cores shows pure high grade cancer (i.e. Gleason score 4+4=8) and the other cores show pattern 3 (3+3, 3+4 or 4+3) cancer. If one reports the grades of each core separately, whereby the highest grade tumour (Gleason score 8) would typically be the one selected by the clinician as the grade of the entire case.
- Others give instead an overall score for the entire case. For example, in a case with Gleason score 4+4=8 on one core with pattern 3 (3+3=6, 3+4=7, 4+3=7) on other cores, the overall score for the entire case would be Gleason score 4+3=7 or 3+4=7, depending on whether pattern 4 or 3 predominated.
- Likewise, it was demonstrated that when one core is Gleason score 4+4=8 with other cores having pattern 3, the pathological stage at radical prostatectomy is comparable to cases with all needle cores having Gleason score 4+4=8. The use of the highest core grade of the given case in cases where there are multiple cores of different grades advocated in current tables and nomograms gives additional support for giving cores a separate grade rather than an overall score for the entire case.
- Consequently, is has been recommended to assign individual Gleason scores to separate cores as long as the cores were submitted in separate containers or the cores were in the same container yet specified by the urologist as to their location (i.e. by different colour inks). In addition, one has the option to also give an overall score at the end of the case.

- In cases where a container contains multiple pieces of tissue and one cannot be sure if is looking at an intact core, it is recommended that one should only give an overall score for that container.

3.5.3 Reporting Gleason Scores in Radical Prostatectomies

- In these specimens one should assign the Gleason score based on the primary and secondary patterns with a comment if present on the tertiary pattern.

Gleason Scores 2–4

- Gleason scores 2–4 are rarely seen as the grade of the main tumour in radical prostatectomies performed for stages T1c or T2 disease. These tumours are typically seen in multifocal incidental adenocarcinoma of the prostate found within the transition zone in transurethral resection (TURP) specimens.
- The situation where Gleason scores 2–4 tumour represents the major tumour at radical prostatectomy performed for tumour incidentally found on TURP (stages T1a and T1b) is uncommon. In one study Gleason score 2–4 was the grade of the main tumour in 2 % of the radical prostatectomy specimens; this represents a disproportionate number of T1a and T1b tumours as compared to what would be currently seen in today's practice. All men with only Gleason scores 2–4 tumour at radical prostatectomy are cured.

Gleason Scores 5–6

- It is important to recognize that the majority of tumours with Gleason scores 5–6 are cured after radical prostatectomy.

Gleason Score 7

- Tumours with a Gleason score of 7 have a significantly worse prognosis than those with a Gleason score of 6. Given the adverse prognosis associated with Gleason pattern 4, one would expect that whether a tumour is Gleason score 3+4 versus 4+3 would influence prognosis. There have been several studies addressing Gleason score 3+4 as compared to Gleason score 4+3 at radical prostatectomy with somewhat conflicting results. In one study they reported no significant survival advantage for Gleason pattern 3+4 over 4+3 but other study showed Gleason score 3+4 versus 4+3 correlated with both stage and progression in men with serum PSA values <10 ng/ml and organ confined disease.
- Several other investigations have shown that Gleason score 4+3 have a worse prognosis. This is an issue in which much work needs to be done.

Gleason Scores 8–10

- Gleason scores 8–10 may account for only 7 % of the grades seen at radical prostatectomy, but these patients have highly aggressive tumours with advanced stage such that they are not amenable to surgical therapy alone. Overall, patients with Gleason scores 8–10 at radical prostatectomy have a 15 % chance of having no evidence of disease at 15 years following surgery.

Percent Gleason Pattern 4/5

- The proportion of high-grade tumour as the preferred method for grading prostate cancer has been proposed as it is predictive for progression at the extremes (greater than 70 % or less than 20 % pattern 4/5). It has been recently demonstrated that classifying tumours based on the combined percent of pattern 4/5 is more predictive than stratifying patients into Gleason score alone. Therefore, it has been recommended being included in the report.

Tertiary Gleason Pattern

- In radical prostatectomy a higher proportion of cases are found to contain more than two grades and over 50 % of them contain at least three different grades. The progression rate of Gleason scores 5–6 tumours with a tertiary component of Gleason pattern 4 is almost the same as those of a pure Gleason score 7 tumours. Gleason score 7 tumours with tertiary pattern 5 experience progression rates following radical prostatectomy approximating pure Gleason 8 tumours. On the other hand, no such significance could be seen in cases of Gleason (4+4) score 8 with tertiary pattern 5; since Gleason score 8 tumours are already aggressive, the existence of pattern 5 elements adds no difference. These tumours should be graded routinely (primary and secondary patterns) with a comment in the report noting the presence of the tertiary element. In the setting of high grade cancer (score 8–10) one should ignore lower grade patterns if they occupy less than 5 % of the area of the tumour.

Tumours with one predominant pattern and a small percentage of higher grade tumour

- Some controversy still exist on how to grade tumours, which are over 95 % of one pattern, where there is only a very small percentage of higher grade tumour. For example, a tumour composed of >95 % Gleason pattern 3 and <5 % pattern 4, some experts would assign a Gleason score 3+3=6, as it has been proposed that one needs over 5 % of a pattern to be present for it to be incorporated within the Gleason score. Others might grade the tumour as Gleason score 3+4=7. It seems like the existence of a high grade component, even it constitutes less than 5 % of the whole tumour has a significant adverse influence.

Radical prostatectomy specimens with separate tumour nodules

- It was recommended that radical prostatectomy specimens should be processed in an organized fashion where one can make some assessment as to whether one is dealing with a dominant nodule or separate tumour nodules. One should assign a separate grade to each dominant tumour nodule(s). With only a couple of exceptions, pathologists within the consensus conference who were authors of large radical prostatectomy series had already adopted this method of grading and the prognostic impact of the Gleason score within these series already reflects this approach. Most often, the dominant nodule is the largest tumour, which is also the tumour associated with the highest stage and highest grade.

3.5.4 Grading Variants and Variations of Adenocarcinoma of the Prostate

- Ductal adenocarcinoma should be graded as Gleason score 4+4=8, while retaining the diagnostic term of ductal adenocarcinoma to denote their unique clinical and pathological features.
- There is no consensus on how mucinous (colloid) carcinoma should be scored. Some authors suggest that a Gleason score of 8 is to be assigned, while others recommend ignoring mucin and grading the tumour based on the underlying architectural pattern. Small cell, sarcomatoid and mucinous signet-ring cell carcinomas should not be assigned a Gleason grade. It has been suggested that the rare pleomorphic giant cell carcinoma of the prostate should be assigned a pattern 5 (Table 3.5).

3.5.5 Correlation Between Needle Biopsy and RP Gleason Scores

- There have been several studies addressing the correlation between Gleason scores in needle biopsies and corresponding radical prostatectomy specimens. Although earlier studies used the thicker (14-guace) needle biopsies, more recent series based on thin-core (18-gauge) needles used in conjunction with biopsy guns attached to trans-rectal ultrasound. Sextant or other modes of systematic sampling is typically performed in the more current series. In a recent compilation of data on 3,789 patients from 18 studies, exact correlation of Gleason scores was found in 43 % of cases and correlation plus or minus one Gleason core unit in 77 % of cases.
- Under-grading of carcinoma in needle biopsy is the most common problem, occurring in 42 % of all reviewed cases. Importantly, over-grading of carcinoma in needle biopsies may also occur, but this was only found in 15 % of cases. In general, adverse findings on needle biopsy accurately predict adverse findings in the radical prostatectomy specimen, whereas favourable findings on the needle biopsy do not necessarily predict favourable findings in the radical prostatectomy specimens in large part due to sampling error.

Sources of discrepancies between needle biopsy and RP Gleason scores

Sampling error

- Perhaps the most important factor is sampling error, which relates to the small amount of tissue removed by thin-core needle biopsies. The average 20-mm, 18-gauge core samples approximately 0.04 % of the average gland volume (40 cc). The most common type of sampling error occurs when there is a higher grade component present within the radical prostatectomy specimen which is not sampled on needle biopsy. This typically occurs when a needle biopsy tumour is graded as Gleason score 3+3=6. In the radical prostatectomy, there exists a Gleason pattern 4 which was not sampled on the biopsy, resulting in a prostatectomy Gleason 3+4=7.
- In some instances, under-grading results from an attempt to grade very tiny areas of carcinoma, so-called minimal or limited adenocarcinoma. Scores of minimal adenocarcinoma in needle biopsies show a reasonably strong correlation with radical prostatectomy scores, but the Gleason scores do not have the same power to predict extra-prostatic extension and positive margin status as they do in non-minimal carcinomas.
- Over-grading can result from sampling error in cases where the high-grade pattern is selectively represented in needle biopsy. It may only represent a very minor element in the radical prostatectomy specimen. Even the same cancer focus may have different grades depending on the area sampled.

Borderline cases

- The other source of discrepancy between biopsy and radical prostatectomy is borderline cases. In the description of the Gleason grading system, there are some cases that are right at the interface between two different patterns where there will be inter-observer variability and possible even intra-observer variability.

Pathology error

- Pathology error is most frequently seen when pathologists assigned a Gleason score of ≤4 on a needle biopsy which in fact was Gleason score 5–6. Many pathologists under-grade needle biopsies by confusing quantitative changes with qualitative changes. When there is a limited focus of small glands of cancer on needle biopsy, by definition this is a Gleason pattern 3. Gleason pattern 3 consists of small glands with an infiltrative pattern. Biopsying truly low-grade adenocarcinoma of the prostate could not result in just a few neoplastic glands but rather would be more extensive, as low-grade adenocarcinoma grows as nodules of closely packed glands rather than infiltrating in and amongst normal glands.
- Under-grading may result from difficulty in recognizing an infiltrative growth pattern or failing to recognize the presence of small areas of gland fusion.

Pathologists' education and experience

- The pathologists' experience in grading thin-core needle biopsies can also influence overall correlation with radical prostatectomy results. With experience, pathologists recognize grading pitfalls; in particular, the fact that Gleason scores of 4 and lower are almost non-existent in needle biopsy situation. Furthermore, small areas of fusion in the presence of a predominantly grade 3 background are recognized and will yield a Gleason score of 7, which often correlates well with radical prostatectomy results.

Intra-observer and inter-observer variability

- Reproducibility studies can be categorized as intra-observer and interobserver. For investigations of intra-observer agreement of Gleason grades, exact agreement was reported in 43–78 % of cases, and agreement within plus or minus one Gleason score unit was reported in 72–87 % of cases. Gleason wrote that he duplicated exactly his previous histological scores approximately 50 % of times.
- Highly variable levels of interobserver agreement on Gleason scores have also

been reported, with range of 36–81 % for exact agreement and 69–86 % observers within plus or minus one Gleason score unit. Improvements in Gleason grading reproducibility can be achieved by recognizing problematic areas and educating physicians via meetings, courses, website tutorials, and publications that specifically focus on the Gleason grading system.

3.5.6 Pathology of the Prostate After Treatment

3.5.6.1 Pathologic Features After Anti-androgen Therapy

Non-neoplastic prostate

- The appearance of hormonally-treated prostates is that of global senescence or involution of the gland. The transition zone shows simplification of the glandular lobules, although the lobular configuration is retained. The ducts and acini are small, ovoid, round or comma-shaped. There is no undulation of the epithelial border.
- The secretory cells have inconspicuous nucleoli, nuclear shrinkage, chromatin condensation and cytoplasmic clearing. The basal cell layer is prominent and focal "immature" squamous and basal cell hyperplasia is seen (Fig. 3.75).
- Within the peripheral and central zones there is inconspicuous branching of the ducts and acini which appear dilated, star-shaped, and lined by flattened atrophic epithelium which is single-layered and seldom double-layered (Table 3.8).

Prostatic intraepithelial neoplasia

- PIN is generally observed within scattered ducts with lower extent of PIN in treated glands. The cell lining shows a basal-cell layer which is marked and recognisable in most instances. A certain degree of secretory cell type stratification is always present. However, crowding is less evident than in the untreated prostate.
- The cells have nuclear shrinkage, chromatin condensation and pyknosis, inconspicuous nucleoli, cytoplasmic clearing. Apoptotic cells are easily identifiable in all the cell type layers (Figs. 3.76 and 3.77).
- The duct and acinar lumen is always rich in cells: some are macrophages, some sloughed secretory cells with degenerative features, while others correspond to apoptotic cells. No post-treatment grading of PIN is possible.
- Blockade of 5-alpha-reductase with finasteride appears to have little or no effect on HGPIN, unlike other forms of androgen deprivation therapy.

Prostate cancer

- Hormonal therapy results in a significant overall reduction in the volume of PCa when compared to untreated PCa in radical prostatectomy samples. Histological response seems to correlate with the tumour patterns and the Gleason grades observed before the androgen ablation therapy is started (Figs. 3.78 and 3.79).
- Residual PCa invading the prostatic capsule, periprostatic soft tissue, seminal vesicle and metastatic to pelvic lymph nodes, shows therapy-induced changes similar to adenocarcinomas confined within the prostate gland.
- The treated tumours, with acinar pattern (primary Gleason grade 1–3) in the biopsy before the androgen ablation therapy, show neoplastic acini which appear shrunken, a decreased frequency of intraluminal crystalloids and areas of individual infiltrating tumour cells separated by abundant connective tissue.
- The epithelial tumour cells have cytoplasmic clearing and enlargement by coalescence of vacuoles and rupture of cell membranes. The nuclear chromatin shows different changes which range from a mild condensation – which barely allows the distinction between coarse chromatin granules (heterochromatin) and finely dispersed chromatin (euchromatin) – to a tightly condensed state close to that observed in apoptosis.
- Apoptotic bodies are easily identifiable in all epithelial cell layers as well as macrophages and sloughed epithelial cells in the lumina.
- The hallmark of all the untreated adenocarcinomas is that the tumour nuclei are frequently multinucleolated, the nucleoli being promi-

nent (mean diameter 1.47 μm), marginated and with a perinuclear halo. By contrary, in the treated cases the nucleoli become inconspicuous, without margination, and have a decreased mean diameter of 1.09 m, the nucleolar diameter being below 1.0 μm in 20 % of the tumours.

- The treated tumours with pre-treatment cribriform and solid/trabecular patterns (primary Gleason grade 4 and 5) show nuclear and cytoplasmic changes which appear less pronounced than in the acinar pattern.
- The stroma shows variable degrees of fibrosis, reduced capillary vascularity and variable density of lymphocytic infiltrates, often intermingled with mast cells, plasma cells, and eosinophilis. Infiltrates of foamy histiocytes, difficult to distinguish from PCa cells with clear cytoplasm, are sometimes present. Periprostatic fibrosis, obscuring the normal cleavage plane and making the operation more difficult, is reported after hormonal therapy. The longer patients receive hormonal therapy prior to surgery, the more fibrosis is observed around the prostate.

Immunohistochemistry

- In some cases residual tumour, consist only of isolated cells or cell clusters within prostatic stroma. Significant difficulty may be encountered in separating minute clusters and single file ribbons of tumour cells from lymphocytes, myocytes and fibroblasts.
- Immunostaining with PSA and prostatic acid phosphatase can detect persisting tumour cells. Immunohistochemistry with a low-molecular-weight cytokeratin, such as CAM 5.2 antibody, will stain residual PCa cells, but the same cells will lack reactivity for high-molecular-weight cytokeratin 34βE12 which highlights basal cells (Fig. 3.80).

Pathological "grading" of treated prostate cancer

- Because of therapy-induced morphologic changes, grading of residual PCa, based on Gleason criteria, is not accurate and, therefore, discouraged. However it may be performed in the situation of that changes related to therapy are not present in a given case.

Pathologic stage and resection margin status of treated prostate cancer

- There is conflicting evidence regarding pathological downstaging, with some studies suggesting benefit and others no benefit of androgen manipulation before radical prostatectomy. Likewise, it seems like neoadjuvant therapy in clinical T2 tumours was associated with 20 % decrease in positive margins in radical prostatectomy specimens.

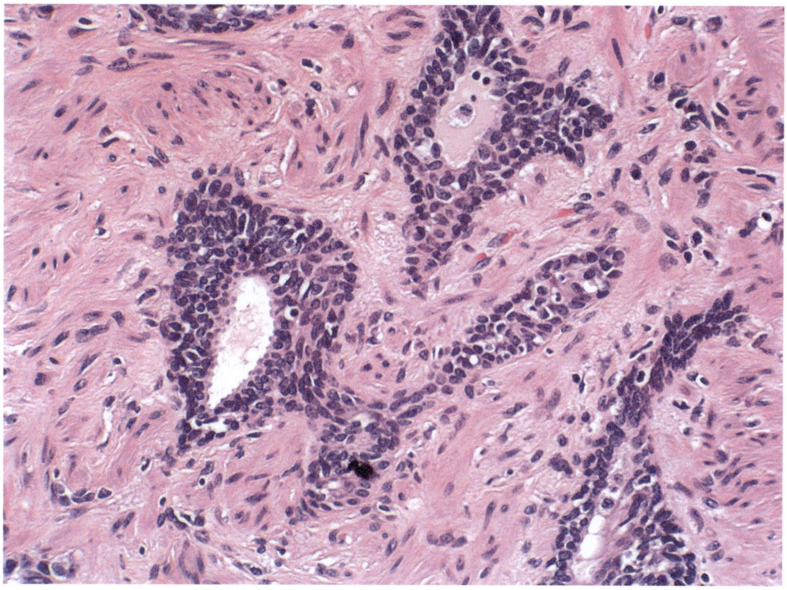

Fig. 3.75 Non-neoplastic prostate after anti-androgen therapy

Table 3.8 Pathologic findings in the prostate following androgen blockade (the changes affect normal prostate, PIN and cancer)

Architecture
Prominent acinar atrophy with loss of hyperplastic glandular architecture in the transition zone
Basal cell prominence and hyperplasia in benign prostate
Squamous metaplasia, including the immature variant
Decrease in extent of PIN
Decrease in extent of prostatic adenocarcinoma with loss of luminal (acinar) architecture
Decreased frequency of intraluminal crystalloids in prostatic adenocarcinoma
Cytology
Cytoplasmic clearing and vacuolisation
Nuclear shrinkage
Nuclear hyperchromasia
Nuclear pyknosis with increased frequency of apoptotic bodies
Lack of mitotic figures
Loss of nucleolar prominence
Stroma
Focal hypercellularity
Focal lymphocytic/histiocytic infiltrate (including foamy, lipid-laden histiocytes)

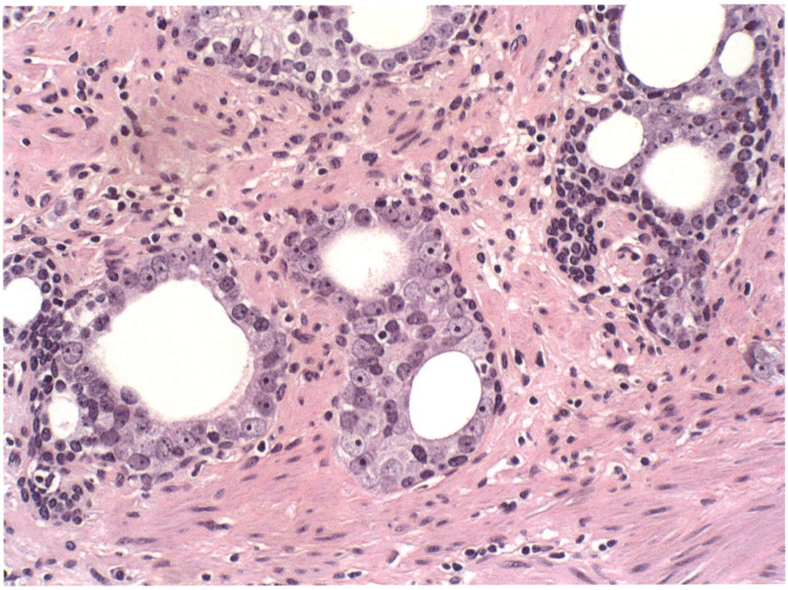

Fig. 3.76 PIN after anti-androgen therapy

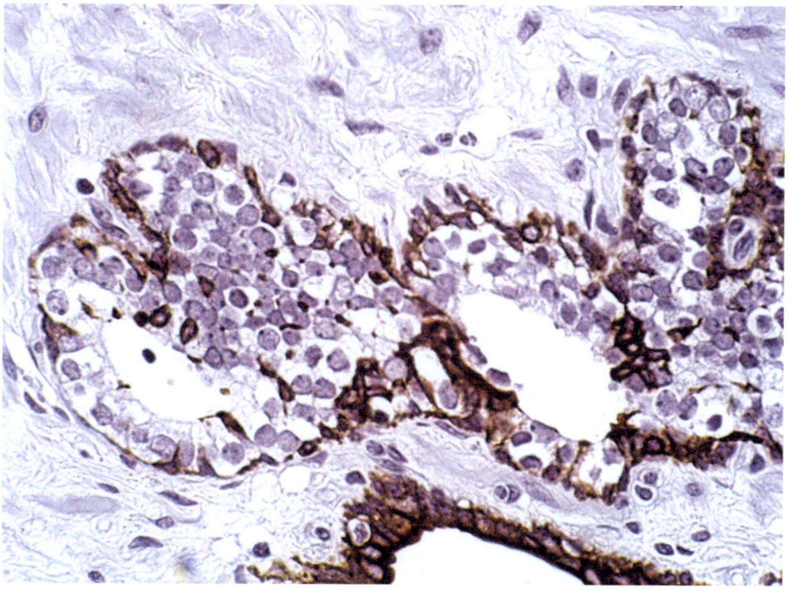

Fig. 3.77 PIN after anti-androgen therapy. Anti-basal cell cytokeratin highlights basal cell layer

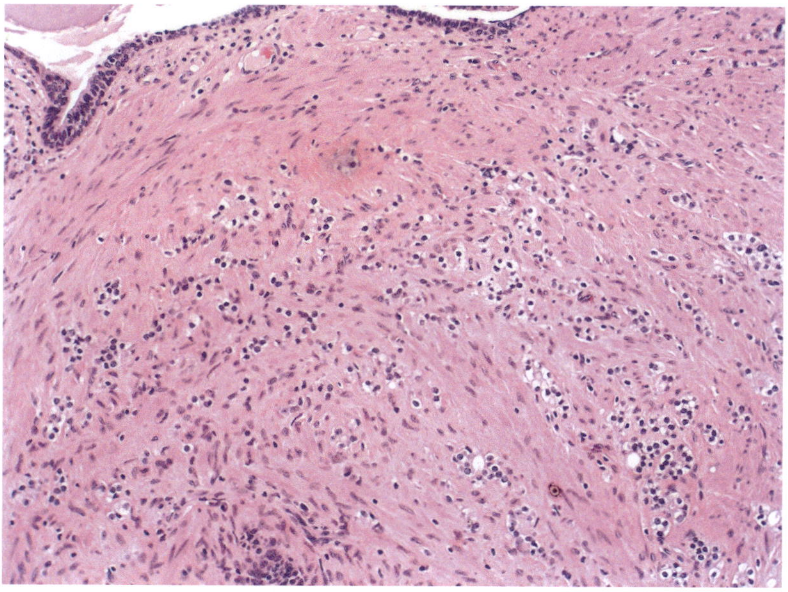

Fig. 3.78 Microscopic features of prostate carcinoma after anti-androgen therapy (low power)

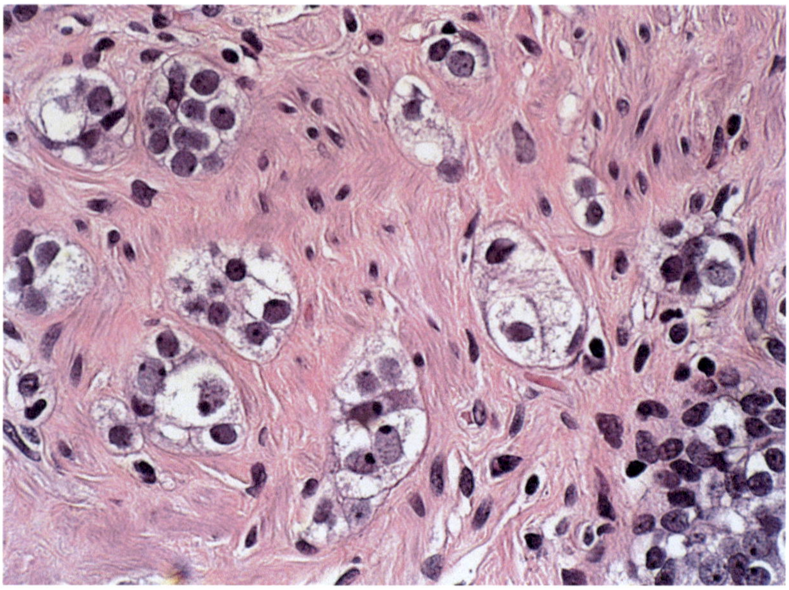

Fig. 3.79 Microscopic features of prostate carcinoma after anti-androgen therapy (high power)

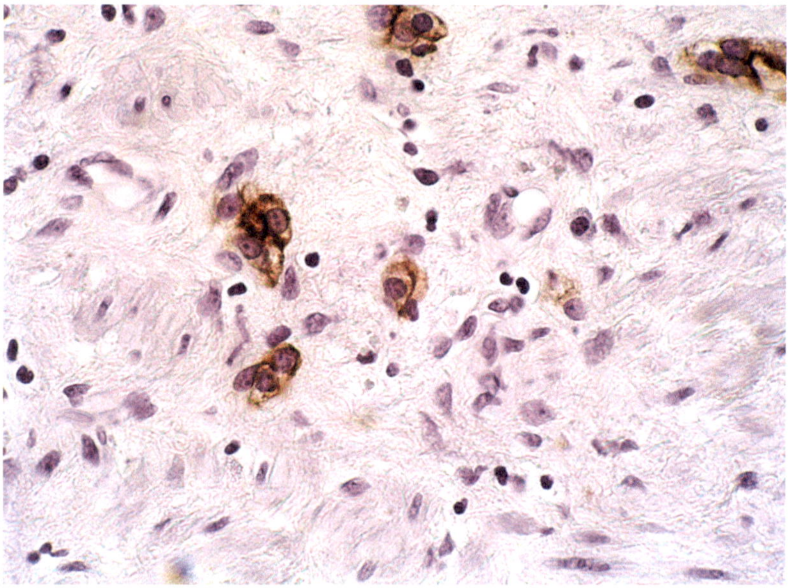

Fig. 3.80 CAM 5.2 immunohistochemistry highlights cancer acini after anti-androgen therapy

3.5.6.2 Pathologic Changes After Radiation Therapy (RT)

Prostatic intraepithelial neoplasia

- PIN identified after RT usually retains the features characteristic of untreated PIN. It is readily recognised in the RP specimens. The salient pathologic features include nuclear crowding, nuclear overlapping and stratification, nuclear hyperchromasia, and prominent nucleoli. The basal cell layer is still present, but fragmented. The most common patterns of PIN are tufting and micropapillary. Basal cell prominence and secretory cell cytoplasm vacuolisation may be seen in PIN after RT (Figs. 3.81 and 3.82).
- In some cases, the use of immunostaining for high-molecular-weight keratin may be helpful in distinguishing atypical basal cell hyperplasia from high-grade PIN.

Prostatic cancer

- The histological effects of RT on the cancer are identical. After radiation therapy the prostate gland is usually small and hard. Radiation therapy affects prostate cancer variably with some glands showing marked radiation effect and others showing no evidence of radiation damage. Architecturally, carcinoma showing treatment effect typically loses their glandular pattern, resulting in clustered cells or individual cells.
- Cytologically, the cytoplasm of the tumour cells is pale, increased in volume and often vacuolated. There is often a greater variation of nuclear size than in non-irradiated prostate cancer and the nuclei may be pyknotic or large with clumped chromatin. Nucleoli are often lost. The stroma is often sclerosed or hyalinised (Figs. 3.83 and 3.84).

Immunohistochemistry

- By immunohistochemistry, tumour cells with treatment effect are usually positive for PAP and PSA. These antibodies along with pancytokeratins are very helpful to detect isolated residual tumour cells, which can be overlooked in H&E stained sections. Immunohistochemistry with antibodies against 34βE12 or p63 is useful to distinguish cancer from normal with effects due to radiation therapy.

Pathologic "grading" of treated adenocarcinoma

- Following radiation therapy, prostatic biopsy should be diagnosed as no evidence of cancer, cancer showing no or minimal radiation effect, or cancer showing significant radiation effect, or a combination of the above. Although there are different systems to grade radiation effects in cancer, these are not recommended for routine clinical practice.

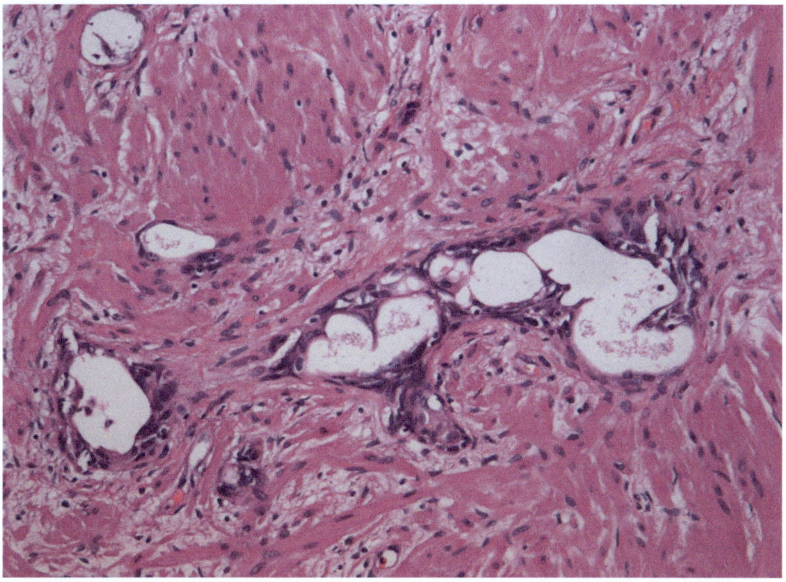

Fig. 3.81 Non-neoplastic prostate after radiation therapy

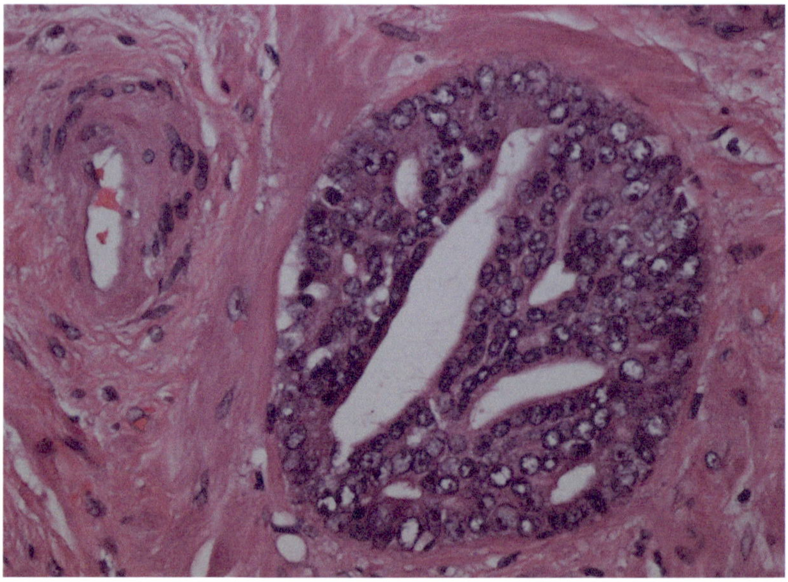

Fig. 3.82 PIN after radiation therapy

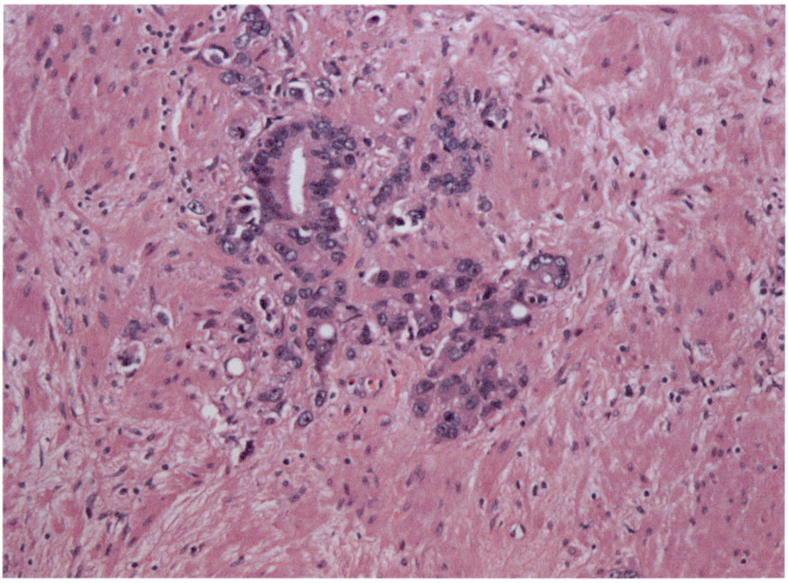

Fig. 3.83 Microscopic features of prostate carcinoma after radiation therapy (low power)

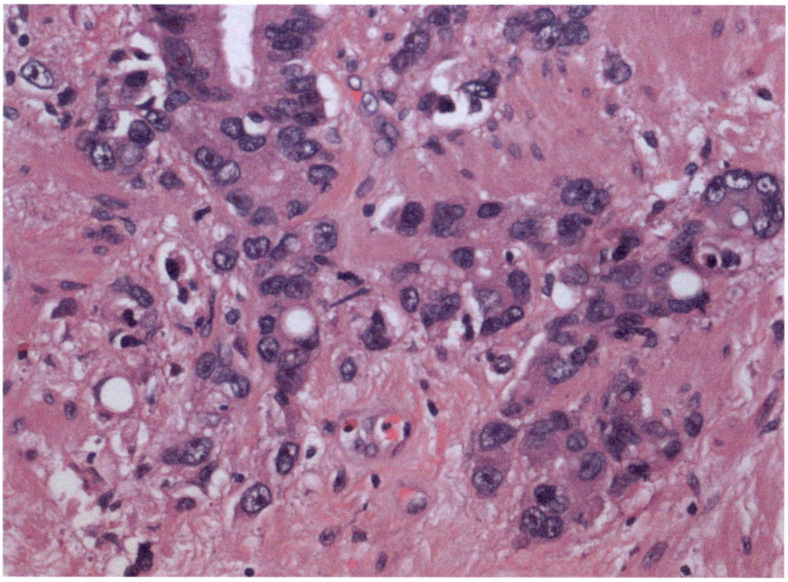

Fig. 3.84 Microscopic features of prostate carcinoma after radiation therapy (high power)

3.6 Pathologic Prognosis of Prostate Cancer

3.6.1 Prostate Biopsy

- The surgical pathology report should thus be comprehensive and yet succinct in providing relevant information to urologists, radiation oncologists and oncologists. Parameters to included are (Table 3.9):

Histological Type

- Since acinar adenocarcinoma is the overwhelming histological type of cancer in needle biopsy specimens, it is not necessary to specify such cancers as acinar or conventional type in biopsy pathology reports.
- Morphologic variations such as atrophic, pseudohyperplastic, hypernephroid, and other are patterns are descriptive terms used to help pathologists recognize potential diagnostic pitfalls but have no known prognostic significance, therefore, do not deserve specific mention in the final diagnostic repoport.
- Several variants of prostate cancer have been described, including ductal, mucinous, signet ring cell, adenosquamous, small cell carcinoma and sarcomatoid carcinoma. The former three are diagnoses tenable only on examination of radical prostatectomy or transurethral resection specimens.
- When present in needle biopsies the diagnostic terminology used must be: adenocarcinoma of prostate with ductal features; adenocarcinoma of prostate with signet ring cell features; and adenocarcinoma of prostate with mucinous differentiation. Small cell carcinoma, sarcomatoid carcinoma and adenosquamous carcinoma may be diagnosed on needle biopsies.

Gleason grade (score)

- The Gleason grading system is recommended as the international standard for grading prostate cancer (see also specific section at pages).

Extent of tumor involvement of needle core

- The amount of tumour in prostate needle cores is an important pathologic parameter that must be reported. The extent of involvement of needle cores by prostatic adenocarcinoma has been shown to correlate with the Gleason score, tumour volume, surgical margins and pathologic stage in radical prostatectomy specimens. The extent of needle core involvement including bilateral involvement has also been shown to predict biochemical recurrence, post-prostatectomy progression and radiation therapy failure in univariate and often in multivariate analysis.

- There is lack of consensus in the literature as to the best method of reporting the extent of tumour involvement. The report should provide the number of involved of cores. In addition, one or both of the following more detailed methods of tumour extent should be performed. One method is to report the linear length of cancer in mm (total tumour length in all biopsies; longest single length of tumour). The other method is to provide a percentage estimate of involvement of each of the cores derived by visual estimation (overall % of cancer in all biopsies, % of each core involved; reporting the percentage of cancer involvement in increments of 5 or 10 % is appropriate).
- One problem encountered with this otherwise straightforward method is when there is extreme fragmentation of the needle biopsy specimen, making assessment of the number of cores and the percentage of cancer within each core difficult. In case of highly fragmented tissue this may be overcome by providing a composite (global) percentage of involvement of cancer in all needle biopsy tissue, and this may be a slightly more accurate correlate of the amount of cancer in the prostate gland itself. Each container submitted needs to receive a separate report including Gleason score and tumor extent is positive cases.
- Bilateral cancer, which indicates multifocality, is indirectly suggestive of greater tumour volume. This parameter is easily deduced from the pathology report findings of each of the cores submitted. In patients not subsequently treated by radical prostatectomy, this is a critical factor in assigning clinical stage (Table 3.10).

Local invasion

- Routine biopsy sampling may occasionally contain extraprostatic fat or seminal vesicle tissue. If cancer is noted to involve these structures, the finding would indicate pT3 disease. The presence of seminal vesicle invasion or extraprostatic fat involvement in the staging biopsy is highly correlative of similar findings at radical prostatectomies. Extraprostatic fat invasion at needle biopsy is highly predictive of biochemical recurrence (78 % compared to 41 % failure rate in cases with extraprostatic extension not detected by needle biopsy).
- Only exceptionally rarely is fat present within the normal prostate. Hence, tumour in adipose tissue in a needle biopsy specimen can safely be interpreted as extraprostatic extension. Ganglion cells and skeletal muscle involvement by tumour is not equivalent to extraprostatic extension as they may both be found frequently within the prostate.
- Distinction between the seminal vesicle epithelium and ejaculatory duct epithelium may be impossible in limited samples, although occasionally the seminal vesicle can be distinguished if its smooth muscle wall is present. In contrast, ejaculatory duct epithelium has a rim of fibrous tissue that is rich in thin blood vessels (Fig. 3.85).
- If the distinction between seminal vesicle tissue/ejaculatory duct is not feasible, diagnostic terminology such as "adenocarcinoma of the prostate with invasion of seminal vesicle/ejaculatory duct tissue" may be used (Fig. 3.86).
- Using immunohistochemistry might be relevant in separating seminal vesicle/ejaculatory ducts from prostate carcinoma. SVs are typically CKAE1/AE3+, p63+, PAX-2+, PSA-, PAP-, P504S-.

Perineural invasion

- Perineural, circumferential or intraneural invasion is defined as the presence of prostate cancer juxtaposed intimately along, around or within a nerve. Other descriptors of perineural invasion that may strengthen the prognostic significance of this parameter include extensive (multifocal) perineural invasion and greater nerve diameter. Involvement of nerves present within adipose tissue (extraprostatic nerves) by cancer indicates extraprostatic extension and deserves notation in the pathology report when present (Figs. 3.87 and 3.88).
- Although perineural invasion in needle biopsy specimens is not an independent predictor of prognosis when the Gleason score, serum PSA and extent of cancer are factored in, most studies indicate that its presence variably cor-

relates with extraprostatic extension is some reports with data suggesting that this finding may independently predict lymph node metastasis and post-surgical progression.

- Some of the data from the radiation oncology literature suggests that it is an independent risk factor for predicting adverse outcome after external beam radiation therapy.

Vascular/lymphatic invasion

- Microvascular invasion consists of tumour cells within endothelial-lined spaces. Also, we do not differentiate between vascular and lymphatic channels because of the difficulty and lack of reproducibility among different observers by routine light microscopic examination. Microvascular invasion may be confused with fixation-associated retraction artifact of acini. Immunohistochemical stains directed against endothelial cells such as CD31, or CD34 may increase the detection rate although this is not necessary in routine work.
- Lymphovascular invasion as studied in radical prostatectomy specimens correlates with lymph node metastasis, biochemical recurrence and distinct metastasis, its presence in the needle biopsy is likely to have similar correlations. This feature is very rarely seen in needle biopsy specimens.

Nuclear DNA content

- DNA ploidy pattern correlates with cancer grade, tumour volume, and stage. Most low-stage tumours are diploid, and high-stage tumours are nondiploid, but many exceptions occur.

Microvessel density

- A significant increase in microvessel density (MVD) occurs in prostatic intraepithelial neoplasia and carcinoma compared with normal prostatic tissue. Mean blood vessel count is higher in tumours with metastases than in those without, and most studies but not all show a correlation with pathologic stage. MVD appears to be an independent predictor of cancer progression in some studies. Some studies suggest that increased MVD contributes to extraprostatic spread of adenocarcinoma.

Table 3.9 Prognostic factors to be reported in prostate biopsies with cancer

Location and distribution of tumour
Histopathologic type
Gleason score including primary and secondary pattern
Extent of involvement (percentage and or cancer extension in millimeters)
Local invasion: extraprostatic extension and seminal vesicle involvement
Perineural invasion: extent (focal vs. multifocal) and diameter of nerve bundles
Lymphovascular invasion

Table 3.10 Diagnostic reporting of amount of tumour in needle cores

Number of cores involved
Amount of cancer in biopsy (either method optional)
Linear measurement in mm (total tumour length in all biopsies, longest single length of tumour)
Percent of sampled tissue (overall % of cancer in all biopsies, % of each core involved)
Bilaterality

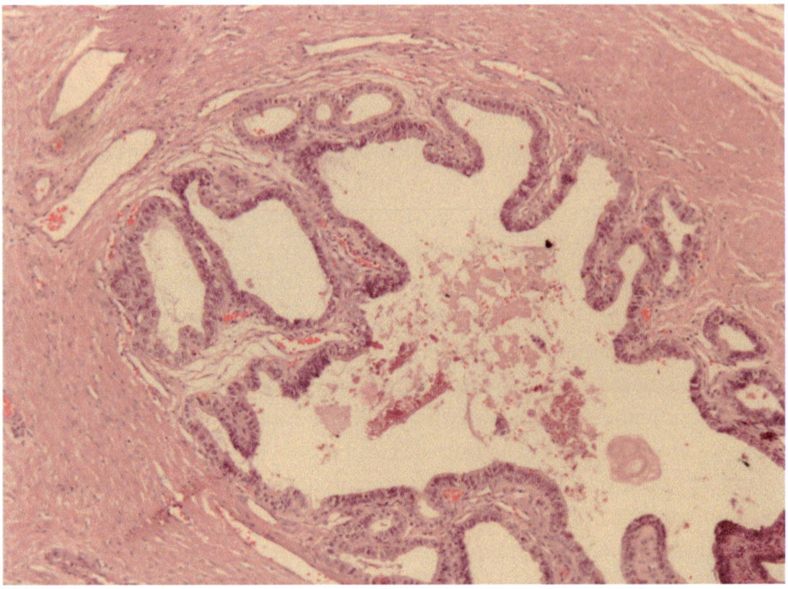

Fig. 3.85 Histology of ejaculatory duct epithelium surrounded by fibrous tissue

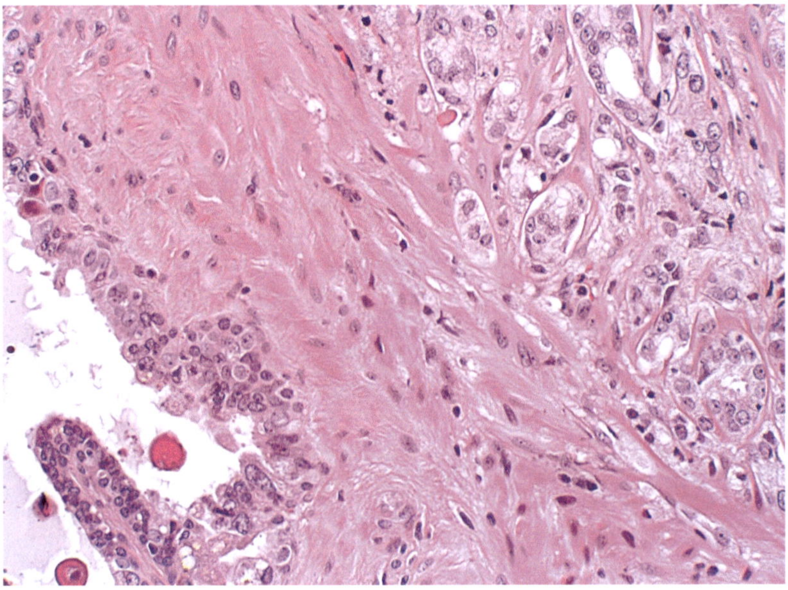

Fig. 3.86 Seminal vesicle infiltration by prostate cancer

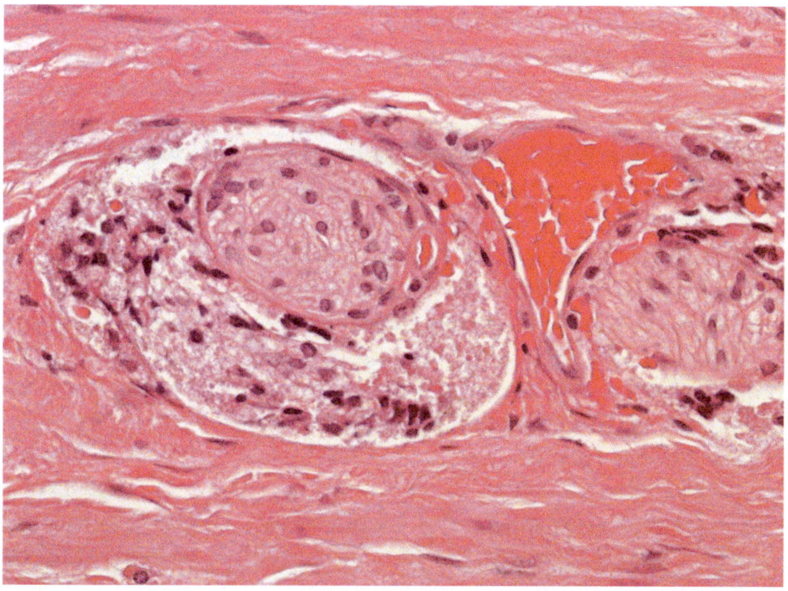

Fig. 3.87 Perineural invasion by prostate cancer with apoptosis-like changes

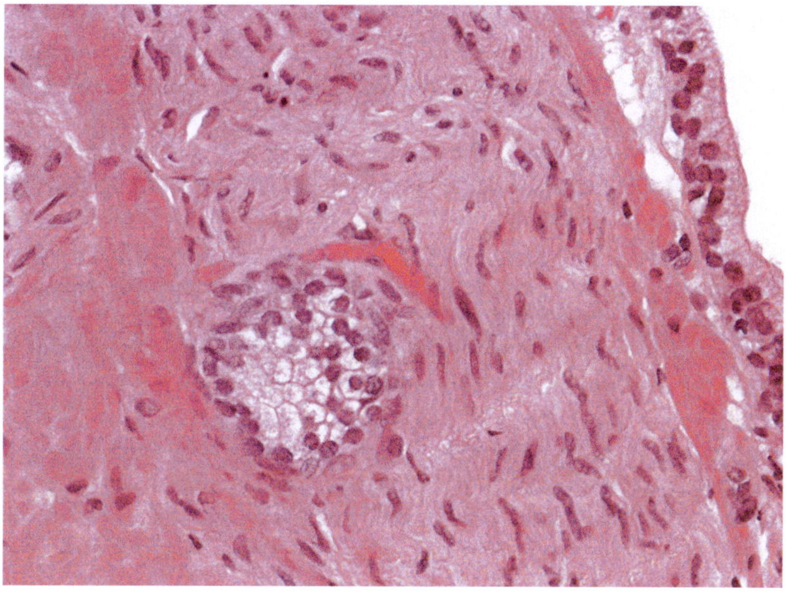

Fig. 3.88 Benign prostate gland juxtaposed to a nerve. This change should not be misdiagnosed as malignancy

3.6.2 Prognostic Factors After Radical Prostatectomy

Histological type of prostatic carcinoma

- Rare and other infrequent histological variants or subtypes of prostatic carcinoma have been identified. These variants represent the spectrum of changes which can occur in adenocarcinoma. The biological behaviour of many of these variants may differ from typical adenocarcinoma and proper clinical management relays on accurate diagnosis and reporting. Mixtures of different histological types should be indicated (Table 3.11).

Histological grade of cancer

- The Gleason score assigned to the tumour at radical prostatectomy is the most powerful predictor of progression following radical prostatectomy (see also specific section at pages).

Staging

- The protocol recommends the use of the most recent revision of the TNM Staging System for carcinoma of the prostate of the American Joint Committee on Cancer (AJCC) and the International Union Against Cancer (UICC).
- Clinical classification (cTNM) is usually carried out by the referring physician before treatment during initial evaluation of the patient or when pathologic classification is not possible. The prefix symbol "p" refers to the pathologic classification of the TNM (pTNM), as opposed to the clinical classification.
- Tumour remaining in a resection specimen following previous treatment of any type (radiation therapy alone, chemotherapy therapy alone, or any combined modality treatment) is codified by the TNM using a prescript "y" to indicate the post-treatment status of the tumour (e.g., ypT1). The classification of residual disease may be a predictor of postoperative outcome.
- Tumour that is locally recurrent after a documented disease-free interval following surgical resection is classified according to the TNM categories but modified with the prefix "r" (e.g., rpT1).

Extent of local invasion

- This includes extraprostatic extension (pT3a) and seminal vesicle involvement (pT3b). Microscopic involvement of bladder neck muscle fibres in radical prostatectomy specimens should also be defined as pT3b. Because the prostate lacks a discrete capsule, the term "extraprostatic extension" (EPE) has replaced "capsular penetration" to describe tumour that has extended out of the prostate into periprostatic soft tissue (Fig. 3.89).
- Histologically, the prostatic capsule is not well defined. In areas there may appear to be a fibrous or fibro-muscular band at the edge of the prostate although in other areas normal prostatic glands extend out to the edge of the prostate without any appearance that there is a capsule.
- Tumour abutting on or admixed with fat constitutes extraprostatic extension. EPE may also be reported when tumour involves perineural spaces in the neurovascular bundles, even in the absence of periprostatic fat involvement.
- Difficulty in diagnosing EPE arises when tumour extends out of the prostatic gland and induces a dense desmoplastic response in the periprostatic adipose tissue. This is most commonly seen in prostatectomy specimens obtained after endocrine neoadjuvant therapy. Because of the desmoplastic response, it can be difficult to judge whether the tumour has extended out of the gland or is within the fibrous tissue of the prostate.
- The best way of assessing whether extraprostatic extension has occurred is to look at the adjacent edge of the prostate on scanning magnification where there is no tumour and follow the edge of the gland to the area in question to see whether the normal rounded contour of the gland has been altered by a protuberance corresponding to extension of tumour into the periprostatic tissue.
- In certain locations, such as the anterior prostate and bladder neck regions, there is paucity of fat. In these locations EPE is determined when the tumour extends beyond the confines of the normal glandular prostate. At the apex, tumour admixed with skeletal muscle elements does not constitute extraprostatic extension.

- The degree of extraprostatic extension varies from only a few glands outside the prostate (focal EPE) to cases with more extensive extraprostatic spread (non-focal or established). The amount of EPE carries prognostic importance.
- Different ways have been used to define the amount of EPE. If it is equal to, or less than two high-power (40×) microscopic fields, then EPE is focal. Any amount in excess of two high-power fields is considered to be either non-focal or extensive.
- Other define focal EPE as extraprostatic tumor occupying less than 1 high power field on ≤2 separate histologic sections.
- Cases showing focal EPE have a progression rate of 20 % versus about 60 % progression for cases with established (non-focal) EPE, a fact that seems to be relevant since organconfined (pT2) disease shows about 13 % progression rate.
- Seminal vesicle invasion is defined as cancer invading into the muscular coat of the seminal vesicle. It has been shown in numerous studies to be a significant prognostic indicator. While in most cases, seminal vesicle invasion occurs in glands with EPE, the latter cannot be documented in a minority of these cases.
- Some of these patients had only minimal involvement of the seminal vesicles, or involve only the portion of the seminal vesicles that is at least partially intraprostatic. Patients in this category were reported to have a favourable prognosis similar to patients without seminal vesicle invasion.
- Histologic patterns of seminal vesicle invasion are:
- Extension up the ejaculatory duct complex;
- Spread across the base of the prostate without other evidence of EPE or involvement from tumour invading the seminal vesicles from the periprostatic and periseminal vesicle adipose tissue
- As an isolated tumour deposit without continuity with the primary prostate cancer tumour focus (Table 3.12).

Positive surgical margins

- Patients with positive margins have a significantly increased risk of progression as compared to those with negative margins. Surgical margins should be designated as "negative" if tumour is not present at the inked margin and is "positive" if tumour cells touch the ink at the margin (Fig. 3.90).
- There are two main causes for positive margins:
- Non-iatrogenic positive margins: positive margins can result from a failure to excise extraprostatic extension of tumour.
- Capsular incision: One cause of a positive resection margin is transection of intraprostatic tumour (capsular incision).
- Positive surgical margins should not be interpreted as extra-prostatic extension. If the surgical margin is positive, the pathologist should state this explicitly in the report. Surgical margin positivity predicts disease progression.
- It is also of importance the location of positive margin since it is not the same a positive margin extraprostatic vs. intra-prostatic.
- The pathologist should be aware of "false positive" margins due to the penetration of ink into cracks present on the external surface.
- The main cause for discrepancy in the definition of a positive margin is seen in situations in which cancer was very close but not clearly touching the inked margin or when the colour used to identify the margin appeared very pale. The apex should be closely examined because of its unusual susceptibility to positive margins.
- The specific locations of the positive margins should be documented since it provides feedback to the urologist, and there should be some indication (e.g. number of positive blocks, linear extent in millimetres) of the extent of margin positivity. It is currently preferred to provide linear extent of positive margins in millimeters, with focal ≤3 mm vs. extensive >3 mm. It is also recommended to report when tumor cells are close (<1 mm) to the inked margin, though is this case surgical margin is still considered negative ad should be reported accordingly.

- The pathology report should also indicate the presence of normal prostate tissue at the resection margin level. This might help the urologist explain why the serum PSA in patients with such a feature remains detectable after radical prostatectomy. In fact, the serum PSA value, even though very low, is not linked to tumour recurrence and persistence but to incomplete resection of the prostate gland.

Vascular Invasion

- It is recommended to report vessel invasion (lymphatic or venous) in prostatic samples even if it remains unclear its independent prognostic significance.

Perineural invasion

- Perineural invasion is one of the major mechanisms by which prostate cancer spreads out of the gland. Perineural invasion is almost ubiquitously present in radical prostatectomy specimens. As with all of the other parameters, the key question is whether the presence of (intra-prostatic) perineural invasion in the prostatectomy specimen is an independent prognosticator. At this time it is not entirely clear whether there are differences in terms of prognosis between intra-prostatic and extra-prostatic perineural invasion.

Volume of cancer

- One of the most controversial aspects of the pathological assessment of radical prostatectomy specimens is the measurement of tumour volume. The critical and controversial question concerns whether tumour volume is an independent prognostic parameters once other routinely assessed variables are accounted for.
- There is one situation where it is important to give some estimate of tumour volume at radical prostatectomy. As a consequence of screening for prostate cancer, we have seen an increase in the resection of prostates harbouring cancers that are so small that they are histologically difficult to identify. These cases currently account for approximately 4 % of radical prostatectomy specimens.
- The pathologist has to specify in the pathology report that these tumours are "small" or "minute" (i.e., less than 0.5 cc) since these tumors carry on low clinical significance. Most of them if not all are cured by surgery.

Biomarkers to predict progression following radical prostatectomy

- The drive to identify prognostic markers in prostate cancer is based on the perceived need to develop "objective" markers to either supplant or supplement more "subjective" markers such conventional histological grading.
- The more established biomarkers are as follows: DNA ploidy, microvessel density (Angiogenesis), KI-67, neuroendocrine differentiation, p53 $P27^{kip1}$, $p21^{WAF1}$, bcl-2, Her-2/neu, E-cadherin, CD44, Retinoblastoma (Rb) proteins, apoptotic index, androgen receptor status, PSA and PSAP expression, nuclear morphometry. Non of them is actually incorporated to the clinic.
- It is important to recognize that these "objective" markers are subject to the same variability as more conventional histological parameters.

Pelvic lymph node assessment

- The adverse prognosis of metastatic disease to the pelvic lymph nodes is universally accepted. The incidence of pelvic lymph node metastases at the time of radical prostatectomy has decreased over the last couple of decades.
- As a consequence of the declining incidence, concerns have been raised as to whether pelvic lymphadenectomy is necessary in all patients, especially those with a low risk of having positive lymph nodes based on pre-operative clinico-pathologic findings. The major factors contributing to this decrease are better patient selection as to who is a good candidate for surgery and the earlier detection of prostate cancer.
- In about 6 % of the cases the only lymph node metastasis is not in a grossly recognized lymph node but in small lymph nodes embedded in the adipose tissue, a finding of uncertain significance that is not included in the current TNM.

Isolated Tumour Cells

- Isolated tumour cells (ITC) are single cells or small clusters of cells not more than 0.2 mm in greatest dimension. Lymph nodes or distant sites with ITC found by either immunohistological examination or non-morphological techniques (e.g., flow cytometry, DNA analysis, polymerase chain reaction [PCR] amplification of a specific tumour marker) should be classified as N0 or M0, respectively. Specific denotation of the assigned N category is suggested for cases in which ITC are the only evidence of possible metastatic disease.

Table 3.11 Reporting of radical prostatectomy specimen

1. Histologic type of carcinoma
2. Gleason Grade (when untreated) (if 3 patterns are present, record the predominant and second most common patterns; the tertiary pattern should be recorded in a comment if higher than primary and secondary patterns)
3. Tumour Location
4. Margin Status
Extent if positive
Focal
Non-focal
Location of positive margins
Specify status of following margins: Bladder neck, Apical, Vas deferentia (optional)
Nature of positive margins
In area of extra-prostatic extension
Iatrogenic (pT2+)
5. Extra-Prostatic Extension (EPE)
Extent of EPE
Focal
Non-focal
Location of EPE
6. Vascular invasion
7. Seminal Vesicle Invasion
8. Tumour volume (optional)
9. Pathologic Staging (pTNM)
10. Comments: Correlation with intraoperative consultation; correlation with other specimens, as appropriate; correlation with clinical information, as appropriate

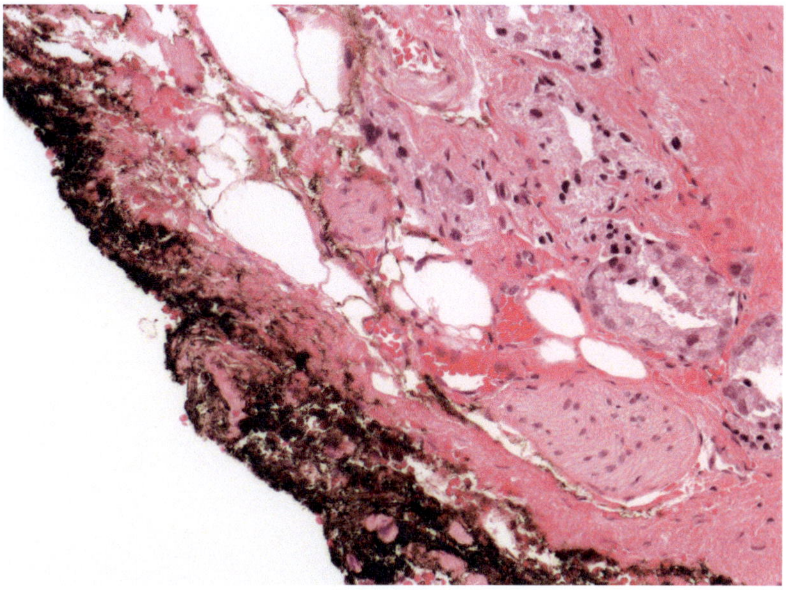

Fig. 3.89 Focal extraprostatic extension

Table 3.12 Primary tumour, pathologic (pT) (2010 revision)

Primary tumor (T) (there is no pathologic T1 category)
pT2: Organ confined
T2a: Tumour involves one half of one lobe or less
T2b: Tumour involves more than half of one lobe, but not both lobes
T2c: Tumour involves both lobes
pT3: Extraprostatic extension
pT3a: Extraprostatic extension
pT3b : Seminal vesicle extension
pT4: Invasion of bladder, rectum
Regional lymph nodes (N)
NX: Regional lymph nodes cannot be assessed
N0: No regional lymph node metastasis
N1: Metastasis in regional lymph node or nodes
Distant metastasis (M) (when more than one site of metastasis is present, the most advanced category (pM1c) is used)
MX: Distant metastasis cannot be assessed
M0: No distant metastasis
M1: Distant Metastasis
M1a: non-regional lymph node(s)
M1b: bone(s)
M1c: other site(s)

Invasion into the prostatic apex or into (but not beyond) the prostatic capsule is not classified as T3, but as T2. Tumour extension into periprostatic soft tissue is T3. Bladder neck invasion is T3

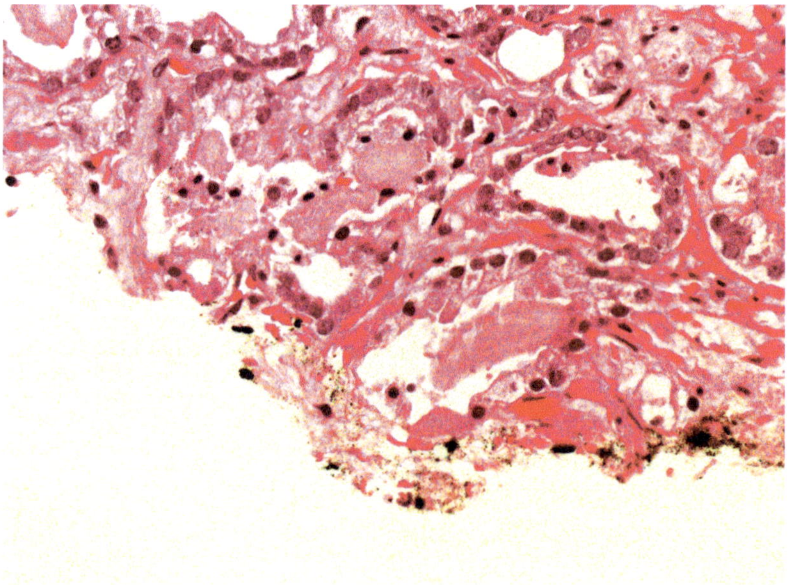

Fig. 3.90 Focal surgical margin positive for malignancy

3.7 Basic Molecular Pathology of Prostate Cancer

Inherited susceptibility

- Currently, the evidence for a strong genetic basis in prostatic carcinoma is compelling: about 9 % of all cases of PCa are thought to have a genetic basis.
- The identification of highly penetrant PCa genes, i.e., genes that markedly increase the risk of cancer, has been particularly difficult for two main reasons. First, due to the advanced age of onset (median 60 years), availability of more than two generations to perform molecular studies on is difficult.
- Second, given the high frequency of PCa, it is likely that cases considered to be hereditary during segregation studies actually represent phenocopies, i.e., sporadic cases in families with high rates of PCa. In addition, hereditary prostate cancer (HPC) does not occur in any of the known cancer syndromes and does not have any clinical (other than a somewhat early age of onset at times) or pathologic characteristics to allow researchers to distinguish it from sporadic PCa. Rearrangement in chromosome 22 between TMPRSS2 and ERG is seen in about 50 % of PCa.
- Hereditary PCa is characterized by Mendelian autosomal dominant or X-linked mode of inheritance, and an early onset of the disease. Based on the family clustering of PCa, a number of groups have worked to identify the genes involved. Generally, they have used linkage analysis of large families affected by PCa. Work over the past decade using genome wide scans in PCa families has identified high-risk loci.

Susceptibility loci

- There are at least 7 susceptibility loci for PCa identified on different chromosomes. Chromosome 1 is of particular interest, with 3 proposed loci. The chromosomal region 1q24-25, designated the locus of the hereditary prostate cancer (HPC1) gene, has been the most thoroughly investigated. Some analyses have confirmed a link between HPC1 and PCa, but others have failed to detect an association. The other two proposed susceptibility loci are 1q42.2-q43 and 1p36.
- Additional loci have been identified on chromosome 16 (16q23.2), chromosome 17 (17p11, or HPC2, i.e., hereditary prostate cancer 2, also called ELAC2), chromosome 20 (20q13 or HPC20), and chromosome X (Xq27-28 or HPCX).

Candidate HPC genes

- Mutations in a growing number of candidate HPC loci and genes have been detected suggesting that defects in critical pathways involving DNA damage response, apoptosis and innate immunity may have a particular important role in the initiation of PCa. The types of alterations associated with such genes are basically represented by base substitutions, deletions and insertions. The following highly penetrant genes probably account for 10 % or less of hereditary PCa cases: *RNASEL* (a candidate tumour suppressor gene within the HPC1 locus located on 1q24-25), *MSR1* (located on 8p22, encodes subunits of class A macrophage-scavenger receptor 1), *CYP17* (located on 10q24.3, encodes cytochrome P-450c17, an enzyme that catalyzes key reactions in sex-steroid biosynthesis), *HPC2/ELAC2* (located on 17p11 and is considered a tumour suppressor gene), *BRCA2* (located on chromosome 13q), and *CHEK2* (encodes an upstream regulator of p53 in the DNA damage signalling pathway) (366). A number of germline variants and mutations of these genes have been associated with increased risk of PCa.
- An increased risk of PCa has been associated with sexually transmitted infections, regardless of the pathogen, suggesting that inflammation, rather than infection, initiates prostatic carcinogenesis. Inflammatory cells elaborate numerous microbiological oxidants than might cause cellular or genomic damage in the prostate. Two of the candidate PCa susceptibility genes identified thus far, *RNASEL* and *MRS1*, encode proteins with critical functions in host response to infections. Mutations in these genes might reduce the ability to eradicate infectious agents, thus resulting in chronic

inflammation. RNASEL is believed to regulate cellular proliferation and apoptosis through the interferon-inducible 2′,5′-oligoadenylate dependent RNA decay pathway. At least 2 mutations inactivating RNASEL have been identified that are potentially responsible for PCa cases in families showing linkage to HPC1. Germline MSR1 mutations have been linked to PCa in some families with early-onset hereditary PCa.
- BRCA2, located on chromosome 13q, is a gene that has been implicated as a prostate cancer susceptibility locus primary due to its analysis in breast cancer families. Studies of families with breast cancer suggest that male carriers of BRCA2 mutations are at increased risk for PCa, particularly at an early age. Inactivating mutations in BRCA2 have been reported in approximately 2 % of men with early onset PCa, conforming the relevance of this gene to PCa susceptibility.

Genetic polymorphisms
- Perhaps even more important in terms of inherited susceptibility for PCa are common polymorphisms in a number of low penetrance alleles of other genes – the so-called genetic modifier alleles. The major pathways currently under examination include those involved in androgen action, DNA repair, carcinogen metabolism, and inflammation pathways. It is widely assumed that the specific combinations of these variants, in the proper environmental setting, can profoundly affect the risk of developing PCa.
- The androgen receptor (AR) gene, a member of the steroid and thyroid hormone receptor gene superfamily, is a transcription factor that mediates the action of androgen in prostate cells. It is located on Xq11-12. The amino-terminal domain encoded by exon 1 contains a variable number of trinucleotide repeats. Decreased transactivation activity and binding affinity for androgen is associated with an increased number of trinucleotide repeats. Shorter CAG repeat lengths have been associated with a greater risk of developing PCa.
- Additional examples of genetic polymorphisms are related to *SRD5A2* – a gene located on 2p23 that encodes a polypeptide that catalyzes the conversion of testosterone to dihydrotestosterone – and to Vitamin D Receptor. Polymorphisms in the former have been reported to confer an increased risk of PCa, particularly in African Americans and Hispanics. The contribution of the Vitamin D Receptor gene polymorphisms to PCa susceptibility remains controversial.

Somatic gene alterations
- Many somatic mutations, gene deletions, gene amplifications, chromosomal rearrangements, and changes in DNA methylation are detectable in PCa cells at the time of diagnosis. These alterations probably accumulate over a period of several decades and the number of changes increases with the stage of the disease. Telomerase activity is frequently upregulated in PCa. This may contribute to genetic instability and promote neoplastic transformation. Although multiple alterations that appear to contribute to disease progression have been suggested, no single key change has been detected. Perhaps the exception is the description of rearrangements in chromosome 22 between TMPRSS2 and ERG seen in about 50 % of PCa.

Gene alterations
- The role of PTEN, CDKN1B, AMACR and TMPRSS2-ERG fusion genes have been investigated in several recent publications.
- PTEN (phosphatase and tensin homologue) is a tumour-suppressor gene encoding a phosphatase active against both protein and lipid substrates. PTEN induces G1 cell cycle arrest via negative regulation of the phosphatidylinositol 3′-kinase/protein kinase B (PI3/Akt) signalling pathway that is essential for cell-cycle progression and cell survival. By inhibiting PI3K/Akt, PTEN can increase the levels of CDKN1B messenger RNA and p27 protein (see below). PTEN is frequently mutated or deleted in PCa cell lines and tumours. PTEN alterations are more common in metastatic deposits than in primary carcinomas. By immunohistochemistry, PTEN is present in normal epithelial cells and PIN. The level of PTEN is frequently reduced in PCa of high

grade or stage. Somatic allelic losses (i.e., haploinsufficiency) in both PTEN and NKX3.1 appear to be common in prostate carcinoma and may promote an abnormal proliferation of prostate cells.

- CDKN1B encodes p27kip1, a cyclin-dependent kinase inhibitor. The p27kip1 protein regulates cell cycle progression from G1 to S phase by its inhibitory interaction with the cyclin E/cdk2 complex. In PCa, p27kip1 expression progressively decreases with increasing tumour grade and stage. Low levels of p27kip1 may be as much a result of CDKN1B alterations as of the PTEN loss whose function is mediated by the PI3K-Akt signalling pathway. A recent paper by Dreher et al dealt with a combined analysis of PTEN and p27kip1 expression in PCa and greatly contributed to the knowledge that activated Akt blocks p27kip1 entry into the nucleus by phosphorylating a residue within the nuclear localisation signal of p27kip1.
- AMACR (Alpha-methylacyl-CoA racemase) encodes an enzyme that plays an important role in the β-oxidation of branched-chain fatty acids and serves as a "caretaker" gene. It has been found consistently upregulated in PCa and high-grade prostatic intraepithelial neoplasia (HGPIN), a direct precursor of PCa.

TMPRSS2 gene fusion in prostate cancer

- About 50 % of pCa show fusion of the TMPRSS2 and ETS gene family; a change that is specific for prostate cancer. ETS transcription factors include ERG, ETV1, ETV4, and ETV5 as 3′ end fusion. ERG is the most common fused gene at 5′ end with TMPRSS2 comprising about 90 % of cases. Fused ERG is under the control of an androgen-regulated promoter, thus causing overexpression. Fusion of these two genes occurs via genetic rearrangements or more rarely by translocation. The most common reported fusion is between exon 1 of TMPRSS2 and exon 4.
- Histologic characteristics of PCa associated with TMPRSS2:ERG include aggressive features like cribriform pattern, intraductal spread, macronucleoli and signet-ring cells.
- The clinical significance of this gene fusion remains unclear due to conflicting reports by different studies.

DNA methylation

- Epigenetic events that can affect gene expression without altering the actual sequence of DNA include phenomena such as DNA methylation, chromatin remodelling, histone modification and RNA interference. Many gene promoters are associated with GC rich regions of the DNA known as CpG islands. Abnormal methylation of CpG islands located within gene promoters is associated with decreased transcriptional activity and it occurs in many types of cancers. Abnormal methylation of genes such as those involved with control of cellular growth or detoxification is believed to have a critical role in early stages of PCa progression. A certain number of genes, such as GSTP1 and E-Cadherin , are commonly methylated in human PCa.
- GSTP1 (pi-class of Glutathione S-transferase), located on 11q13, probably serves as a caretaker gene. It defends prostate cells against genomic damage mediated by carcinogens or various oxidants. GSTP1 demonstrates hypermethylation in more than in 90 % of prostate carcinomas, thus preventing expression of this protective gene.
- E-Cadherin, located on 16q22.1, encodes a Ca2+-dependent cell adhesion molecule that is important in normal cell growth and development and is considered a suppressor of neoplastic invasion. E-Cadherin is methylated in approximately 50 % of cases. Decreased expression of E-cadherin has been detected in several primary and metastatic prostate carcinomas.

Androgen receptors

- Many somatic alterations of androgen receptors (AR) have been detected in those PCas that progress despite hormonal treatment. At the same time, prostate tumour cells appear to have several possible mechanisms by which they could become androgen refractory.
- Mutations of the AR could allow it to respond to other steroids or even to anti-androgens. In particular, mutations in the ligand-binding domain of AR could not only increase sensi-

tivity to normal ligands, such as adrenal androgens, which are present at low levels, but also may cause the AR to be responsive to other molecules, such as antiandrogens, which are not normal ligands.
- Mutations in the AR hormone-binding domain or amplification of the AR gene could also increase tumour cell sensitivity to androgens. In fact, the increased levels of AR DNA are associated with an increase in AR messenger RNA. Increased levels of AR protein associated with AR gene amplification have been implicated in the ability of cells to more effectively use the low levels of androgens that are produced by the adrenal glands and that are still available during androgen deprivation therapy.
- Alterations in the expression or function of genes in regulatory pathways involving peptide growth factors or cytokines could cause inappropriate activation of the AR. For instance, growth factors serve as ligands for receptor tyrosine kinases and activate downstream intracellular kinase cascades. Receptor tyrosine kinases may also be involved in the progression to androgen-refractory PCa through an interaction with the AR. The receptor tyrosine kinase Her2/neu is expressed at low levels in normal epithelial cells. Several studies have demonstrated Her2/Neu protein overexpression and/or gene amplification in a subset of PCa patients.
- The AR could be bypassed entirely, possibly as a result of constitutive activation of regulatory molecules downstream of the AR. For instance, PTEN inactivation, p53 mutations, bcl-2 pathway alterations, neuroendocrine factors, and alternative growth factor regulation and utilization could potentially bypass the need for activation of the AR in some tumors.

3.8 Rare Forms of Prostatic Tumours

Basal cell carcinoma and basal cell proliferations of the prostate
- Basal cell proliferations in the prostate gland exhibit a morphologic continuum ranging from basal cell hyperplasia in the setting of nodular hyperplasia to malignant basal cell lesions that resemble, to a certain degree, basal cell carcinoma of the skin and adenoid cystic carcinoma of the salivary gland. A large number of terms have been used for these neoplasms and related growths (Tables 3.13, 3.14, 3.15 and 3.16).

Histology
- A spectrum of basal cell proliferations ranging from hyperplasia to carcinoma exists in the prostate. These are usually located in the transition zone.

Ordinary (Usual, typical or classical) basal cell hyperplasia (BCH)
- Consists of numerous small to normal-sized, round basophilic acini with several layers of basal cells (glandular architectural type) or solid nests either arranged in a lobular configuration or seldom “infiltrating” the stroma.
- None of the cases of ordinary BCH, by definition, contains either prominent nucleoli (their mean diameter is less than 1 μm) or polymorphism; however, rare cases may show the presence of hyper-chromatic nuclei, enlarged nuclei, and rare mitotic figures. BCH resembles prostate acini seen in the fetus. BCH may be composed of basal cell nests with areas of luminal differentiation resembling similar lesions of the salivary gland. This is denoted as the adenoid basal form of BCH.
- Histologic features may include intracytoplasmic globules (these stain for alpha-fetoprotein and alpha-1 antitrypsin), calcifications, squamous features, and cribriform morphology; changes not seen in other prostatic lesions and therefore useful in differential diagnosis.
- BCH may have a florid appearance (i.e., florid basal cell hyperplasia) showing compact glandular proliferation with solid nests; the cytology in some areas looks disturbing because the cells have a moderately enlarged nucleus, often with a prominent nucleolus; a few mitotic figures are present; the intervening stroma is scant and cellular; the lesions is not well circumscribed and are intermingled with the surrounding glands, giving the false

impression of "infiltration". Florid basal cell hyperplasia is also being defied as extensive proliferation of basal cells involving more than 100 small crowded acini (in a given section) forming a nodule.

- BCH may have prominent nucleoli (i.e., basal cell hyperplasia with prominent nucleoli; basal cell hyperplasia with atypia), but is otherwise identical to ordinary BCH. The nucleoli are round to oval and lightly eosinophilic, similar to those seen in acinar adenocarcinoma of the prostate (their mean diameter is 1.96 μm). There is chronic inflammation in most cases, suggesting that prominent nucleoli are a reflection of reactive atypia.
- BCH with prominent nucleoli may be mistaken for high-grade prostatic intraepithelial neoplasia (PIN). Although occasionally the distinction between these two entities may be difficult, usually they are distinct. The nuclei in BCH tend to be round whereas, at times, the cells form small solid basal cell nests. In contrast, the cells in PIN tend to be more pseudostratified and columnar and do not occlude the glandular lumina. Within areas of BCH, atypical looking basal cells can be seen underling the overlying benign appearing secretory cells. PIN has full thickness cytological atypia with the nuclei oriented perpendicular to the basement membrane. The use of antibody against either 34betaE12 or p63 can help in difficult cases. In BCH immunohistochemistry shows multilayered staining of the basal cells, whereas an interrupted immuno-reactive basal cell layer is seen in PIN. Immunostaining for alpha-methylacyl-coenzyme racemase (i.e., P504S) is negative in florid BCH and positive in HGPIN and adenocarcinoma. Immunostaining for glutathione-s-transferase pi (GST-pi) is positive in florid BCH and negative in adenocarcinoma.
- BCH, mainly with a glandular architecture or when florid, may be confused with adenocarcinoma. BCH can be distinguished from adenocarcinoma by its very basal cell appearance. The glands appear basophilic at low power due to multilayering of basal cells which have scant cytoplasm. In contrast, gland-forming adenocarcinoma of the prostate almost always has more abundant cytoplasm resulting in a more eosinophilic appearance to the glands. Utilization of immunohistochemistry with basal cell specific antibodies (34betaE12 or p63) can differentiate between these two lesions.
- If florid BCH is the direct precursor of basal cell carcinoma remains as an open question.

Basal cell adenoma

- Is identical to ordinary BCH, although the proliferating basal cell masses are usually large and circumscribed, with nodular or adenoma-like pattern. In contrast to basal cell carcinoma, basal cell adenoma is well circumscribed, lack necrosis, and the stroma between the basal cell nests is similar to that of the surrounding normal prostatic stroma. Occasionally, BCH is multifocal (also known as adenomatosis). The terms basal cell adenoma and adenomatosis are very rarely used.

Basal cell carcinoma (basal cell carcinoma/adenoid cystic carcinoma)

- It is characterized by proliferation of cells arranged in various architectural patterns. Two morphological variants of basal cell carcinomas can be recognized in the prostate. Similar to basal cell carcinoma of the skin, it is characterized by islands and cords of basaloid cells with peripheral palisading. The second type, also called adenoid cystic carcinoma-like, is composed of nests of infiltrating tumour cells with an adenoid cystic pattern, morphologically similar to the adenoid cystic carcinoma of the salivary glands. Focal squamous differentiation and clear cell change may be focally present (Figs. 3.91, 3.92, 3.93, 3.94, 3.95, 3.96 and 3.97).
- The diagnostic criteria for malignancy in basal cell carcinoma include:

1. Extensive infiltration between normal prostate glands
2. Extension out of the prostate
3. Perineural invasion
4. Variable tumor necrosis

- The differential diagnosis of basal cell carcinoma includes poorly differentiated (mostly Gleason's grade 5) adenocarcinoma (basal cell carcinoma may occur, rarely, in combination with conventional adenocarcinoma) and urothelial carcinoma. Poorly differentiated adenocarcinoma may growth in solid nests and, similarly to basal cell carcinoma, is not reactive for PSA. Lack of immuno-reactivity for p63 and 34betaE12, however, is helpful in recognizing conventional adenocarcinoma, though it has been reported that this tumour may occasionally express p63. Most basal cell carcinomas express diffusely bcl-2 by immunohistochemistry.

- Similarly to basal cell carcinoma, urothelial carcinoma may exhibit a solid growth pattern with peripheral palisading and central necrosis and may express high level of p63. However, urothelial carcinoma expresses CK20 and CK7 in most cases. Basal cell carcinoma is positive for CK7 and negative for CK20.

Natural history of basal cell carcinoma

- There is limited information regarding basal cell carcinoma. Patients are generally elderly, presenting with urinary obstruction, TURP being the most common tissue source of diagnosis. Rare cases may occur in younger patients.
- The outcome for patients diagnosed with basal cell carcinoma of the prostate is uncertain, since most cases have been reported with a short follow-up. Overall, basal cell carcinoma of the prostate is viewed as a low grade carcinoma with a 20 % rate of metastases.

Immunohistochemistry of basal cell proliferations

- Immunohistochemistry clearly indicates that they have the same immuno-phenotype of the basal cells present in normal ducts and acini. The cells are positively and strongly stained with 34betaE12 and p63. These are the two consolidated markers for the basal cells in the prostate, and their absence is in favour of prostate adenocarcinoma.
- The cells that are located in the center of the nests and those lining the small lumina stain positively with AE1/AE3, whereas the basaloide cells are negative but positive for basal cell markers.
- Another interesting feature is that the basal cell proliferations express two markers usually seen in neoplasias of other sites and organs. The first is the demonstration of laminin both in the stroma surrounding the cell nests and in small eosinophilic globules surrounded by the cells. This feature is usually seen in tumours of the salivary glands. The other is represented by the expression of HER2-neu onco-protein, similar to that seen in breast cancer. The presence of a small proportion of cells with neuroendocrine differentiation, as documented by chromogranin immunostaining has also been reported.

Urothelial carcinoma of the prostate

- The frequency of primary urothelial carcinoma ranges from 0.7 to 2.8 % of prostatic tumours in adults. In patients with invasive bladder carcinoma, there is involvement of the prostate gland in up to 45 % of cases.
- Primary urothelial carcinoma is usually located within the proximal prostatic ducts. Many cases are locally advanced at diagnosis and replace the prostate gland. Primary urothelial carcinoma presents like other prostatic masses including urinary obstruction and hematuria. Most cases are diagnosed by transurethral resection or by needle biopsy (Fig. 3.98).
- Digital rectal examination is abnormal in the majority of cases.

Tumour spread and prognosis

- In situ urothelial carcinoma can spread along ducts and involve acini or may spread along ejaculatory ducts and into seminal vesicles. Invasion of prostatic stroma (subepithelial connective tissue as pT1 or with established stromal invasion as pT2) is most relevant feature.
- Local spread beyond the confines of the prostate may occur. Metastases are to regional lymph nodes and bone. Bone metastases are osteolytic. These tumours are staged as urethral tumours. The full range of histological types and grades of urothelial neoplasia can be seen in primary and secondary urothelial neoplasms of the prostate.
- The single most important prognostic parameter is the presence of prostatic stromal inva-

sion. With stromal invasion or extension beyond the confines of the prostate prognosis is poor.

Squamous cell neoplasms of the prostate

- Squamous cell carcinomas may originate either in the periurethral glands or in the prostatic glandular acini. Approximately 50 % of adenosquamous carcinomas may arise in prostate cancer patients subsequent to endocrine therapy or radiotherapy. The incidence of squamous cell carcinoma of the prostate is less than 0.6 % of all prostate cancers. Adenosquamous carcinoma of the prostate is even less frequent (Figs. 3.99 and 3.100).
- Most, if not all pure squamous cell carcinomas become clinically manifest by local symptoms such as urinary outflow obstruction, occasionally in association with bone pain and hematuria. Adenosquamous carcinomas may be detected by increased serum PSA, but more typically by obstruction of the urinary outflow, requiring transurethral resection. Both squamous cell carcinomas and adenosquamous carcinomas tend to metastasize rapidly with a predilection for the skeletal bones.

Histology

- By definition pure squamous cell carcinomas do not contain glandular features and they are identical to squamous cell carcinomas of other organs. Primary prostatic squamous cell carcinomas must be distinguished on clinical grounds from secondary involvement of the gland by bladder or urethral squamous carcinomas. Histologically, squamous cell carcinoma must be distinguished from squamous metaplasia as may occur in infarction or after hormonal therapy. Histologically, squamous metaplasia associated to prostatic infarction may be very atypical and therefore a challenging diagnosis. One must pay attention to necrotic or fibrotic background. Usually squamous metaplasia associated to infarction is frequently associated to basal cell proliferation and has a lobular configuration, a rare finding in squamous carcinoma which shows an infiltrative appearance.
- Adenosquamous carcinomas are defined by the presence of both glandular (acinar) and squamous carcinoma components. The glandular tumour component generally expresses PSA and PAP, whereas the squamous component displays high molecular weight cytokeratins.

Adenocarcinoma arising from the prostatic urethra

- Even rarer are cases of in-situ and infiltrating mucinous adenocarcinoma arising from the prostatic urethra with invasion into the prostate. The histological growth pattern found in these tumours were identical to mucinous adenocarcinoma of the bladder consisting lakes of mucin lined by tall columnar epithelium with goblet cells showing varying degrees of nuclear atypia and in some of these cases, mucin-containing signet cells. These tumours have been negative immunohistochemically for PSA, PAP and other markers of prostatic origin.

Neuroendocrine tumours of the prostate

- Neuroendocrine differentiation in prostatic carcinoma has five forms:

1. Focal neuroendocrine differentiation in acinar prostatic adenocarcinoma
2. Adenocarcinoma with Paneth-cell like neuroendocrine differentiation
3. Carcinoid tumour
4. Small cell carcinoma
5. Large cell neuroendocrine carcinoma

Focal neuroendocrine differentiation in acinar prostatic adenocarcinoma

- Conventional acinar prostatic adenocarcinoma may present variable neuroendocrine differentiation when evaluated with immunohistochemistry. The cells may react with antibodies to chromogranin, serotonin or many other markers in about 50 % of cases, most of times without clinical evidence of endocrine activity. Androgen-deprivation therapy is associated with an increased number of neuroendocrine cells. Frequently these cells are androgen-receptor negative. It remains controversial if neuroendocrine differentiation in conventional carcinoma worsens prognosis.

Adenocarcinoma with Paneth-cell like neuroendocrine differentiation

- The term Paneth cell-like has been used to describe chromogranin positive, eosinophilic, and granular neuroendocrine cells basally located, in PIN and conventional prostatic carcinoma. Most frequently these cells are seen isolated, patchy in small solid nests or diffusely involving glands. Gleason grading of these tumors should be assigned only to the areas of conventional adenocarcinoma. Paneth cell-like change seems not to be related to aggressiveness of the tumor.

Carcinoid tumour

- True carcinoid tumours of the prostate are exceedingly rare, and most lesions reported as carcinoid tumors represent prostatic adenocarcinoma with focal neuroendocrine differentiation. Most of them are positive for prostatic markers and behave as conventional carcinomas (Figs. 3.101 and 3.102).
- The term "carcinoid-like tumors" has been applied by some authorities to label these carcinomas. True carcinoid tumours of the prostate show classic cytological features of carcinoid tumour seen elsewhere, are reactive for neuroendocrine markers and negative for PSA and PAP. The prognosis is uncertain due to the small number reported (Fig. 3.103).

Small cell carcinoma

- Prostate small cell carcinoma is rare and might represent less than 2 % of prostatic carcinomas. It is most frequently in elderly patients with obstructive symptoms. Some cases may present paraneoplastic symptoms due to ACTH or ADH overproduction. Serum PSA is variable with some cases having normal PSA even in metastatic disease. Most are of advanced stage at time of diagnosis and the prognosis is dismal with survival of less than 2 year, in most cases.

Histology

- Histologically are similar to those arising in the lung with tumor cells showing scant cytoplasm and round, oval or spindled nuclei usually smaller than 3 times the size of lymphocytes. Chromatin is finely granular, and nucleoli are absent to inconspicuous. Other cases show intermediate cells with larger cytoplasm and more visible nucleoli (Figs. 3.104, 3.105 and 3.106).
- About half of small cell carcinoma cases arising in the prostate are pure with the remaining cases admixed with prostatic adenocarcinoma, most frequently of Gleason score 8–10.

Immunohistochemistry

- In addition to the positivity of neuroendocrine markers (synaptophysin, chromogranin, CD56), focal positivity for PSA or PSMA is seen in some cases. TTF1 and AMACR are frequently positive, and p63, CK7, CK20 and 34βE12 are typically negative. CKAE1/AE3 is usually positive showing a dot-like (paranuclear) pattern. Ki67 is present in >70 % of cells. Some reports suggest that CD44 is positive in small cell carcinoma of prostate and negative in non-prostatic small cell carcinoma.

Differential diagnosis

- Small cell carcinoma arising in the prostate are diagnosed based on morphologic. Immunohistochemistry is useful in equivocal cases, in particular those with intermediate type of cells are likely to be underdiagnosed and may benefit of immunohistochemistry. Main differential diagnosis includes Gleason 5+5 conventional adenocarcinoma. Immunohistochemistry can be helpful. Synaptophysin may be focally seen in conventional adenocarcinoma; therefore, it is advisable to use a panel also including additional neuroendocrine markers. Single cell pattern of infiltrative growth, prominent nucleoli, abundant cytoplasm, negative CD44, strong positivity for prostatic markers and diffuse 34βE12 expression favours poorly differentiated adenocarcinoma.

Large cell neuroendocrine carcinoma

- There is limited experience on this type of neuroendocrine carcinoma since it is extremely rare in the prostate. Most cases are diagnosed after long-standing hormonal therapy (mean 4 years). Large cell neuroendocrine carcinomas are aggressive tumor that usually present at advanced stage and metastatic disease.

Histology

- Sheets and ribbons of amphophilic cells with large nuclei, high mitotic rate and foci of tumor necrosis are characteristically present. The cells strongly react with neuroendocrine markers with focal or negative PSA and

PAP expression. AMACR may be positive (Fig. 3.107).

Cystadenoma (multilocular cyst)

- Patients present with obstructive symptoms with normal or elevated PSA and abnormal digital rectal examination. Some are attached to the prostate by a pedicle and may be as large as 20 cm in diameter.
- Histologically, the cysts are lined by atrophic prostatic epithelium which reacts with prostate markers and lack of basal cells (Fig. 3.108).

Table 3.13 Basal cell proliferations of the prostate

Ordinary (usual) basal cell hyperplasia (including basal cell adenoma and adenomatosis)
Florid basal cell hyperplasia
Basal cell hyperplasia with prominent nucleoli (or atypical basal cell hyperplasia)
Basal cell carcinoma (adenoid cystic carcinoma)

Table 3.14 Basal cell hyperplasia (ordinary, florid and with nucleoli): differential diagnoses

High-grade PIN
Acinar adenocarcinoma
Sclerosing adenosis
Benign seminal vesicle/ejaculatory duct epithelium
Squamous metaplasia
Transitional cell metaplasia

Table 3.15 Basal cell carcinoma: diagnostic criteria for malignancy

Extensive infiltration between normal prostate glands
Extension out of the prostate
Perineural invasion
Necrosis

Table 3.16 Basal cell carcinoma: differential diagnoses

Poorly differentiated adenocarcinoma (mostly Gleason's grade 5)
Transitional cell (urothelial) carcinoma
Neuroendocrine carcinoma
Basaloid carcinoma of the rectum

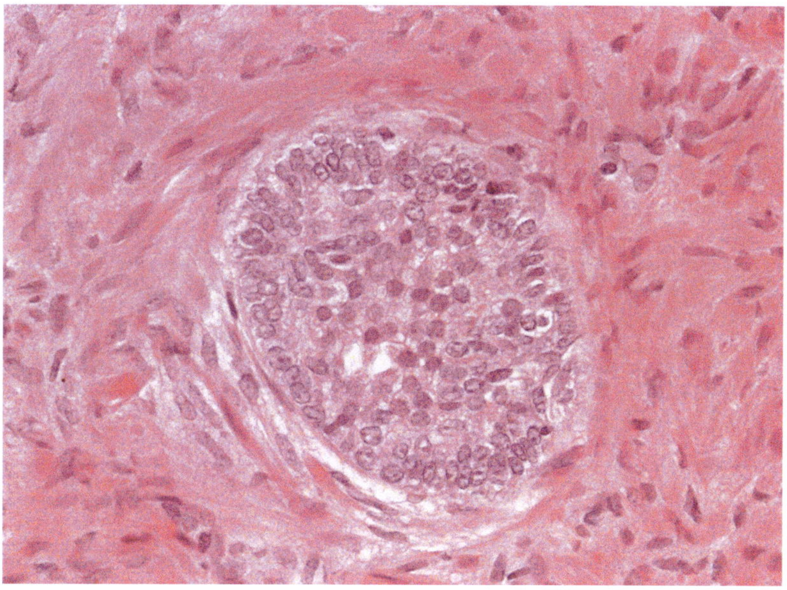

Fig. 3.91 Basal cell hyperplasia, solid nest pattern

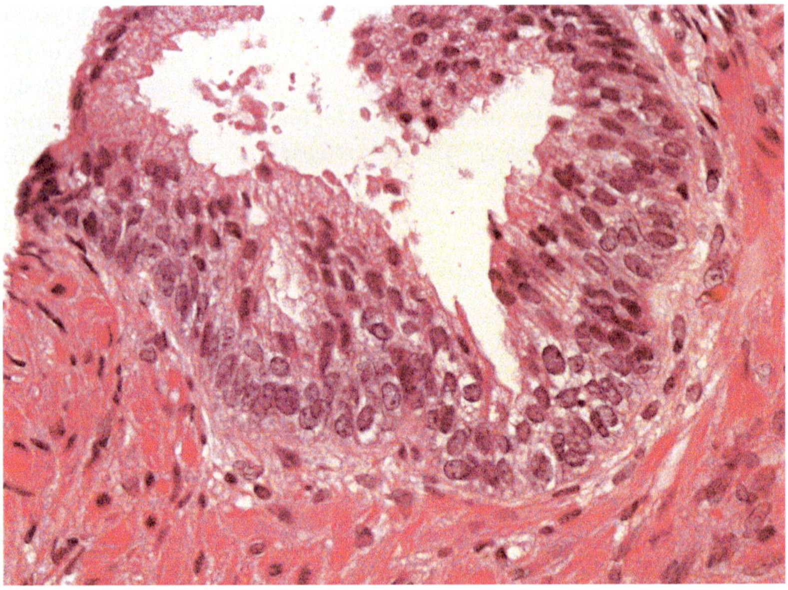

Fig. 3.92 Basal cell hyperplasia with nucleoli

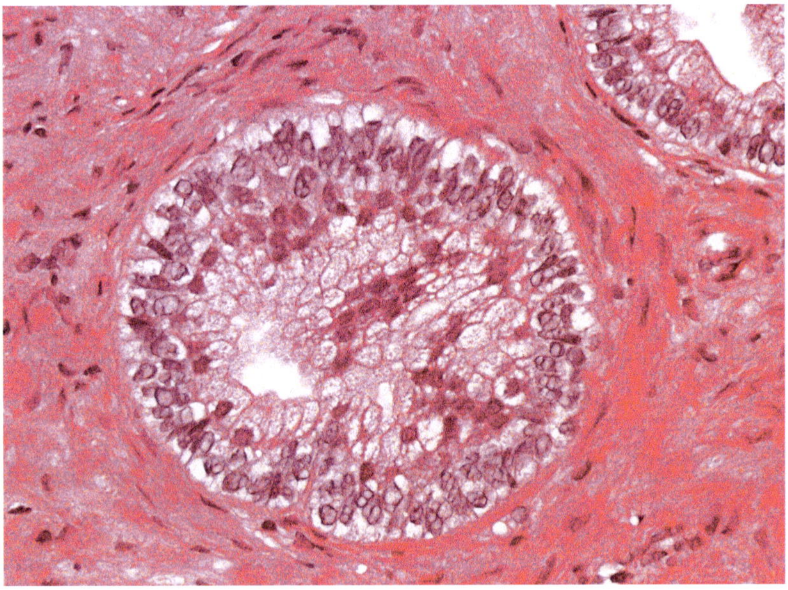

Fig. 3.93 Basal cell hyperplasia with nucleoli and clear cell features

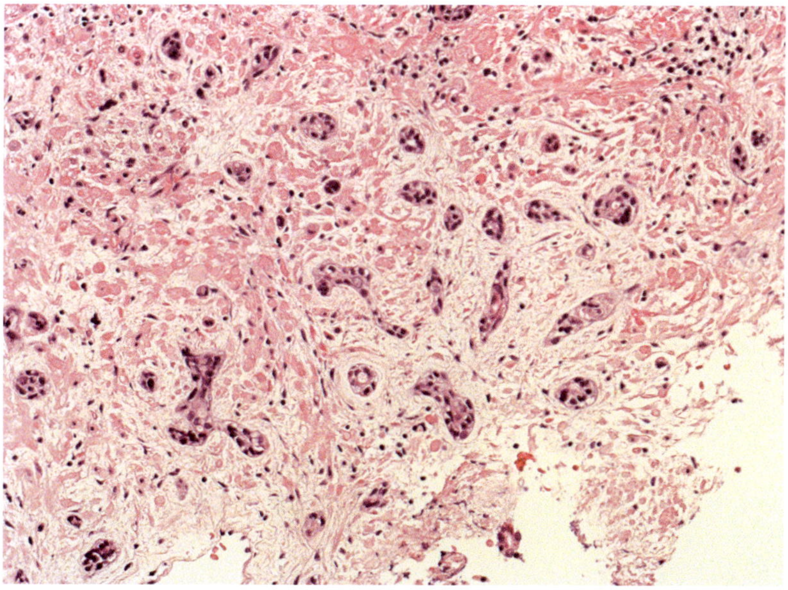

Fig. 3.94 Basal cell carcinoma with small infiltrating nests

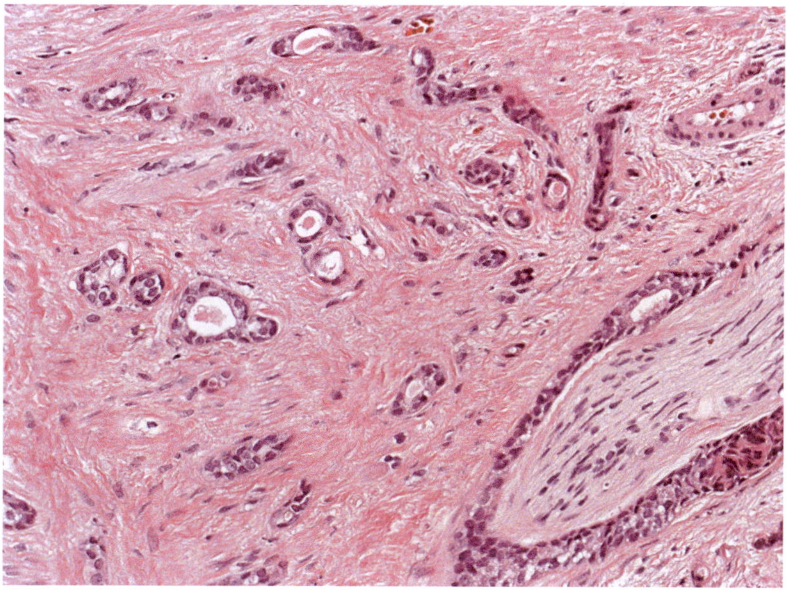

Fig. 3.95 Basal cell carcinoma with small infiltrating nests and perineural invasion

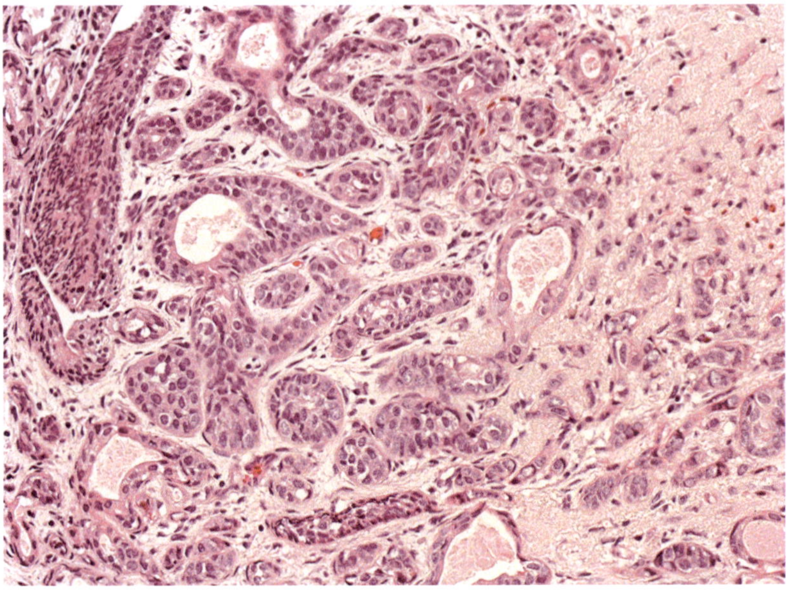

Fig. 3.96 Basal cell carcinoma with variable sized acini and ducts

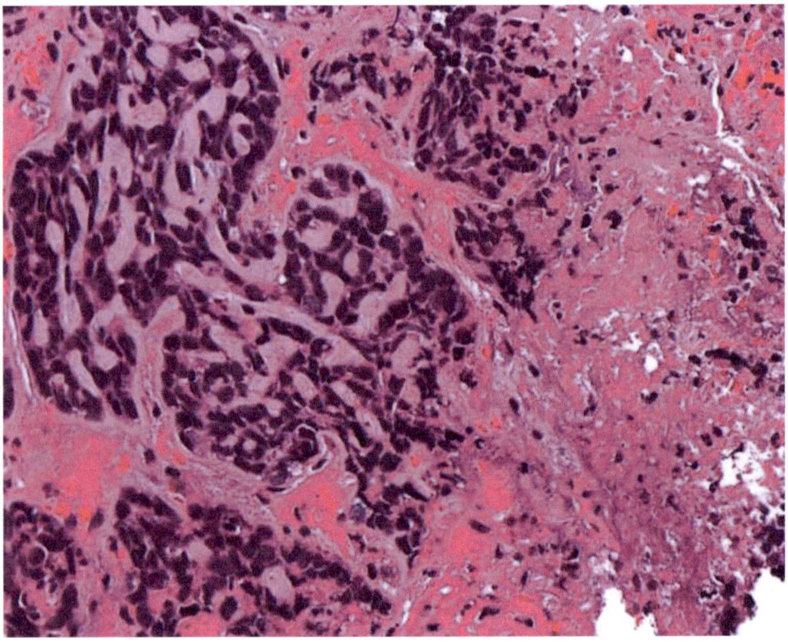

Fig. 3.97 Basal cell carcinoma with adenoid-cystic-like features

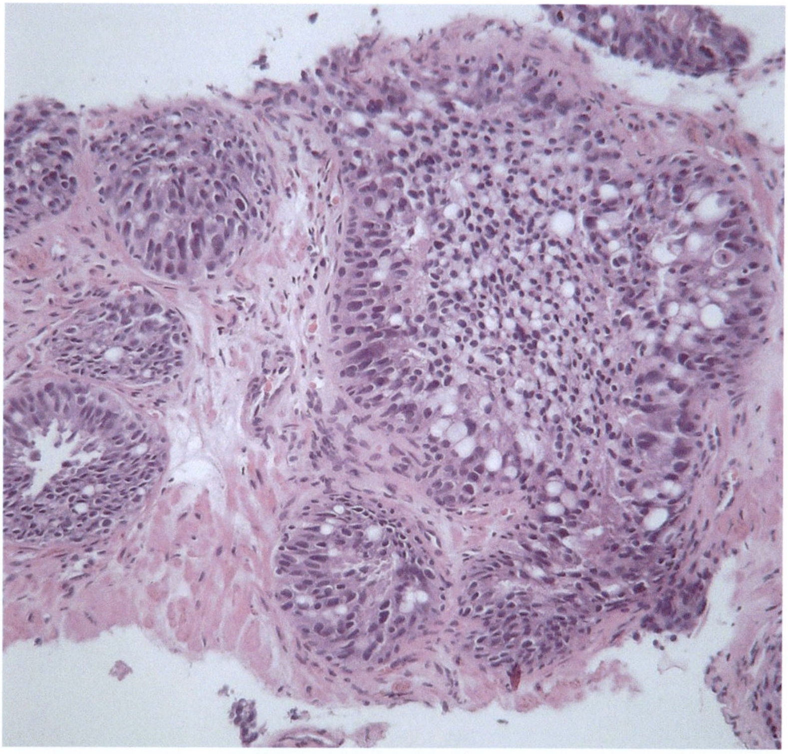

Fig. 3.98 Urothelial carcinoma of the prostate

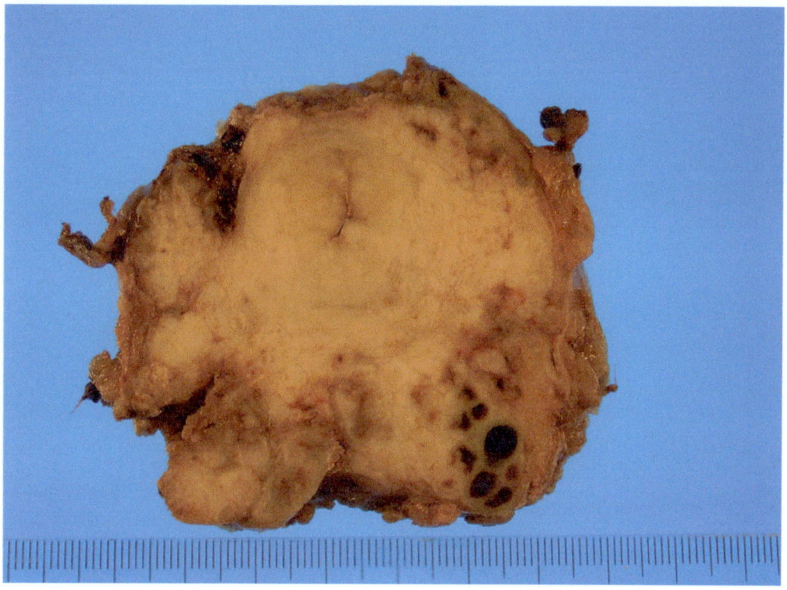

Fig. 3.99 Adenosquamous carcinoma of the prostate with extraprostatic extension

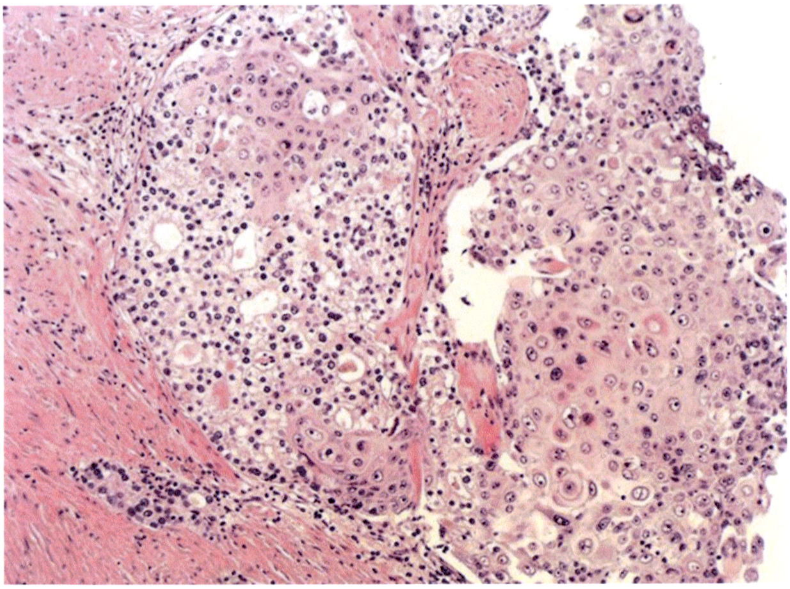

Fig. 3.100 Microscopic features of adenosquamous carcinoma of the prostate

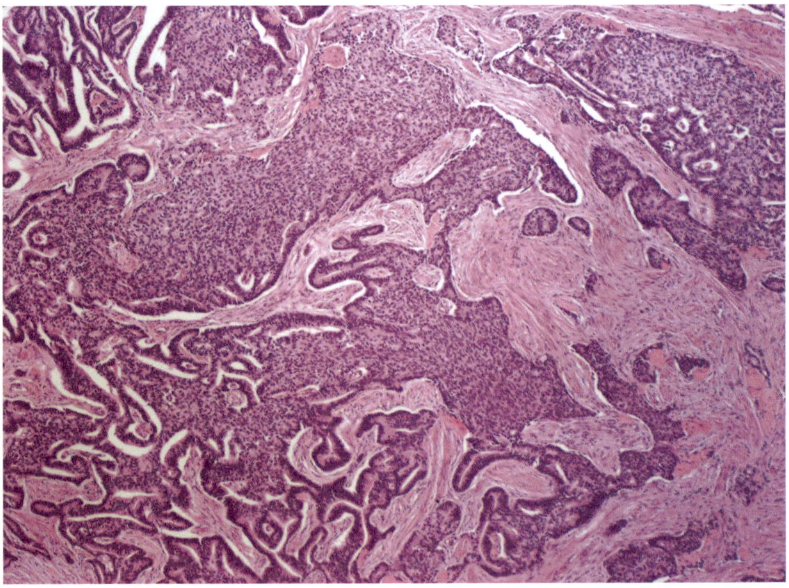

Fig. 3.101 Prostate adenocarcinoma with focal neuroendocrine differentiation (H&E)

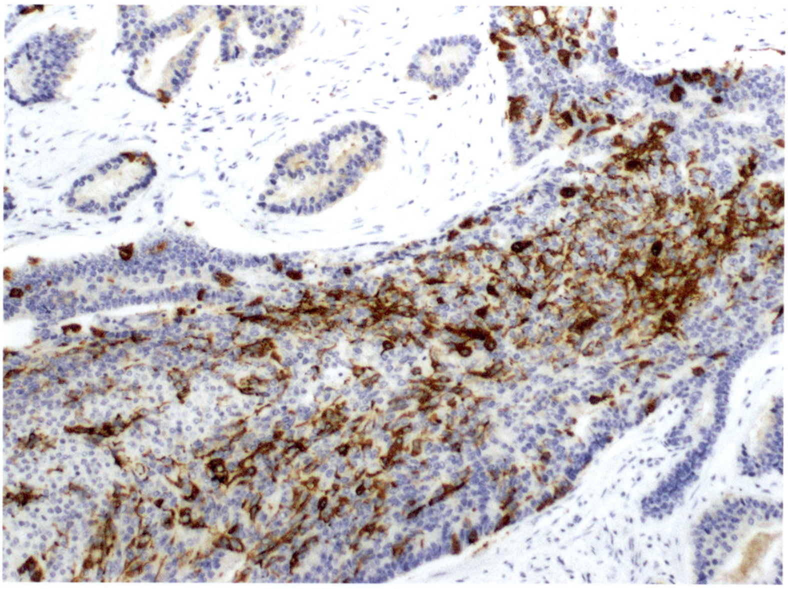

Fig. 3.102 Prostate adenocarcinoma with focal neuroendocrine differentiation as seen by synaptophisin immunohistochemistry

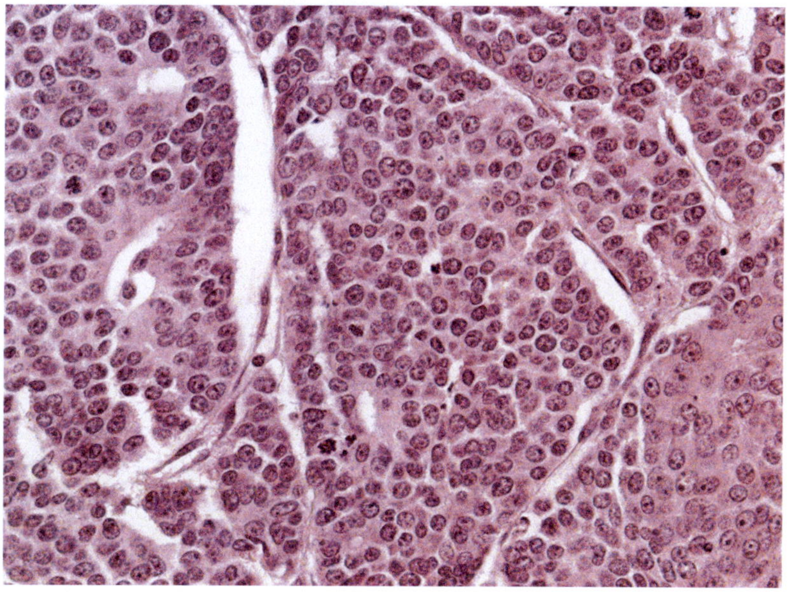

Fig. 3.103 Carcinoid tumor of the prostate

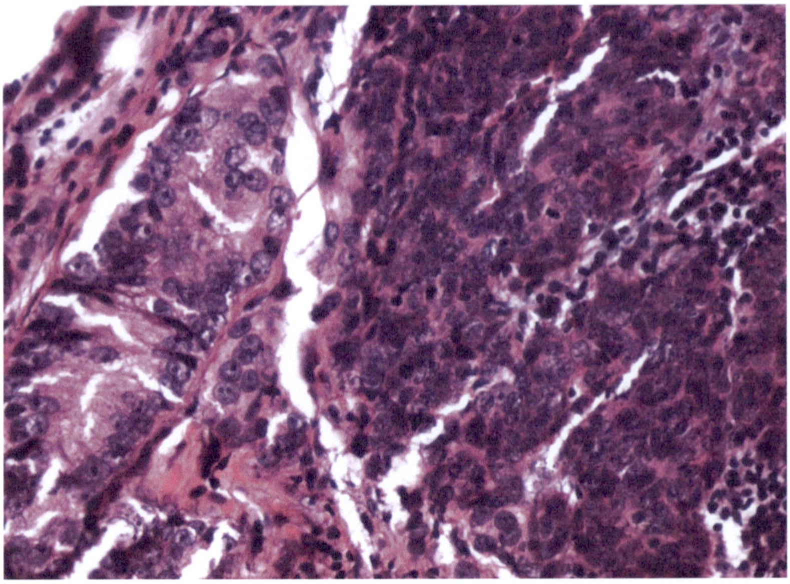

Fig. 3.104 Small cell carcinoma of the prostate admixed with acinar prostatic adenocarcinoma (*left*)

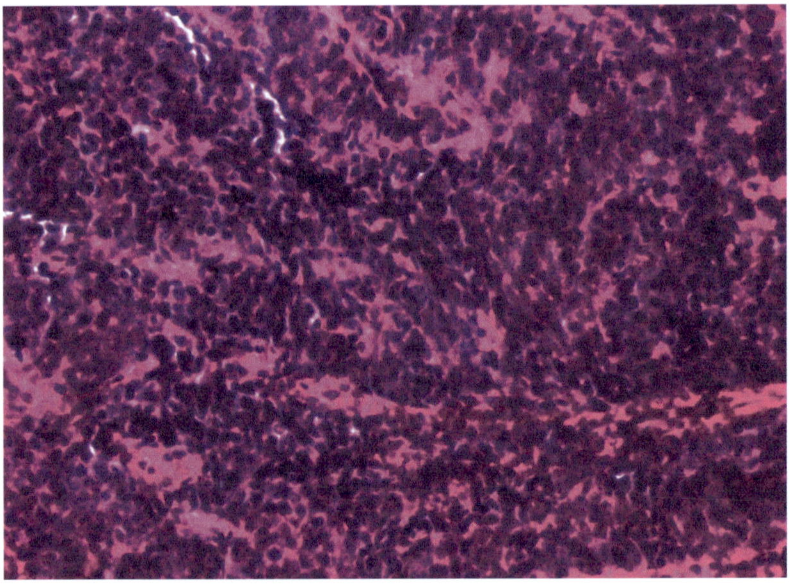

Fig. 3.105 Pure small cell carcinoma

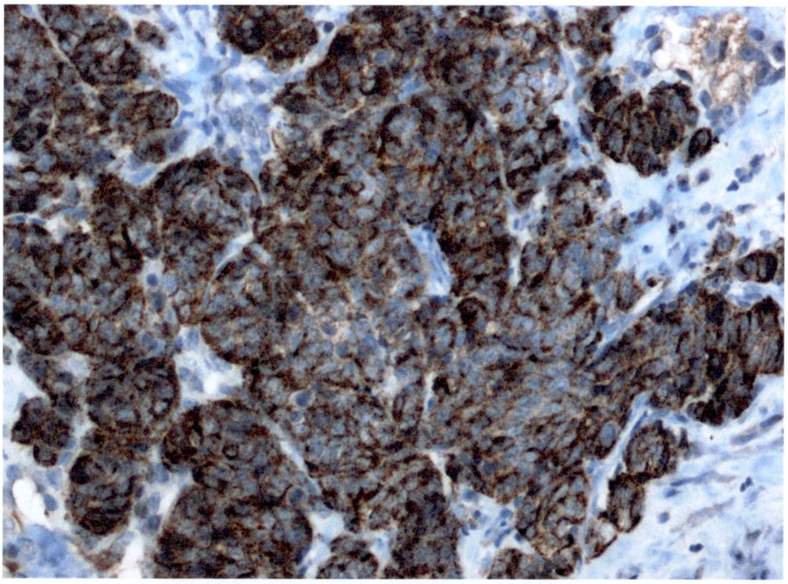

Fig. 3.106 Chromogranin expression in small cell carcinoma of the prostate

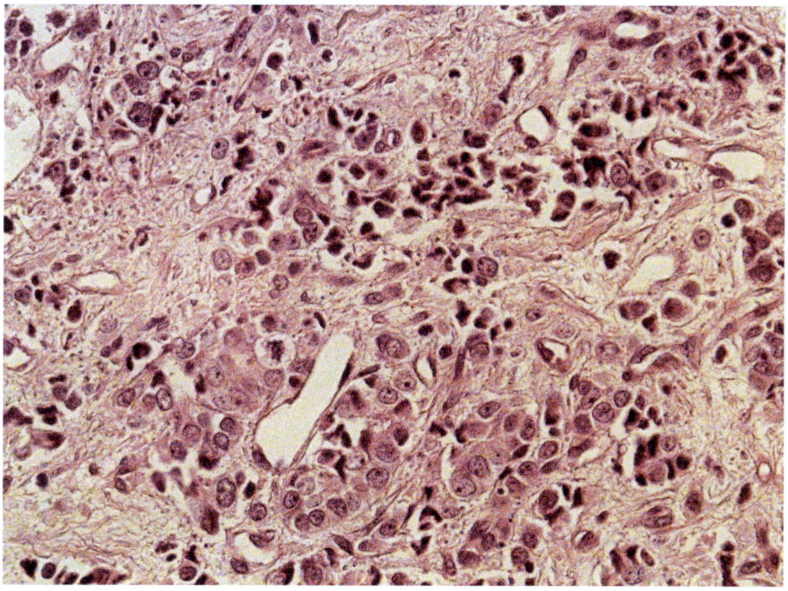

Fig. 3.107 Mixed large and small cell carcinoma

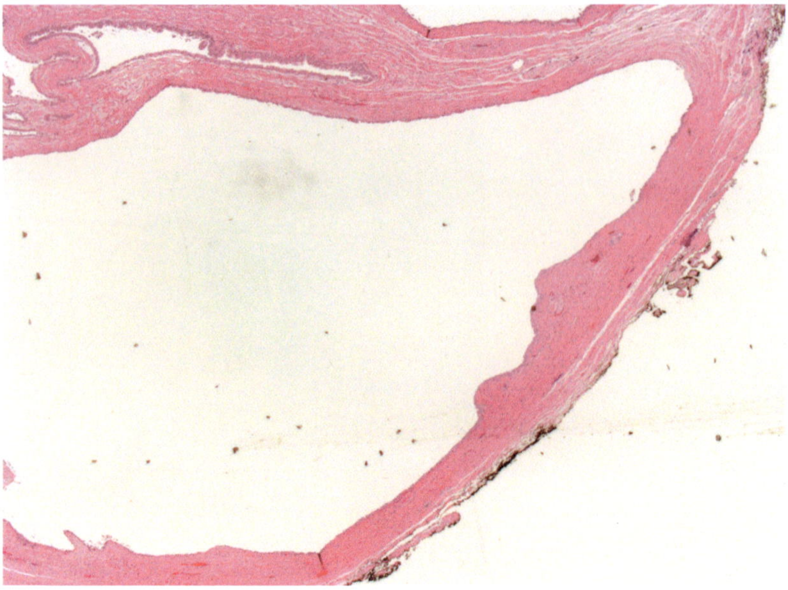

Fig. 3.108 Large cyst lined with atrophic epithelium suggesting of cytadenoma

3.9 Tumors and Tumor-Like Conditions of the Prostate Stroma

- A wide variety of soft tissue lesions occur in the prostate, including reactive stromal proliferations, benign neoplasms and sarcomas. Although many of these tumours are distinguished easily, considerable diagnostic difficulty may be encountered with some of the rare and newly identified lesions. Patient age and clinical history are essential in this setting. The serum PSA concentration is usually not significantly elevated (Table 3.17).
- The most common lesion is represented by benign prostatic hyperplasia, which is easy to recognise because of the usual association with areas of glandular proliferation. Pure stromal nodules may be challenging because the presence of myxoid stroma with spindle cells. They lack mitosis and infiltrative borders (Fig. 3.109).
- Inflammatory myofibroblastic tumor may arise in the prostate mimicking sarcomas. Sarcomas in the prostate are rarely reported and represent 0.1 % of prostatic malignant neoplasms.
- The most common sarcomas are rhabdomyosarcoma and leiomyosarcoma. The former is more common in children and bears a very poor prognosis, whereas the latter is seen in adults, and follows a slower course, but generally recurs after initial therapy.

Pseudosarcomatous spindle cell proliferations

- Reactive, nonneoplastic fibrous lesions of soft tissue that, because of their clinical presentation, gross appearance, growth pattern, and light microscopic features, may be mistaken for a malignancy, usually a sarcoma, often are referred to as pseudosarcomas. These lesions can be divided into two groups distinguished by differences in etiology and morphological appearance, e.g., postoperative spindle cell nodule and inflammatory myofibroblastic tumour.

Postoperative spindle cell nodule

- Also called postsurgical inflammatory myofibroblastic tumour, is a rare benign reparative process occurring within few months of surgery and consists of nodules of spindle cells arranged in fascicles with a variable number of mitotic figures. The cells have abundant cytoplasm; the nucleus is centrally located and elongated to ovoid in shape; small prominent nucleoli are present (Fig. 3.110).
- The features that can be used to distinguish postoperative spindle cell nodule from a sarcoma are:

1. lack of significant nuclear pleomorphism and of atypical mitoses,
2. plexiform pattern of blood vessels
3. presence of chronic inflammation
4. small size of the nodule
5. lack of recurrence after conservative excision.

Inflammatory myofibroblastic tumour

- Is a rare benign pathological entity of unknown etiology occurring in the prostate, urethra, bladder and other sites without a history of prior surgery.
- Histologically, this lesion resembles granulation tissue with variable cellularity. Cells are more haphazard in their distribution than postoperative spindle cell nodules. Lesions often show a densely cellular spindle cell pattern admixed with a very myxoid component. Cells resemble those seen in nodular fasciitis with a tissue culture appearance.
- Occasionally there may be prominent nucleoli with infrequent, moderately pleomorphic and hyperchromatic cells. These lesions show myofibroblastic differentiation with expression of smooth-muscle markers and focal keratin expression. About 60 % of cases may express ALK-1 by immunohistochemistry with gene translocation by FISH. This finding is useful in differential diagnosis with sarcomatoid carcinoma and leiomyosarcoma which are ALK-1 negative by immunohistochemistry.
- The features that can be used to distinguish inflammatory myofibroblastic tumour from a sarcoma are:
  1. areas of the lesion resembling granulation tissue
  2. mitotic figures infrequent
  3. less pleomorphism
  4. prominent myxoid change
  5. recurrence rare following incomplete excision.

Atypical stromal cells

- Pleomorphic, hyperchromatic nuclei may be seen in the prostatic stroma cells between the epithelial elements in otherwise unremarkable cases of benign prostatic hyperplasia, in circumscribed benign fibromuscular nodules in which smooth muscle typically predominates, and in leiomyoma (Fig. 3.111).
- It is important to be aware that malignant neoplasms of the prostate, such as sarcomas and mixed epithelial-stromal tumours, may contain atypical stromal cells similar to those that can be seen either in nodular hyperplasia or fibromuscular nodules. The distinction of the latter two entities from the former depends on:
  1. the absence of a mass
  2. the lack of stromal hypercellularity or phyllodes-type architecture
  3. the degenerative nuclear appearance with smuggled chromatin
  4. the lack of mitoses.
- Distinction of degenerative stromal atypia from the atypicality seen with neoplasms may be very difficult in a limited sampling, and, it has been suggested the designation "prostatic stromal proliferation of uncertain malignant potential" to alert the clinician to this uncertainty.

Prostatic stromal proliferation of uncertain malignant potential and stromal sarcomas

- This lesions is also known as atypical stromal hyperplasia, phyllodes type of atypical stromal hyperplasia, phyllodes tumor, or cystic epithelial-stromal tumor.
- Prostatic stromal tumors arising from specialized prostatic stroma are rare and distinct exhibiting diverse histologic patterns of growth. Currently the preferred terminology include prostatic stromal proliferation of uncertain malignant potential (STUMPs) and stromal sarcomas (Table 3.17).
- Most reported cases of STUMP occur in patients aged 25–80 years with obstructive symptoms and abnormal digital rectal examination. Serum PSA may be normal or elevated. Stromal sarcomas tend to occur at a younger population, most frequently before the age of 50 years. STUMP and stromal sarcoma may coexist.

STUMPs

- Four histologic patterns, seen as pure or mixed forms, have been described:
  1. Hypercellular stroma with degenerative-type nuclear atypia admixed with benign prostate glands (most common pattern)
  2. Hypercellular stroma with bland fusiform eosinophilic admixed with benign glands

3. Leaf-like hypocellular fibrous stroma covered by benign-appearing prostatic epithelium (similar to phyllodes tumor of the breast) (Figs. 3.112 and 3.113).
4. Myxoid stroma containing bland stromal cells often lacking admixed glands

Stromal sarcomas

- Solid growth of neoplastic stromal cells, which may have fibrosarcomatous, storiform, epithelioid, or more rarely leaf-like pattern of growth. Stromal sarcomas may show hypercellularity, cellular atypia, necrosis and mitosis. Stromal sarcomas have been subclassified as low or high grade based on the degree of pleomorphism, hypercellularity, number of mitosis and the presence of tumor necrosis (Fig. 3.114).
- Immunohistochemistry is not useful in differentiating STUMP from stromal sarcoma which relies on morphologic grounds alone. Both types of lesions are positive for vimentin, SMA, desmin, progesterone receptor and CD34. S100 and CD117 are negative.
- Differential diagnosi may include sarcomatoid carcinoma (cytokeratin and p63 positive), leiomyosarcoma (SMA, desmin and caldesmon positive) or GIST (CD117 positive)

Leiomyoma

- Unusual prostatic spindle cell lesion. Histologically the lesion is composed of a well-circumscribed mass of smooth muscle cell proliferation in prostatic or juxtaprostatic tissue that is devoid of epithelial elements and reaches 1 cm or more in diameter.
- No specific histological criterion exists to differentiate a leiomyoma from a leiomyosarcoma of the prostate as opposed to smooth muscle tumours of the uterus.
- The definition of "atypical leiomyoma" of the prostate is used by some authors to refer to well-circumscribed lesions with a variable amount of nuclear atypia and scattered mitotic activity. Although most atypical leiomyomas have shown no evidence of disease with short follow-up, a few have recurred. Because smooth-muscle tumours of the prostate are rare, the criteria for distinguishing between leiomyosarcoma and leiomyoma in these cases with borderline features have not been elucidated.

Leiomyosarcoma

- Sarcomas of the prostate are very rare and aggressive tumors accounting less than 0.2 % of all malignant prostatic tumors. Leiomyosarcoma is the most common sarcoma involving the prostate in adults.
- Microscopically, leiomyosarcoma is hypercellular composed of intersecting bundles of spindle cells with moderate to severe atypia (Figs. 3.115, 3.116 and 3.117).
- Most reported cases are high grade with high mitotic count and frequent tumor necrosis. Low grade cases are even rarer. Leiomyosarcoma commonly express actin, desmin, caldesmon, and vimentin. Some may focally express cytokeratin and progesterone receptor.

Rhabdomyosarcoma

- Most frequent in pediatric population, may rarely arise as primary prostatic sarcoma. Histologically most are of the embryonal subtype. Histologically are similar to those seen in other organs.
- Proliferating cells vary from primitive cells with scant cytoplasm to more well differentiated tumor cells with more abundant eosinophilic cytoplasm in which cross striations may be seen by conventional H&E staining and light microscopy. Some tumors may have spindle cell appearance or exhibit myxoid growth pattern.

Solitary fibrous tumour of the prostate (SFTs)

- SFTs involving the prostate are uncommon with only isolated cases reported in the literature. Owing to their relative rarity and lack of long-term follow-up, the clinical behaviour of prostatic SFTs is difficult to predict. Complete resection of tumour is currently the single main prognostic factor.
- At low-power magnification, SFTs have a smoothly contoured periphery surrounded by normal prostatic tissue. Lesional tissue shows a low to moderately cellular process set in a densely sclerotic collagenous matrix interrupted by pockets of edematous stroma. The tumour consisted of short spindled cells possessing with eosinophilic cytoplasm and bland nuclei with uniformly distributed chromatin

and inconspicuous nucleoli. The mitotic rate is low (2/ 10 HPF). No necrosis is identified

- Separation of the cells from the dense collagen focally imparted a "pseudoangiomatous" appearance. Paucicellular foci with increased sclerotic or edematous stromal matrices are observed. The vascular element consisted of capillary-sized vessels with muscular walls. The vessels had either a rounded configuration or more commonly were ectatic with an irregular contour, resulting in an angiofibromatous appearance.
- The tumour also features scattered cellular zones exhibiting cells arranged in a haphazard pattern. The cells exhibited nuclear atypia in the form of mild hyperchromasia and variation in the nuclear size and shape.
- The tumour cells were immunoreactive to CD34 and bcl-2, and negative for CD117 (c-kit), ALK-1, smooth muscle actin, and progesterone receptors.

Gastrointestinal stromal tumor (GIST)

- Most cases present with obstructive symptoms and abnormal rectal examination. GIST are typically large masses arising from rectum or perirectal space that compress but do not invade the prostate. They can be diagnosed by needle biopsy and are morphologically similar to those found within the gastrointestinal tract. CD117 is uniformly expressed in all cases and CD34 is frequently positive (Figs. 3.118 and 3.119).
- Main differential diagnosis includes neural and smooth muscle tumors, SFTs and STUMP.

Prostatic blue nevus

- It is a rare spindle cell proliferation containing melanin within prostatic stroma. This histological appearance is reminiscent of the common blue nevus of the skin (Fig. 3.120).
- It is believed that this lesion does not transform into melanoma, in contrast to the cellular blue nevus, which occasionally undergoes malignant transformation.
- The terms blue nevus and melanosis of the prostate are occasionally used interchangeably, although most authors refer to as melanosis when melanin is present within both the glandular and stromal melanocytes.

Table 3.17 Classification of prostatic non-epithelial tumour-like conditions and tumours

Tumour-like proliferations and inflammatory pseudotumours
Postoperative spindle cell nodules
Inflammatory myofibroblastic tumour
Blue nevus
Granulomatous prostatitis
Variants of prostatic hyperplasia
Stromal hyperplasia with atypia
Fibroadenoma-like foci in benign hyperplasia
Phyllodes-like hyperplasia
Cystoadenoma
Mixed epithelial-stromal tumours (phyllodes tumour)
STUMPs
Stromal Sarcoma
Stromal tumours
Benign
Leiomyoma, including its variants (atypical leiomyoma, cellular leiomyoma, and leiomyoblastoma)
Others
Malignant
Leiomyosarcoma
Rhabdomyosarcoma
Others

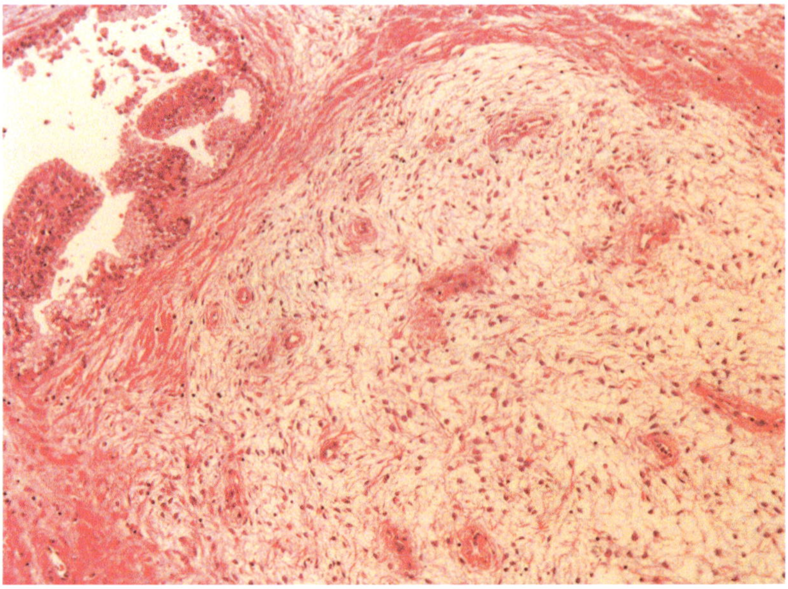

Fig. 3.109 Pure stromal nodule in benign prostate hyperplasia

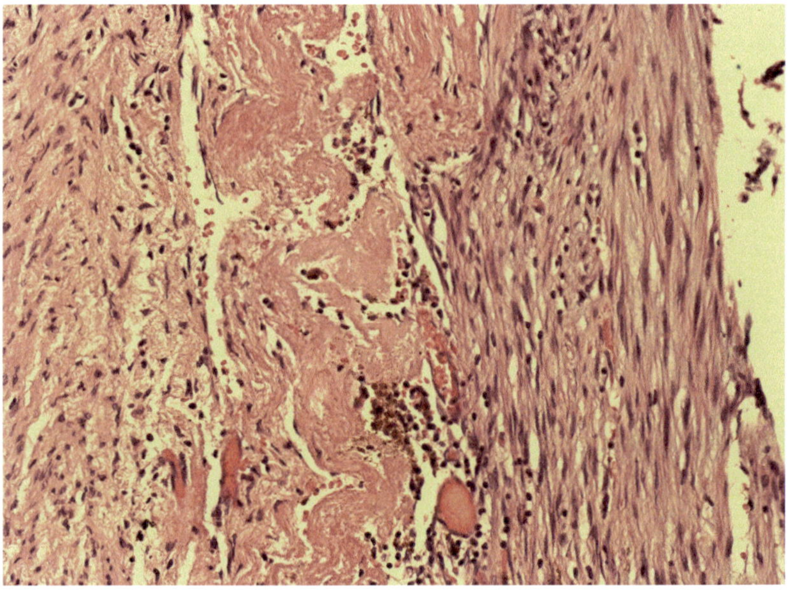

Fig. 3.110 Postoperative spindle cell nodule in a prostate that received previous transurethral resection

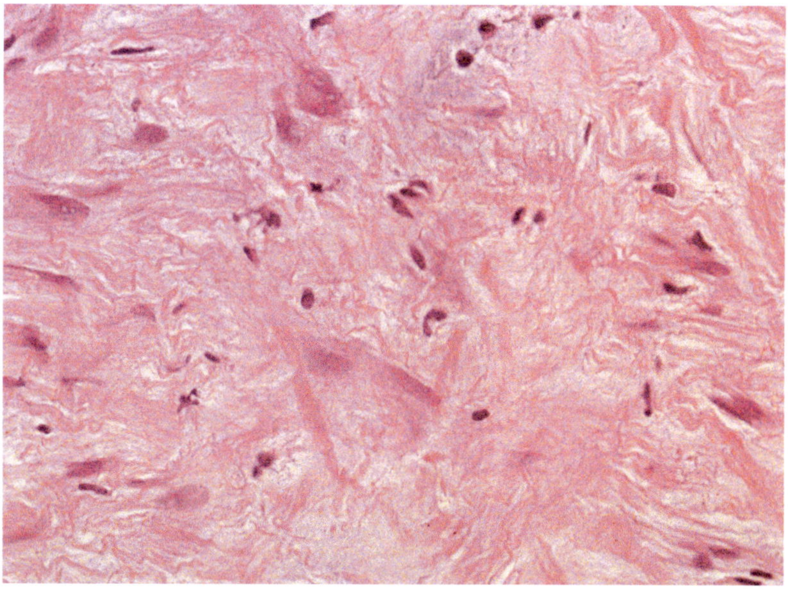

Fig. 3.111 Atypical prostatic stroma cells seen in cases of benign prostatic hyperplasia

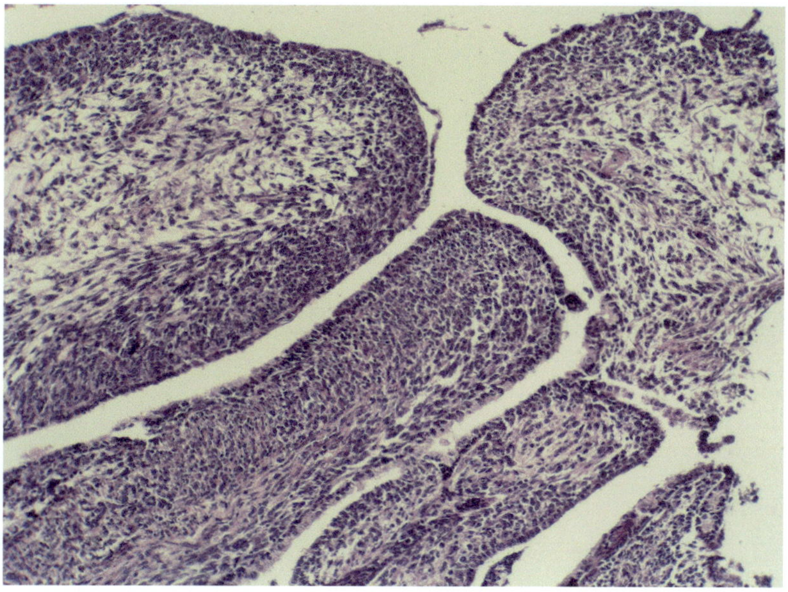

Fig. 3.112 Phyllodes tumor (STUMP) of the prostate showing leaf-like fibrous stroma covered by benign-appearing prostatic epithelium

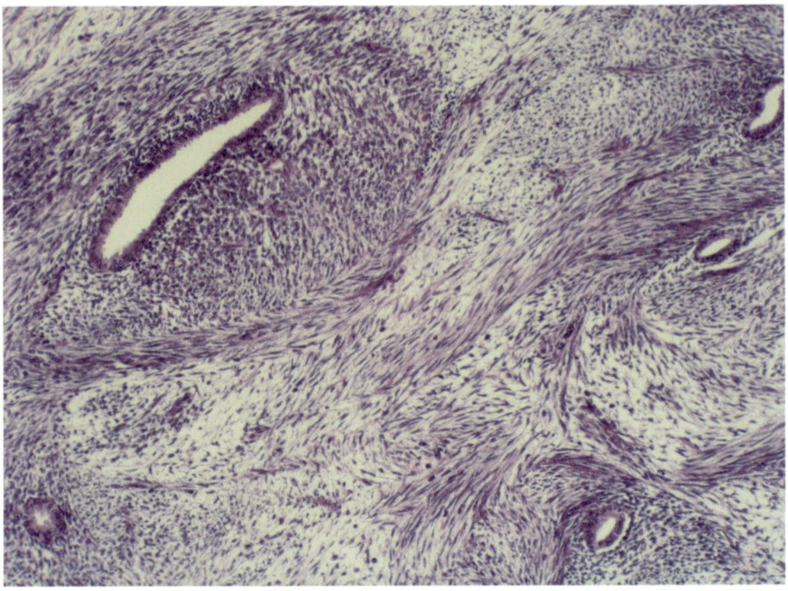

Fig. 3.113 Phyllodes tumor (STUMP) of the prostate showing myxoid stroma

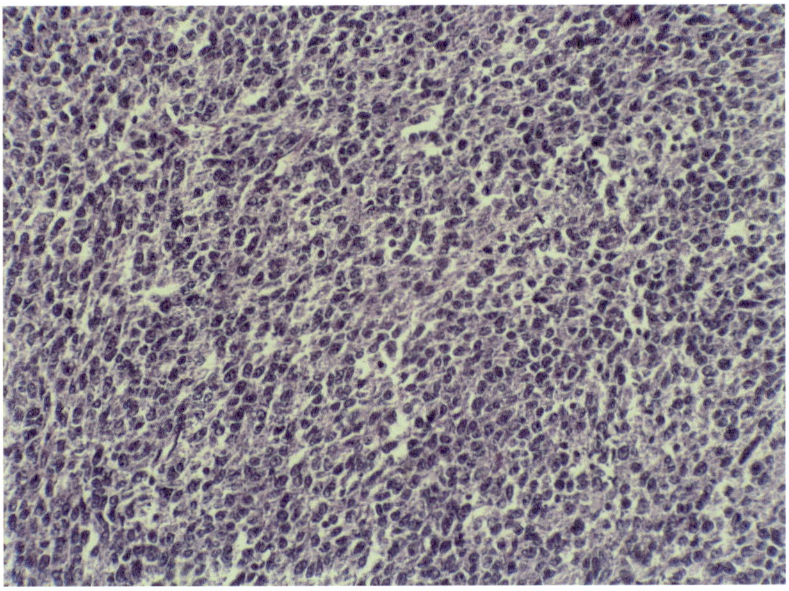

Fig. 3.114 Stromal sarcoma of the prostate with monotonous cell proliferation and low mitotic index

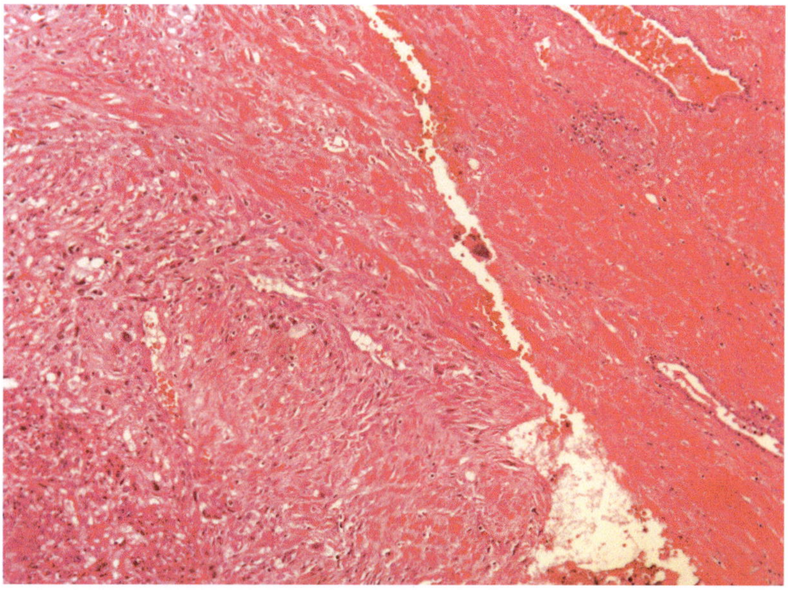

Fig. 3.115 Leiomyosarcoma of the prostate (low power)

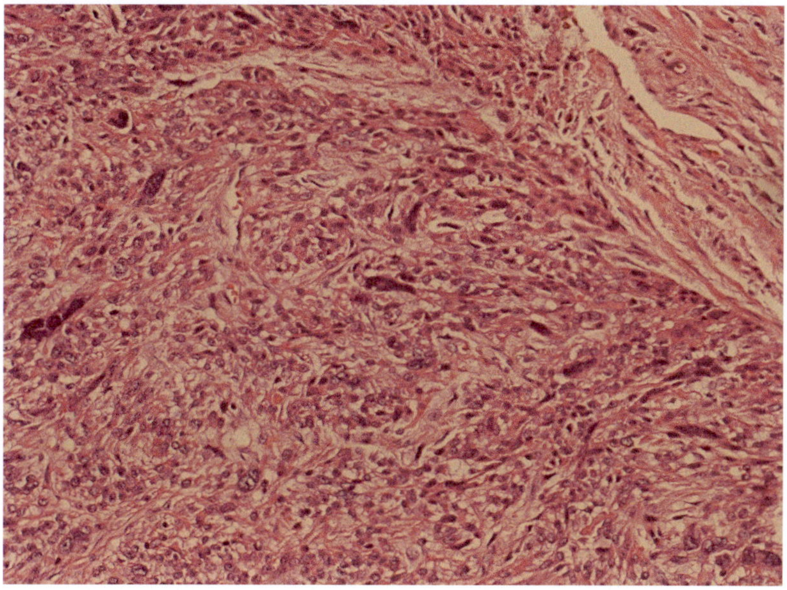

Fig. 3.116 Leiomyosarcoma of the prostate with atypical spindle cells (high power)

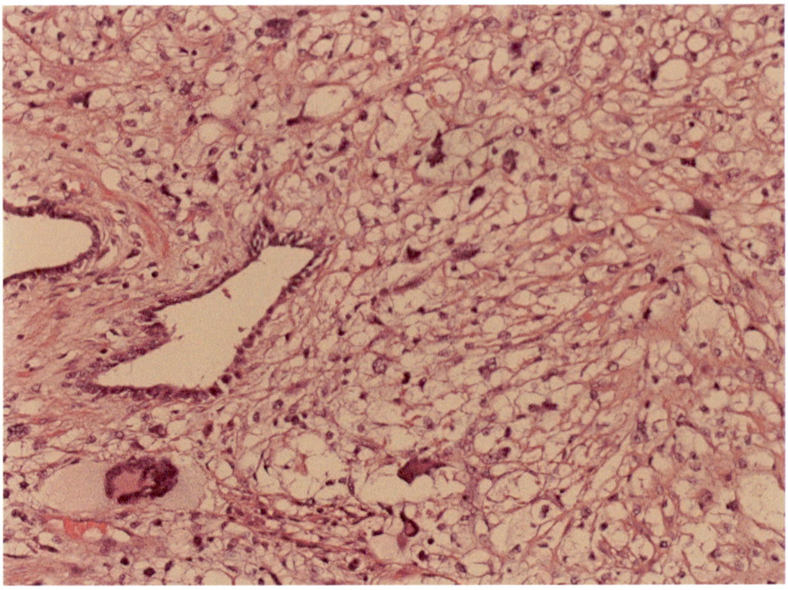

Fig. 3.117 Leiomyosarcoma of the prostate with focal myxoid change

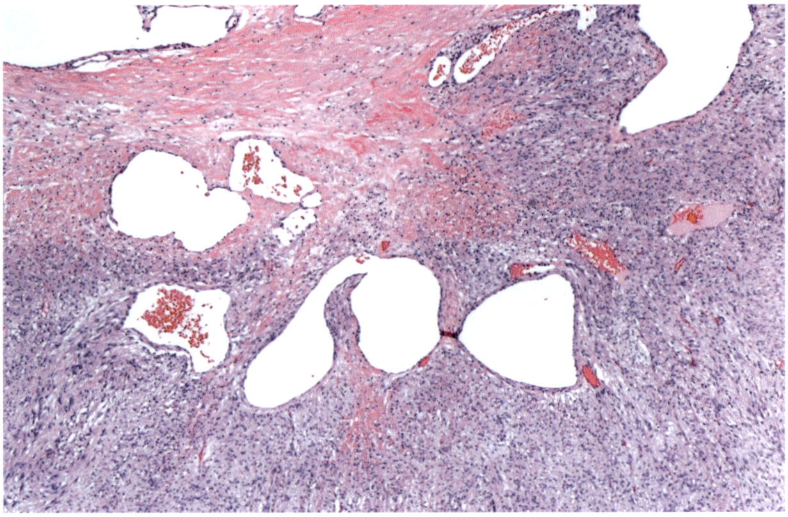

Fig. 3.118 Gastrointestinal stromal tumor involving the prostate

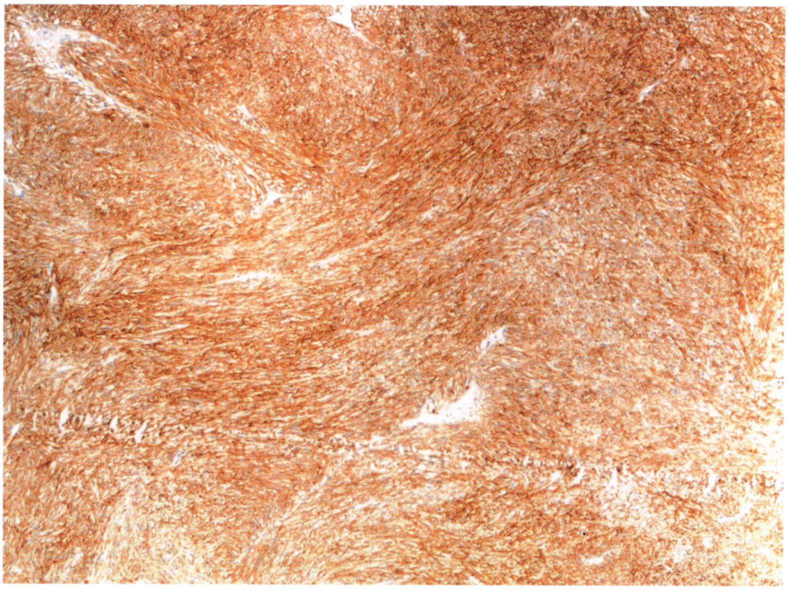

Fig. 3.119 CD117 expression in gastrointestinal stromal tumor

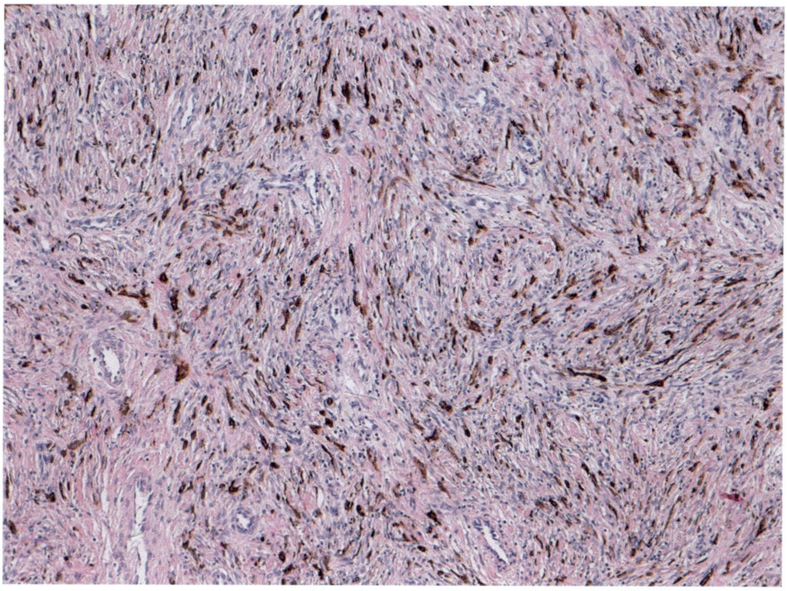

Fig. 3.120 Blue nevus arising in the prostate

3.10 Miscellaneous Primary Tumours of the Prostate

- This is a very heterogeneous group of tumours which are very rarely observed in the prostate: Wilms' tumour (nephroblastoma), Malignant rhabdoid tumour, Tubulo-cystic clear cell adenocarcinoma, Melanoma of the Prostate, Paraganglioma, hemangioma (mostly arising in the prostatic urethra) and Neuroblastoma, Malignant perivascular epithelioid cell tumor (pecoma), malignant mixed germ cell tumors, endodermal sinus tumor, renal-type clear cell carcinoma.
- The most common sarcomas are rhabdomyosarcoma and leiomyosarcoma. Rare cases of malignant fibrous histiocytoma, angiosarcoma, osteosarcoma, chondrosarcoma, malignant peripheral nerve sheath tumours, ectomesenchymoma with rhabdmyosarcoma and ganglioneuroma, PNET, and synovial sarcoma, chondroma, schwannoma, granular cell tumor, neurofibroma, or hemagiopericytoma have been reported.

Lymphoid tumours of the prostate

- The prostate is a rare site of extranodal lymphoma which accounts for only 0.1 % of all newly diagnosed lymphoma. Typically present in older men. Rarely Hodgkin's lymphoma and mucosa-associated lymphoid tissue (MALT) lymphoma were reported.
- Most reported non-Hodgkin's lymphomas are diffuse large B-cell followed by small lymphocytic lymphoma. Most frequent symptoms are those related to lower urinary obstruction. Rare cases of myeloma and T-cell lymphoma are on record. The entire spectrum of lymphoma seen in other sites my become manifest in the prostate.
- Of patients with chronic lymphocytic leukemia, 20 % are reported to have prostate involvement at autopsy.

3.11 Secondary Tumours Involving the Prostate

- Prostate involvement by a secondary tumour occurs either as a metastasis or by direct extension. Metastases from gastrointestinal tract, lung, skin (melanoma), and endocrine glands are on record. Prostatic metastases from other genitor-urinary primaries, such as kidney and testis, have been rarely cited. They are reported in 0.1 and 2.9 % of all postmortems and in 0.2 % of all surgical prostatic specimens. The more common occurrence of secondary involvement of prostate by a bladder urothelial carcinoma can be diagnostically challenging in needle biopsy specimens.

Prostate involvement from bladder urothelial carcinoma

- Attention to subtle histological features such papillary or solid growth, the relatively higher degree of nuclear pleomorphism, brisk mitotic activity, the occasional squamoid cytoplasm should raise the possibility of urothelial carcinoma (UC) (Figs. 3.121, 3.122 and 3.123).
- Another helpful feature is the identification of pre-existing prostatic duct/acini distended by the malignant urothelial cells with occasional pagetoid or undermining pattern of spread. Some of the latter structures can be surrounded by concentric fibrosis even in the absence of stromal prostatic invasion.
- The differential diagnosis for the intraductal spread of UC into the prostate should include high-grade prostatic intraepithelial neoplasia, prostatic ductal adenocarcinoma and "intraductal" prostatic adenocarcinoma. Unlike UC, the latter lesions demonstrate positive reactivity for prostate specific markers, i.e., PSA, prostate-specific membrane antigen (PSMA) and P504S and are negative for high molecular weight cytokeratins (34betaE12). Furthermore, intraductal UC spread into prostate is positive for uroplakin, thrombomodulin and/or p63.
- Intraductal UC spread into prostate could be extensive and can involve the peripheral prostate zone and rarely the seminal vesicle through the ejaculatory duct. The latter should be distinguished from invasion into prostatic stroma which usually have a more infiltrative pattern, displaying irregular rather than smooth bordered urothelial nests and is associated with desmoplastic response.
- In cases of advanced urinary bladder UC, direct extension into the prostate through

transmural bladder wall penetration may be seen. Given the significant difference in management of the two diseases their distinction is crucial.

- Even in poorly differentiated PCa, there is relatively little pleomorphism or mitotic activity compared to poorly differentiated UC. A subtler finding is that the cytoplasm of prostatic adenocarcinoma is often foamy and pale imparting a “soft” appearance. The findings of infiltrating cords of cells or focal cribriform glandular differentiation are other features more typical of prostatic adenocarcinoma than transitional cell carcinoma (Figs. 3.124 and 3.125).
- In the differential diagnosis of high grade Pca. vs. urothelial carcinoma (UC), the primary option is to use PSA as a first test to identify Pca. and GATA3 to identify UC. If GATA3 is not available, then HMWCK and p63. If the tumor is PSA positive with intense staining and HMWCK and p63 negative, the findings are diagnostic of Pca. If the tumor is equivocal/weak/negative for PSA and negative/focal for p63 and HMWCK, then one needs to do P501S, NKX3.1 and GATA3. Some experts also include PAP in this second round of staining. If the tumor is negative for PSA and diffusely strongly positive for p63 and HMWCK, the findings are diagnostic of UC. If the tumor is negative for PSA and moderate-strong positive for GATA3, it is diagnostic of UC.

Prostate involvement from colorectal carcinoma

- A source of secondary tumour extension into prostate is the topographically adjacent colorectal tract. Attention to some characteristic morphologic features should raise the possibility of a secondary spread on prostate needle biopsy specimen. The presence of goblet/columnar cell differentiation, pseudo-stratified nuclei, and characteristic “dirty necrosis” are more likely encountered in colorectal carcinoma.
- One should be cautioned that single infiltrating glands of prostatic duct adenocarcinoma can resemble infiltrating colonic adenocarcinoma. The differentiation between prostatic duct adenocarcinoma and secondary involvement of the prostate by colorectal carcinoma can be facilitated by finding more typical prostatic duct adenocarcinoma elsewhere within the biopsy.
- An immunohistochemical profile of positive nuclear CDX2 staining, positive nuclear (cytoplasmic staining can occur in PCa), β-catenin and villin, and positive staining for CK20 in the face of negative reactivity for prostate specific antigen (PSA) and prostatic acid phosphatase (PAP), prostate-specific membrane (PSMA), can be used to confirm the diagnosis of colorectal carcinoma spread.

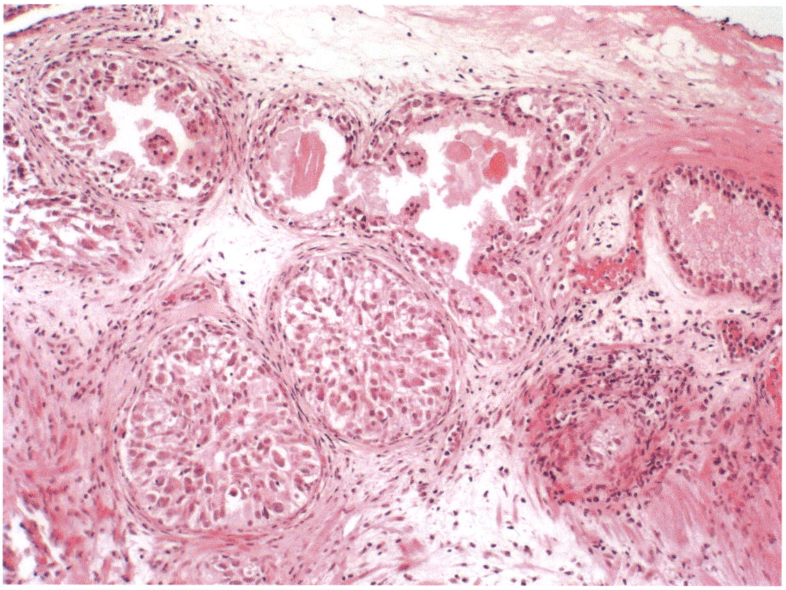

Fig. 3.121 Prostate involvement from urothelial carcinoma without stromal invasion

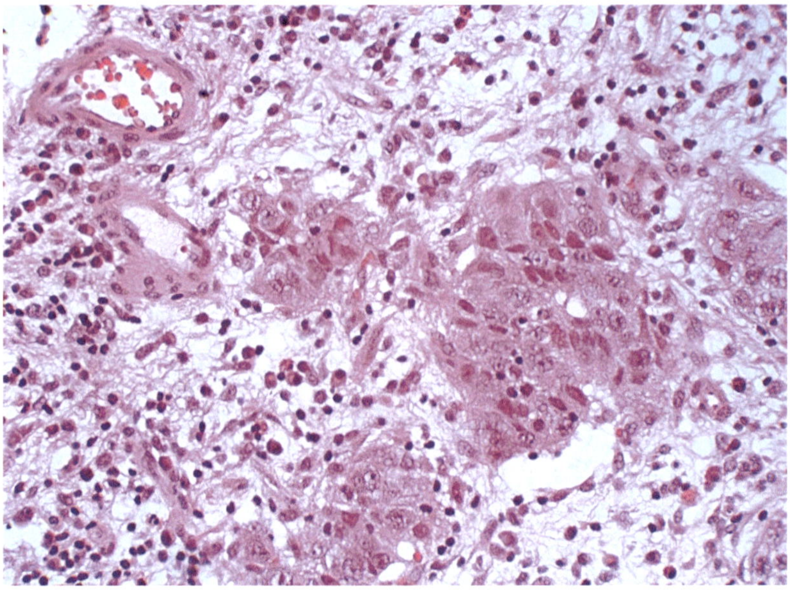

Fig. 3.122 Prostate involvement from urothelial carcinoma with stromal invasion

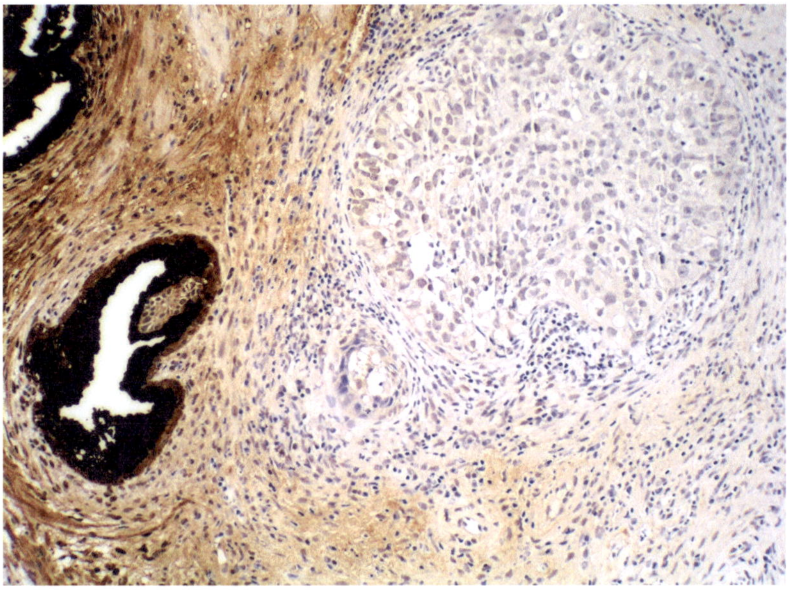

Fig. 3.123 PSA expression in prostate glands and negative in urothelial carcinoma

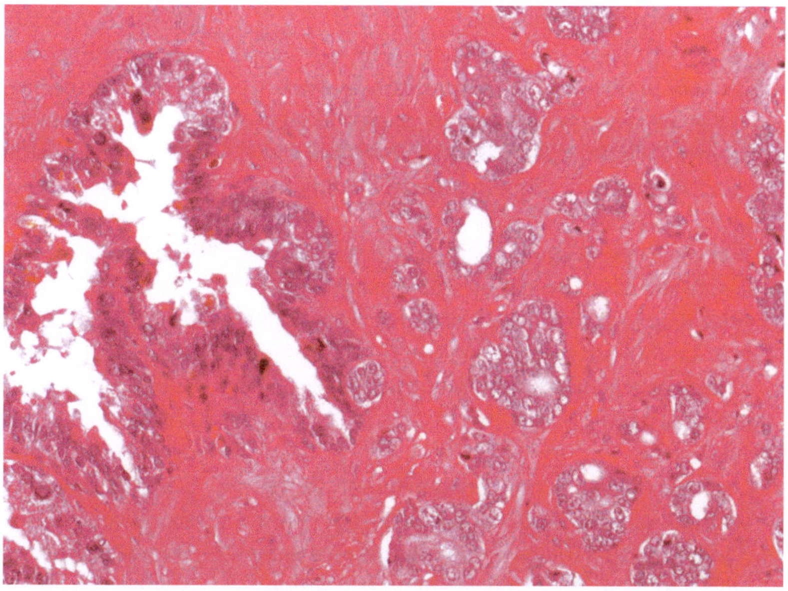

Fig. 3.124 Seminal vesicle invasion by prostate carcinoma

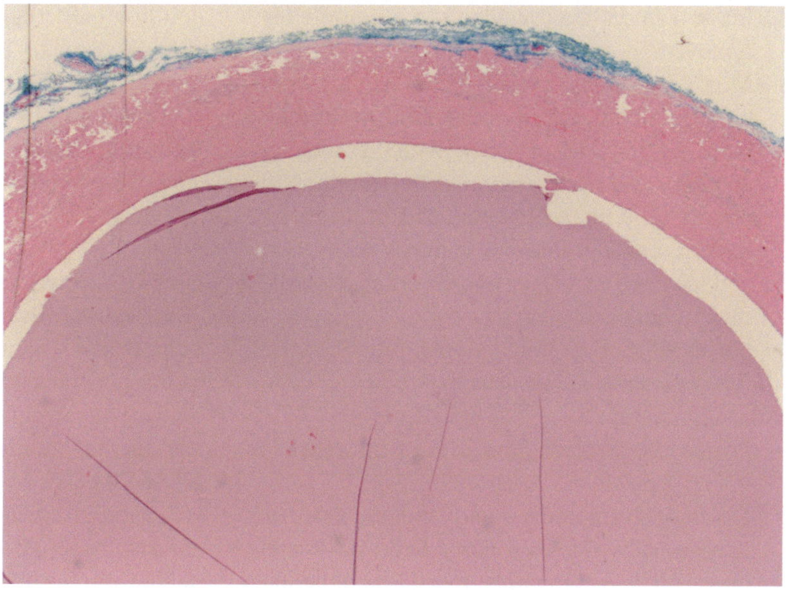

Fig. 3.125 Unilocular cyst of the seminal vesicle (low power)

3.12 Seminal Vesicles

- Primary tumors arising in the seminal vesicles (SVs) are extremely rare with anecdotal case reported (Table 3.18). Pelvic pain, urinary or rectal obstructive symptoms are frequently the onset of disease.
- Some may be asymptomatic, and detected by digital rectal examination and imaging, but final diagnosis frequently requires biopsy. It may be difficult to ascertain the site of origin of a given tumor when adjacent pelvic organs are involved.

Cystadenoma

- Cystadenoma is a rare benign tumor of the seminal vesicles. Patients range in age from 37 to 66 years. They may be asymptomatic or have symptoms of bladder outlet obstruction. Imaging reveals a complex, solid-cystic pelvic mass. Tumors may recur when incompletely removed.
- Microscopically, cystadenoma is a well-circumscribed tumor containing variable-sized glandular spaces with branching contours and cysts separated by spindle cell stroma. The glands are grouped in a lobular pattern, contain pale intraluminal secretions, and are lined by one or two layers of cuboidal to columnar cells.
- No significant cytologic atypia, mitotic activity, or necrosis are present.

Adenocarcinoma

- Primary adenocarcinoma is rare with less than 100 acceptable cases reported.
- Presenting symptoms usually include obstructive uropathy due to a non-tender peri-rectal mass and, less commonly, hematuria or hematospermia. Serum carcinoembryonic antigen may be elevated. Most are in older men (mean 62 years), but may occur under the age 40 years.
- Strict criteria for the diagnosis of this lesion require the exclusion of a concomitant prostatic, bladder, or rectal carcinoma. Suggested criteria include: (i) Tumor located primarily in the SVs, (ii) No evidence of carcinoma in the prostate, bladder or rectum, (iii) histology of adenocarcinoma with papillary, sheet-like growth or mucinous differentiation, (iv) in situ adenocarcinoma in the adjacent seminal epithelium (criteria yet undefined), (v) cytoplasmic immunoreactivity for CEA, (vi) absence of staining for PSA and PAP.
- The tumors are usually large (3–5 cm) and often invade the bladder, ureter, or rectum. Tumors can show a mixture of glandular, papillary, and trabecular features with varying degrees of differentiation. Tumors with a colloid pattern have been described.
- Tumor cells cytoplasm may show clear cell or hobnail morphology. It is important to exclude a prostatic adenocarcinoma.
- Carcinoembryonic antigen (CEA) and CK7 are detectable in normal seminal vesicle. Tumor of the SVs should be positive for CK 7 (unlike many prostatic adenocarcinomas), CEA, and for CA125 (unlike carcinoma arising in a mullerian duct cyst) and negative for CK 20 (unlike bladder and colonic carcinoma), PSA and PAP.
- The prognosis of primary seminal vesicle adenocarcinoma is poor. Since most patients present with metastases at diagnosis, overall survival in 95 % of patients is less than 3 years.

Secondary carcinoma

- The seminal vesicle is involved by secondary tumors much more frequently than it contains primary adenocarcinoma. Most frequent secondary involvement is from prostate adenocarcinoma, but urothelial carcinoma may also invade de SVs by direct extension (stage T4) or mucosal spread from the urethra, in this case as pagetoid spread or mucosal replacement from in situ urothelial carcinoma.
- Rectal adenocarcinoma occasionally invades SVs (Fig. 3.124)
- Other metastases to SVs and /or retrovesical space may originate in renal cell carcinoma, hepatocellular carcinoma, thymoma, seminoma.

Differentiating prostate gland, seminal vesicle and ejaculatory duct

- Occasionally, uropathologists face a differential diagnosis between prostate tissue, seminal vesicle or ejaculatory duct in the setting of needle biopsies.

- Seminal vesicle wall consists of a thick circumferential coat of smooth muscle and the ejaculatory ducts are surrounded by a collagenous stroma. SVs are CKAE1/AE3+, p63+, PAX-2+, PSA-, PAP-, P504S-.
- The use of a panel based on the P504S/p63 one-color cocktail is a practical and cost-effective stain to differentiate prostatic carcinoma that involves the seminal vesicle from seminal vesicle epithelium. It is superior to PSA and PAP since these cannot distinguish benign from malignant glands.
- More recently, the use of nuclear PAX-2 immunoreactivity has been suggested as robust marker in this setting. PAX-2 is typically positive in epithelium of the seminal vesicle and ejaculatory duct; but the intensity of staining is less in the ejaculatory duct.
- No reactivity for PAX-2 is seen in prostatic adenocarcinoma or prostatic intraepithelial neoplasia.

Angiosarcoma

- Reported patients present with pelvic pain and died of distant metastasis within 4 months after the diagnosis.

Hemangiopericytoma

- Anecdotal cases of malignant hemangiopericytoma of the seminal vesicle have been reported with patients died of disseminated disease after surgery.

Leiomyosarcoma

- Imaging methods show a large pelvic mass in the region of the SVs. Most reported patients with seminal vesicle leiomyosarcoma presented with pelvic pain and obstructive symptoms.
- Resection of the tumor mass by radical prostatectomy and vesiculectomy is the therapy of choice. This approach may result curative in some cases although another may developed metastasis. Morphologically it is identical to leiomyosarcoma of other locations.

Liposarcoma

- Only rare cases of liposarcoma of the SVs have been described. One case had associated prostatic carcinoma.

Malignant fibrous histiocytoma (undifferentiated sarcoma)

- This tumor is exceedingly rare in the seminal vesicle. The therapy should be the complete surgical resection.

Leiomyoma

- It is usually asymptomatic with smaller tumors seen incidentally at time of prostatectomy. Larger tumors may be detected on digital rectal examination or imaging.
- Leiomyoma ranges 0.5–5 cm, and local excision yields no recurrence.

Solitary fibrous tumor

- Anecdotal cases have been reported in the seminal vesicle, most frequently in the right organ. The origin of the tumor was established by imaging methods. The clinical presentation includes pelvic pain and/or hematuria. Complete local excision appears to be curative.

Other

- Rare examples of fibroma, schwannoma, paraganglioma, mammary-type myofibroblastoma, fibrosarcoma, osteosarcoma, rhabdomyosarcoma, pleomorphic sarcoma, malignant myoblastoma, PNET, carcinoid, and GIST are on record.
- Rare primary germ cell (choriocarcinoma, seminoma) tumors have been reported in the SVs
- A case of primary squamous cell carcinoma arising in a patient with seminal cyst, and few lymphoma cases are on record
- Recently, a unique case of an intraepithelial abnormality in pre-existing ducts and acini in the left SV of a patient 73-year-old patient with prostatic adenocarcinoma have been reported. The case shows morphological and immunohistochemical features similar to those of basal cell hyperplasia of the prostate.
- The epithelial lining was thicker than the surrounding normal ducts with obliteration of the acinar lumen, and there was some degree of cell stratification.
- PSA, PSAP, PSMA, Prostein (P501S), AMACR, as well as GATA3 were negative. p63, 34betaE12, CK5/6 and p53 were positive in cells in a basal and suprabasal position, whereas CA-125 was expressed in the luminal cells. The clinical significant of this lesion is not known.

Benign and malignant mixed epithelial–stromal tumors

- There have been about 25 acceptable cases reported on this category
- The criteria for the diagnosis of mixed epithelial–stromal tumors are:
- They arise from the seminal vesicle. (i) There is no normal seminal vesicle within the tumor. (ii) They do not invade the prostate (with rare exceptions). (iii) They have a less conspicuous and less cellular stromal component than cystadenoma. (iv) They are not immunoreactive for prostatic markers.

Fibroadenoma and adenomyoma

- These tumors have been reported in men aged 39–66 years, and presented with pain and voiding symptoms. These lesions are grossly solid and cystic, ranging from 3.5 to 16 cm.
- The distinction from epithelial–stromal tumor of low-grade (below) is based on stromal characteristic (bland cytology) and inconspicuous to absent mitotic activity.
- Some cases referred to as low-grade phyllodes tumor or benign mesenchymoma.

Malignant epithelial–stromal tumors

- The reported cases occurred in men aged 48–63 years who had urinary obstruction, painful ejaculation, constipation or abdominal pain. Most patients treated with cystoprostatectomy had pelvic recurrence or developed lung metastasis; likewise, some cases appear to be cured with surgery alone.
- Macroscopically, the tumors are either multicystic or solid and cystic. Microscopically, the stroma is at least focally densely cellular and tends to condense around distorted glands lined by cuboidal to focally stratified epithelium.
- The tumors are categorized as low-grade or high-grade, depending on mitotic activity, atypia, and necrosis.
- Rare cases referred to as high-grade phyllodes tumor (Cystosarcoma phyllodes) suggesting that features predictive of malignant behavior might be similar phyllodes tumors of the breast.

Tumor-like conditions

- Rare infections, ectopic tissues, age-related changes and cysts may occasionally present as tumor-like lesions.
- With age the columnar epithelium is replaced by flattened cuboidal cells and the muscular stroma becomes hyalinized and fibrotic. Lipochrome pigment is frequently present in SVs epithelium. Occasionally, stromal hyaline bodies may be present. The epithelium shows highly atypical cells with large, hyperchromatic nuclei with prominent nucleoli. Multinucleated cells may be present. Mitotic figures are absent. When present in needle biopsies, this should not be mistaken as prostate cancer.
- Ectopic prostate tissue may be seen in the SVs, frequently in the wall of a vesicle cyst. Urothelial or squamous metaplasia has been reported rarely arising in the SVs.
- Cysts may be congenital or acquired. Congenital ones are usually diagnosed between 17 and 42 years of age and are usually unilateral, unilocular, contains viscous white fluid, and are lined by cuboidal or flattened epithelium with a fibrous wall. Intracystic papillary adenoma may be rarely seen (Figs. 3.125 and 3.126)
- Acquired cysts are associated with inflammation and obstruction of the ejaculatory ducts and/or SVs. Often contains blood cells and spermatozoa. The epithelial lining is inflamed or sloughed. Cystadenoma may enter in differential diagnosis. Hydatidic cyst has been described in retrovesicular space.
- SVs amyloidosis (localized amyloidosis) which is Congo Red+ with apple-green polarization birefringence.
- Fibrosis associated with retroperitoneal and mediastinal fibrosis.
- Chronic or acute seminal vesiculitis including SVs abscess, tuberculosis, BCG therapy related granuloma, seminal schistosomiasis (usually secondary to Schistosoma haematobium infection from unrinary bladder), malakoplakia, virosis, and SVs wall calcification or calculi (Fig. 3.127).
- Androgen deprivation therapy in patients with prostate cancer may result in shrinkage of the SVs, and radiation therapy causes atrophy and fibrosis f the SVs.

Table 3.18 Tumors of the seminal vesicles

Epithelial tumors
Cystadenoma
Adenocarcinoma (primary)
Mesenchymal tumors (benign and malignant)
Angiosarcoma
Hemangiopericytoma
Leiomyoma
Leiomyosarcoma
Liposarcoma
Malignant fibrous histiocytoma
Solitary fibrous tumor
Mixed epithelial stromal tumors (benign and malignant)
Fibroadenoma
Adenomyoma
Malignant epithelial–stromal tumors
Lowgrade
High-grade
Other
Germ cell tumors

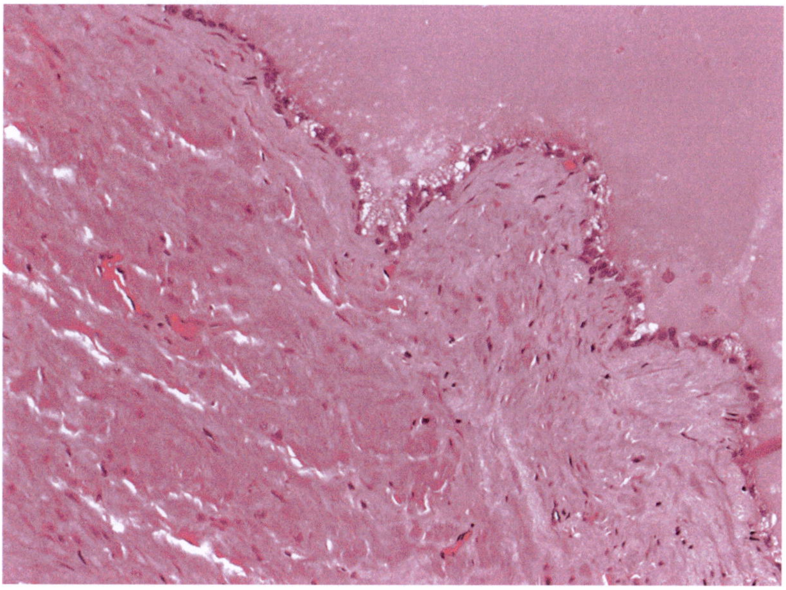

Fig. 3.126 Unilocular cyst of the seminal vesicle (high power)

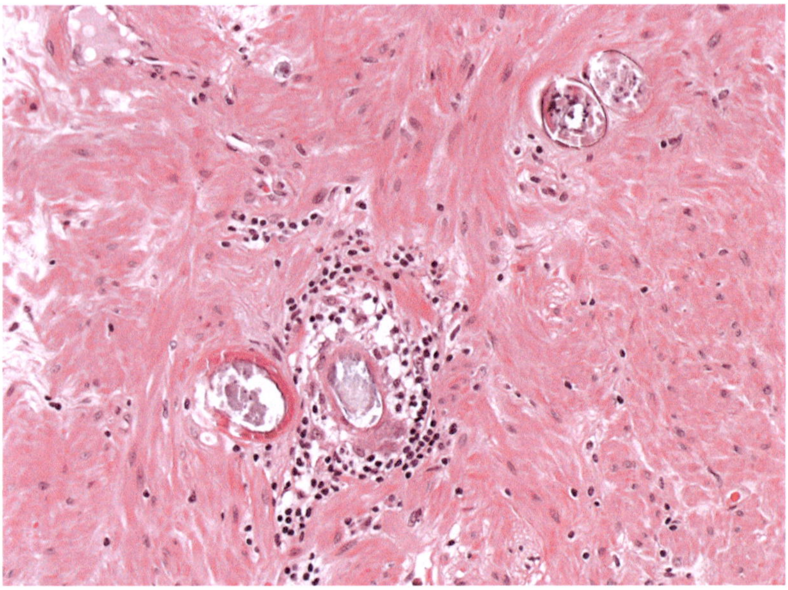

Fig. 3.127 Schistosoma hematobium in seminal vesicle muscle wall

Suggested Reading

Arya M, Hayne D, Brown RS, O'Donnell PJ, Mundy AR. Hemangiopericytoma of the seminal vesicle presenting with hypoglycemia. J Urol. 2001;166:992.

Berney DM, Algaba F, Camparo P, Compérat E, Griffiths D, Kristiansen G, Lopez-Beltran A, Montironi R, Varma M, Egevad L. Variation in reporting of cancer extent and benign histology in prostate biopsies among European pathologists. Virchows Arch. 2014a;464:583–7.

Berney DM, Algaba F, Camparo P, Compérat E, Griffiths D, Kristiansen G, Lopez-Beltran A, Montironi R, Varma M, Egevad L. The reasons behind variation in Gleason grading of prostatic biopsies: areas of agreement and misconception among 266 European pathologists. Histopathology. 2014b;64(3):405–11. doi:10.1111/his.12284. Epub 2013 Nov 6.

Biermann K, Montironi R, Lopez-Beltran A, Zhang S, Cheng L. Histopathological findings after treatment of prostate cancer using high-intensity focused ultrasound (HIFU). Prostate. 2010;70(11):1196–200.

Brimo F, Montironi R, Egevad L, Erbersdobler A, Lin DW, Nelson JB, Rubin MA, van der Kwast T, Amin M, Epstein JI. Contemporary grading for prostate cancer: implications for patient care. Eur Urol. 2013;63(5):892–901. doi:10.1016/j.eururo.2012.10.015.

Camparo P, Egevad L, Algaba F, Berney DM, Boccon-Gibod L, Compérat E, Evans AJ, Grobholz R, Kristiansen G, Langner C, Lopez-Beltran A, Montironi R, Oliveira P, Vainer B, Varma M. Utility of whole slide imaging and virtual microscopy in prostate pathology. APMIS. 2012;120(4):298–304. doi:10.1111/j.1600-0463.2011.02872.x. Review.

Capitanio U, Cheng L, Lopez-Beltran A, Scarpelli M, Freschi M, Montorsi F, Montironi R. The importance of interaction between urologists and pathologists in incidental prostate cancer management. Eur Urol. 2011;60(1):75–7.

Cheng L, Bishop E, Zhou H, Maclennan GT, Lopez-Beltran A, Zhang S, Badve S, Baldridge LA, Montironi R. Lymphatic vessel density in radical prostatectomy specimens. Hum Pathol. 2008a;39(4):610–5.

Cheng L, Foster SR, MacLennan GT, Lopez-Beltran A, Zhang S, Montironi R. Inflammatory myofibroblastic tumors of the genitourinary tract–single entity or continuum? J Urol. 2008b;180(4):1235–40.

Cheng L, MacLennan GT, Abdul-Karim FW, Lopez-Beltran A, Montironi R. Eosinophilic metaplasia of the prostate: a newly described lesion distinct from other eosinophilic changes in prostatic epithelium. Anal Quant Cytol Histol. 2008c;30(4):226–30.

Cheng L, MacLennan GT, Lopez-Beltran A, Montironi R. Anatomic, morphologic and genetic heterogeneity of prostate cancer: implications for clinical practice. Expert Rev Anticancer Ther. 2012a;12(11):1371–4. doi:10.1586/era.12.127. No.

Cheng L, Montironi R, Bostwick DG, Lopez-Beltran A, Berney DM. Staging of prostate cancer. Histopathology. 2012b;60(1):87–117. doi:10.1111/j.1365-2559.2011.04025.x. Review.

Cheng L, Davidson DD, Maclennan GT, Lopez-Beltran A, Montironi R, Wang M, Tan PH, Baldridge LA, Zhang S. Atypical adenomatous hyperplasia of prostate lacks TMPRSS2-ERG gene fusion. Am J Surg Pathol. 2013;37(10):1550–4. doi:10.1097/PAS.0b013e318294e9bc.

De Marzo AM, Platz EA, Epstein JI, Ali T, Billis A, Chan TY, Cheng L, Datta M, Egevad L, Ertoy-Baydar D, Farre X, Fine SW, Iczkowski KA, Ittmann M, Knudsen BS, Loda M, Lopez-Beltran A, Magi-Galluzzi C, Mikuz G, Montironi R, Pikarsky E, Pizov G, Rubin MA, Samaratunga H, Sebo T, Sesterhenn IA, Shah RB, Signoretti S, Simko J, Thomas G, Troncoso P, Tsuzuki TT, van Leenders GJ, Yang XJ, Zhou M, Figg WD, Hoque A, Lucia MS. A working group classification of focal prostate atrophy lesions. Am J Surg Pathol. 2006;30(10):1281–91.

Egevad L, Algaba F, Berney DM, Boccon-Gibod L, Compérat E, Evans AJ, Grobholz R, Kristiansen G, Langner C, Lockwood G, Lopez-Beltran A, Montironi R, Oliveira P, Schwenkglenks M, Vainer B, Varma M, Verger V, Camparo P. Interactive digital slides with heat maps: a novel method to improve the reproducibility of Gleason grading. Virchows Arch. 2011;459(2):175–82. Epub 2011 Jun 23.

Egevad L, Ahmad AS, Algaba F, Berney DM, Boccon-Gibod L, Compérat E, Evans AJ, Griffiths D, Grobholz R, Kristiansen G, Langner C, Lopez-Beltran A, Montironi R, Moss S, Oliveira P, Vainer B, Varma M, Camparo P. Standardization of Gleason grading among 337 European pathologists. Histopathology. 2013;62(2):247–56. doi:10.1111/his.12008.

Epstein JI, Allsbrook WC, Amin MB, Egevad LL, Bastacky S, Lopez-Beltran A, et al. The 2005 International society of urological pathology (ISUP) consensos conference on Gleason grading of prostatic carcinoma. Am J Surg Pathol. 2005;29:1228–42.

Fain JS, Cosnow I, King BF, Zincke H, Bostwick DG. Cystosarcoma phyllodes of the seminal vesicle. Cancer. 1993;71:2055–61.

Galosi AB, Mazzucchelli R, Scarpelli M, Lopez-Beltran A, Cheng L, Muzzonigro G, Montironi R. Solitary fibrous tumour of the prostate identified on needle biopsy. Eur Urol. 2009;56(3):564–7.

Gentile AT, Moseley HS, Quinn SF, Franzini D, Pitre TM. Leiomyoma of the seminal vesicle. J Urol. 1994;151:1027–9.

Harvey AM, Grice B, Hamilton C, Truong LD, Ro JY, Ayala AG, Zhai QJ. Diagnostic utility of P504S/p63 cocktail prostate-specific antigen, and prostatic acid phosphatase in verifying prostatic carcinoma involvement in seminal vesicles a study of 57 cases of radical prostatectomy specimens of pathologic stage pT3b. Arch Pathol Lab Med. 2010;134:983–8.

Hodges KB, Abdul-Karim FW, Wang M, Lopez-Beltran A, Montironi R, Easley S, Zhang S, Wang N, MacLennan GT, Cheng L. Evidence for transformation of fibroadenoma of the breast to malignant phyllodes tumor. Appl Immunohistochem Mol Morphol. 2009;17(4):345–50.

Juhasz J, Kiss P. A hitherto undescribed case of 'collision' tumour: liposarcoma of the seminal vesicle and prostatic carcinoma. Int Urol Nephrol. 1978;10:185–93.

Lamont JS, Hesketh PJ, de las Morenas A, Babayan RK. Primary angiosarcoma of the seminal vesicle. J Urol. 1991;146:165–7.

Laurila P, Leivo I, Makisalo H, Ruutu M, Miettinen M. Mullerian adenosarcomalike tumor of the seminal vesicle. A case report with immunohistochemical and ultrastructural observations. Arch Pathol Lab Med. 1992;116:1072–6.

Lee S, Han JS, Chang A, Ross HM, Montironi R, Yorukoglu K, Lane Z, Epstein JI. Small cell-like change in prostatic intraepithelial neoplasia, intraductal carcinoma, and invasive prostatic carcinoma: a study of 7 cases. Hum Pathol. 2013;44(3):427–31. doi:10.1016/j.humpath.2012.06.008.

Lopez-Beltran A, Qian J, Montironi R, Luque RJ, Bostwick DG. Atypical adenomatous hyperplasia (adenosis) of the prostate: DNA ploidy analysis and immunophenotype. Int J Surg Pathol. 2005a;13:167–73.

Lopez-Beltran A, Eble JN, Bostwick DG. Pleomorphic giant cell carcinoma of the prostate. Arch Pathol Lab Med. 2005b;129:683–5.

Lopez-Beltran A, Mikuz G, Luque RJ, Mazzucchelli R, Montironi R. Current practice of Gleason grading of prostate carcinoma. Virchows Arch. 2006;448(2):111–8.

Lopez-Beltran A, Cheng L, Prieto R, Blanca A, Montironi R. Lymphoepithelioma-like carcinoma of the prostate. Hum Pathol. 2009;40(7):982–7.

Lopez-Beltran A, Cheng L, Blanca A, Montironi R. Cell proliferation and apoptosis in prostate needle biopsies with adenocarcinoma Gleason score 6 or 7. Anal Quant Cytol Histol. 2012a;34(2):61–5.

Lopez-Beltran A, Vidal A, Montironi R, Kirkali Z, Muñoz E, Blanca A, Cheng L. Lymphocytic vasculitis of the prostate transition zone. BJU Int. 2012b;110:1775–80. doi:10.1111/j.1464-410X.2012.11079.x.

Lunardi A, Ala U, Epping MT, Salmena L, Clohessy JG, Webster KA, Wang G, Mazzucchelli R, Bianconi M, Stack EC, Lis R, Patnaik A, Cantley LC, Bubley G, Cordon-Cardo C, Gerald WL, Montironi R, Signoretti S, Loda M, Nardella C, Pandolfi PP. A co-clinical approach identifies mechanisms and potential therapies for androgen deprivation resistance in prostate cancer. Nat Genet. 2013;45(7):747–55. doi:10.1038/ng.2650. Epub 2013 Jun 2.

Maheshkumar P, Harper C, Sunderland GT, Conn IG. Cystic epithelial stromal tumour of the seminal vesicle. BJU Int. 2000;85:1154.

Marks RA, Koch MO, Lopez-Beltran A, Montironi R, Juliar BE, Cheng L. PMID: 17509394 [PubMed – indexed for MEDLINE] Related Articles, Links The relationship between the extent of surgical margin positivity and prostate specific antigen recurrence in radical prostatectomy specimens. Hum Pathol. 2007;38(8):1207–11.

Mazur MT, Myers JL, Maddox WA. Cystic epithelial-stromal tumor of the seminal vesicle. Am J Surg Pathol. 1987;11:210–7.

Mazzucchelli R, Lopez-Beltran A, Cheng L, Scarpelli M, Kirkali Z, Montironi R. Rare and unusual histological variants of prostatic carcinoma: clinical significance. BJU Int. 2008;102(10):1369–74.

Mazzucchelli R, Morichetti D, Lopez-Beltran A, Cheng L, Scarpelli M, Kirkali Z, Montironi R. Neuroendocrine tumours of the urinary system and male genital organs: clinical significance. BJU Int. 2009a;103(11):1464–70. Epub 2009 Feb 27. Review.

Mazzucchelli R, Scarpelli M, Cheng L, Lopez-Beltran A, Galosi AB, Kirkali Z, Montironi R. Pathology of prostate cancer and focal therapy ('male lumpectomy'). Anticancer Res. 2009b;29(12):5155–61.

Mazzucchelli R, Nesseris I, Cheng L, Lopez-Beltran A, Montironi R, Scarpelli M. Active surveillance for low-risk prostate cancer. Anticancer Res. 2010;30(9):3683–92.

Mazzucchelli R, Barbisan F, Santinelli A, Lopez-Beltran A, Cheng L, Scarpelli M, Montironi R. Immunohistochemical expression of prostate tumor overexpressed 1 in cystoprostatectomies with incidental and insignificant prostate cancer. Further evidence for field effect in prostatic carcinogenesis. Hum Pathol. 2011;42(12):1931–6.

Mazzucchelli R, Scarpelli M, Lopez-Beltran A, Cheng L, Montironi R. Spectrum of prostatic nonepithelial tumors and tumorlike conditions with spindle cell features. Anal Quant Cytol Histol. 2012a;34(3):139–44.

Mazzucchelli R, Scarpelli M, Lopez-Beltran A, Cheng L, Di Primio R, Montironi R. A contemporary update on pathology reporting for urinary bladder cancer. Int J Immunopathol Pharmacol. 2012b;25(3):565–71.

Mazzucchelli R, Scarpelli M, Lopez-Beltran A, Cheng L, Di Primio R, Montironi R. Treatment effects in prostate cancer following traditional and emerging therapies. Int J Immunopathol Pharmacol. 2013a;26(2):291–8. Review.

Mazzucchelli R, Scarpelli M, Barbisan F, Santinelli A, Lopez-Beltran A, Cheng L, Montironi R. Immunohistochemical expression of prostate tumour overexpressed 1 (PTOV1) in atypical adenomatous hyperplasia (AAH) of the prostate: additional evidence linking (AAH) to adenocarcinoma. Cell Oncol (Dordr). 2013b;36(1):37–42. doi:10.1007/s13402-012-0111-7.

Montironi R, Vela Navarrete R, Lopez-Beltran A, Mazzucchelli R, Mikuz G, Bono AV. Histopathology reporting of prostate needle biopsies. 2005 update. Virchows Arch. 2006a;449(1):1–13.

Montironi R, Scattoni V, Mazzucchelli R, Lopez-Beltran A, Bostwick DG, Montorsi F. Atypical foci suspicious but not diagnostic of malignancy in prostate needle biopsies (also referred to as "atypical small acinar proliferation suspicious for but not diagnostic of malignancy"). Eur Urol. 2006b;50(4):666–74.

Montironi R, Mazzucchelli R, Lopez-Beltran A, Cheng L, Scarpelli M. Mechanisms of disease: high-grade prostatic intraepithelial neoplasia and other proposed preneoplastic lesions in the prostate. Nat Clin Pract Urol. 2007;4(6):321–32.

Montironi R, Cheng L, Mazzucchelli R, Lopez-Beltran A. Pathological definition and difficulties in assessing positive margins in radical prostatectomy specimens. BJU Int. 2009a;103(3):286–8.

Montironi R, Cheng L, Lopez-Beltran A, Mazzucchelli R, Scarpelli M, Kirkali Z, Montorsi F. Joint appraisal of the radical prostatectomy specimen by the urologist and the uropathologist: together, we can do it better. Eur Urol. 2009b;56(6):951–5.

Montironi R, Mazzucchelli R, Lopez-Beltran A, Cheng L. Words of wisdom. Re: peripheral zone prostate cancers: location and intraprostatic patterns of spread at histopathology. Eur Urol. 2010a;58(1):180–2.

Montironi R, Cheng L, Lopez-Beltran A, Scarpelli M, Mazzucchelli R, Mikuz G, Kirkali Z, Montorsi F. Original Gleason system versus 2005 ISUP modified Gleason system: the importance of indicating which system is used in the patient's pathology and clinical reports. Eur Urol. 2010b;58(3):369–73.

Montironi R, Lopez-Beltran A, Cheng L, Scarpelli M. Cervical-type squamous metaplasia and myoepithelial cell differentiation in stromal tumor of the prostate. Am J Surg Pathol. 2011a;35(11):1752–4. No abstract available.

Montironi R, Mazzucchelli R, Lopez-Beltran A, Scarpelli M, Cheng L. Prostatic intraepithelial neoplasia: its morphological and molecular diagnosis and clinical significance. BJU Int. 2011b;108(9):1394–401. doi:10.1111/j.1464-410X.2011.010413.x. Epub 2011 Aug 26. Review.

Montironi R, Lopez-Beltran A, Scarpelli M, Mazzucchelli R, Cheng L. Handling of radical prostatectomy specimens: total embedding with whole mounts, with special reference to the Ancona experience (Letter). Histopathology. 2011c;59(5):1006–10.

Montironi R, Cheng L, Lopez-Beltran A, Mazzucchelli R, Scarpelli M. Editorial comment to When should we expect no residual tumor (pT0) once we submit incidental T1a-b prostate cancers to radical prostatectomy? Int J Urol. 2011d;18(2):153–4. doi:10.1111/j.1442-2042.2010.02717.x.

Montironi R, Lopez Beltran A, Mazzucchelli R, Cheng L, Scarpelli M. Handling of radical prostatectomy specimens: total embedding with large-format histology. Int J Breast Cancer. 2012a;2012:932784. Epub 2012 Jul 10.

Montironi R, Scarpelli M, Cheng L, Lopez-Beltran A, Zhou M, Montorsi F. Do not misinterpret intraductal carcinoma of the prostate as high-grade prostatic intraepithelial neoplasia! Eur Urol. 2012b;62(3):518–22. Epub 2012 Jun 5.

Montironi R, Scarpelli M, Mazzucchelli R, Cheng L, Lopez-Beltran A, Montorsi F. Extent of cancer of less than 50 % in any prostate needle biopsy core: how many millimeters are there? Eur Urol. 2012c;61(4):751–6. Epub 2012 Jan 5. No abstract available.

Montironi R, Cheng L, Lopez-Beltran A, Mazzucchelli R, Scarpelli M. Combined handling of prostate base/bladder neck and seminal vesicles in radical prostatectomy specimens: our approach with the whole mount technique. Histopathology. 2013a;63(3):431–5. doi:10.1111/his.12158. Epub 2013 Jun 24. No abstract available.

Montironi R, Lopez-Beltran A, Cheng L, Montorsi F, Scarpelli M. Central prostate pathology review: should it be mandatory? Eur Urol. 2013;64(2):199–201;

discussion 202–3. doi:10.1016/j.eururo.2013.04.002. Epub 2013 Apr 16. No abstract available.

Montironi R, Scarpelli M, Cheng L, Lopez-Beltran A, Montorsi F, Kirkali Z. Somatostatin receptor expression in prostate carcinoma: the urological pathologist's role in the era of personalised medicine. Pathology. 2013c;45(1):93–6. doi:10.1097/PAT.0b013e32835bae76. No abstract available.

Montironi R, Lopez-Beltran A, Cheng L, Galosi AB, Montorsi F, Scarpelli M. Seminal vesicle intraepithelial neoplasia versus basal cell hyperplasia in a seminal vesicle. Eur Urol. 2014;66(4):623–7. doi:10.1016/j.eururo.2014.02.054.

Montironi R, Cheng L, Lopez-Beltran A, Montironi MA, Galosi AB, Scarpelli M. A low grade PIN-like neoplasm of the transition zone immunohistochemically negative for basal cell markers: a possible example of low grade adenocarcinoma with stratified epithelium. Pathology. 2014b;46(1):88–91. doi:10.1097/PAT.0000000000000036.

Morichetti D, Mazzucchelli R, Lopez-Beltran A, Cheng L, Scarpelli M, Kirkali Z, Montorsi F, Montironi R. Secondary neoplasms of the urinary system and male genital organs. BJU Int. 2009;104(6):770–6.

Muentener M, Hailemariam S, Dubs M, Hauri D, Sulser T. Primary leiomyosarcoma of the seminal vesicle. J Urol. 2000;164:2027.

Ormsby AH, Haskell R, Ruthven SE, Mylne GE. Bilateral primary seminal vesicle carcinoma. Pathology. 1996;28:196–200.

Ormsby AH, Haskell R, Jones D, Goldblum JR. Primary seminal vesicle carcinoma: an immunohistochemical analysis of four cases. Mod Pathol. 2000;13:46–51.

Quick CM, Gokden N, Sangoi AR, Brooks JD, McKenney JK. The distribution of PAX-2 immunoreactivity in the prostate gland, seminal vesicle, and ejaculatory duct: comparison with prostatic adenocarcinoma and discussion of prostatic zonal embryogenesis. Hum Pathol. 2010;41:1145–9.

Rao Q, Williamson SR, Lopez-Beltran A, Montironi R, Huang W, Eble JN, Grignon DJ, Koch MO, Idrees MT, Emerson RE, Zhou XJ, Zhang S, Baldridge LA, Cheng L. Distinguishing primary adenocarcinoma of the urinary bladder from secondary involvement by colorectal adenocarcinoma: extended immunohistochemical profiles emphasizing novel markers. Mod Pathol. 2013;26(5):725–32. doi:10.1038/modpathol.2012.229. Epub 2013 Jan.

Santos LD, Wong CS, Killingsworth M. Cystadenoma of the seminal vesicle: report of a case with ultrastructural findings. Pathology. 2001;33:399–402.

Scarpelli M, Mazzucchelli R, Barbisan F, Santinelli A, Lopez-Beltran A, Cheng L, Montironi R. Is there a role for prostate tumour overexpressed-1 in the diagnosis of HGPIN and of prostatic adenocarcinoma? A comparison with alpha-methylacyl CoA racemase. Int J Immunopathol Pharmacol. 2012;25(1):67–74.

Schelling LA, Williamson SR, Zhang S, Yao JL, Wang M, Huang J, Montironi R, Lopez-Beltran A, Emerson RE, Idrees MT, Osunkoya AO, Man YG, Maclennan GT, Baldridge LA, Compérat E, Cheng L. Frequent TMPRSS2-ERG rearrangement in prostatic small cell carcinoma detected by fluorescence in situ hybridization: the superiority of fluorescence in situ hybridization over ERG immunohistochemistry. Hum Pathol. 2013;44(10):2227–33. doi:10.1016/j.humpath.2013.05.005. Epub 2013 Jul 12.

Seipel AH, Delahunt B, Samaratunga H, Amin M, Barton J, Berney DM, Billis A, Cheng L, Comperat E, Evans A, Fine SW, Grignon D, Humphrey PA, Magi-Galluzzi C, Montironi R, Sesterhenn I, Srigley JR, Trpkov K, van der Kwast T, Varma M, Zhou M, Ahmad A, Moss S, Egevad L. Diagnostic criteria for ductal adenocarcinoma of the prostate. Interobserver variability among 20 expert uropathologists. Histopathology. 2014. doi:10.1111/his.12382.

Smith SC, Palanisamy N, Zuhlke KA, Johnson AM, Siddiqui J, Chinnaiyan AM, Kunju LP, Cooney KA, Tomlins SA. HOXB13 G84E-related familial prostate cancers: a clinical, histologic, and molecular survey. Am J Surg Pathol. 2014;38(5):615–26.

Ukimura O, Coleman JA, de la Taille A, Emberton M, Epstein JI, Freedland SJ, Giannarini G, Kibel AS, Montironi R, Ploussard G, Roobol MJ, Scattoni V, Jones JS. Contemporary role of systematic prostate biopsies: indications, techniques, and implications for patient care. Eur Urol. 2013;63(2):214–30. doi:10.1016/j.eururo.2012.09.033.

Valerio M, Ahmed HU, Emberton M, Lawrentschuk N, Lazzeri M, Montironi R, Nguyen PL, Trachtenberg J, Polascik TJ. The role of focal therapy in the management of localised prostate cancer: a systematic review. Eur Urol. 2013. pii: S0302-2838(13)00557-5. doi:10.1016/j.eururo.2013.05.048.

Varinot J, Drouin S, Rouprêt M, Montironi R, Lopez-Beltran A, Compérat E. Prostate cancer with clear cell features and an unusual nested-like pattern of growth: a case report. Anal Quant Cytol Histol. 2012;34(5):289–92.

Varma M, Berney DM, Algaba F, Camparo P, Compérat E, Griffiths DF, Kristiansen G, Lopez-Beltran A, Montironi R, Egevad L. Prostate needle biopsy processing: a survey of laboratory practice across Europe. J Clin Pathol. 2013;66(2):120–3. doi:10.1136/jclinpath-2012-200993.

Wagner DG, Yao JL, di Sant'Agnese PA, Cheng L, Lopez-Beltran A, Montironi R, Huang J. Soft tissue tumors of the prostate: a review. Anal Quant Cytol Histol. 2007;29(6):341–50.

Wang X, Jones TD, Zhang S, Eble JN, Bostwick DG, Qian J, Lopez-Beltran A, Montironi R, Harris JJ, Cheng L. Amplifications of EGFR gene and protein expression of EGFR, Her-2/neu, c-kit, and androgen receptor in phyllodes tumor of the prostate. Mod Pathol. 2007;20(2):175–82.

Westra WH, Grenko RT, Epstein J. Solitary fibrous tumor of the lower urogenital tract: a report of five cases involving the seminal vesicles, urinary bladder, and prostate. Hum Pathol. 2000;31:63–8.

Williamson SR, Zhang S, Yao JL, Huang J, Lopez-Beltran A, Shen S, Osunkoya AO, MacLennan GT,

Montironi R, Cheng L. ERG-TMPRSS2 rearrangement is shared by concurrent prostatic adenocarcinoma and prostatic small cell carcinoma and absent in small cell carcinoma of the urinary bladder: evidence supporting monoclonal origin. Mod Pathol. 2011;24(8):1120–7. doi:10.1038/modpathol.2011.56.

Williamson SR, Bunde PJ, Montironi R, Lopez-Beltran A, Zhang S, Wang M, Maclennan GT, Cheng L. Malignant perivascular epithelioid cell neoplasm (PEComa) of the urinary bladder with TFE3 gene rearrangement: clinicopathologic, immunohistochemical, and molecular features. Am J Surg Pathol. 2013;37(10):1619–26. doi:10.1097/PAS.0b013e318293729d.

Yossepowitch O, Briganti A, Eastham JA, Epstein J, Graefen M, Montironi R, Touijer K. Positive surgical margins after radical prostatectomy: a systematic review and contemporary update. Eur Urol. 2014;65(2):303–13. doi:10.1016/j.eururo.2013.07.039. Epub 2013 Aug 3.

Zhang C, Montironi R, MacLennan GT, Lopez-Beltran A, Li Y, Tan PH, Wang M, Zhang S, Iczkowski KA, Cheng L. Is atypical adenomatous hyperplasia of the prostate a precursor lesion? Prostate. 2011;71(16):1746–51. doi:10.1002/pros.21391. Epub 2011 Apr 7.

Testis and Paratesticular Structures

4

Contents

4.1 **Basic Anatomy and Histology** 312

4.2 **Classification of Tumors and Tumor-Like Conditions** 313
4.2.1 Germ Cell Tumors 314
4.2.2 Intratubular Germ Cell Neoplasia, Unclassified (IGCNU) 315
4.2.3 Germ Cell Tumors of One Histologic Type 316
4.2.4 Seminoma 316
4.2.5 Spermatocytic Seminoma 320

4.3 **Non-seminomatous Germ Cell Tumors (NSGCTs)** 322
4.3.1 Embryonal Carcinoma 322

4.4 **Yolk Sac Tumor** 326
4.4.1 Pathology 326
4.4.2 Immunohistochemistry 327
4.4.3 Genetics 330

4.5 **Polyembryoma** 331

4.6 **Choriocarcinoma and Other Types of Throphoblastic Neoplasia** 331
4.6.1 Pathology 331
4.6.2 Morphologic Variants 332
4.6.3 Immunohistochemistry 333
4.6.4 Genetics 334

4.7 **Teratoma** 334
4.7.1 Pathology 334
4.7.2 Variants 334
4.7.3 Genetics 335

4.8 **Burned Out GCTs** 335

4.9 **Tumors of More than One Histologic Type (Mixed Forms)** 335
4.9.1 Pathology 336
4.9.2 Prognostic Factors 337

4.10 **Tumors of Sex Cord/Gonadal Stroma** 338

4.11 **Benign and Malignant Leydig Cell Tumors** 339
4.11.1 Pathology of Benign Tumors 339
4.11.2 Pathology of Malignant Tumors 339
4.11.3 Genetics 342

4.12 **Benign and Malignant Sertoli Cell Tumors** 342
4.12.1 Pathology of Benign Tumors 342
4.12.2 Pathology of Malignant Tumors 346
4.12.3 Genetics 346

4.13 **Large Cell Calcifying Sertoli Cell Tumor (LCCST)** 346
4.13.1 Pathology 346

4.14 **Granulosa Cell Tumor of Adult Type** 347

4.15 **Granulosa Cell Tumor of Juvenile Type** 347

4.16 **Thecoma–Fibroma Type Tumors** 347

4.17 **Mixed or Incompletely Differentiated (Undifferentiated) Gonadal Stromal Tumors** 348

4.18 **Mixed Germ Cell/Sex Cord Stromal Tumor** 348
4.18.1 Gonadoblastoma 348
4.18.2 Germ Cell Sex Cord/Gonadal Stromal Tumor, Unclassified 350

4.19 **Other Tumors of the Testis** 350
4.19.1 Carcinoid 350
4.19.2 Nephroblastoma 350
4.19.3 Lymphoma and Plasmacytoma 350
4.19.4 Leukemia 351

4.20 **Other Rare Tumors** 352

4.21 **Testicular Metastases** 353

4.22 **Tumors of the Paratesticular Region** 355

A. Lopez-Beltran et al., *Rare Tumors and Tumor-like Conditions in Urological Pathology*,
DOI 10.1007/978-3-319-10253-5_4,

4.23 **Tumors of Ovarian (Müllerian) Epithelial Types** . . . 355

4.24 **Tumors of Collecting Ducts and Rete Testis** . . . 355
4.24.1 Adenoma . . . 355
4.24.2 Adenocarcinoma of Rete Testis . . . 355

4.25 **Epithelial Tumors of the Epididymis** . . . 356
4.25.1 Papillary Cystadenoma of the Epididymis . . . 356
4.25.2 Adenocarcinoma of the Epididymis . . . 357
4.25.3 Adenomatoid Tumor . . . 358

4.26 **Mesothelioma of the Tunica Vaginalis Testis** . . . 358
4.26.1 Pathology . . . 359

4.27 **Melanotic Neuroectodermal Tumor of Infancy** . . . 360

4.28 **Desmoplastic Small Round Cell Tumor** . . . 360

4.29 **Soft Tissue Tumors of the Spermatic Cord** . . . 361

4.30 **Tumor-Like Conditions** . . . 362
4.30.1 Intratesticular Hemorrhage . . . 362
4.30.2 Segmental Testicular Infarction . . . 362
4.30.3 Organized Testicular Hematocele . . . 362
4.30.4 Inflammatory Lesions . . . 362

4.31 **Meconium Periorchitis** . . . 363

4.32 **Sperm Granuloma** . . . 364

4.33 **Sclerosing Lipogranuloma** . . . 364

4.34 **Cysts** . . . 364
4.34.1 Epidermoid Cyst . . . 364
4.34.2 Tubular Ectasia of the Rete Testis . . . 364
4.34.3 Epididymal Cysts and Spermatoceles . . . 364
4.34.4 Spermatic Cord Cysts . . . 365

4.35 **Ectopic Tissues** . . . 365
4.35.1 Ectopic Adrenocortical Tissue . . . 365
4.35.2 Splenic-Gonadal Fusion . . . 365
4.35.3 Lipomatosis Testis . . . 365

4.36 **Testicular Appendages** . . . 366

4.37 **Other Tumor-Like Lesions** . . . 366
4.37.1 Fibrous Pseudotumor . . . 366
4.37.2 Amyloidosis . . . 366
4.37.3 Polyorchidism . . . 366
4.37.4 Sertoli Cell Hyperplasia . . . 366
4.37.5 Leydig Cell Hyperplasia . . . 366
4.37.6 Hyperplasia of the Rete Testis . . . 366
4.37.7 Cribriform Hyperplasia and Atypical Nuclei in the Epididymis . . . 367
4.37.8 Reactive Mesothelial Hyperplasia . . . 367
4.37.9 Vasitis/Epididymitis Nodosa . . . 367
4.37.10 Proliferative Funiculitis . . . 367
4.37.11 Embryonic Remnants . . . 367

Suggested Reading . . . 367

4.1 Basic Anatomy and Histology

- The adult testis is an egg-shaped organ that hangs in the scrotum from the spermatic cord, the retro-epididymal surface, and the scrotal ligament. Mean testicular diameter is 4.6 cm for the longest axis.
- The tunica albuginea consists of three connective tissue layers: an outer layer containing a mesothelial lining that rests on a basal lamina (tunica vaginalis), a middle layer of dense fibrous tissue, and an inner layer of loose connective tissue (tunica vascularis) with nerves, and blood and lymphatic vessels. The thickness of tunica albuginea increases with age. Myofibroblasts are common in the tunica albuginea.
- The seminiferous tubules comprise about 80 % of testicular volume. The tubular lining of germ cells and Sertoli cells is surrounded by a lamina propria. Sertoli cells are columnar cells that extend from the basal lamina to the tubular lumina.
- Sertoli cell nucleus is located near de basal lamina, and is triangular with indented outline. The nucleolus is central and voluminous and that differentiates Sertoli cells from germinal cells (show coarse chromatin granules and variable number of nucleoli) in routine histologic sections.
- Charcot-Botcher crystals are often seen in the cytoplasm. Sertoli cells also produce several components of the seminiferous tubule wall, including type IV collagen, laminin, and heparin sulfate-rich proteoglycans.

- The germs cells include spermatogonia, primary and secondary spermatocytes, and spermatids (primary and secondary). These can be recognized on conventional histologic evaluation.
- The interstitium between the seminiferous tubules contains Leydig cells, macrophages, mast cells, fibroblasts (CD34+), neuron-like cells, myofibroblasts, blood and lymphatic vessels, and nerves. Leydig cells have spherical eccentric nuclei with one or two nucleoli. The eosinophilic cytoplasm is abundant, and it contains lipofuscin granules. Reinke crystalloids are seen only in Leydig cells of adults.
- The testis is supplied by the testicular artery, which arises from abdominal aorta.
- The inner two thirds of the testis parenchyma is drained by centripetal veins that follow interlobular septa to the mediastinum testis. The out third is drained by centrifugal veins that lead to the tunica albuginea. Both types of veins anastomose, and leave the testis by the veins from pampiniform plexus which drains de tested via the spermatic cord.
- Lymphatic vessels are poorly developed in the testes. Afferent nerve endings form corpuscles similar to those of Meissner and Pacini seen in the tunica albuginea. Efferent innervation is mainly supplied by neurons of the pelvic ganglia.
- The rete testis is a network of channels and cavities that connect the seminiferous tubules with the ductuli efferentes. The epithelium of the mediastinal rete testis consists of flattened cells interspersed with small areas of columnar cells. Both cell types have numerous microvilli and a single cilium on their free surface and contain keratin and vimentin filaments.
- The fetal testis has three types of germ cells known as gonocytes (OCT4+, CD117+), intermediate germ cells (OCT4 +/–, CD117–), or spermatogonia (OCT4–, CD117–). The prepubertal testis develops into three phases:
  - (i) Newborn and perinatal period showing solid tubules with centrally located Sertoli cells and gonocytes. At the age of 6 months there are no gonocytes since they have been transformed in spermatogonia. Leydig cells are similar to those seen in adults.
  - (ii) In infants, after the age of 6 months the testis remains at rest after the age of 3 years. Then it is observed a margination of the cells imparting a pseudo-luminal appearance to the tubules. These include Sertoli and undifferentiated cells and some spermatogonia. Leydig cells have decreased and there is low level of testosterone.
  - (iii) In boys, from age 9 years but mainly between the age of 13 and 15 years, interstitial stromal cells are transformed in adult Leydig cells that produce testosterone under LH stimulation. LH also stimulates development of germ cells, growth of tubules, and development of central lumen.
- Undescended testis is frequently smaller than contralateral descended testes. Histologically may present slight alterations only (histology or prepubertal testis), or may present testes with marked germinal hypoplasia showing spermatogonia irregularly distributed, frequently within the same lobule.

  In severe cases, the testes show severe germinal hypoplasia with giant spermatogonia, dark nuclei and edematous interstitium.
- With age and decreasing hormonal levels, changes of atrophy are frequent after the age of 70 years. After the age of 80 years, there is always certain degree of fibrosis in the tubular wall, but some degree of spermatogenesis persists.

4.2 Classification of Tumors and Tumor-Like Conditions

- Testicular tumors are classified according to the WHO (2004) classification (Table 4.1) and represent a heterogeneous group of neoplasms. Although rare, germ cell tumors have always been of great interest and nowadays can be cured in more than 90 % of cases.

Table 4.1 WHO 2004 classification of testicular tumors

Germ cell tumors
Intratubular germ cell neoplasia, unclassified
Other types
Tumors of one histologic type (pure forms)
Seminoma
Seminoma with syncytiotrophoblastic cells
Spermatocytic seminoma
Spermatocytic seminoma with sarcoma
Embryonal carcinoma
Yolk sac tumor
Trophoblastic tumors
Choriocarcinoma
Trophoblastic neoplasms other than choriocarcinoma
Monophasic choriocarcinoma
Placental site trophoblastic tumor
Teratoma
Dermoid cyst
Monodermal teratoma
Teratoma with somatic type malignancies
Tumors of more than one histologic type (mixed forms)
Mixed embryonal carcinoma and teratoma
Mixed teratoma and seminoma
Choriocarcinoma and teratoma/embryonal carcinoma
Others
Sex cord/gonadal stromal tumors
Pure forms
Leydig cell tumor
Malignant Leydig cell tumor
Sertoli cell tumor
Sertoli cell tumor lipid rich variant
Sclerosing Sertoli cell tumor
Large cell calcifying Sertoli cell tumor
Malignant Sertoli cell tumor
Granulosa cell tumor
Adult type granulosa cell tumor
Juvenile type granulosa cell tumor
Tumors of the thecoma/fibroma group
Thecoma
Fibroma
Sex cord/gonadal stromal tumor incompletely differentiated
Sex cord/gonadal stromal tumor, mixed forms
Malignant sex cord/gonadal stromal tumor
Tumors containing both germ cell and sex cord/gonadal stromal element Gonadoblastoma
Germ cell–sex cord/gonadal stromal tumor, unclassified

(continued)

Table 4.1 (continued)

Miscellaneous tumors of the testis
Carcinoid tumor
Tumors of ovarian epithelial types
Serous tumor of borderline malignancy
Serous carcinoma
Well-differentiated endometrioid carcinoma
Mucinous cystadenoma
Mucinous cystadenocarcinoma
Brenner tumor
Nephroblastoma
Paraganglioma
Hematopoietic tumors
Tumors of collecting ducts and rete
Adenoma
Carcinoma
Tumors of paratesticular structures
Adenomatoid tumor
Malignant mesothelioma
Benign mesothelioma
Well-differentiated papillary mesothelioma
Cystic mesothelioma
Adenocarcinoma of the epididymis
Papillary cystadenoma of the epididymis
Melanotic neuroectodermal tumor
Desmoplastic small round cell tumor
Mesenchymal tumors of the spermatic cord and testicular adnexae
Secondary tumors of the testis (metastases)

4.2.1 Germ Cell Tumors

4.2.1.1 Overview

- Carcinoma in situ (CIS) cells develop from primordial germ cells and early gonocytes. Placenta-like alkaline phosphatase (PLAP) was the first marker described in CIS and seminoma. Of greater importance for an understanding germ cell oncogenesis was the discovery of factors essential for maintaining pluri-potency and self-renewal capability of embryonic stem cells CD117 (c-KIT) and OCT-3/4 (OCT-4).
- The best support for the theory of the common origin of the germ cell tumors (GCTs) is the presence of the iso-chromosome i(12p), a chromosome with four short arms present in about 80 % of GCTs regardless of

their morphology. Non-seminomatous GCTs (NSGCTs) usually have more i(12p) copies of than Seminomas.

- GCTs are rare tumors and account for only 1–2 % of malignant tumors in males. White men living in Western industrialized countries show the highest incidence rates, whereas black men in Africa show the lowest. The incidence in Asiatic men lies somewhere between both extremes.
- Well-established epidemiologic causes of GCTs are listed in Table 4.2. The average age of patients at presentation significantly correlates with the pathologic type of GCTs (Table 4.3).

Table 4.2 Causes of germ cell tumors and the relative risk

Cryptorchidism	2–17-fold
Contralateral GCT	25-fold
Familial GCT	3.8–7.6-fold
Male infertility	1.6–10-fold
Gonadal dysgenesis	30–50-fold
Testicular atrophy	2.7–12.7-fold
Surgery (trauma)	Low risk
Occupational exposure	1.1–14.7-fold
Mother older than 30 years old	Low risk
Mother breast cancer	Low risk
Birth weight <2.5 kg	1–13.5-fold
High socioeconomic status, microlithiasis, infectious diseases	probably no risk

Table 4.3 The typical age presentation of patients with germ cell tumors

Seminoma	35–40 y
	Extremely rare before puberty
Spermatocytic seminoma	Average 52 y
	Rare after 70 y
Embryonal carcinoma	Average age 30 y
	Rare before puberty and after 50 y
Teratoma (pure form)	Average age in children 20 months
	Rare after the age of 4 y
	Adults 20–30 y
Choriocarcinoma	Average age 25–30 y
Yolk sac tumor (pure form)	Average age 25–30 y
	15–40 % of GCTs in children
Mixed forms	33 y if seminoma prevails
	28 y if NSGCT prevails

y years

4.2.2 Intratubular Germ Cell Neoplasia, Unclassified (IGCNU)

4.2.2.1 Overview

- Intratubular germ cell neoplasia (IGCNU) is the official name of the lesion, better known as *carcinoma* in situ of the testis or testicular intratubular neoplasia. The adjective “unclassified” is utilized to emphasize that the morphology of the tumor cells does not permit an assignment to a definite type of GCT.
- If the intratubular tumor cells can be definitely recognized, the adjective intratubular is used in connection with the respective name of the GCT (i.e. intratubular embryonal carcinoma or intratubular seminoma). The prevalence of IGCNU in healthy men is estimated 0.4–0.8 % and about 1 % in infertile men. In cryptorchid testes of adults the frequency is 2–4 %. With the exception of spermatocytic seminoma, atypical germ cells are constantly found (in 98 % of the healthy tissue surrounding invasive GCTs of adults (Table 4.4).

4.2.2.2 Pathology

- The IGCNU cells are attached to the usually thickened basement membrane and push the Sertoli cells towards the lumen of the seminiferous tubules. The cytoplasm is clear because of the large amount of glycogen (PAS+). The nuclei are bigger than those of spermatogonia and contain one or more nucleoli (Fig. 4.1).
- Mitoses are frequent but may be overlooked. IGCNU can also spread in a ‘pagetoid’ pattern into the rete testis or present as microinvasive lesion. Lymphocytic infiltration of the interstitial tissue surrounding the affected, mostly clearly narrowed tubules is frequent.

Table 4.4 Prevalence of intratubular germ cell neoplasia unclassified

Infertile men	1.0 %
Healthy men	0.4–0.9 %
Intersex	20 %
Cryptorchid testis of adults	2–4 %
Retroperitoneal ‘extragonadal’ GCT	49 %
Patients with germ cell tumor–contralateral testis	4–6 %

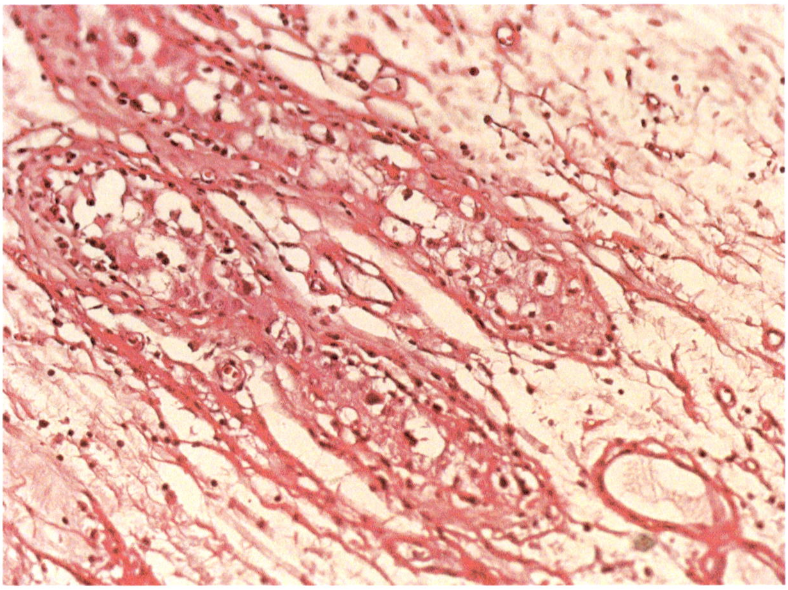

Fig. 4.1 Intratubular germ cell neoplasia unclassified

4.2.2.3 Immunohistochemistry

- PLAP, c-KIT (CD117), and OCT 3/4 antibodies are positive, and can thus easily be distinguished from non-reacting normal spermatogonia, which are PAS-. IGCNU are aneuploidy and gain i(12p) copies only shortly before they become microinvasive.

4.2.3 Germ Cell Tumors of One Histologic Type

- Seminoma is the most common pure germ cell tumor followed by embryonal carcinoma. Pure yolk sac tumor occurs almos exclusivelly in infants. Main clinico-pathologic characteristics of these tumors follow.

4.2.4 Seminoma

- About half of intrascrotal tumors are seminomas. Patients are on average 30–34 years of age. Most common GCT in its pure form.

4.2.4.1 Pathology

- The affected testis is usually enlarged, but can be normal or even atrophic. The tumor is uniform, cream-coloured or pink, and always well-circumscribed. The cut surface is lobulated and the consistency varies from soft to firm, depending on the amount of tumor stroma. Nowadays in the majority of cases the tumors are confined to the testis, but extension to the epididymis and spermatic cord can occur and were very frequent (43 %) in old series. In large tumors necrosis may occur (Fig. 4.2).
- Hemorrhage is not frequent and can indicate the presence of a non-seminomatous tumor component. Small hemorrhagic spots are very characteristic of seminoma with syncytiotrophoblastic giant cells.

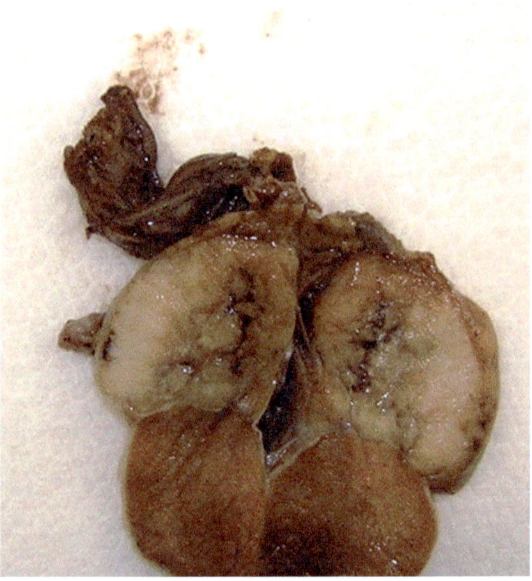

Fig. 4.2 Gross features of testicular seminoma

- Seminoma cells are rather uniform with a rounded shape and a mostly clear, glycogen- (PAS-positive) and lipid-rich cytoplasm. In 'classical' seminomas tumor cells typically grow in cords and/or nests separated by more or less delicate trabeculae. In some cases, however, small nests of tumor cells are surrounded by abundant fibrotic tissue (Figs. 4.3, 4.4, 4.5, 4.6 and 4.7; Table 4.5).
- Lymphocytic infiltration of tumor stroma is a typical feature of about 90 % of seminoma and can be used as a diagnostic criterion in poorly preserved, improperly processed surgical specimens.
- The amount of lymphatic infiltration varies from some few lymphocytes to heavy infiltration and formation of lymphoid follicles. Furthermore, in about one-third of seminomas, epithelioid granulomas also develop.
- Lymphocytic infiltrates probably represent a true immunologic reaction directed against the tumor. In fact, in old series, observed before the introduction of new therapy protocoling, lymphocyte rich seminomas

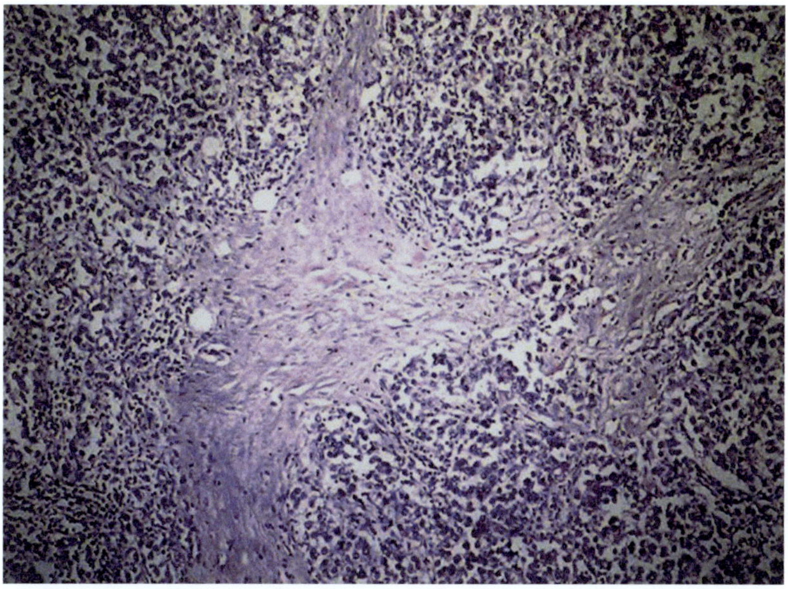

Fig. 4.3 Seminoma. Low power microscopic features of neoplastic seminoma cells with mild lymphocytic infiltration

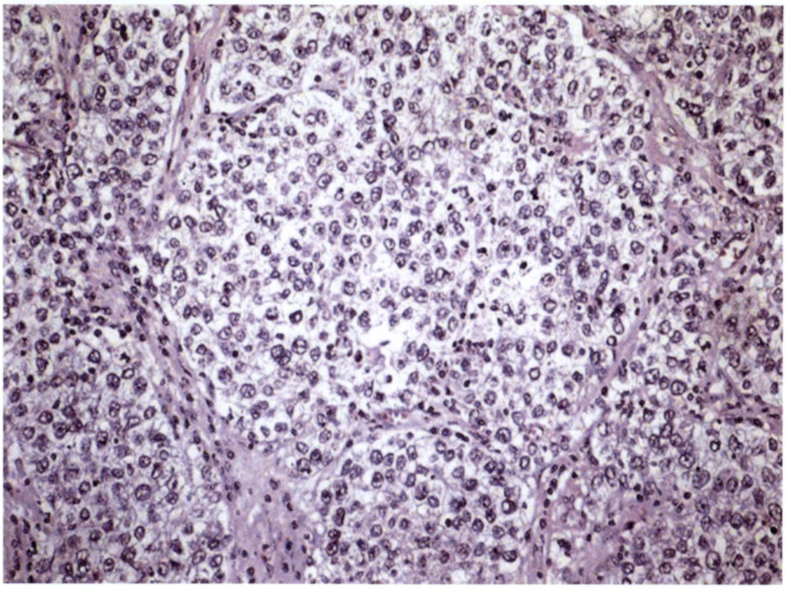

Fig. 4.4 Seminoma. Large nests of neoplastic seminoma cells showing clear cytoplasm and scarce connective tissue

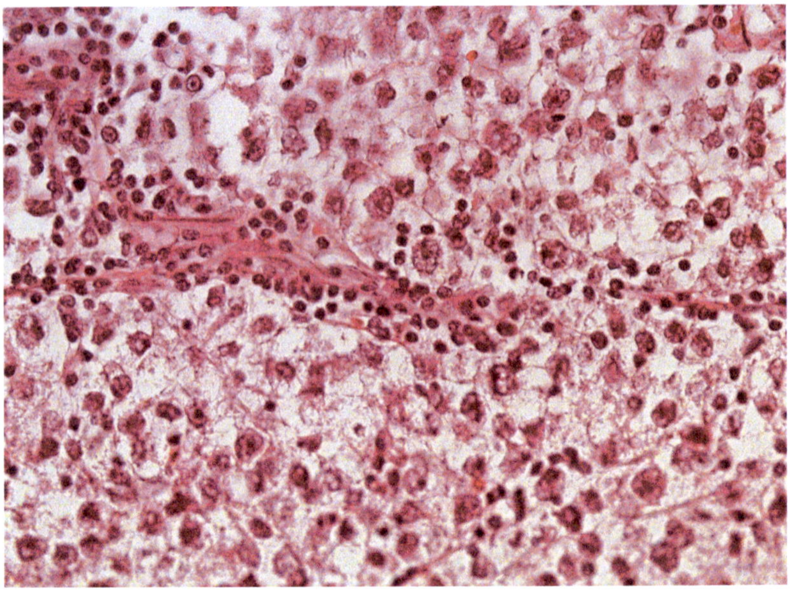

Fig. 4.5 Lymphocytes in stroma are common in some seminomas

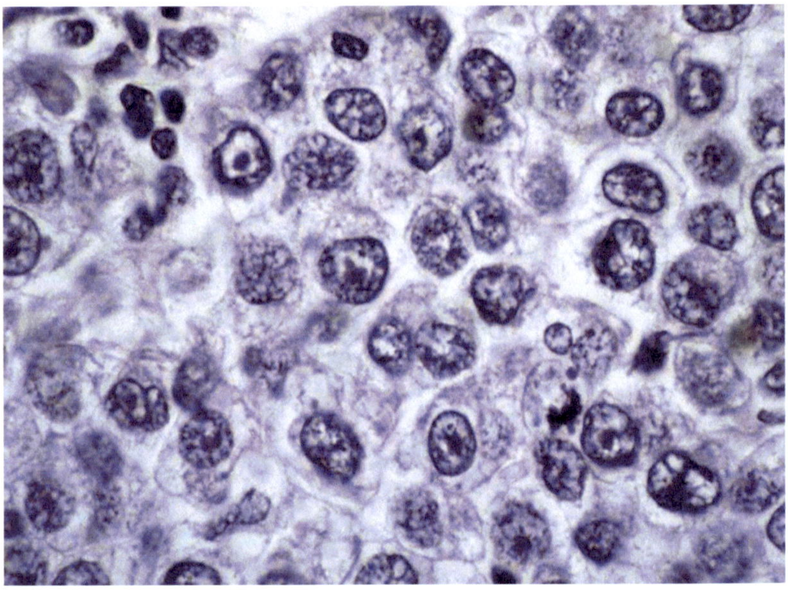

Fig. 4.6 High power view of seminoma cells

did significantly better than those without lymphocytes.

4.2.4.2 Morphologic Variations

- Seminoma with syncytiotrophoblastic cells: using H&E staining multinucleated giant cells are detected in about 7 % of seminomas, mostly in the surroundings of vessels. With immunohistochemistry against hCG, however, positive cells are present in about 25 % of all cases. The presence of hCG cells should not be confused with true choriocarcinomas.
- Accumulation of edematous fluid in interstitial tissue gives the tumor a microcystic or cribriform (seminoma) appearance.
- In pseudoglandular and tubular seminoma, tumor cells form small gland-like clefts.
- The name intratubular or interstitial seminoma derives from the predominant way the tumor cells spread.

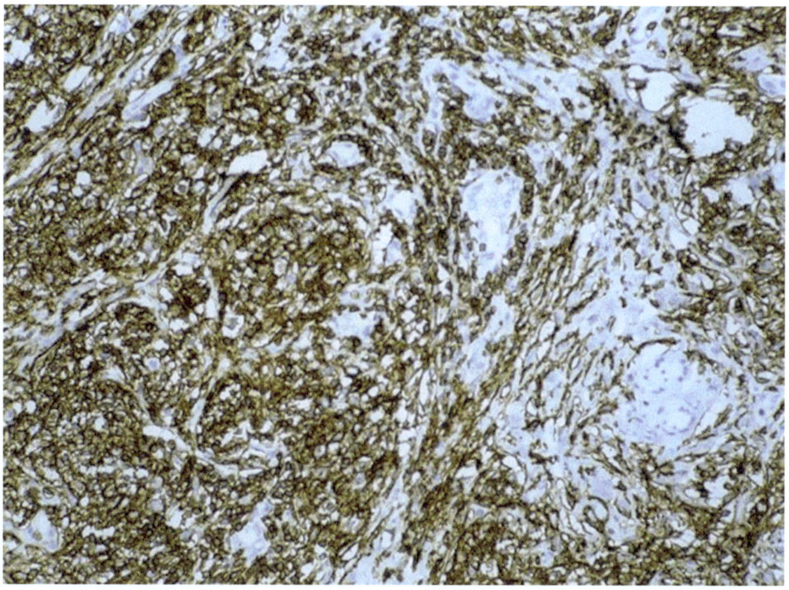

Fig. 4.7 PLAP expression in seminoma

Table 4.5 Different pathologic variants of seminoma

Intratubular seminoma
Interstitial seminoma
Tubular seminoma
Cribriform seminoma
Pseudoglandular seminoma
Microcystic seminoma
Seminoma with high mitotic rate

- The formerly anaplastic or atypical seminomas have been renamed as seminomas with high mitotic rate, which is indeed more appropriate because the degree of cellular anaplasia is not higher than in the classical type. High proliferative activity measured by counting mitoses or cells positive for proliferation markers (Ki 67) does not, however, negatively influence the course of the disease (Table 4.5).

4.2.4.3 Immunohistochemistry

- Seminoma cells react with many different antibodies. For diagnostic purposes, however, only a few are really important. The most frequent misdiagnosis is to confound seminoma with embryonal carcinoma, which usually happens when the surgical specimen is improperly fixed.
- Seminoma cells stain with CD 117 (c-kit) and do not react with CD 30 antibodies, whereas the cells of embryonal carcinoma are CD117-negative and CD30-positive.
- In some rare seminomas, single tumor cells are cytokeratin- and CD 30-positive. OCT4 is typically positive in seminoma and embryonal carcinoma. Likewise, yolk sac tumor, spermatocytic seminoma, and choriocarcinoma are all OCT4 negative. Almost all seminomas (and cases of IGCNU) express podoplanin on the cytoplasmic membranes, whereas embryonal carcinomas are either negative or, in about 30 % of the cases, show limited reactivity that is restricted to the apical surfaces of the cells. SOX1 occurs in about 95 % of seminomas and is negative in embryonal carcinoma. CD 30 positive reactivity occurs in 93–100 % of embryonal carcinomas but the other germ cell tumors, including seminoma, are either negative or show only rare positive cells.
- Rarely, these tumors are mistaken for lymphoma. This typically spread interstitially among the entrapped, atrophic seminiferous tubules.

4.2.4.4 Genetics

- Seminomas are, without exception, aneuploid tumor with low copy number of i(12p).

Table 4.6 Prognostic factors predictive of metastasis in seminoma

Diameter >40 mm	Strong evidence
Age <30 years	Equivocal
Invasion of rete testis	Strong evidence
Vascular invasion	Equivocal

4.2.4.5 Prognostic Factors

- The most important prognostic factors are the diameter of the tumor and the invasion of the rete testis, whereas vascular invasion seems not to have the same prognostic importance as in NSGCT (Table 4.6)

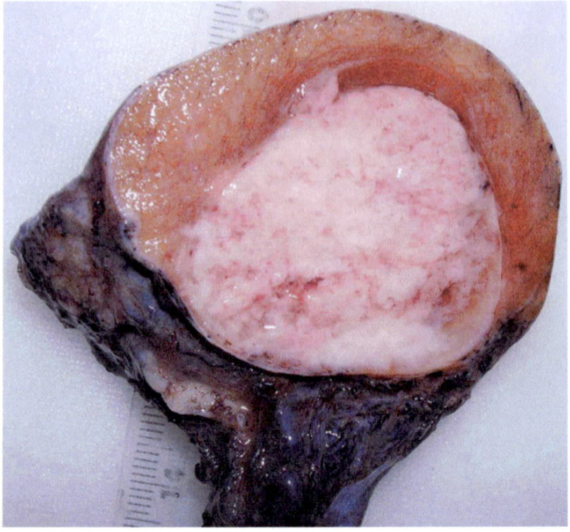

Fig. 4.8 Gross features of spermatocytic seminoma

4.2.5 Spermatocytic Seminoma

- It arises only in the male gonad and represents 1–4 % of seminomas. Patients are older (average 52 years) than those with other types of GCTs. Asynchronous bilateral occurrence is also more frequent (9 %) than in other TGCTs.
- There are no racial differences or causal relationships with cryptorchidism.

4.2.5.1 Pathology

- The cut surface is described as mucoid, gelatinous or edematous showing cystic, necrotic, and even hemorrhagic areas. The tumor tissue is yellowish or cream-colored, well circumscribed and can be multinodular. The tumor grows in an expansive and not infiltrative manner.
- Microscopically, the tumor borders are sharp. Three different tumor cell types are present. The large (15–20 μm) cells with rather regular round nucleus predominate. The small cells (6–8 μm) resemble lymphocytes and the single scattered giant cells (50–150 μm). All have nuclei with a coarse chromatin.
- Lymphocytes are scanty and in the neighboring tubules IGCNUs cells are missed. Intratubular spread of tumor cells is frequent. The polymorphous micromorphology with many mitotic figures gives the impression of an extremely aggressive tumor (Fig. 4.8, 4.9 and 4.10).
- The so-called anaplastic spermatocytic seminoma contains a monomorphous population of large cells with big nucleoli that has no prognostic significance. Spermatocytic seminoma combined with sarcoma, mostly rhabdomyosarcoma, has been described and is a very aggressive disease.

4.2.5.2 Immunohistochemistry

- The tumor cells are negative for all markers which are commonly found in GCTs. The PLAP reaction is, with very few exceptions, negative. Forty percent of spermatocytic seminomas are CD117+ and some few show a dot-like focal perinuclear reaction for low molecular-weight cytokeratin (CAM 5.2). Spermatocytic seminoma is OCT4 negative, a fact that can be used to differentiate from seminoma and embryonal carcinoma in selected cases, since both are positive.

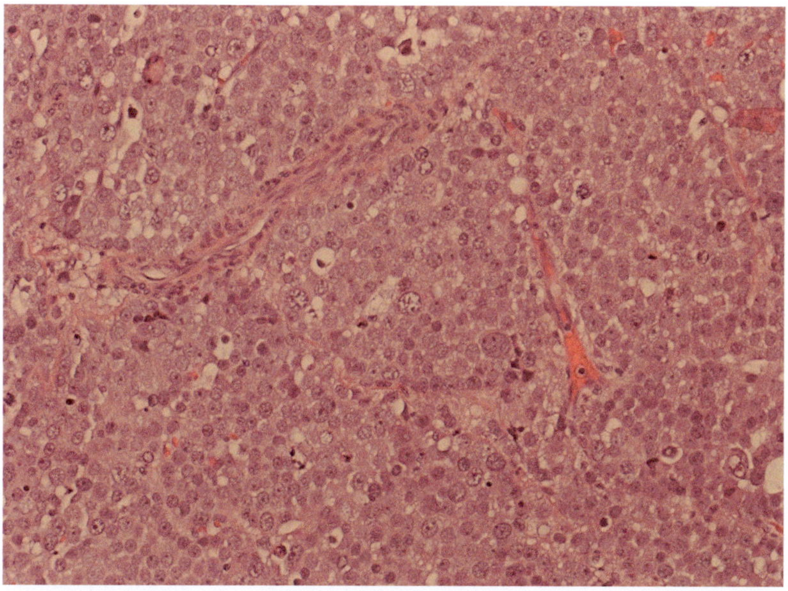

Fig. 4.9 Microscopic features of spermatocytic seminoma

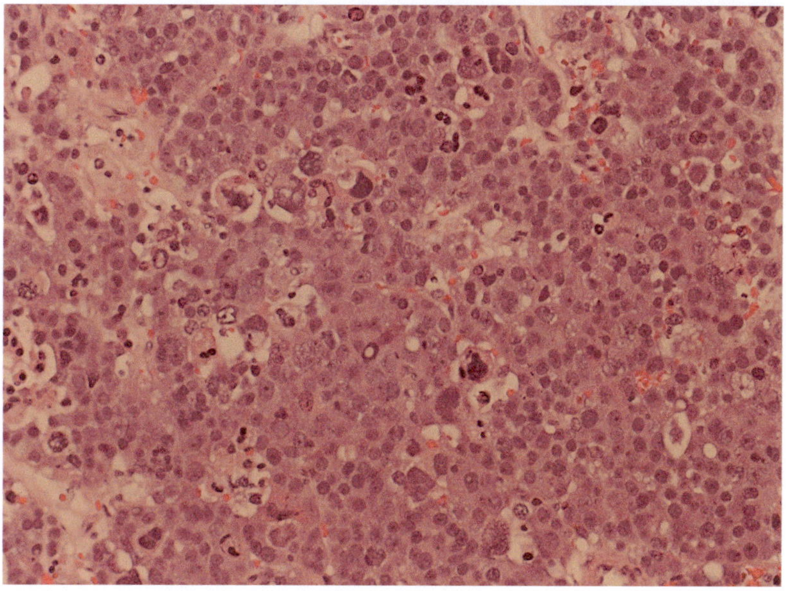

Fig. 4.10 Three cell type characteristic of spermatocytic seminoma

4.2.5.3 Genetics

- The tumor cells are polyploid or aneuploid. Gain of chromosome 9 combined with an unchanged chromosome 12 seems to be specific for this tumor.

4.2.5.4 Prognostic Factors

- Usually these tumors are confined to the testis and never relapse and only rarely metastasize. The sarcoma component in mixed tumors metastasizes primarily to the lung and may be responsible of patient dead.

4.3 Non-seminomatous Germ Cell Tumors (NSGCTs)

4.3.1 Embryonal Carcinoma

- The pure form of embryonal carcinoma (EC) accounts only for 2–10 % of all GCTs, but is very frequent (80 %) in mixed neoplasms with more than one germ cell component. The patients are on average 30 years old.

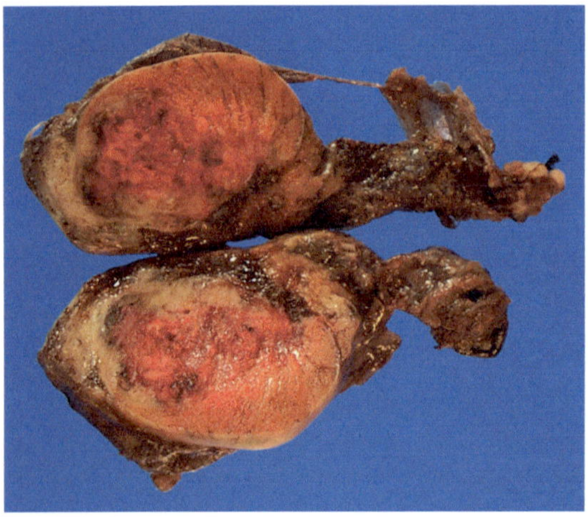

Fig. 4.11 Gross features of embryonal carcinoma of the testes

4.3.1.1 Pathology

- The tumors are usually small and the cut surface is granular. Necrosis and small hemorrhagic spots give the grayish colored tumor. The growth pattern can be solid, papillary, glandular, or tubular (predominant architectural pattern occupying at least 50 %). Less common primary patterns include nested, anastomosing glandular, micropapillary, sieve-like glandular, pseudopapillary, and blastocyst-like. Rarely, embryonal carcinoma develops in the context of polyembryoma-like (Fig. 4.11, 4.12, 4.13, 4.14, 4.15, 4.16, 4.17, 4.18 and 4.19).
- Occasionally, EC may present significant chronic inflammation and granulomatous lesion suggesting seminoma. Also, features suggesting endodermal sinus tumor or teratoma may be seen.
- The tumor cells are large primitive epithelial cells with a cytoplasm varying from amphophilic to basophilic or clear (seminoma-like cells). Finding intratubular spreading tumor masses with central necrosis is common.
- The large pleomorphic and hypercromatic nuclei contain one or more large eosinophilic nucleoli. Mitoses are abundant. Syncytiotrophoblast giant cells may be present. Half of cases show vascular invasion.

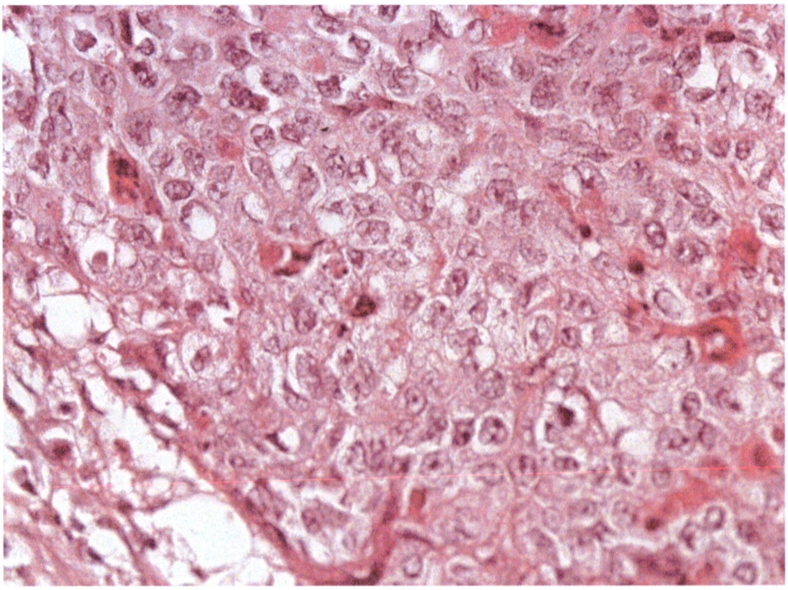

Fig. 4.12 Embryonal carcinoma of the testes showing solid growth

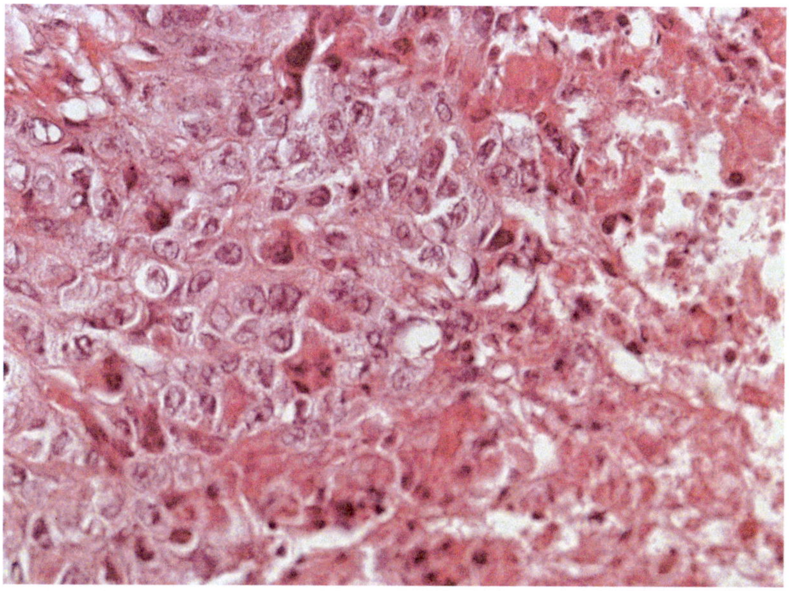

Fig. 4.13 Embryonal carcinoma of the testes showing solid growth and focal tumor necrosis

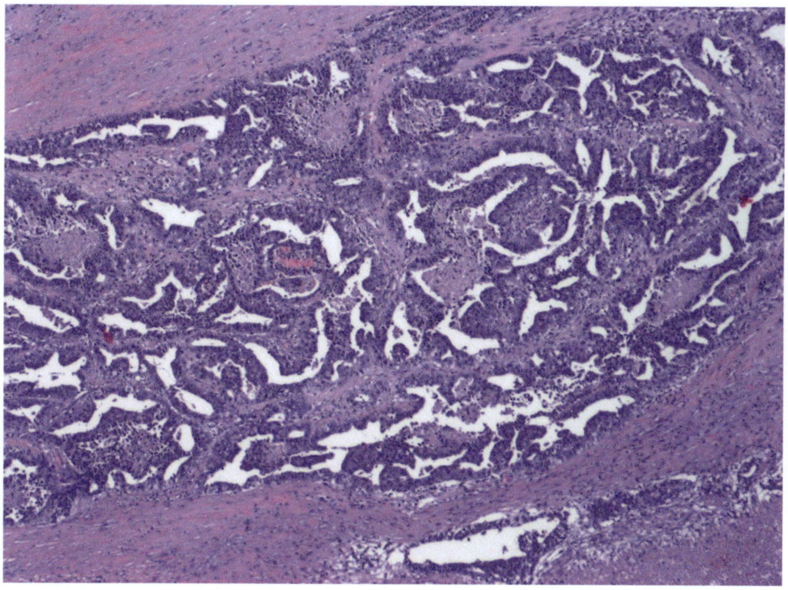

Fig. 4.14 Embryonal carcinoma showing anastomosing glandular architecture

4.3.1.2 Immunohistochemistry

- The positive staining with cytokeratin antibodies (AE1/AE3; CAM 5.2) confirms the epithelial nature of these tumors. Unlike with seminomas, the PLAP reaction is only focally positive.
- The strong and specific staining with CD 30 (Ki 1, Ber-H2) can lead to a wrong diagnosis of giant cell (immunoblastic) lymphoma. Nuclear expression of OCT4 and SALL4 is common in EC. As already mentioned, ECs are negative for CD 117, whereas seminomas do not react with cytokeratin antibodies and CD 30. SOX1 occurs in about 95 % of seminomas and is negative in embryonal carcinoma.

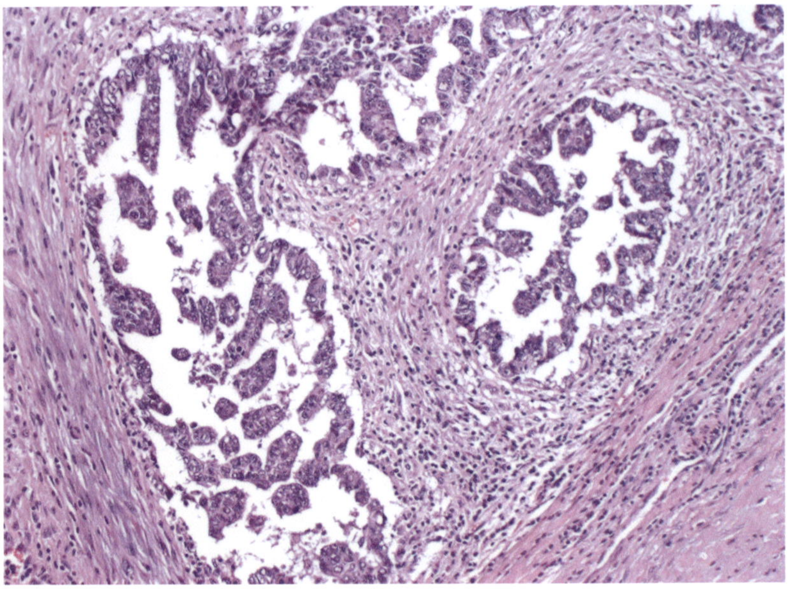

Fig. 4.15 Embryonal carcinoma showing glandular and micropapillary architecture

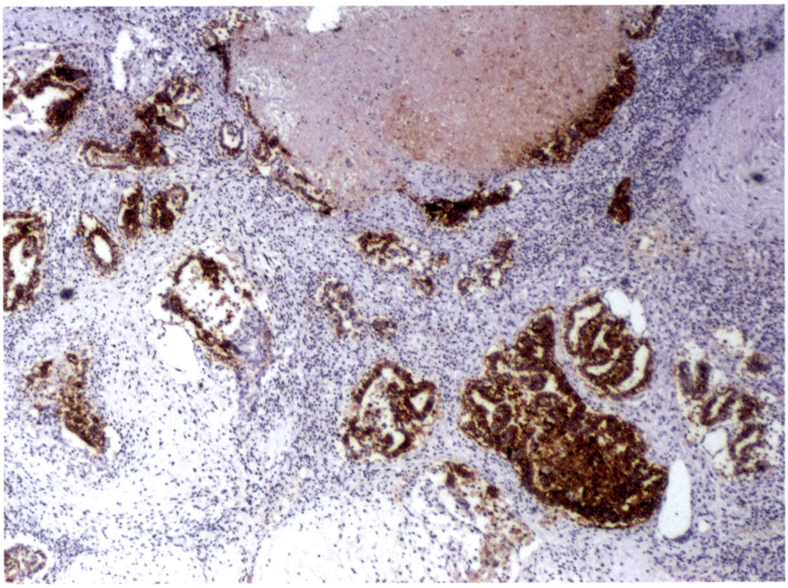

Fig. 4.16 CD30 is positive in embryonal carcinoma

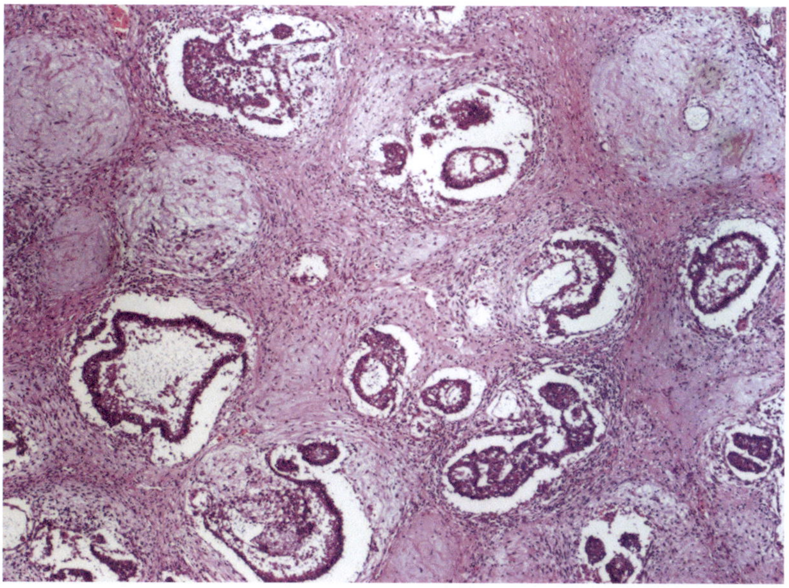

Fig. 4.17 Embryonal carcinoma showing tubular architecture

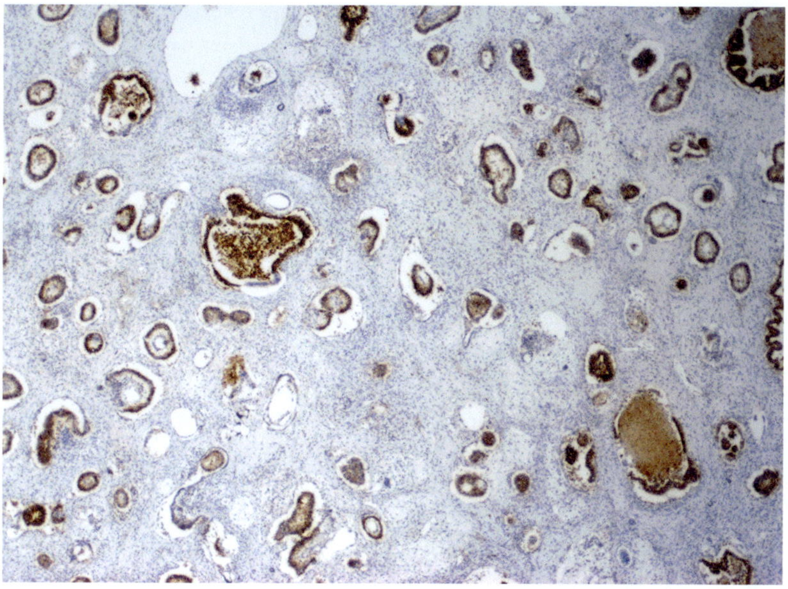

Fig. 4.18 Tubular structures highlighted with anti-CD30 immunhistochemistry

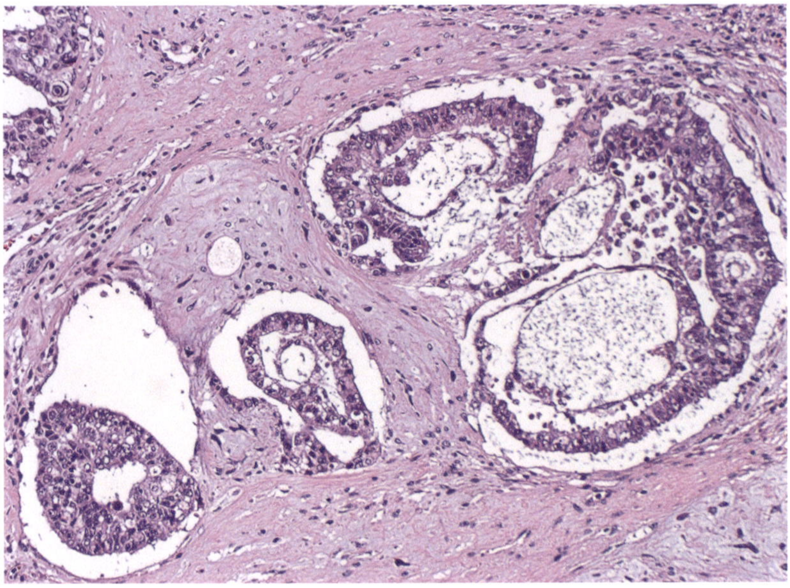

Fig. 4.19 Embryonal carcinoma showing blastocyst-like features

4.3.1.3 Genetics

- The aneuploid or even triploid tumor cells show manifold chromosomal aberrations, most constant being the presence of i(12p). The number of i(12p) copies seems to correlate with the aggressiveness of the EC.

4.4 Yolk Sac Tumor

- The pure form of yolk sac tumor (YST) is the most frequent (80 %) GCT of childhood. The average patient age is about 18 months, since most tumors arise in the first 2 years of life. In adults, YST is a frequent (40 %) component of mixed GCT, but rare in pure form.

4.4.1 Pathology

- The tumor is not encapsulated and is yellow or white in color. Tissue consistency is usually soft, but can also be firm. Necrosis and hemorrhages are present, especially in large tumors of adults. Cystic changes are common.

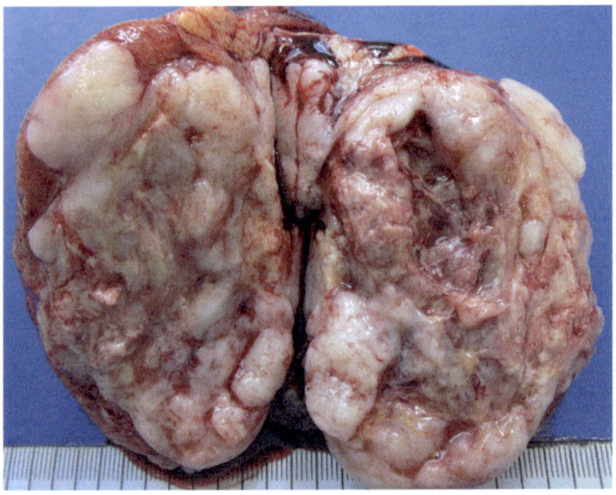

Fig. 4.20 Gross view of pure yolk sac tumor

- The microscopic picture is that of a confusing variety of cells and patterns, but in sporadic cases the tumor is composed of one single cell type or only one histologic pattern.
- Microcystic, papillary, and solid, spindle cell, and mucoid areas can alternate in the different parts of the tumor and produce a meshwork with spaces appearing to be empty or glandular and pseudoglandular structures (Figs. 4.20, 4.21, 4.22, 4.23, 4.24, 4.25, 4.26, 4.27, 4.28 and 4.29).

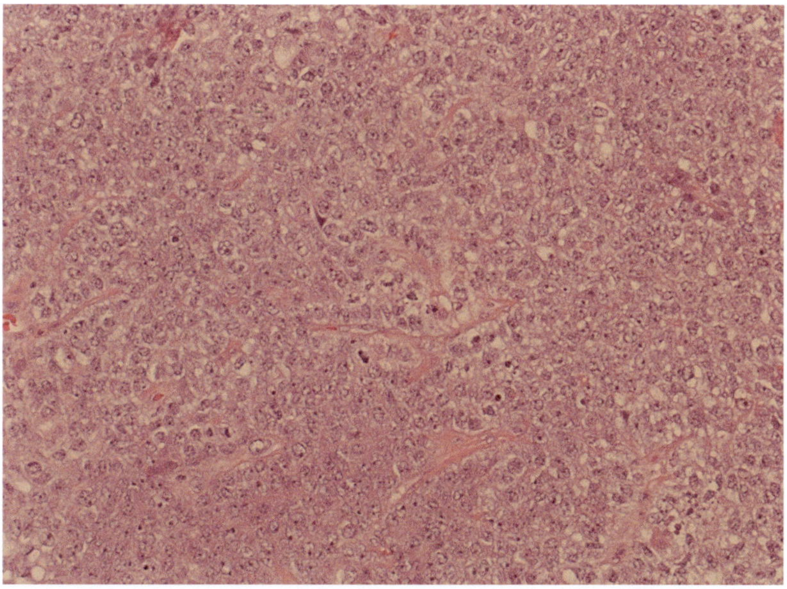

Fig. 4.21 Solid growth pattern of yolk sac tumor

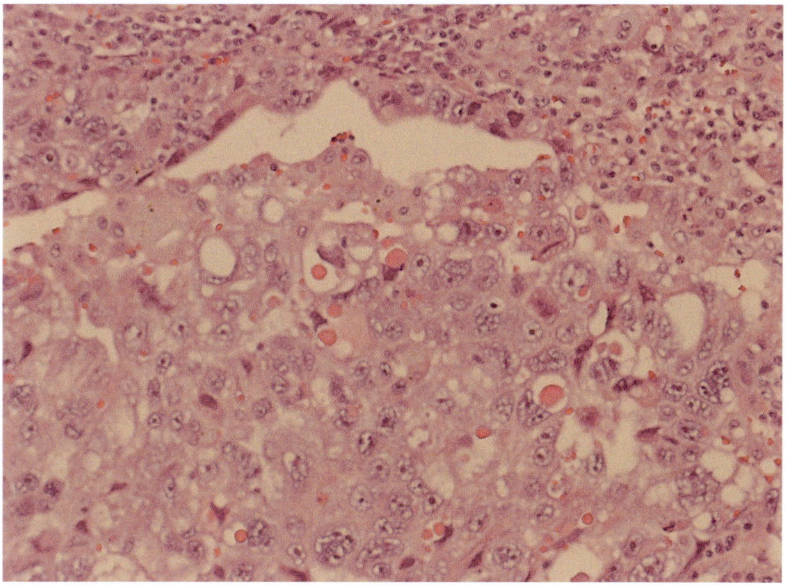

Fig. 4.22 Solid microscopic pattern of yolk sac tumor with hyaline globules

- Structures resembling yolk sac (vitelline) are not always present. Characteristic Schiller–Duval bodies simulate the endoderm with cuboidal cells covering a vascularized stalk of connective tissue. PAS+ (diastase-resistant) hyaline globules are common. Histologic growth patterns (Table 4.7) lack any clinical significance.

4.4.2 Immunohistochemistry

- Immunohistochemically all tumor cells react strongly positive with cytokeratin antibodies, and, unlike embryonal carcinoma, is negatively with CD 30. AFP is positive in 74–100 % of cases.

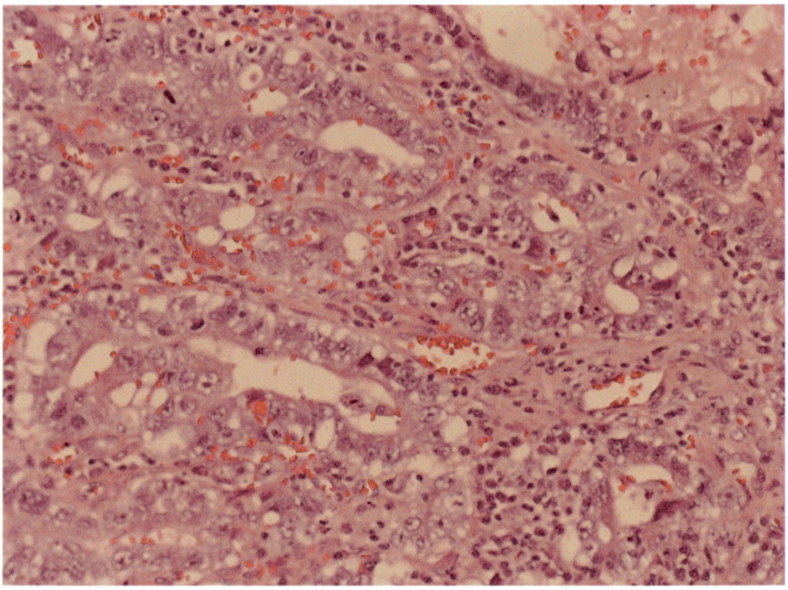

Fig. 4.23 Glandular pattern of yolk sac tumor

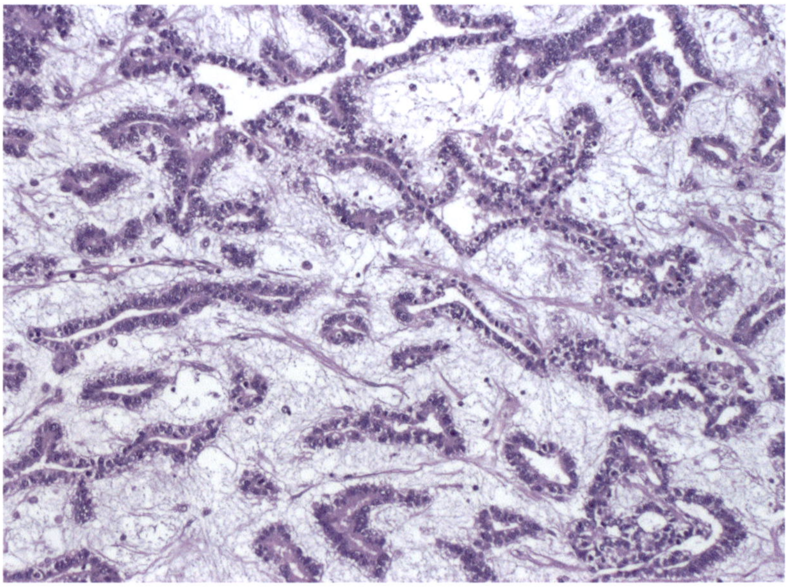

Fig. 4.24 Glandular pattern of yolk sac tumor with myxoid stroma

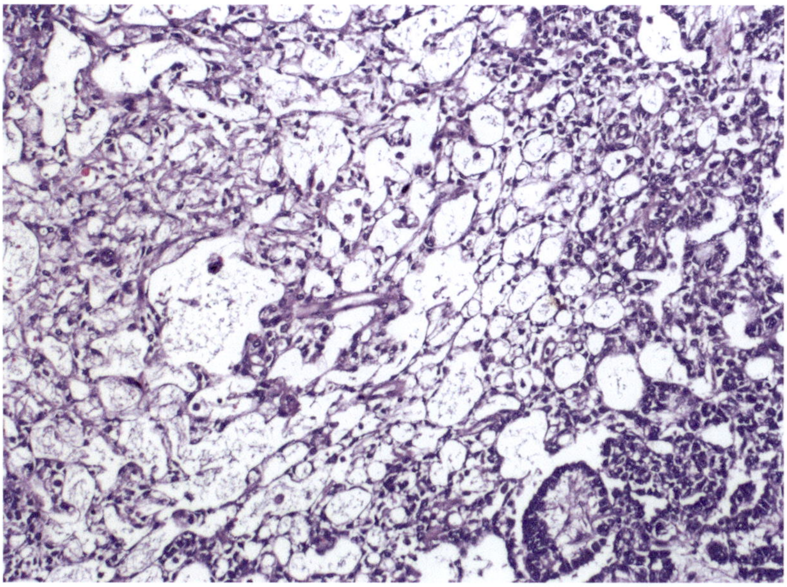

Fig. 4.25 Microcystic pattern of yolk sac tumor

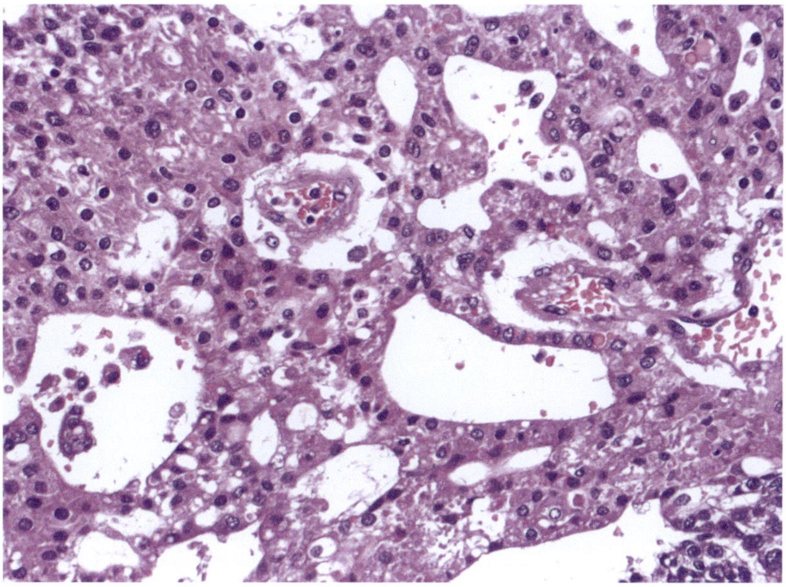

Fig. 4.26 Hepatoid pattern of yolk sac tumor

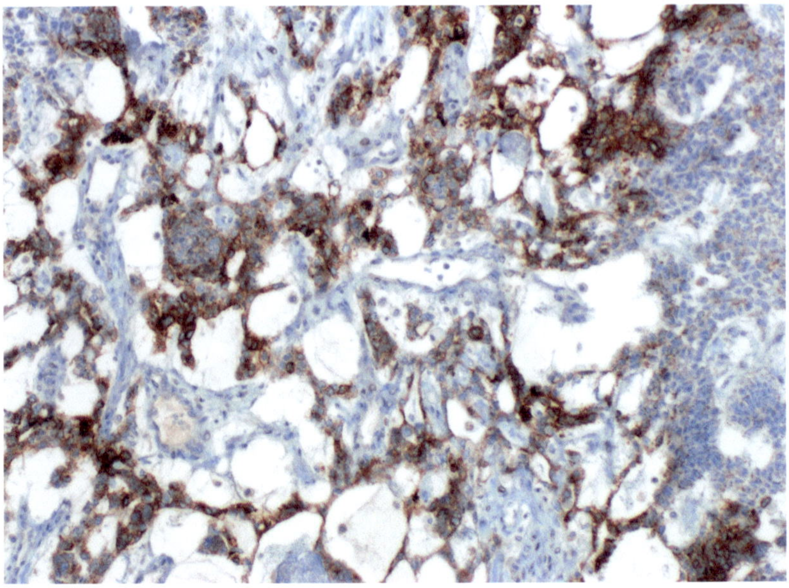

Fig. 4.27 Glypican-3 expression in hepatoid yolk sac tumor

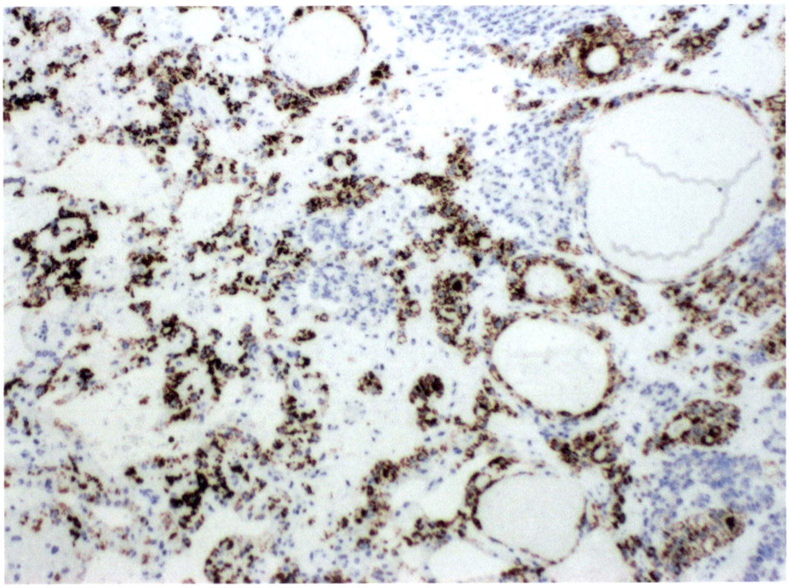

Fig. 4.28 Heppar-1 expression in hepatoid yolk sac tumor

- In children completely negative or patchy positive tumors can be observed. To avoid wrong diagnosis, awide sampling is advisable; also because AFP-positive tumor cells are encountered in one-third of ECs. Expression of SALL4 and glypican 3 but not OCT4 is characteristic of YST.

4.4.3 Genetics

- Loss of 1p and 6q is rather typical for infantile YST.

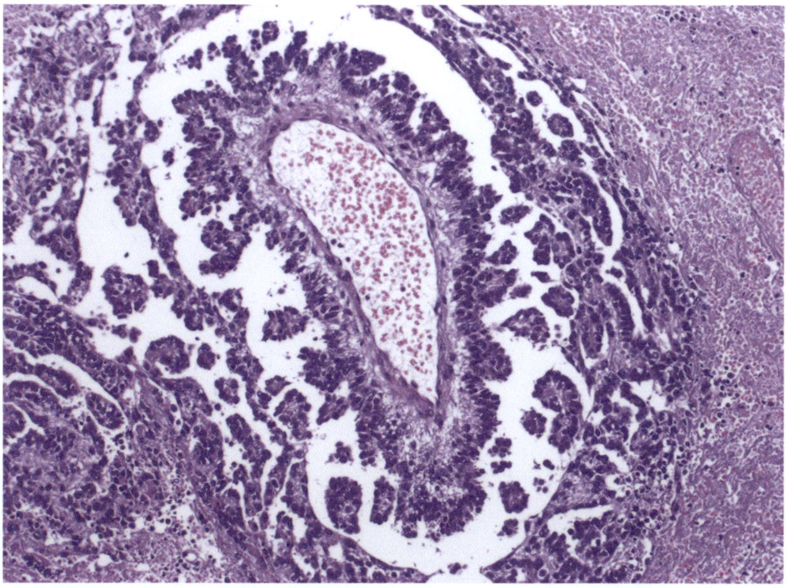

Fig. 4.29 Schiller–Duval bodies in yolk sac tumor

Table 4.7 Pathologic patterns of yolk sac tumor

Microcystic–reticular
Macrocystic
Papillary
Endodermal sinus
Solid pattern
Myxomatous
Glandular–alveolar
Sarcomatoid–spindle cell
Vitelline
Hepatoid
Parietal

4.5 Polyembryoma

- This tumor never occurs in pure form and invariably represents only a microscopically detectable structure, which is part of a NSGCT, frequently of a teratoma (Fig. 4.30).
- The 'embryoid body' roughly resembles a presomitic embryo of about 14 days old. The 'embryoid bodies' are embedded in a myxomatous stroma and rare among other components of NSGCT.

4.6 Choriocarcinoma and Other Types of Throphoblastic Neoplasia

- Choriocarcinomas are the rarest GCT. The pure form accounts for less than 0.2 % of all GCTs.
- The patients are young, with a peak incidence between 25 and 30 years, and about 70 % of patients have metastatic disease at the time of diagnosis. Lung (100 %), liver (86 %), gastrointestinal tract (71 %), and brain (56 %) are the commonest, whereas the retroperitoneal lymph nodes are not involved.

4.6.1 Pathology

- Grossly the tumor is a small, hemorrhagic nodule sometimes surrounded by a rim of whitish preserved tumor tissue. The tumor masses are surrounded by blood and are located close to small vessels.
- The tumor consists of three cellular components: the cytotrophoblast, the intermediate trophoblast, and the syncytiotrophoblastic

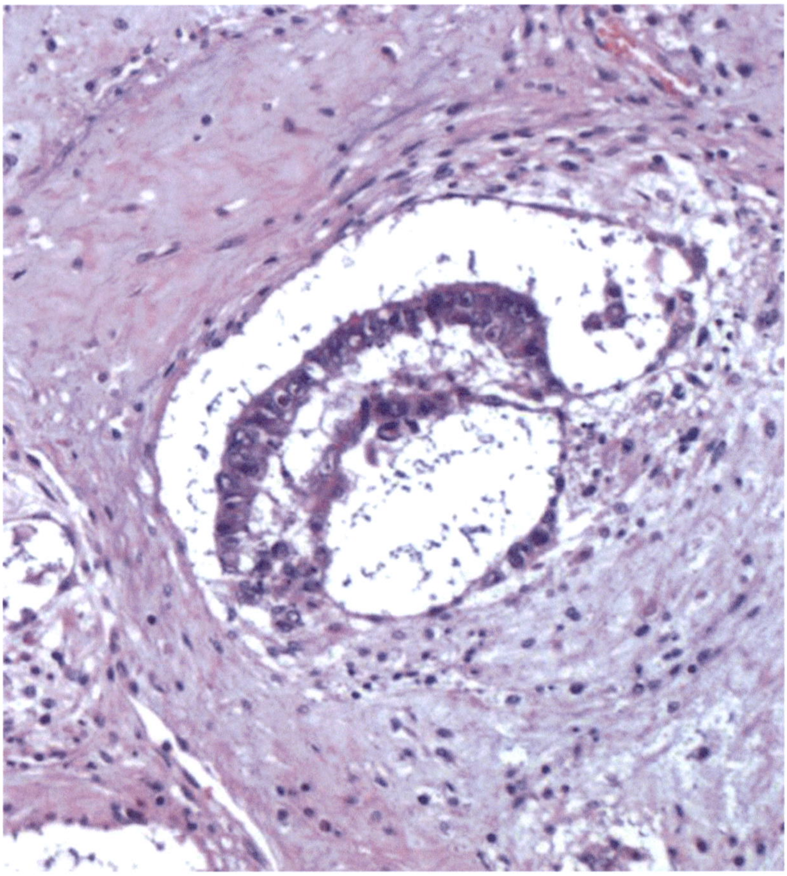

Fig. 4.30 Histologic features of embryoid body in Polyembryoma

giant cells, with cytotrophoblast being the most common cell and shows a water-clear cytoplasm; 'intermediate trophoblast' cells show more eosinophilic cytoplasm. The syncytiotrophoblastic giant cells lie on the surface of the cytotrophoblast (Figs. 4.31, 4.32 and 4.33).

4.6.2 Morphologic Variants

- Monophasic choriocarcinoma are tumors composed only of cytotrophoblasts (p63 +) lacking the syncytiotrophoblast giant cells. Tumors made out of solely intermediate cytotrophoblasts (p63 –) are called, as in the uterus, placental site trophoblastic tumor.

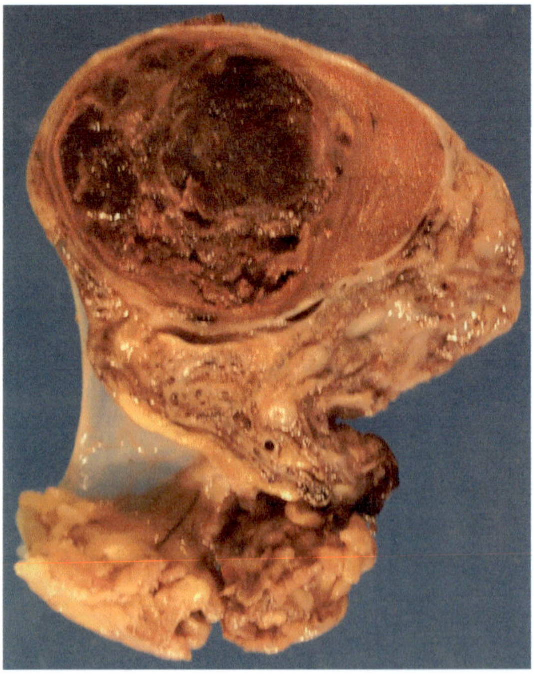

Fig. 4.31 Gross features of choriocarcinoma of the testes showing necrosis and hemorrhage

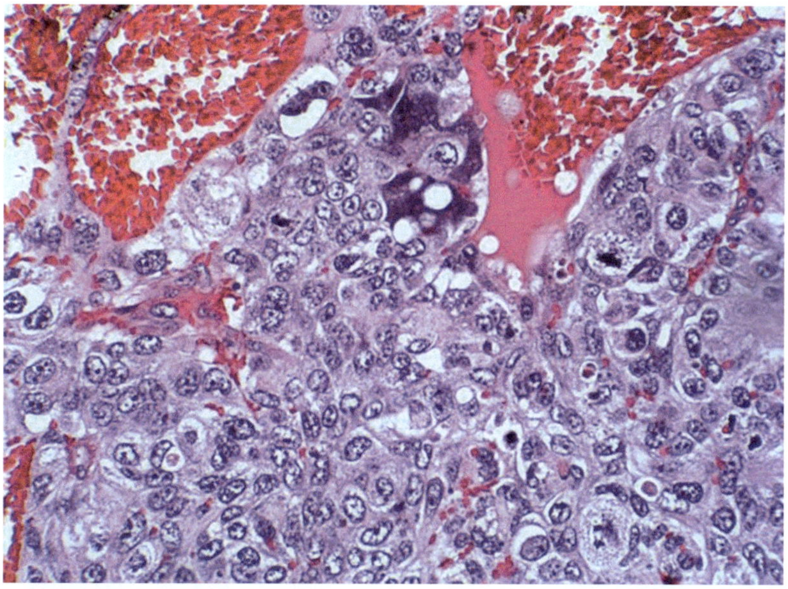

Fig. 4.32 Microscopic features of choriocarcinoma

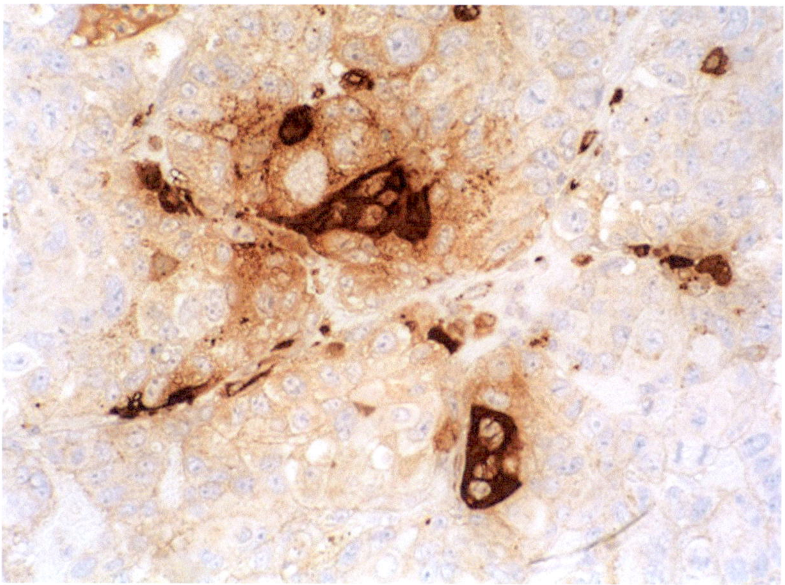

Fig. 4.33 Syncytiotrofoblast giant cells highlighted with anti-B-HCG immunohistochemistry

- Cystic trophoblastic variants have been described in metastatic sites post chemotherapy. Currently, it is regarded as variant of teratoma (Table 4.8).

Table 4.8 Cystic testicular lesions in childhood

Teratoma
Epidermoid cyst
Yolk sac tumor
Dermoid cyst
Ovarian type cystadenoma
Cystic lymphangioma
Juvenile granulosa cell tumor
Simple cysts
Cystic dysplasia of the rete testis

4.6.3 Immunohistochemistry

- All types of cytotrophoblast react immunohistochemically with cytokeratin antibodies

(CK 7, 8, 18, 19, CAM5.2, AE1/AE3) and with human placental lactogen.

- Syncytiotrophoblast giant cells obviously react strongly positive with β-hCG antibodies, and also express epithelial membrane antigen and α-inhibin. OCT4 is negative in choriocarcinoma. Monophasic choriocarcinoma is positive for p63. PLAP is variable positive. Cytotrophoblast may be β-hCG negative. Placental site tumor may react with EMA.

4.6.4 Genetics

- Some may exhibited the typical i(12p).

4.7 Teratoma

- Teratomas are, after YST, the second most frequent (14–20 %) GCT in infancy, with an average age of 20 months. In adults pure teratomas account for 3–7 % of GCTs but they are a component in more than half of the mixed germ cell tumors (Table 4.8).
- The tumor is benign in childhood, whereas in adults only epidermoid and dermoid cysts do not metastasize or relapse. In adults they are typically metastatic to the retroperitoneal lymph nodes

4.7.1 Pathology

- Composed of tissue components deriving from all three germinal layers–endo-, ecto-, and mesoderm. Thus, the gross morphology depends on the distribution and amount of single tumor components (Fig. 4.34).
- On the cut surface, glassy nodules representing cartilaginous areas, small cysts filled either with mucus or with laminated keratin, and pigmented areas can be recognized. In children the appearance is usually multicystic. Compared with other GCTs the consistency is always significantly more firm.

4.7.2 Variants

- Mature teratomas contain cysts lined by squamous or glandular epithelium of enteric type or ciliated respiratory type epithelium, and cysts can be filled with mucus or keratin. Organoid structures mimicking gut or bronchous are made of the corresponding epithelium encircled by smooth muscle. Neuroendocrine cells may be present.
- Mesodermal tissue is always represented by smooth muscle and mostly also by hyaline cartilage; bone with or without hematopoietic

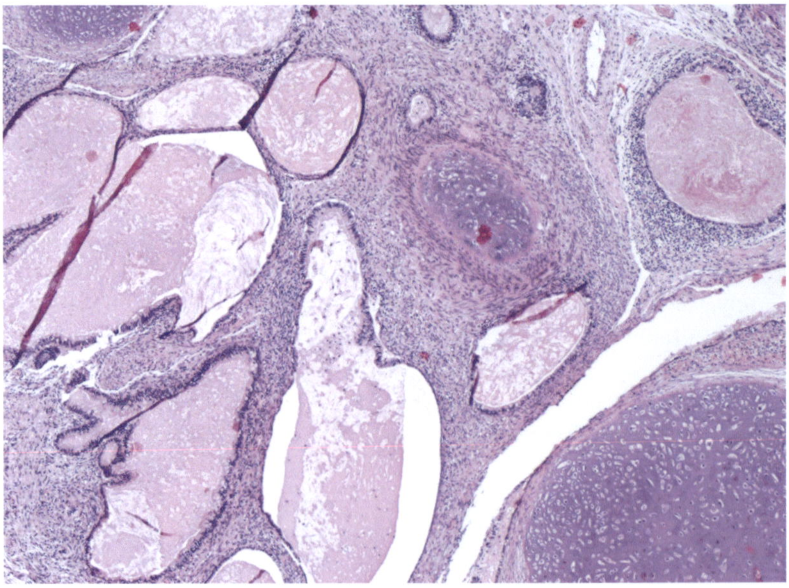

Fig. 4.34 Microscopic features of testicular teratoma showing cartilaginous areas and small cysts lined by glandular epithelium

marrow is less common. Differentiated liver, prostate, pancreas, and thyroid are rarities Neuroglia with ependymal differentiation is also a rather common component. Pigmented retinal epithelium can occasionally be seen.

- Immature teratomas contain an undifferentiated spindle cell mesenchymal stroma and small immature glands. Also the squamous epithelium is arranged in solid nests without keratinization. Other components are primitive neuroepithelium, renal blastema resembling Wilms tumor, rhabdomyoblasts, and fetal adipose tissue with lipoblasts.
- Dermoid cyst consists of cysts lined by epidermis with skin, hair follicle, and sebaceous glands. This teratoma type is common in the ovary but remains extremely rare in the testis and some authors challenge it malignant potential.
- Monodermal teratomas are those tumors in which a tissue component deriving from one germinal layer overgrows the other. The most frequent form is the primitive neuroectodermal tumor (PNET).
- The most common monodermal differentiated tumor is the epidermoid cyst which accounts for 1 % of all intrascrotal tumors and can arise at any age. They have a thin whitish wall and are filled with horny material arranged in a laminated layer (onionskin-like).
- The cyst is lined by an epidermis-like layer of squamous epithelium. Some authors regard the cyst as a teratoma only in cases when the surrounding testicular tissue presents IGCNU cells. Otherwise the cyst is considered to be a tumor-like lesion.
- If a non-germ cell tumor arises from a somatic tissue component, it is classified as teratoma with somatic type malignancy. Such malignancies become clinically important only if the somatic malignancy reaches a field of view by low magnification (4× objective).
- Sarcomas, in particular rhabdomyosarcoma, are the most common. But PNET tumors and squamous and adenocarcinomas have also been observed. Somatic type differentiation is seen in 4 % of patients with metastatic disease (Table 4.9).

Table 4.9 Somatic type malignancies seen in testicular teratoma

Rhabdomyosarcoma
Chondrosarcoma
Osteosarcoma
PNET
Adenocarcinoma
Malignant Schwannoma
Wilms tumor (Nephroblastoma)
Neuroendocrine carcinoma
Carcinoid
Squamous carcinoma

4.7.3 Genetics

- Teratomas are diploid in children and hypotriploid in adults. The only specific aberration is the iso-chromosome i(12p).

4.8 Burned Out GCTs

- So-called extragonadal germ tumors arising isolated in mediastinum and pineal regions are, with few exceptions, true primaries.
- Primary retroperitoneal germ cell tumors should be considered metastases of a small occult viable or completely regressed ('burned out') germ cell tumor located in the testis. In an autopsy series of metastasizing GCTs, burned out tumors represented approximately 10 % of all cases.
- The testes involved can appear normal or show a circumscribed scar, which is also the most common histologic finding. Normal appearing or fibrotic areas show foci of atrophic, hyalinized, or collapsed seminiferous tubules, which frequently (49 %) contain IGCNUs cells. Macrophages, plasma cells and/or calcification may be present (Figs. 4.35 and 4.36).

4.9 Tumors of More than One Histologic Type (Mixed Forms)

- These tumors are almost as frequent as pure seminomas.

4.9.1 Pathology

- The gross aspect and the histology strongly depend on the amount of the single histologic components which are randomly mixed; nevertheless, certain combinations are significantly more frequent than others.
- Embryonal carcinoma is the most frequent (80 %) single component, but teratoma and YST are also common. Seminoma is a component of about 15 % of all mixed TGCTs, preferentially combined with embryonal carcinoma. In the past, the combination of teratoma and embryonal carcinoma was called teratocarcinoma (Figs. 4.37, 4.38, 4.39 and 4.40).

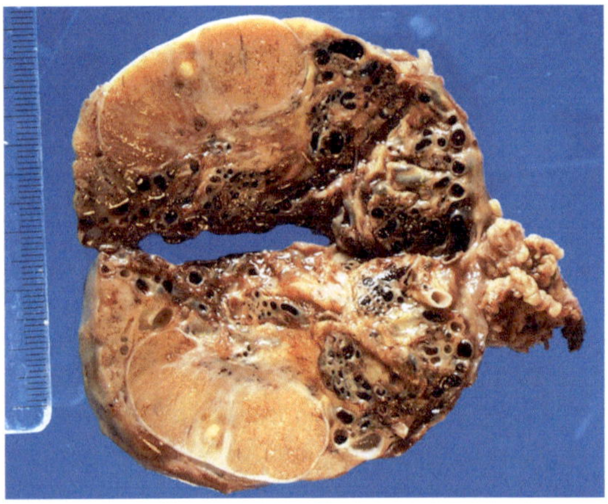

Fig. 4.35 Gross features of burned out germ cell tumor

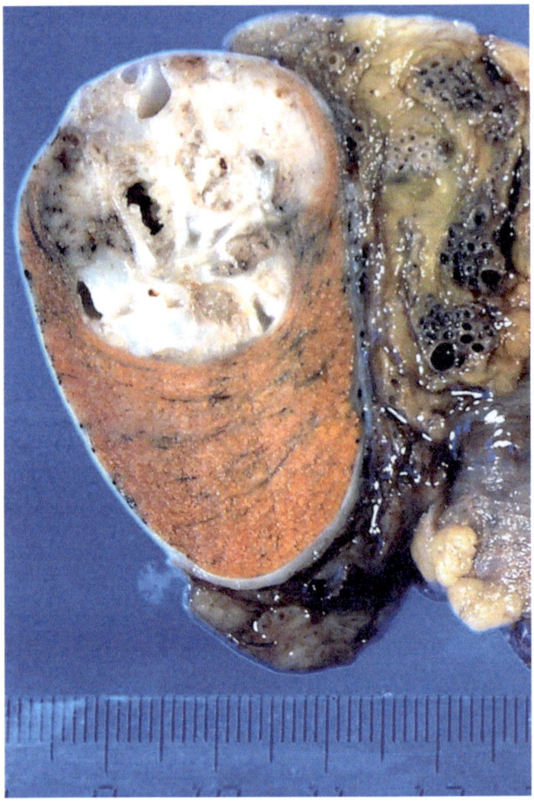

Fig. 4.37 Gross appearance of a mixed germ cell tumor incorporating teratoma and embryonal carcinoma (teratocarcinoma)

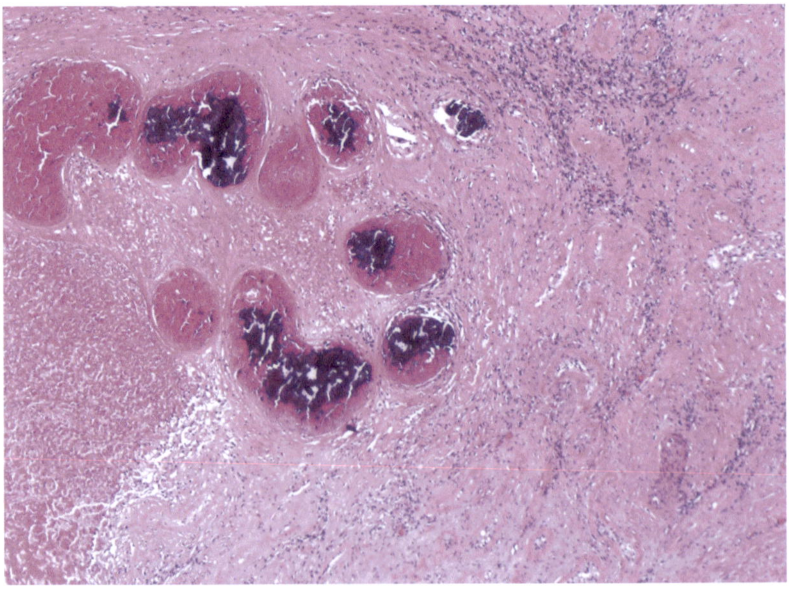

Fig. 4.36 Microscopic appearance of completely regressed ('burned out') germ cell tumor showing necrotic and calcified tubules

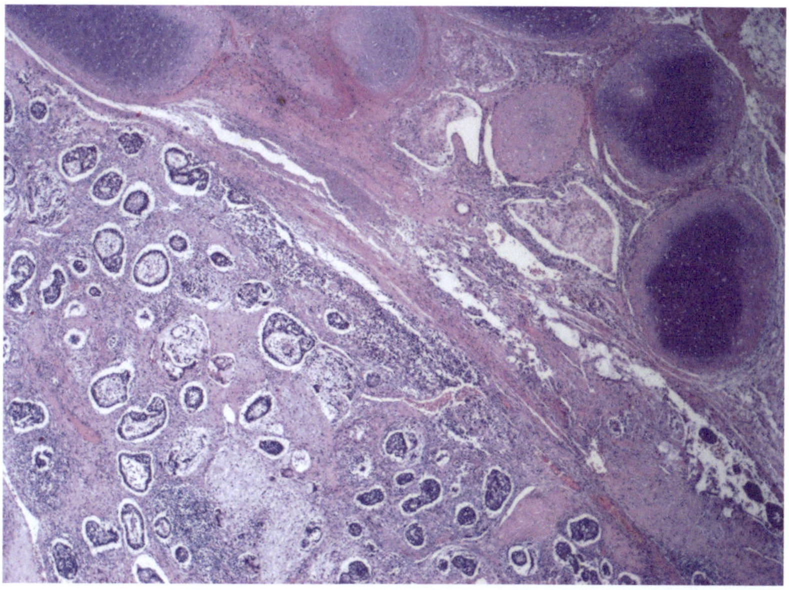

Fig. 4.38 Microscopic features of a mixed germ cell tumor with teratoma and embryonal carcinoma

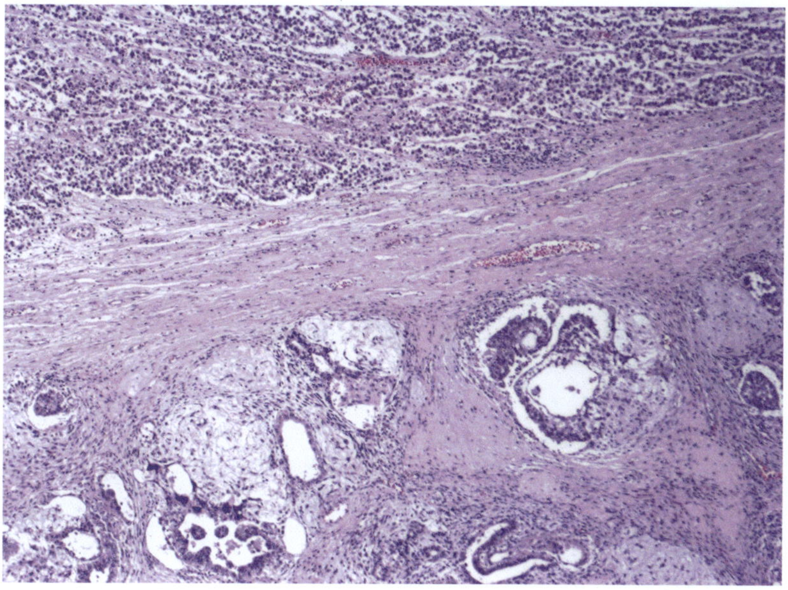

Fig. 4.39 Microscopic features of a mixed germ cell tumor with embryonal carcinoma and seminoma

4.9.2 Prognostic Factors

- In NSGCTs, the invasion of lymph and/or blood vessels (pT2) is the most powerful predictor of relapse or retroperitoneal metastases. Vascular invasion is very frequent in embryonal carcinomas and in fact, when frequent in a mixed germ cell tumor negatively influence the prognosis.
- The pathology report should therefore incorporate a rough estimate of the relative amount as a percentage of tumor type present.
- Teratoma and/or YST presence in the tumor are markers of a favorable prognosis.
- With the exception of hematogenous metastasizing choriocarcinoma, all other NSGCTs primarily metastasize to the retroperitoneal lymph nodes (Tables 4.10 and 4.11).

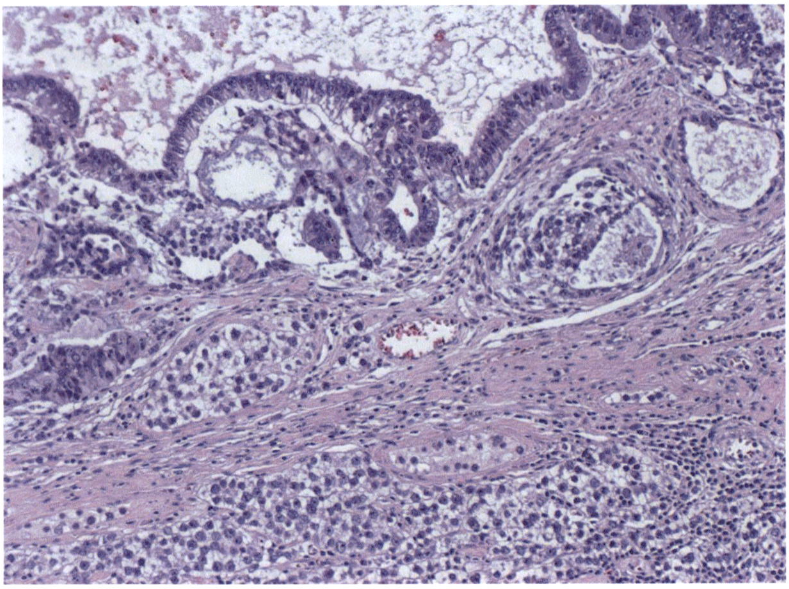

Fig. 4.40 Microscopic features of a mixed germ cell tumor with teratoma and seminoma

Table 4.10 Prognostic factors in mixed NSGCTs

Vascular/lymphatic invasion	Unfavorable
High amount (%) of embryonal carcinoma	Unfavorable
In absence of embryonal carcinoma	S-phase fraction >29 % unfavorable
Presence of yolk sac tumor	Favorable
Presence of teratoma	Favorable

Table 4.11 pTNM (2010) definitions on Testis cancer (after radical orchiectomy)

Primary tumor	
pTX	Primary tumor cannot be assessed
pT0	No evidence of primary tumor (e.g. histologic scar in testis)
pTis	Intratubular germ cell neoplasia (carcinoma in situ)
pT1	Tumor limited to th testis and epididymis without vascular/lymphatic invasion; tumor may invade into the tunica albuginea but not the tunica vaginalis.
pT2	Tumor limited to the testis and epididymis with vascular/lymphatic invasion, or tumor extending through the tunica albuginea with involvement of the tunica vaginalis
pT3	Tumor invades the spermatic cord with or without vascular/lymphatic invasion
pT4	Tumor invades the scrotum with or without vascular/lymphatic invasion

Table 4.11 (continued)

Regional lymph nodes (pN)	
pNX	Regional lymph node cannot be assessed
pN0	No regional lymph node metastasis
pN1	Metastasis with a lymph node mass 2 cm or less in greatest dimension and less than or equal to five nodes positive, none more than 2 cm in greatest dimension
pN2	Metastasis with a lymph node mass more than 2 cm but not more than 5 cm in greatest dimension; or more than five nodes positive
pN3	Metastasis with a lymph node mass more than 5 cm in greatest dimension

Distant metastasis (M)	
M0	No distant metastastasis
M1	Distant metastasis
M1a	Nonregional nodal or pulmonary metastasis
M1b	Distant metastasis other than M1a

4.10 Tumors of Sex Cord/Gonadal Stroma

- These are very rare tumors which may account for 1.6–6 % of adult testicular tumors, are somewhat more frequent in children, and derive from Leydig, Sertoli, granulosa, and theca cells. In the current WHO

(Table 4.1) classification pure forms with one cell type, mixed forms composed of two cell types, and incompletely differentiated tumors are listed.

4.11 Benign and Malignant Leydig Cell Tumors

- Leydig cell tumors (LCTs), represent 1–3 % of all testicular neoplasms, are the most frequent type in this category and represent 4–9 % of all primary testis tumors in prepubertal males.
- The age of the patients ranges 2–90 years. May be associated with cryptorchidism. About 3 % of tumors are bilateral. In adults approximately 10 % of LTCs are malignant, but in children the tumor is always benign.

4.11.1 Pathology of Benign Tumors

- LCTs are usually well-circumscribed, yellow-brownish tumors with a thin capsule. They can be lobulated by fibrous septa and show foci of necrosis or small hemorrhages (25 %). The average diameter in the large series was 2.6 cm and extension to the rete testis or spermatic cord was observed in 10–15 % of cases. Tumor cells arranged in a solid formation with scanty fibrous stroma is the most common growth pattern (Figs. 4.41 and 4.42)
- The tumor cells are large and polygonal with abundant eosinophilic cytoplasm which occasionally can be granulated or vacuolated. Spindle cell differentiation is rare. In one-third of cases, the cytoplasm contains Reinke crystals and, in 15 %, lipochrome pigment.
- The nuclei are usually perfectly round and contain a visible nucleolus. The mitotic activity is, with some exceptions, generally low. In a few cases, a marked variation of size and shape occur. Trabecular or pseudotubular structures with prominent fibrous stroma and psammoma-like calcification have been rarely observed. Confusion with lymphomas or plasmocytomas is possible. The use of immunohistochemistry can help.
- Leydig cells typically react with α-inhibin, melan-A, calretinin, WT1 and vimentin. Cytokeratins and S100 are negative of focally positive. CD30, CD117, OCT4, and PLAP are negative.
- A marked Leydig cell hyperplasia in atrophic testis of the Klinefelter syndrome can also easily be confused with LCT if the pathologist does not know the clinical history. However, true LCTs have been described in a Klinefelter testis.
- Also, the tumors of the adrenogenital syndrome may be mistaken as LCT. These are more common in adults and present with large polygonal eosinophilic cytoplasm arranged in nests, sheets and cord, embedded in a fibrous (keloid-like bands) or myxoid stroma. Calcification may be present.
- Immunohistochemistry does not help to separate from LCTs, therefore, clinicopathological correlation is mandatory.

4.11.2 Pathology of Malignant Tumors

- The most reliable criterion of malignancy is the size of the tumor, usually greater than 5 cm (average 4.7 cm versus 2.6 cm for benign tumors). There is no significant histologic difference between benign and malignant Leydig cells, but atypical mitotic figures are more frequent and the mitotic index is significantly higher in malignant tumors. Also, ki67 proliferation index is higher in malignant tumors (mean 18.6 % vs 1.2 %).
- Vascular invasion, infiltrative margins, and necrosis are also associated with malignancy, but are not reliable as a single criterion.
- Metastatic LCTs commonly involve the retroperitoneal lymph node (72 %). Blood-born metastases are located in the lung (43 %), the liver (38 %), and the bones (28 %).

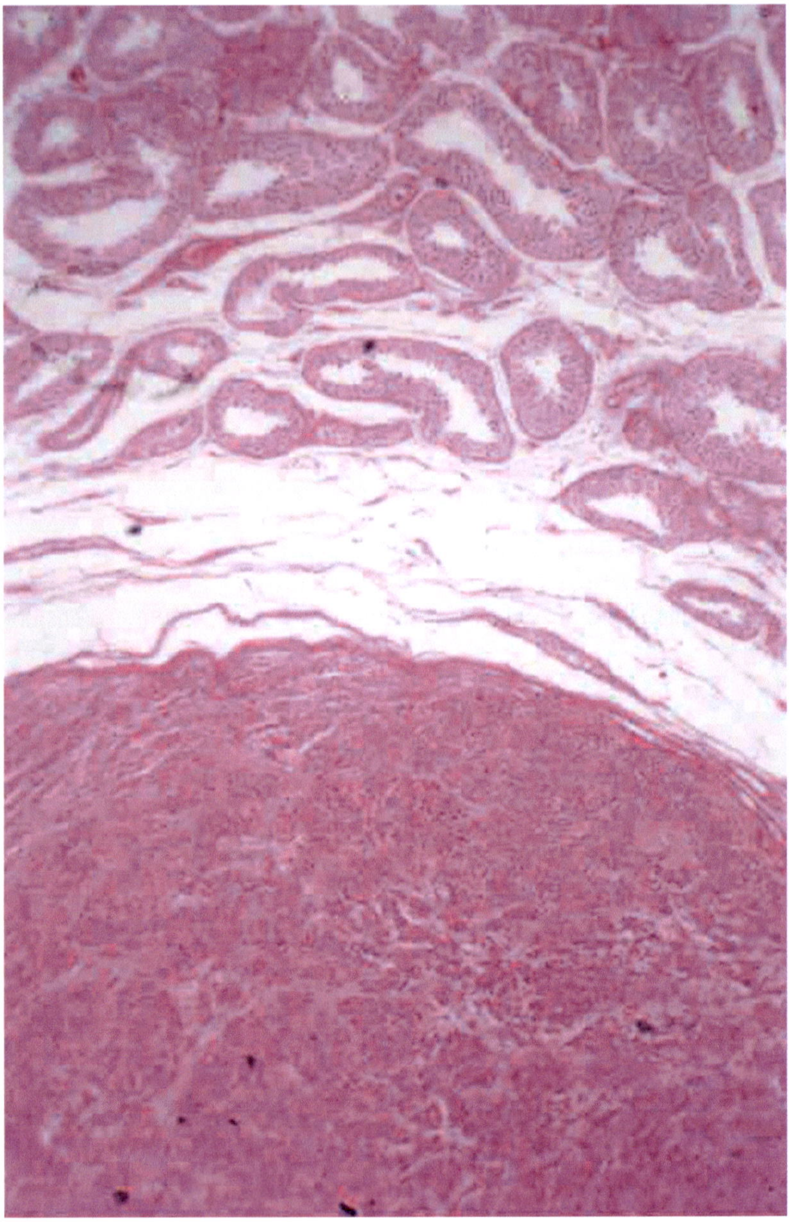

Fig. 4.41 Microscopic features of benign Leydig cell tumor

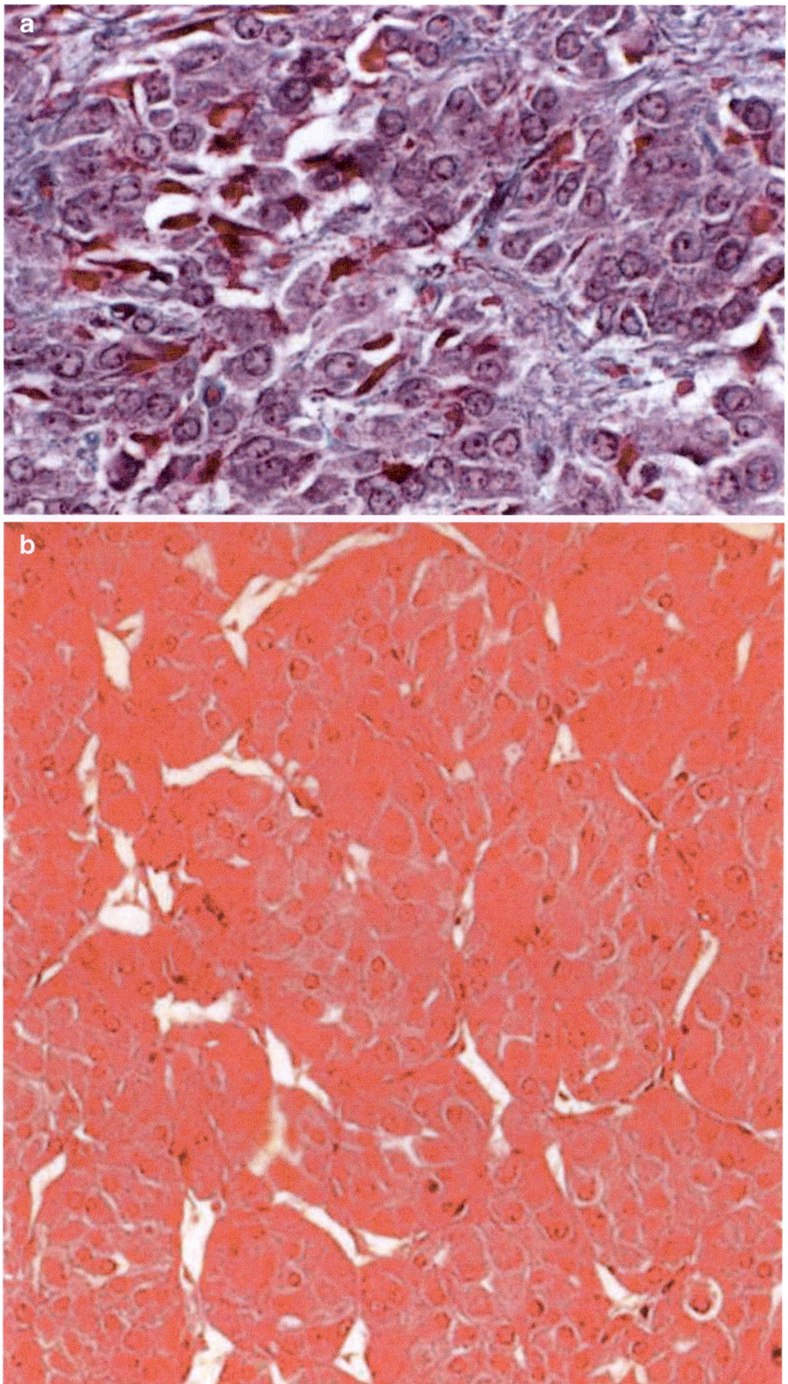

Fig. 4.42 (**a**) Microscopic features of benign Leydig cell tumor with Reinke crystals. (**b**) Close view of Leydig cell tumor. (**c**) Cellular characteristics of Leydig cell tumor. (**d**) Slight nuclear atypia is present in this Leydig cell tumor

Fig. 4.42 (continued)

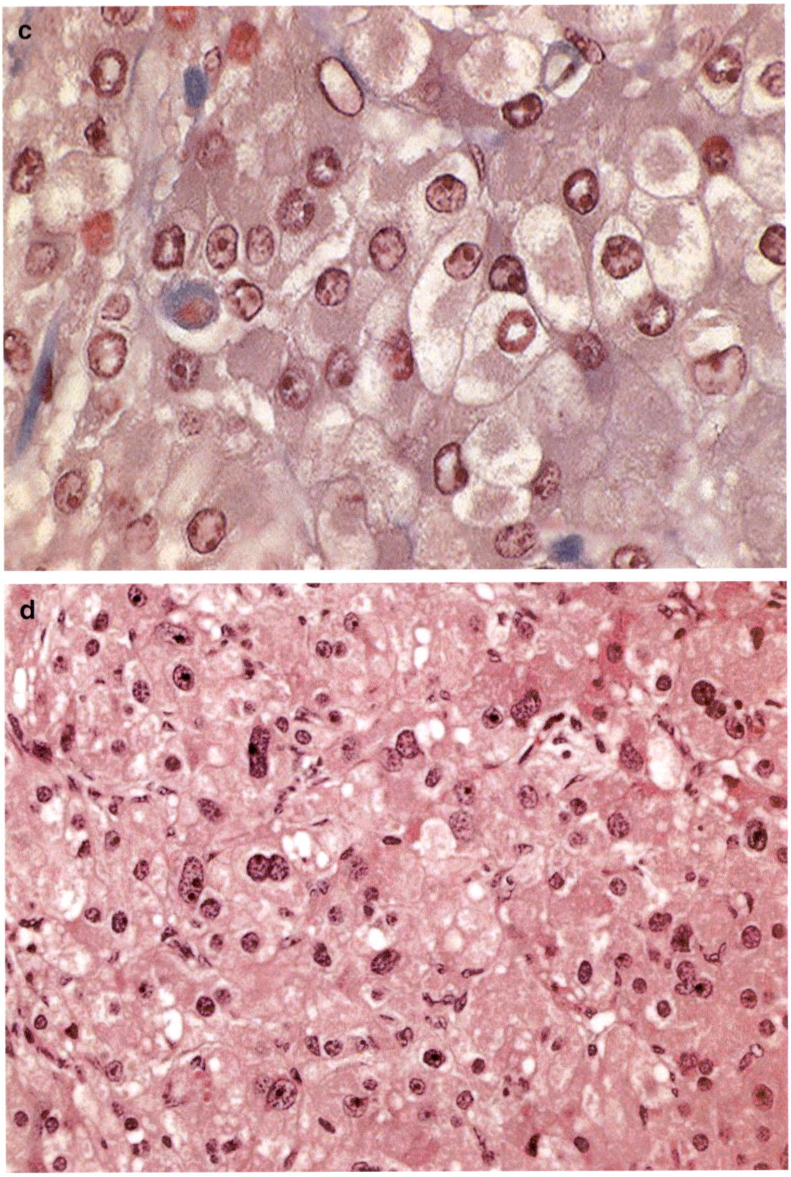

4.11.3 Genetics

- All metastasizing LCTs and one-third of benign ones are DNA aneuploidy, with gain of the X as the only chromosomal aberration.

4.12 Benign and Malignant Sertoli Cell Tumors

- Sertoli cell tumors (SCTs) occur significantly less frequently than LTCs and account for 1 % of all testicular tumors. At an average age of 45 years, the patients are as old as those with LTCs. SCTs are extremely rare in men younger than 20 years.

4.12.1 Pathology of Benign Tumors

- The tumors are usually well circumscribed and a tan-gray, white, or yellow color. Necrotic areas are infrequent but hemorrhagic spots can be seen in some cases.
- Size ranges 0.3–15 cm, but the average diameter is 3.6 cm. Histology varies from

well-differentiated, easily recognizable Sertoli cells to less-differentiated forms which are recognized primarily through their typical arrangement in hollow or solid tubules. The cells grow in solid cords, trabeculae, or small nodules surrounded by a fibrous or hyaline stroma. Usually the cytoplasm is eosinophilic, but sometimes it contains large amount of lipids (lipid-rich variant) (Fig. 4.43 and 4.44).

- Exuberant sclerotic stroma is the morphologic hallmark of a distinct variant called sclerosing Sertoli cell tumor (Fig. 4.45).
- SCTs need to be differentiated from Sertoli cell nodules frequently present in cryptorchid but also in normal descended testes. The nodules consist of small aggregates of seminiferous tubules with a prominent, thick basement membrane and lined solely by Sertoli cells.
- Also adenomatoid tumors, extremely rare in the testis, can be mistaken for SCTs. The cells of adenomatoid tumors as well as Sertoli cells react positively with cytokeratin and vimentin antibodies.

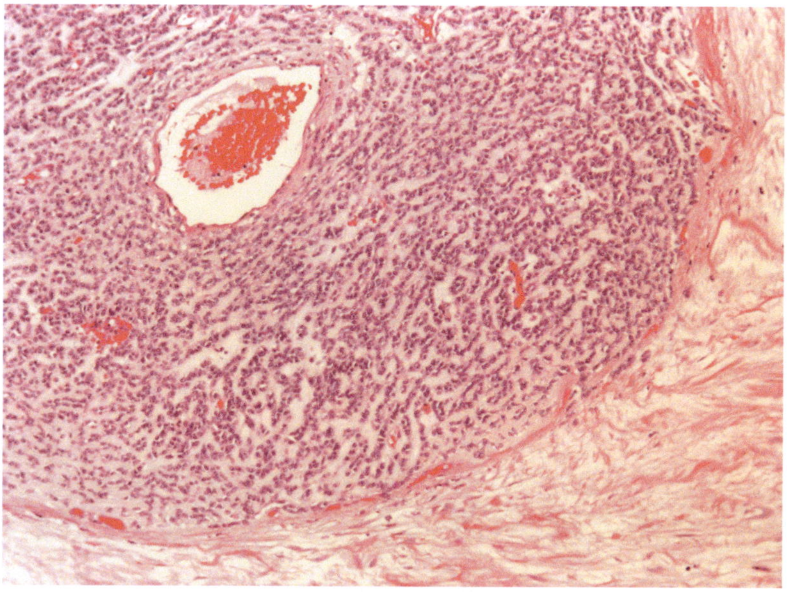

Fig. 4.43 Microscopic features of benign Sertoli cell tumor with solid cords surrounded by a hyaline stroma (low power)

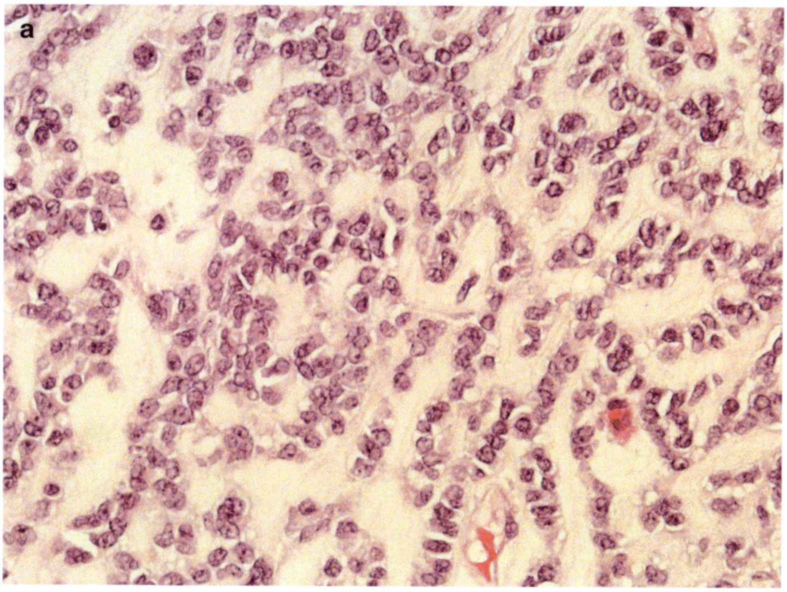

Fig. 4.44 (**a**) Microscopic features of benign Sertoli cell tumor with solid cords surrounded by a hyaline stroma (medium power). (**b**). Closed view of Sertoli cells. (**c**) Microscopic features of Sertoli tumor. (**d**) Sertoli cell with lipidic cytoplasm. (**e**) Large cell calcifying Sertoli cell tumor

Fig. 4.44 (continued)

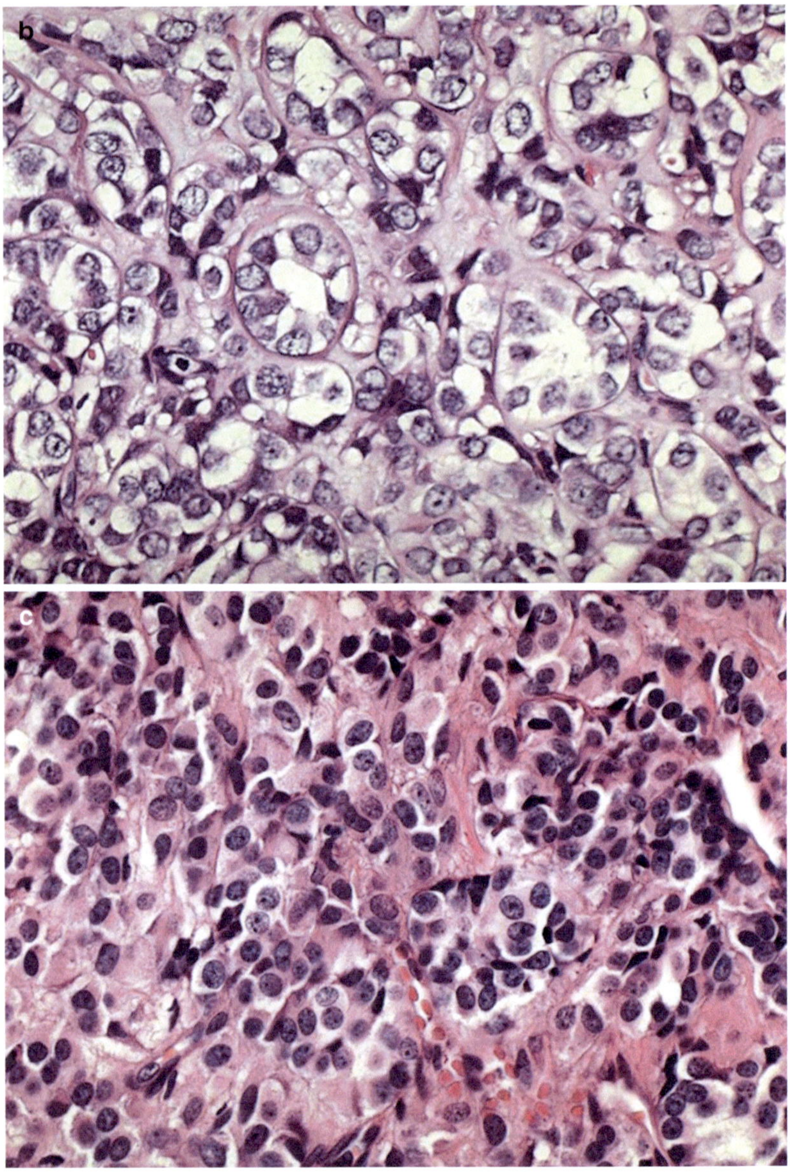

Fig. 4.44 (continued)

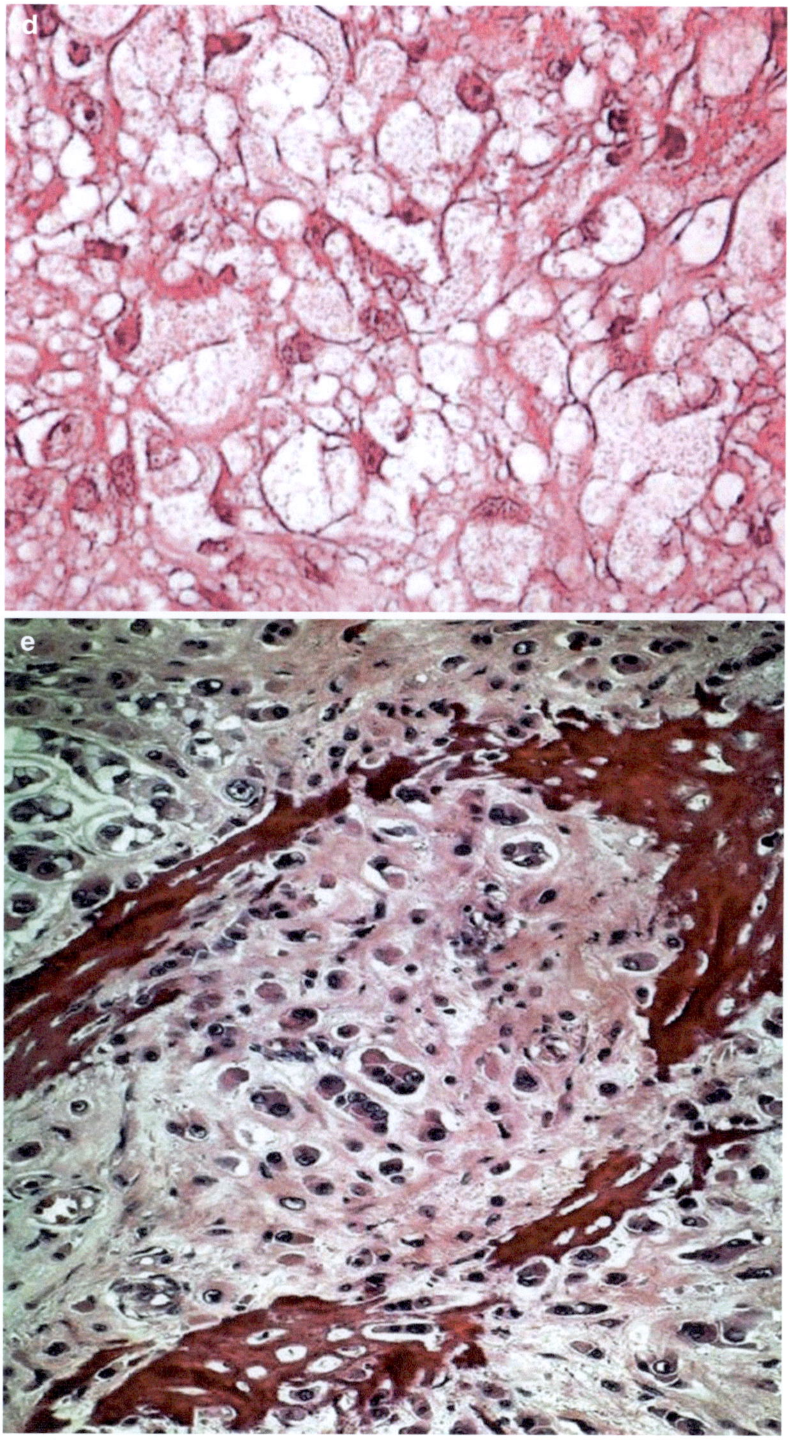

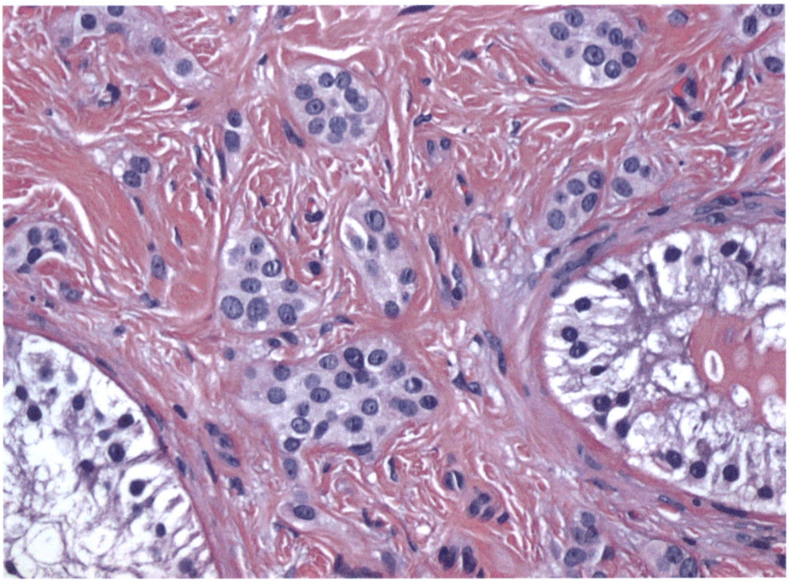

Fig. 4.45 Microscopic features of sclerosing Sertoli cell tumor

- However, SCTs also react with α-inhibin (50 %), CD99, and S-100 (30 %), and adenomatoid tumors does not. SCT are negative with PLAP.

4.12.2 Pathology of Malignant Tumors

- Malignant SCTs differ from their benign counterpart mainly in size, on average >5 cm. Necrosis and hemorrhage are also more frequent. Microscopically the cells show a marked nuclear atypia and high mitotic index. Lymphovascular invasion is common.

4.12.3 Genetics

- Common gain of chromosome X and by loss of the entire or part of chromosome 2.

4.13 Large Cell Calcifying Sertoli Cell Tumor (LCCST)

- Occur at any age in phenotypically normal men or associated with hormonal or genetic disorders like Peutz–Jeghers and Carney syndromes.
- Patients with benign LCCST are 17 years old on average (range 2–38 years), and those with malignant counterpart are on average 39 years old (range 28–74 years).

4.13.1 Pathology

- Benign tumors are usually multifocal and bilateral in 28 % of cases, but malignant are solitary and unilateral. Benign tumors remain confined to the testis; malignant ones can extend to the neighboring organs. Benign LCCSTs are small (0.8–2.3 cm) whereas malignant ones tend to be larger (>4 cm) and can replace the entire testicular parenchyma. Foci of necrosis and hemorrhage are typical in malignant LCCSTs.
- The color varies from gray to tan-white or yellow; grossly apparent calcifications are identified in benign and malignant tumors.
- Large, irregularly shaped and confluent calcification, and even ossification, is the microscopic hallmark. Typical tumor cell have abundant eosinophilic cytoplasm and round nuclei more closely resembling the Leydig than the Sertoli cell. The cells are arranged in solid nests or cords embedded in a myxomatous stroma.
- Malignant LCCSTs have a brisk mitotic activity (4–14 mitoses/10 HPF). Metastases are regarded as an objective sign of malignancy.

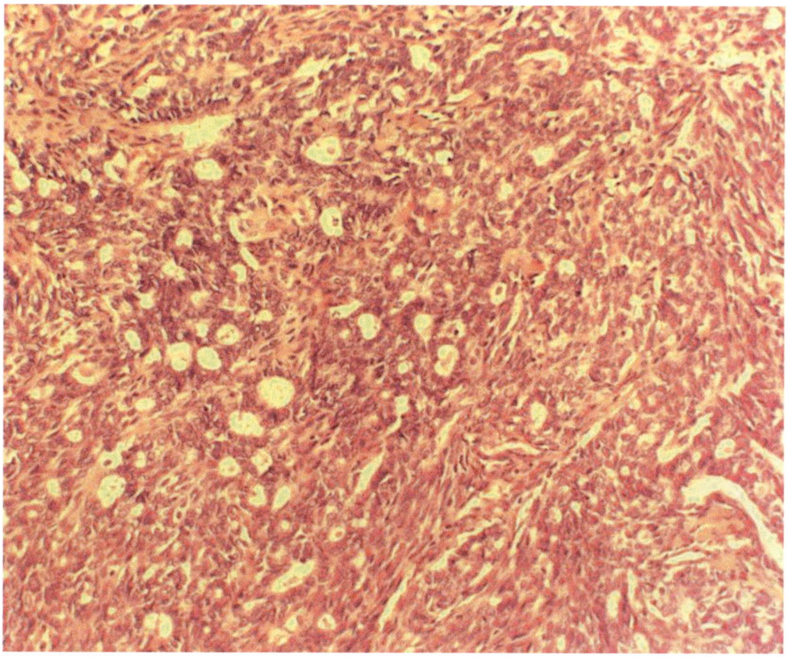

Fig. 4.46 Granulosa cell tumor, adult type

4.14 Granulosa Cell Tumor of Adult Type

- Granulosa cell tumor of adult type is one of the rarest tumor arising in the testis. It ranges 15–60 years. The morphology does not differ from those arising in the ovary. It ranges 0.8–13 cm in size and the color is yellow. The cut surface is lobulated with small cysts. Histologically the patterns are diffuse or microfollicular, with characteristic Call Exner bodies.
- The cells have scanty cytoplasm and the nuclei are all grooved like coffee beans. Gynecomastia is important symptom together with slow growing. Morphologic criteria of malignancy are unclear (Fig. 4.46).

4.15 Granulosa Cell Tumor of Juvenile Type

- The juvenile type is the most common testicular tumor in the first 6 months of life and accounts for 6 % of all prepubertal testicular tumors. The cut surface of the tumor is microcystic. Microscopically, the cysts are lined by cells resembling granulosa cells Among the cysts, tubules with proliferated Sertoli cells form bizarre structures.
- The high mitotic count can erroneously suggest malignancy. It can be mistaken as YST which is tragic since the juvenile granulosa tumor is benign. Some cases are located in an intra-abdominal cryptorchid testis and 20 % of children have ambiguous genital organs. Numerical aberrations of the XY chromosomes (mosaic 45X/46XY) or structural anomalies of Y chromosome may be present.

4.16 Thecoma–Fibroma Type Tumors

- Rare benign tumor in men in their fourth to fifth decade. The tumors are firm, white, and well circumscribed with about 2 cm in diameter.
- The spindle cells resemble cortical ovary with focal storiform growth pattern.
- Usually are immunoreactive for steroid receptors (ER/PR), calretinin, inhibin, Melan-A, pan keratin, bcl-2, S100, CD34, muscle-specific actin and desmin (Fig. 4.47).

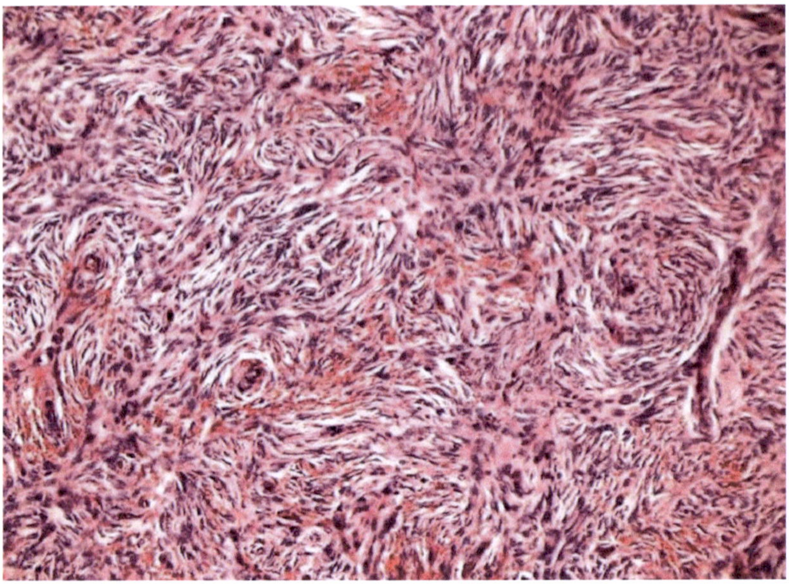

Fig. 4.47 Fibroma-thecoma of the testes

4.17 Mixed or Incompletely Differentiated (Undifferentiated) Gonadal Stromal Tumors

- Mixed tumors usually contain well-differentiated Leydig cells and less-differentiated Sertoli cells, but combinations with granulosa cells also occur.
- The incompletely differentiated cells consist of spindle or more epithelioid cells. Single cells can react with α-inhibin, but usually they are positive only for smooth muscle actin and S-100 protein. Large size is an important predictor of aggressive behaviour. Patient age ranges from 6 months to 60 years. Gynecomastia may be present in some cases.
- In childhood the tumors are benign, whereas some adult tumors metastasized to the retroperitoneal lymph nodes and/or abdominal organs.

4.18 Mixed Germ Cell/Sex Cord Stromal Tumor

- Two types of mixed tumors of germ and gonadal stroma cells. The most common is gonadoblastoma, that affects only dysgenetic gonads. The other one, first observed in the ovary, is called 'mixed germ cell sex cord–stromal tumor, unclassified' and is not related to intersexuality.

4.18.1 Gonadoblastoma

- Gonadoblastoma arises more commonly in individuals who are phenotypically female (80 %) than in those who are phenotypically men. Most of these tumors are diagnosed in the first three decades of life (Figs. 4.48 and 4.49).

4.18.1.1 Pathology

- The tumors have a yellow cut surface and in one-quarter of cases can be detected only microscopically, some replacing the entire testicular parenchyma. The histology is unique with small nests of seminoma and embryonal carcinoma cells, which are wreath-like, surrounded by Sertoli and granulosa cells.
- Leydig cells may also be present. Immunohistochemically staining the germ cells with PLAP or vice versa of the stromal cells with α-inhibin confers on these formations a characteristic appearance. The center of the nests can contain

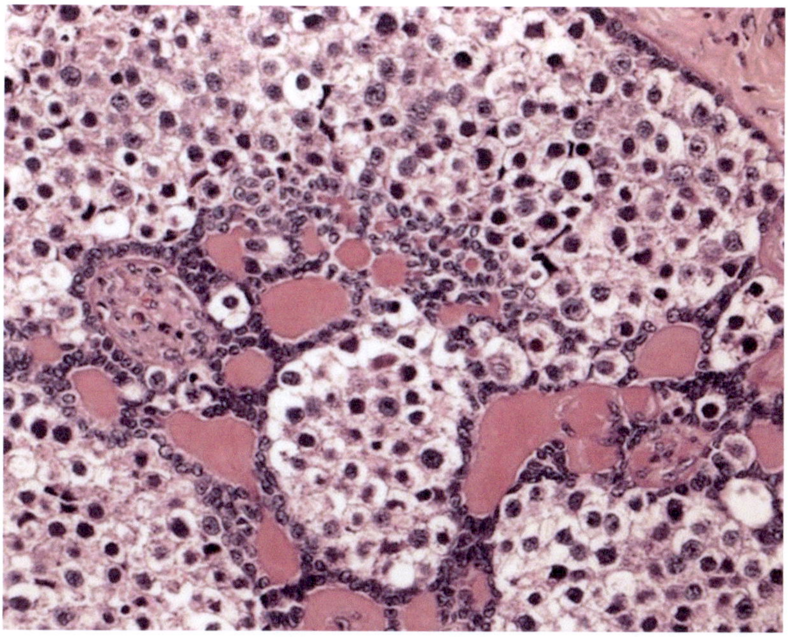

Fig. 4.48 Gonadoblastoma

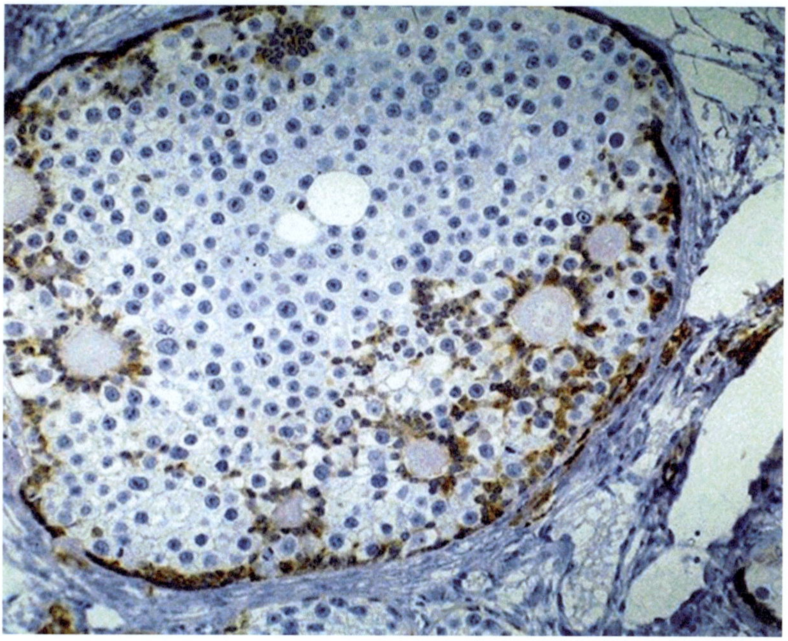

Fig. 4.49 Inhibin is positive in Gonadoblastoma

hyaline nodules, which can calcify and give the tumor a gritty consistency.
- In case the tumor is not removed in time, the germ cell component will overgrow the stromal cells and an overt seminoma or, rarely, a NSGCT will develop.

4.18.1.2 Genetics

- Gonadoblastoma arises only in intersex patients with a Y chromosome.
- The highest risk for gonadoblastoma is in patients with gonadal dysgenesis (46XY,46X/46XY) with intra-abdominal dysgenetic testes.

4.18.2 Germ Cell Sex Cord/Gonadal Stromal Tumor, Unclassified

- This is the official name for mixed germ cell and gonadal stromal tumors which arise in geno- and phenotypically normal adult male individuals. Our knowledge is limited because of its rarity. The reported tumors presented as slow growing testicular masses of up to 7 cm in diameter.
- The tumors are well-circumscribed white masses, which can totally replace the testicular parenchyma.
- The tumors consist of germ cells with clear cytoplasm, which are dissimilar from those of seminomas or embryonal carcinomas. These cells are arranged in small clusters surrounded by the predominant stromal component with α-inhibin-positive small, undifferentiated often spindled cells. Germ cells do not react with the classical seminoma markers PLAP, CD117, OCT4, SALL4 or podoplanin.

4.19 Other Tumors of the Testis

4.19.1 Carcinoid

- Carcinoids arising in teratoma are classified as 'teratomas with somatic type malignancies'. In case remnants of a germ cell tumor cannot be detected, it should be diagnosed as a distinct entity. Moreover, gut carcinoids can metastasize to the testis.
- Carcinoid account for 0.2–1 % of all tumors of the testis. Patients' ages ranged from 20 to 80 years. Carcinoid syndrome is rare.
- The tumors measure 0.5–13 cm and the colour is yellow to tan and the cut surface solid.
- The typical carcinoid cells are arranged in islets of tumor cells surrounded by thin fibrous septa.
- Tumor cells are immunoreactive for the classical neuroendocrine markers chromogranin A, synaptophysin. CD56 is of limited value because of lack of specificity.

4.19.2 Nephroblastoma

- Nephroblastoma (Wilms tumor) can arise in testicular teratomas or intrascrotally in heterotopic renal anlage. Clinically they behave like kidney tumors.

4.19.3 Lymphoma and Plasmacytoma

- Lymphomas are the most frequent testicular tumors in men older then 50 years. Primary testicular lymphomas represents up to 5 % of testicular neoplasms or 1–2 % of all non-Hodgkin-lymphoma (NHLs).
- Children, usually between the ages of 3 and 10, are affected less frequently. Some are bilateral. The spread to the adjacent epididymis or spermatic cord is a common occurrence.
- Plasmacytomas are even less common with a wide age range (26–89 years).

4.19.3.1 Pathology

- Lymphomas are bulky, fleshy, whitish-gray or pink colored tumors with yellow necrotic areas. In contrast to the quite similar seminomas, lymphatic tumors infiltrate the adjacent epididymis (60 %) and/or spermatic cord (40 %). Plasmacytomas are not fleshy but can be soft and tan to tan-white with hemorrhagic areas.
- Lymphoma and plasmocytoma cells spread intertubularly in the interstitium of the testicular parenchyma. Some few seminiferous tubules are always more or less well preserved; others are invaded by the tumor cells. Diffuse sclerosis is a common finding (Figs. 4.50, 4.51, 4.52 and 4.53)
- More than 80 % of NHL belong to the diffuse large B cell type with or without sclerosis. Other types of the B lineage are follicular, mantle cell, and Burkitt type lymphomas.

Natural killer (NK)/T cell lymphomas which are typical for the facial area ('nasal type'), MALT type or Hodgkin disease affecting the testis, have been reported.

- Testicular lymphomas can rarely be mistaken for germ cell tumors. Nevertheless it happens that lymphomas are confused with spermatocytic seminomas, classic seminomas, and even embryonal carcinomas. At immunohistochemistry, lymphoma are negative for PLAP, and cytokeratins, but may be focally positive for OCT4. Anaplastic large cell lymphoma is likely to express CD30.

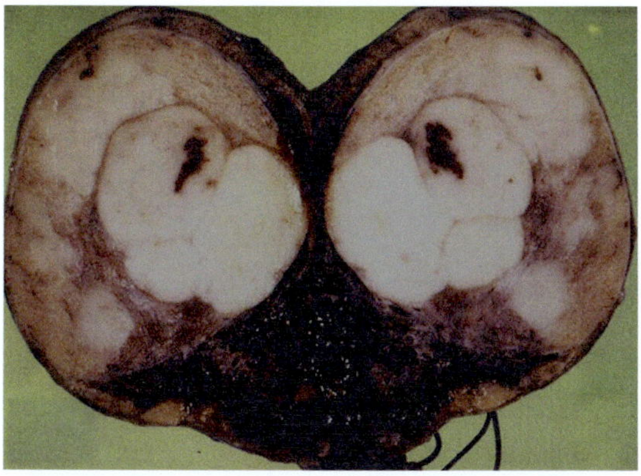

Fig. 4.50 Gross features of a lymphoma of the testes

4.19.4 Leukemia

- Primary leukemia cases (granulocytic/myeloid sarcoma) of the testis are very rare. In children with acute leukemia, regardless whether myeloid or lymphocytic, the testis is more frequently affected; especially after therapy, one-third of relapses occur in the testis.
- Extramedullary myeloid tumors (granulocytic sarcoma, chloroma) can also appear as a first clinical manifestation in the testis. Intertubular spread of the leukemia cells are not different from lymphoma. Common germ cell markers will be negative.

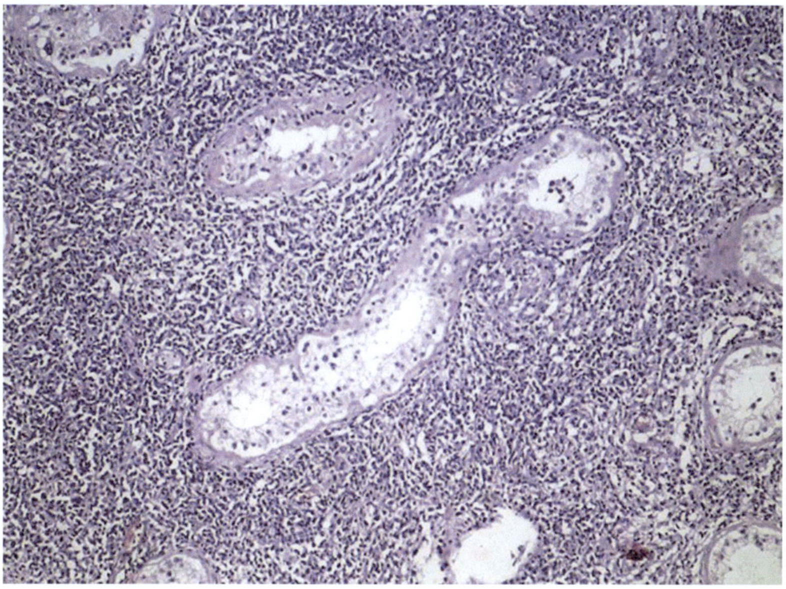

Fig. 4.51 Microscopic appearance of a lymphoma of testes with preservation of tubules

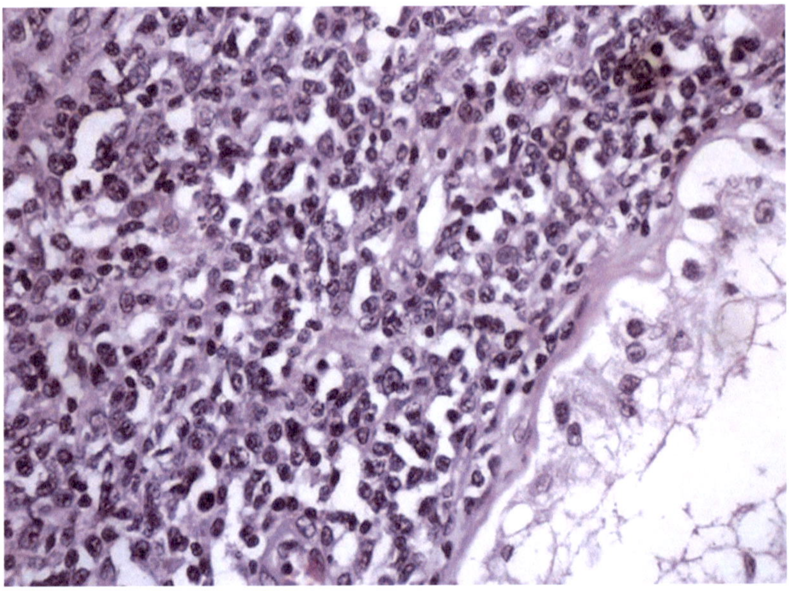

Fig. 4.52 Microscopic appearance of a diffuse B cell lymphoma (high power)

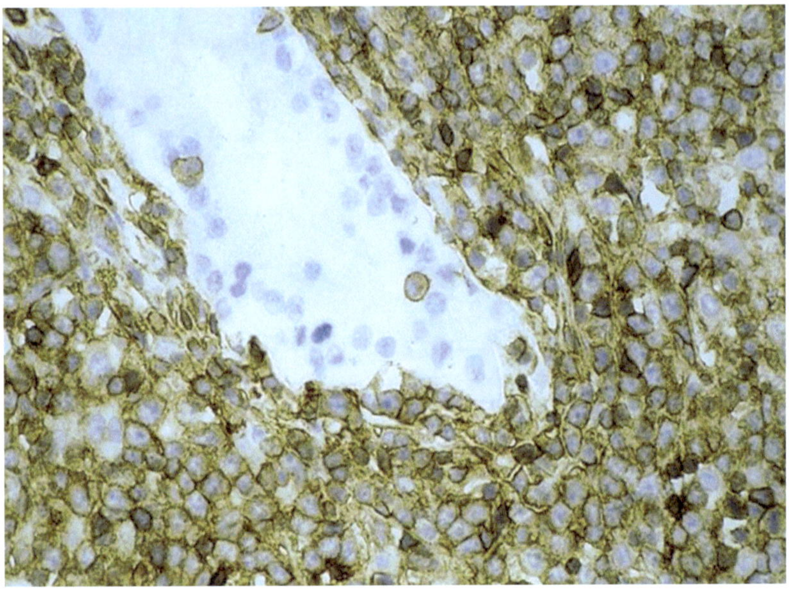

Fig. 4.53 CD 20 positive lymphoma cells

4.20 Other Rare Tumors

- Unusual tumors of the testis are always suspected to be secondary and not primary. Nevertheless, cases of soft tissue primary tumors arising in the testis are reported sporadically in the medical literature. Fibromas of the tunica albuginea and hemangioma are the typical benign tumors in this location.

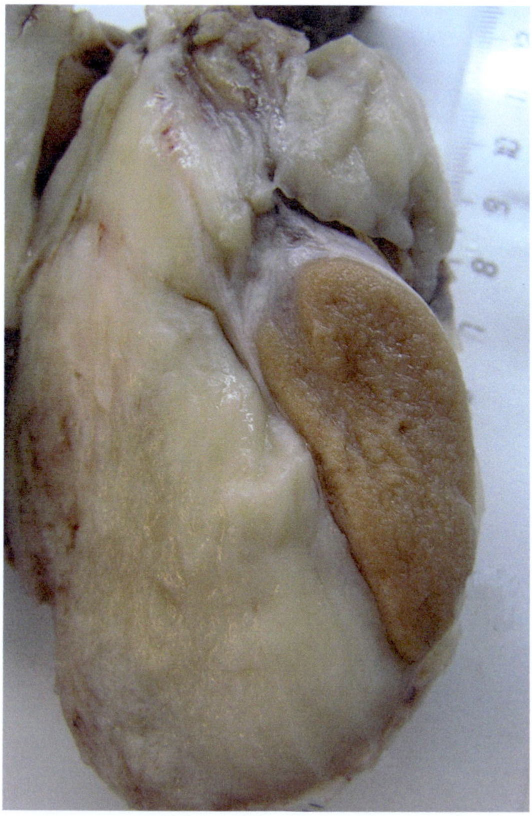

Fig. 4.54 Gross appearance of paratesticular embryonal rhabdomyosarcoma diagnosed in a 15 years old boy

- Sporadically different kinds of sarcomas including rhabdomyosarcoma, osteo- and chondrosarcomas have been reported (Figs. 4.54, 4.55, 4.56 and 4.57).
- Angiosarcoma can be primary or the consequence of radio-chemotherapy of GCTs.

4.21 Testicular Metastases

- It is rather surprising that men dying of widespread cancer only rarely have metastases in the testes. In post-mortem studies the frequency varies from 0.06 to 3.6 %. In orchidectomy specimens metastases are more frequent, however in the epididymis rather than in the testis. The highest frequencies (6 %) were shown in therapeutic orchidectomies in prostate cancer.
- In 6–7 % of cases it presents as the initial evidence of disease as a palpable mass. Bilaterality occurs in 15–20 %. Other tumors which tend to metastasize to the testis are: lung carcinoma, melanoma, intestinal carcinomas, Merkel cell tumor, and kidney cancer. Numerous case reports document, however,

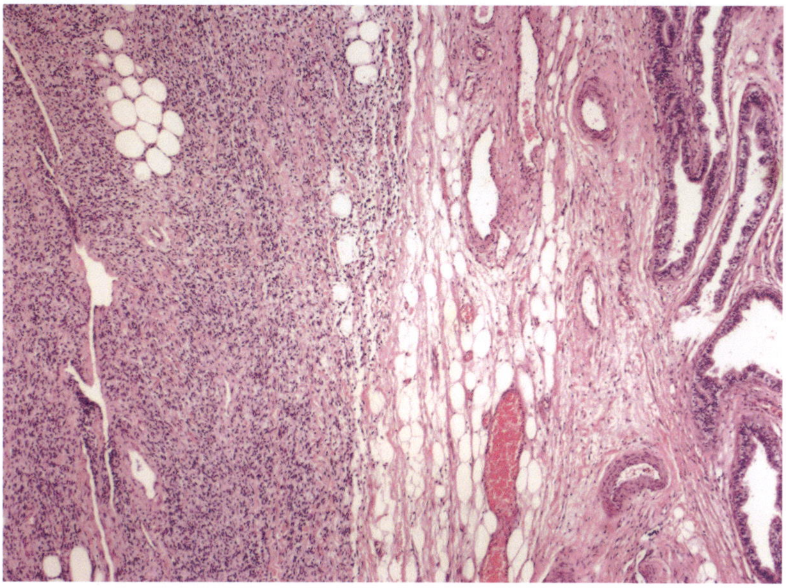

Fig. 4.55 Microscopic features of paratesticular embryonal rhabdomyosarcoma (low power)

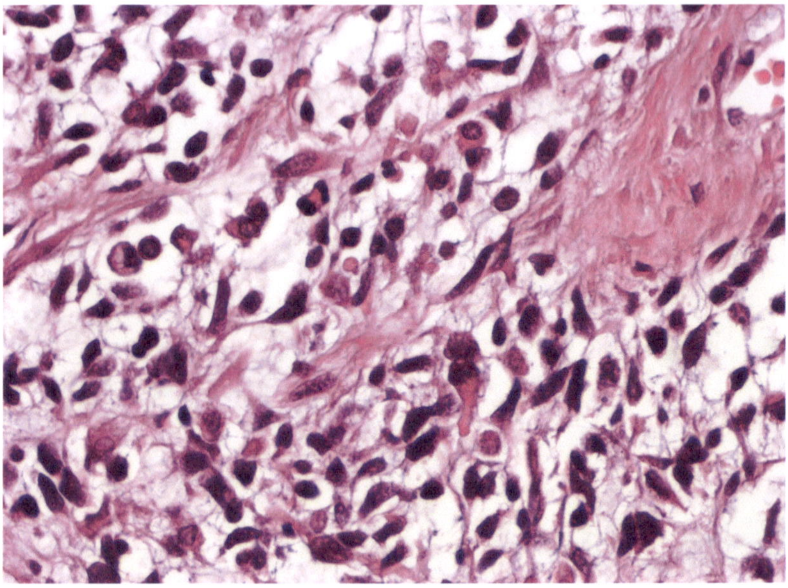

Fig. 4.56 Microscopic features of paratesticular embryonal rhabdomyosarcoma (high power)

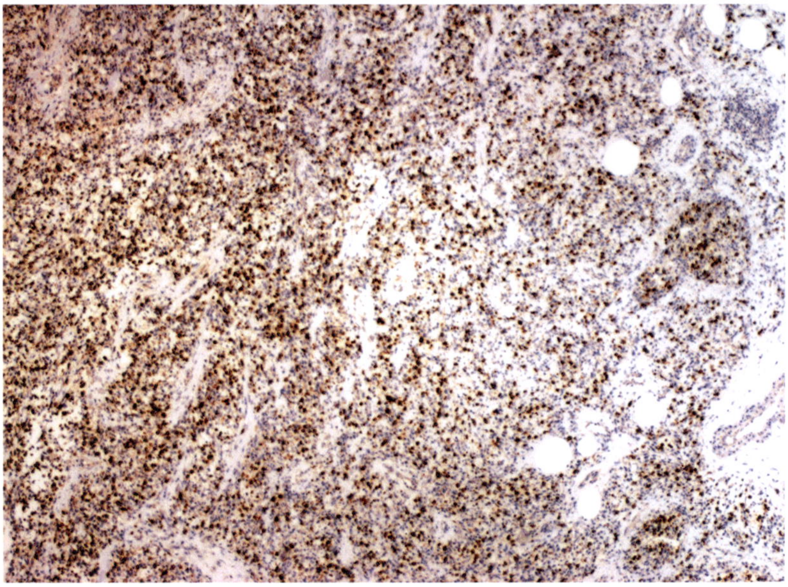

Fig. 4.57 Cells are immunoreactive for myogenin

that any tumor can sporadically metastasize to the testis.

- Metastases appear as single or multiple nodules. The microscopic spread is intertubular as in lymphomas, but invasion of the tubules may be seen. Typical cancer cells are seen in the lumen of the blood vessels (Table 4.12).

Table 4.12 Metastatic tumors to the testis

Prostate	35–60 %
Melanoma	9–15 %
Lung	5–15 %
Kidney	4–9 %
Stomach	4 %
Colon	4–9 %
Other	1–10 %

4.22 Tumors of the Paratesticular Region

- Several rare tumors may occur in the paratesticular region. Main clinicopathologic features follow in the next sections of this chapter.

4.23 Tumors of Ovarian (Müllerian) Epithelial Types

- The entire spectrum of ovarian epithelial tumors has also been described in the testis. They can originate from the appendix testis, which is a Müllerian rest, or from Müllerian metaplasia of the tunica vaginalis testis.
- They are rare and arise in adults with an average age of 55 for the serous and 11–70 years for the mucinous types. Serous tumors are more frequent.
- Benign and borderline tumors are cystic; carcinomas tend to be firm. Depending on the lining epithelium, the cysts contain either a serous fluid or a gelatinous material. In serous tumors the epithelia form small papillae protruding in the lumen.
- Serous cystadenomas and cystadenocarcinomas are lined by a columnar, frequently ciliated epithelium which is bland in benign tumors and more atypical with a variable amount of mitotic figures in borderline lesions. Papillae and psammoma bodies are typical for serous differentiation. Invasion of the capsule could be a sign of malignancy.
- Mucinous cystadenomas are lined by columnar cells with basally situated nuclei. Borderline tumors and mucinous cystadenocarcinomas are lined by intestinal-type cells, which produce large amounts of mucin. Extravasated mucin and dystrophic calcifications are further hallmarks of borderline or malignant cases.
- Rarities include endometrioid carcinoma, clear cell carcinoma, squamous carcinoma and Brenner tumors.
- Müllerian tumors are not easy to distinguish from mesothelioma of the testicular tunics.
- The epithelia of the serous tumors are immunoreactive for CA 125, WT1+, and CD117, those of the mucinous tumors for CEA and cytokeratin 20. Mesothelia react with cytokeratin antibodies but not with CEA and CD117. Other markers for mesothelioma include WT1+, calretinin+, CK7+, CK20–, LeuM1–.

4.24 Tumors of Collecting Ducts and Rete Testis

- The deep part of the rete testis–the tubuli recti–connect the two ends of the seminiferous tubule loops to the rete testis, whose channels lead to the ductuli efferentes in the caput epididymis.
- The channels are lined by ciliated columnar epithelium. The anatomy is the clue to the diagnosis of tumors of the collecting ducts–they must have an anatomic relationship to this small area.

4.24.1 Adenoma

- Rare cases of adenoma, cystadenoma, and papillary cystadenoma have been reported. Actually, only the location distinguishes rete adenomas from tumors of the epididymis or from a Sertoli cell tumor. Hyperplasia of rete testis encountered in cryptorchid testes and in other diseases can mimic an adenoma, the lesion, however, shows a clear continuity with the rete.

4.24.2 Adenocarcinoma of Rete Testis

- Rete testis carcinoma is rare and aggressive. Age range is 17–91 years with a mean of 54 years and a peak incidence around the 70s. Tumors are never bilateral. The prognosis is poor with an overall 5-year survival rate of 12 %.

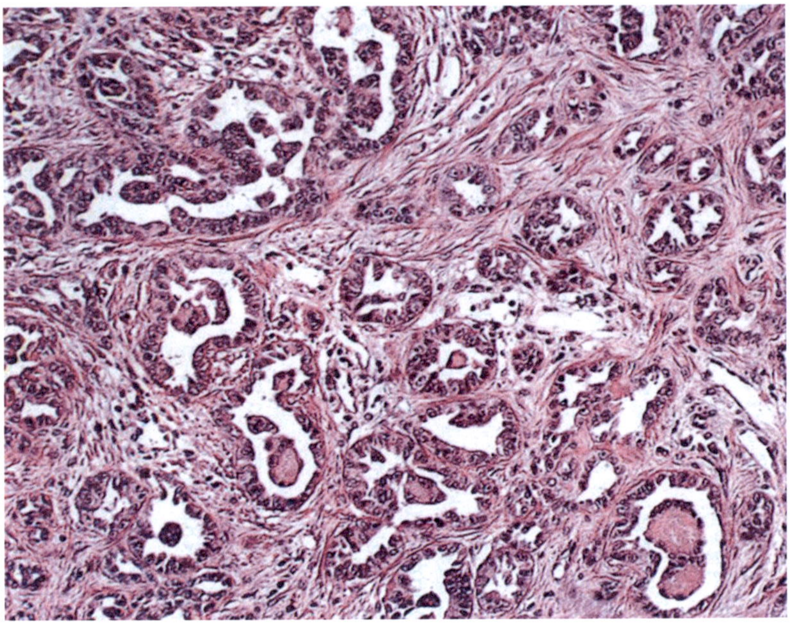

Fig. 4.58 Histologic features of rete testis carcinoma

- A significant prognostic factor is the size of the tumor; 75 % of patients with tumors <5 cm survive 5 years.

4.24.2.1 Pathology

- The diameter of the tumors ranges from 1 to 12 cm; many are multifocal and/or extending to the tunica and to the spermatic cord. Two main types of adenocarcinoma of the rete testis can be distinguished grossly and microscopically.
- The solid lesions tend to be firm and rubbery, usually show a whitish cut surface, and characteristically penetrate the testis and surrounding structures. Cystic lesions recall papillary serous cystadenocarcinomas arising in the ovary and peritoneum, and they can also be multiloculated.
- The morphologic criteria required for diagnosis include: (i) involvement of testicular mediastinum, (ii) transition from normal rete testis epithelium to neoplasia, (iii) intact parietal tunica vaginalis, and (iv) absence of any other primary tumor (Fig. 4.58).

4.24.2.2 Immunohistochemistry

- Immunohistochemistry is not specific for adenocarcinoma of rete testis but help excluding other tumors such mesothelioma or papillary serous carcinoma.
- Adenocarcinoma of the rete are diffusely positive for cytokeratin, CD10 and EMA, and are negative for hCG, AFP, S100, Leu-M1, PLAP, or PSA. Malignant mesotheliomas are positive for calretinin, Ck5/6, WT1, and negative for CEA, LeuM1, BerEP4. Serous carcinoma is positive for CA125 and WT1.

4.25 Epithelial Tumors of the Epididymis

4.25.1 Papillary Cystadenoma of the Epididymis

- Papillary cystadenoma is a cystic tumor reaching the size of 5 cm in diameter. The cysts are lined by columnar cells with water-clear, glycogen-rich cytoplasm. The cells form papillae protruding in the lumen of the cysts filled with a colloid-like fluid (Fig. 4.59).
- Affected men seek help because of sterility. The tumor is rather common (18 %) in men suffering from the Hippel–Lindau diseases, but it is extremely rare in sporadic cases. Mutations of VHL gene (3p25) in tumors can be seen in some cases. Immunohistochemistry is unnecessary in these tumors.

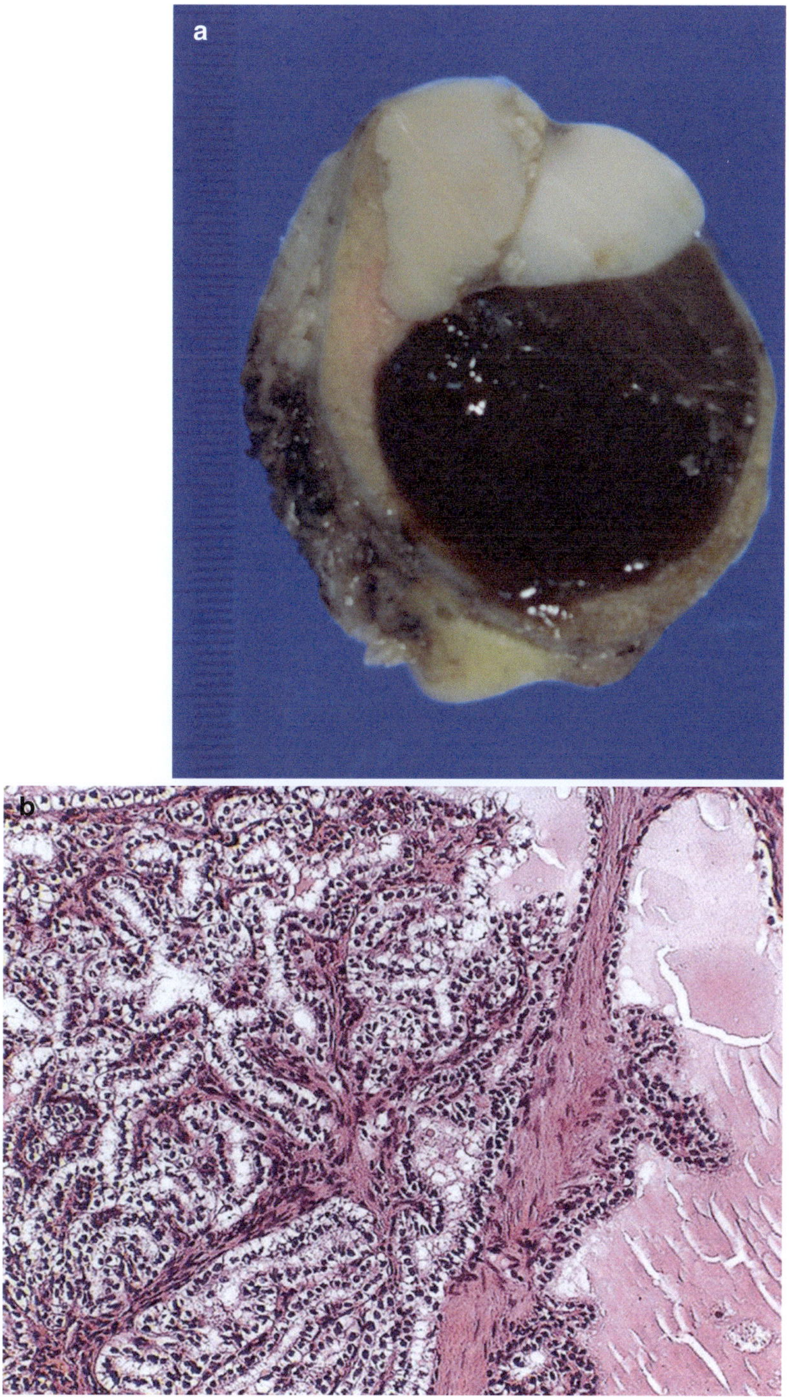

Fig. 4.59 (**a**) Gross features of papillary cystadenoma of the epididymis. (**b**) Microscopic features of papillary cystadenoma of the epididymis

4.25.2 Adenocarcinoma of the Epididymis

- Is one of the rarest malignancies and occur 25–80 years ranging 1–15 cm. Adenocarcinomas of the epididymis also have a tubulopapillary structure and clear cells like the adenomas. It is not associated to VHL. Immunohistochemistry shows cytokeratin+ and EMA+.

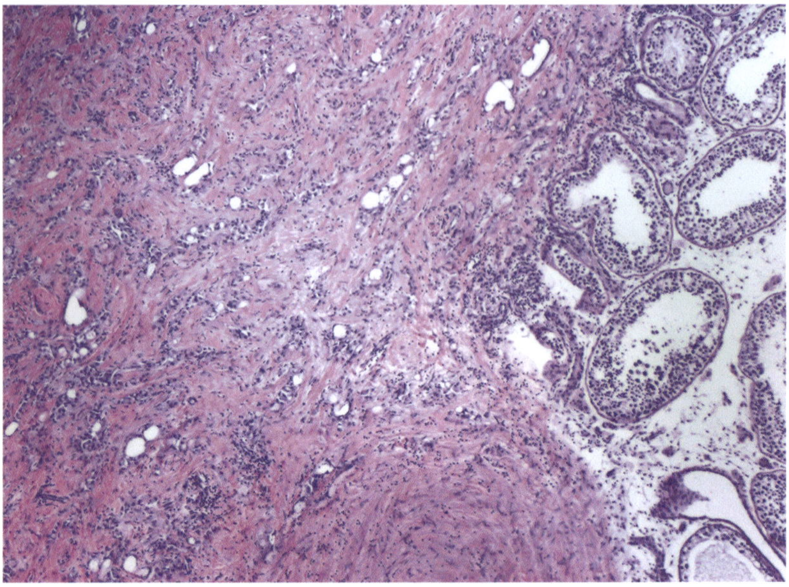

Fig. 4.60 Microscopic features of adenomatoid tumor

4.25.3 Adenomatoid Tumor

(Synonym: benign mesothelioma of the genital tract)

- Adenomatoid tumors are benign proliferations of mesothelial origin. Adenomatoid tumor accounts for 30 % of all paratesticular neoplasms and is the second most common tumor after lipoma in this location.
- Most reported cases arise from the epididymis, but rare cases arise in the testicular tunica, spermatic cord, ejaculatory ducts, prostate, and suprarenal recess. Intratesticular localization is very rare.
- Adenomatoid tumors occur in both sexes and are also found in the ovary, uterus, and fallopian tubes of the female genital tract. It occurs in men with a wide range of ages, with a peak incidence between 20 and 50 years.

4.25.3.1 Pathology

- Spherical tumors are markedly firm and whitish-yellow colored. The tumor size varies from a few millimeters up to 5 cm. The cuboidal tumor cells with intracytoplasmic vacuoles grow in solid cords or form pseudoglandular structures which can be mistaken for hemangioma or even for a Sertoli cell tumor.
- Like all mesothelia the tumor cells are immunoreactive for all types of cytokeratin antibodies, calretinin, WT1, and vimentin. (Figs. 4.60 and 4.61)

4.26 Mesothelioma of the Tunica Vaginalis Testis

- Mesothelioma derives from mesothelia, the cells that line the serous cavities. Irrespective of the primary location, there is a well-documented association with asbestos exposure and with exceptionally poor prognoses. Mesothelioma of the tunica vaginalis testis is an extremely rare tumor.
- The current WHO classification of the mesotheliomas of the tunic vaginalis testis distinguishes between benign and malignant types; the benign form is further subdivided into papillary and cystic types, respectively. Likewise, a clear distinction and prediction of the biological behavior are not always possible.
- Malignant mesothelioma of the tunica vaginalis testis can arise at any age; the range of the reported cases was 7–87 years. A form of mesothelioma of uncertain malignant potential has also been reported.

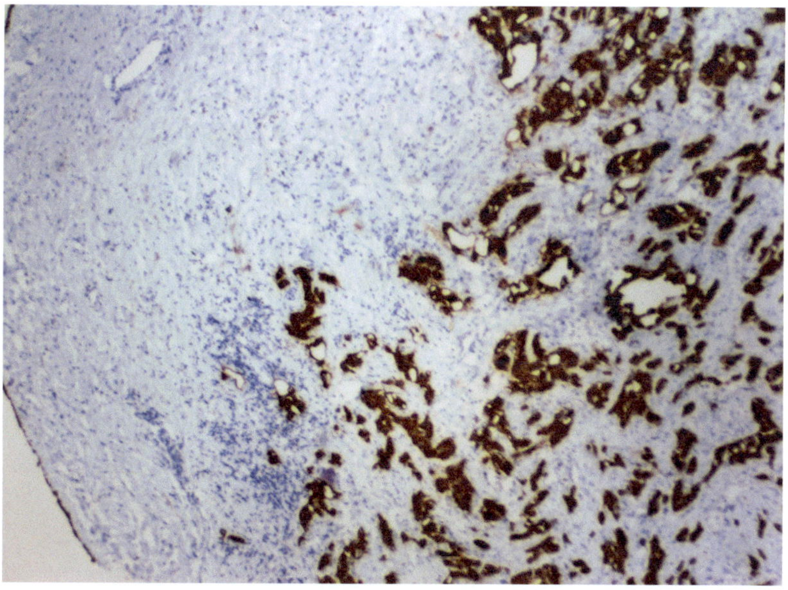

Fig. 4.61 The cells are positive for anti-CK antibodies

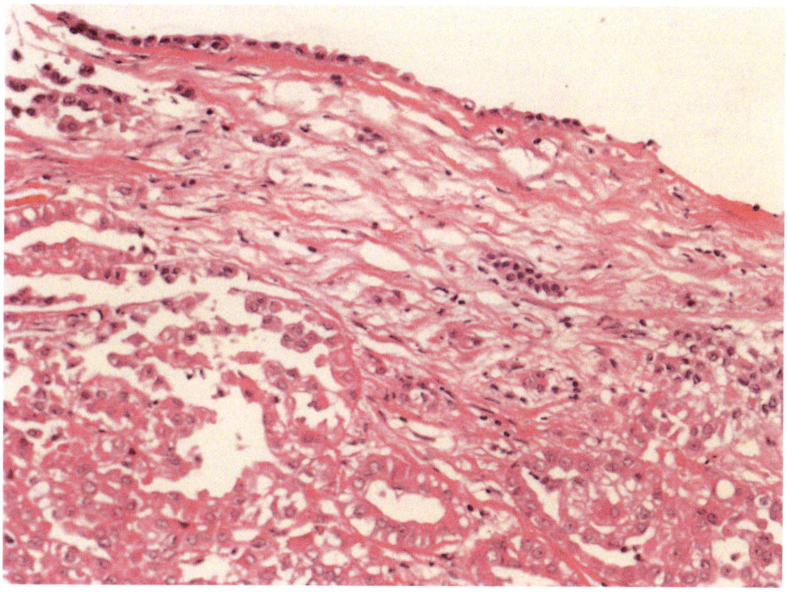

Fig. 4.62 Microscopic aspect of epithelioid mesothelioma of the tunica vaginalis

4.26.1 Pathology

- Most of the mesotheliomas of the tunica vaginalis present as a papillary exophytic in the lumen of a hydrocele sac growing tumor or shows only a more or less pronounced thickening of the tunica vaginalis with formation of small nodules.
- Generally there are three types of mesoteheliomas: the epithelial, the fibrous or sarcomatous, and a mixture of these two types, the biphasic type. In the tunica vaginalis the epithelial type accounts for 60 % and the biphasic type for 36 %, respectively. Sarcomatous mesothelioma is very rare (Figs. 4.62 and 4.63).

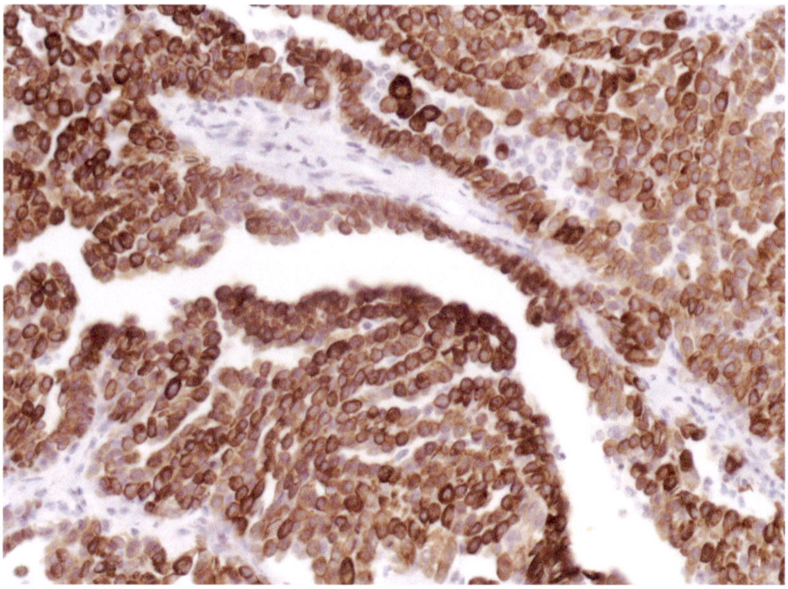

Fig. 4.63 Cells are positive for calretinin

- Even so-called benign papillary mesotheliomas show the invasion of the wall of the tunic in one-quarter of cases, and another fifth infiltrate to the testis. The only benign mesothelioma is the cystic type, which consists of a multilocular cyst lined by mesothelia.
- Benign reactive mesothelial proliferations in hydroceles may look histologically worrisome and are one of the main differential diagnoses. Such proliferations are nonetheless circumscribed, never macroscopically visible, and always microscopically discovered in the wall of a resected hydrocele.
- Mesotheliomas, on the other hand, are always macroscopically visible. As already mentioned, epithelial mesotheliomas can also be mistaken for ovarian type cystadenomas or carcinomas, which, however, have another anatomic location and a different immunophenotype. Malignant mesotheliomas are positive for calretinin, Ck5/6, WT1, and negative for CEA, LeuM1, BerEP4 (CD30).

4.27 Melanotic Neuroectodermal Tumor of Infancy

(Synonyms: congenital melanocarcinoma, retinal anlage tumor, pigmented congenital epulis, melanotic progonoma)

- Melanotic neuroectodermal tumor of infancy (MNTI) is a rare neoplasm. Most commonly, the lesion affects the maxilla of infants during the first year of life, but it may also occur in the mandible, skull, brain, epididymis, testis, and other rare locations
- The patients are young (range 4 months to 18 years)
- The tumor is circumscribed and cream-colored with black spots and shows two cell types: small immature neuroblast-like cells and large columnar or cuboidal epithelial-like cells with or without melanin granules. Some cases metastasize to lymph nodes. CK, HMB45 and EMA are positive in pigmented cells.

4.28 Desmoplastic Small Round Cell Tumor

- Desmoplastic small round cell tumor is a rare, primarily intra-abdominal tumor that has a poor outcome. Rare cases are located either in the tunica vaginalis or in the recess between the rete testis and epididymis. The tumor is firm and tan.
- Microscopically the tumor consists of the typical 'small round blue' cells which means that they have a prominent round nucleus with finely dispersed chromatin and a small rim of cytoplasm.

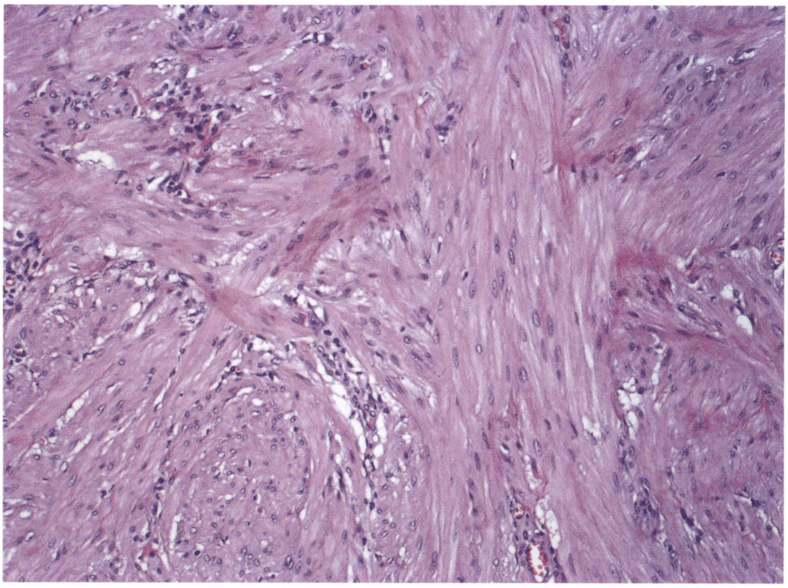

Fig. 4.64 Histologic features of leiomyoma of the spermatic cord

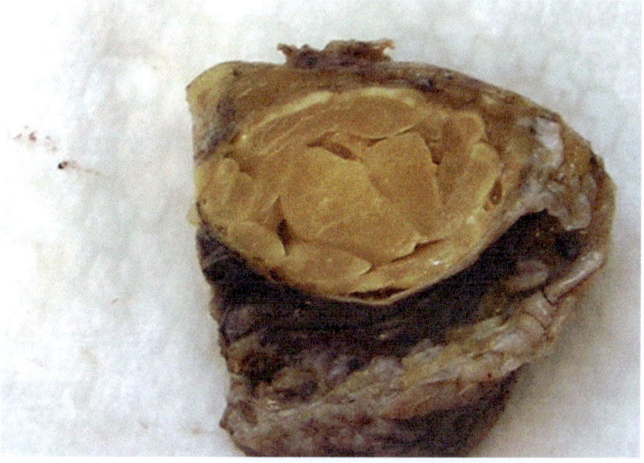

Fig. 4.65 Gross appearance of lipoma of the spermatic cord

- Tumor cell nests are surrounded by desmoplastic stroma. There is a distinctive immunophenotype, specifically positive for keratin, vimentin, desmin, and neuron-specific enolase, as well as a characteristic chromosomal abnormality, the EWS/WT-1 fusion transcript t(11,22)(p13,q12).
- The tumor metastasizes intra-abdominally and to the lung.

4.29 Soft Tissue Tumors of the Spermatic Cord

- Any type of soft tissue tumor can arise in the spermatic cord; nevertheless, they are rare. Lipomas, leiomyomas, hem- and lymphangiomas as well as, less frequently, neurofibromas are benign tumors encountered in this region. Lipo and leiomyosarcomas are the malignant counterpart affecting adult men (Figs. 4.64 and 4.65).
- Of juvenile rhabdomyosarcomas, 25 % (average age 6 years) arise in this location. The spindle cell type has a predilection for the paratesticular region (Fig. 4.66).
- Aggressive angiomyxoma is a rare, locally infiltrative tumor usually arising in the pelvic and perineal soft tissues of young women. Some cases involving scrotum, spermatic cord, inguinal region, and perineum of men have recently been described.
- Aggressive angiomyxoma has a high rate of local recurrence because of its infiltrative growth and anatomic location, making complete excision with wide margins difficult. Angiomyofibroblastoma is rarely observed.

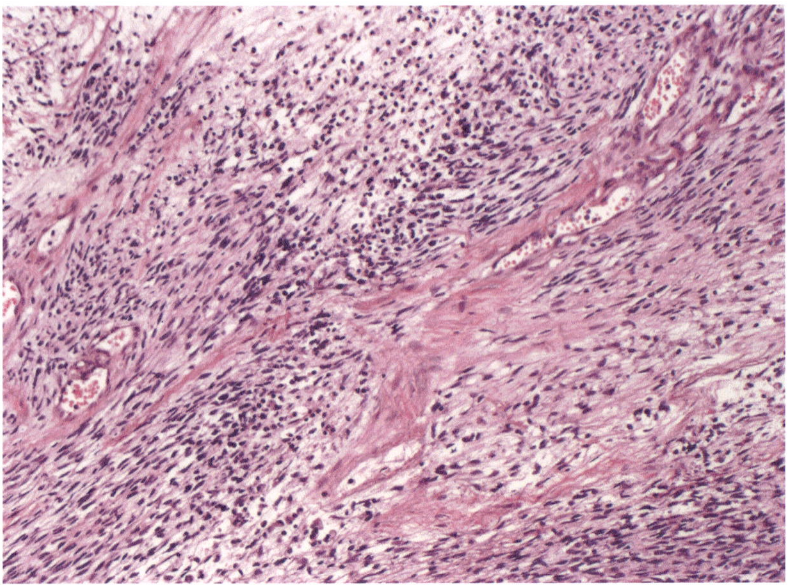

Fig. 4.66 Spindle cell type of juvenile rhabdomyosarcoma

4.30 Tumor-Like Conditions

- Pseudotumors or tumor-like proliferations and benign mimickers (non-neoplastic proliferations) are rare in the testis and paratesticular structures (Table 4.13).
- These lesions are a heterogeneous group relevant in terms of differential diagnosis and originate as vascular, inflammatory, idiopathic, cysts, ectopic tissues, embryonic remnants or hyperplastic lesions.

4.30.1 Intratesticular Hemorrhage

- Occurs spontaneously or in the context of anticoagulation treatment and may occasionally simulate a tumor at ultrasound examination.

4.30.2 Segmental Testicular Infarction

- Clinically characterized by slight local pain unrelated to any acute episode and seems to be associated with systemic vasculitis with morphology of polyarteritis nodosa, giant cell vasculitis, or Wegener granulomatosis.
- Other cases are seen in the context of a hematological disease (sickle cell anemia) or associated to unspecific perivascular fibrosis. Any of the phases of an infarction can be observed at microscopy, from acute (hemorrhagic) to healing stage

4.30.3 Organized Testicular Hematocele

- Like other vaginal hemorrhages are rarely confused with a neoplasia, but this can happen occasionally in long standing cases due to the fibrous thickening with cholesterol granuloma formation in the tunica vaginalis.
- Exceptionally, a true testicular neoplasia presents clinically as hematocele.

4.30.4 Inflammatory Lesions

4.30.4.1 Non-specific Infectious Inflammatory Lesions

- Inflammatory tumor-like presentation that are frequently chronic processes evolving into a progressive fibrosis and result clinically or at ultrasound examination with a diagnosis of neoplasia.

Table 4.13 Tumor-like lesions of testis and paratesticular structures

Vascular lesions
Intratesticular hemorrhage
Segmental testicular infarction
Organizad testicular hematocele
Cholesterol granuloma of the tunica vaginalis
Inflammatory and granulomatous lesions
Non-specific infectious inflammatory lesions
Specific infectious inflammatory lesions
Non-infectious inflammatory lesions
Idiopathic inflammatory lesions
Idiopathic granulomatous orchitis
Testicular malakoplakia
Lymphocitic orchitis (Testicular pseudolymphoma)
Rosai-Dorfman disease
Testicular sarcoidosis
Meconium periorchitis
Sperm granuloma
Sclerosing lipogranuloma
Cysts
Testicular cysts
Albuginea cysts
Parenchymal cysts (epidermoid cysts)
Rete-testis cysts- Cystic displasia of the rete testis
Epididymal cysts and Spermatoceles
Spermatic cord cysts.
Ectopic tissues
Adrenal cortical rests
Spleno-gonadal fusion
Lipomatosis testis
Testicular appendages
Other lesions
Fibrous pseudotumors (fibromatous periorchitis, nodular periorchitis)
Amyloidosis
Polyorchididm
Sclerosing lipogranuloma
Sertoli cell hyperplasia (Pick's adenoma)
Hamartomatous proliferation testicular feminization syndrome
Interstitial cell hyperplasia
Leydig cell hyperplasia
Testicular "tumor" of the adrenogenital syndrome
Hyperplasia of the rete testis (adenomatoid hyperplasia)
Crbriform hyperpsia and atypical nuceli in the epididymis
Mesotelial hyperplasia
Vasitis/epididymitis nodosa
Inflammatory pseudotumor
Other

- Rarely a testicular, epididymal or vas deferens abscess may appear as a neoplasia. Very occasionally testicular neoplasia can clinically present as an acute inflammatory process.

4.30.4.2 Specific Infectious Inflammatory Lesions

- The entities of this group that with greatest frequency have been confused with neoplasias are granulomatous diseases and were described in tuberculosis, brucellosis, syphillis, fungal infections, and parasite diseases.

4.30.4.3 Non-infectious (Idiopatic) Inflammatory Lesions

- Idiopathic granulomatous orchitis, malakoplakia, a lesion that shows fusion of the phagolysosomes with bacterial rests that produces the characteristic Michaelis-Gutman bodies in the macrophages cytoplasm (von Hansemann cells) and exceptionally, it may affect the epididymis only; Sarcoidosis in the testes is usually due to involvement in a systemic sarcoidosis
- Lymphocitic orchitis or testicular pseudolymphoma characterized by a lymphocytic and plasmocelular polyclonal reaction that can be confused with a lymphoma.
- Rosai-Dorfman disease, that may appears as a testicular/paratesticular mass with an inflammatory lesion comprising lymphocytes, plasma cells and sheets of pale staining histiocytes containing lymphocytes within their wide cytoplasm. Histiocytes are CD68+, S100 +, CD1a–.
- Rare cases of sclerosing igG4 have been described in this anatomic region.

4.31 Meconium Periorchitis

- This is an infrequent situation that can be presented in the first months of life; most times there is a clinical history with obstetric problem that has caused the passing of meconium towards the testicular surrounding structures.
- The macroscopic appearance is a mixoid material with calcified pearls resulting from the calcification of squamous cells. The suspicion of

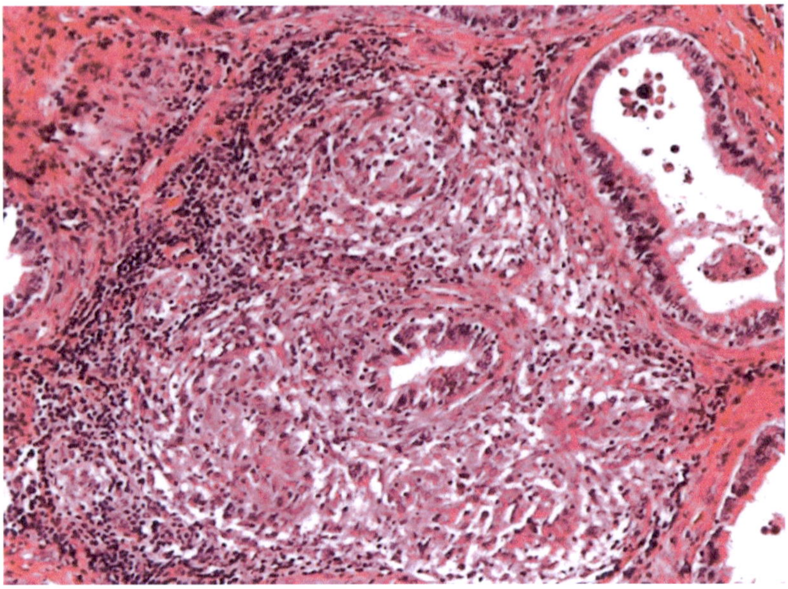

Fig. 4.67 Microscopic view of sperm granuloma

a neoplasia, although in this period of life it is very infrequent, it is consequence of the scrotal mass with detectable calcifications at ultrasound.

4.32 Sperm Granuloma

- This granulomatous lesion with few giant cells is the consequence of extravasation of spermatozoa generally post-vasectomy. When it produces a tumor-like lesion, usually is in the deferent duct or the epididymis; occasionally shows cysts formation (Fig. 4.67).

4.33 Sclerosing Lipogranuloma

- Injection of lipids resulted in granulomatous lesion in the scrotum (see also page 427, Chap. 5), spermatic cord or the epididymis.

4.34 Cysts

- Most cysts with a tumor-like presentation are paratesticular s, but may occasionally occur in the testicle where can be confused with a neoplasia. Most frequently occur in the tunica albuginea or testicular parenchyma.

4.34.1 Epidermoid Cyst

- It represents 1 % of the tumor masses of the testes and must be composed of mature squamous epithelium only. It is recommended to evaluate the specimen "in toto" to avoid any area of teratoma (especially among postpuberal patients), or of intratubular germ cell neoplasia; Recent genetic studies have shown that there is not chromosome 12p abnormality, thus supporting its distinction from true teratoma.

4.34.2 Tubular Ectasia of the Rete Testis

- Usually related to obstruction is generally located at the mediastinum testes and bilateral and histologically different to cystic dysplasia of the rete testis, a congenital lesion with complete testicular parenchyma substitution.

4.34.3 Epididymal Cysts and Spermatoceles

- Relatively frequent and the majority are in relation to the inflammatory processes. The differential diagnosis with other entities are

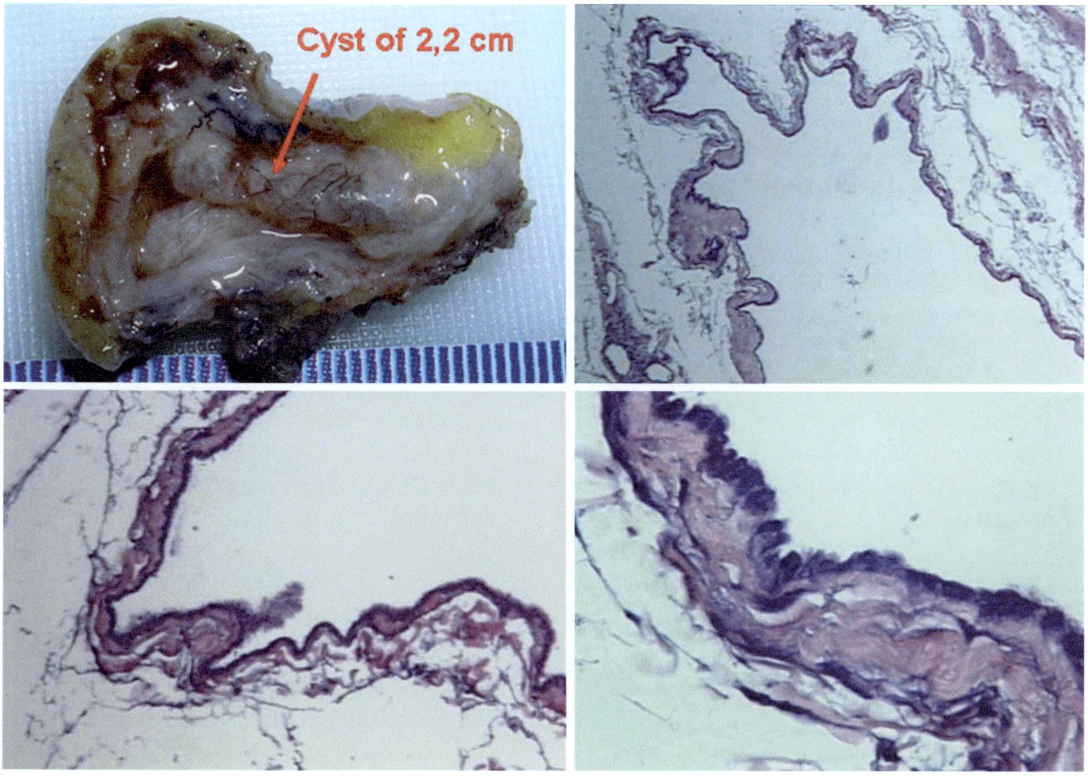

Fig. 4.68 Gross and microscopic features of an epididimal cyst

related to its size and similarities to the other cystic formations (Fig. 4.68).

4.34.4 Spermatic Cord Cysts

- The majority of these cysts do not cause any diagnostic difficulties, but occasionally the epidermoid cyst can simulate a neoplasia. These cysts can be unilocular or multilocular and those of multilocular appearance must be distinguished from the exceptional cystadenomas of probably müllerian origin.

4.35 Ectopic Tissues

4.35.1 Ectopic Adrenocortical Tissue

- Relatively frequent in tunica albuginea, rete testis, epididymis and spermatic cord, and occasionally reaches the size to be symptomatic.
- It is made up of mature adrenal cortical tissue of about 5 mm in diameter surrounded by a connective band.

4.35.2 Splenic-Gonadal Fusion

- Is the fusion of spleen and gonad, it is more frequent on the left side. Morphologically, the ectopic splenic tissue can be in close relation to the head of the epididymis or the upper pole of the testis.

4.35.3 Lipomatosis Testis

- Is a rare condition seen in Cowden disease defined by multiple hamartomatous growths and a high risk of cancer development. The syndrome is inherited as an autosomal dominant. The PTEN/MMAC1/TEP1 tumor suppressor gene on chromosome 10q23.3 contains a germ line mutation. Microscopically, multiple foci of mature fat tissue occupy the testicular interstitium.

4.36 Testicular Appendages

- There are five testicular appendages but for the purpose of the surgical pathologist, only three are of interest (Appendix testis or hydatid of Morgagni, Appendix epididymis, Paradidymis or organ of Giraldes).
- In rare cases of large-sized cysts, they may present as a paratesticular mass. Rarely, ectopic epididymal tissue may be seen in testicular appendages.

4.37 Other Tumor-Like Lesions

4.37.1 Fibrous Pseudotumor

(Synonyms: chronic periorchitis, Fibromatous periorchitis, Nodular periorchitis, Fibrous proliferation of the tunica, Nonspecific paratesticular fibrosis, Granulomatous periorchitis, Nodular fibrous pseudotumor, Fibrous pseudotumor, Inflammatory pseudotumor, Fibroma, or Reactive periorchitis)

- This name refers to a fibrosis phenomenon with hipocellular hyalinized collagen presenting as nodular (single or multiple) or diffuse lesion of the testicular tunics.
- Sometimes a nodule can be free (scrotal mouse). Some cases have previous history of trauma or infection, and on occasion, an inflammatory component can be observed and granulation tissue suggesting the possibility that there might be the healing of an inflammatory pseudotumor.

4.37.2 Amyloidosis

- It is usually bilateral and present in a patient with a prior history of amyloidosis but rarely it is a primary form that simulates a testicular tumor.

4.37.3 Polyorchidism

- Supernumerary testes is a rare condition, easy to recognize, but on occasions can simulate a tumor-like condition.

4.37.4 Sertoli Cell Hyperplasia

- Non-encapsulated nodules of Sertoli cells can be found, especially known in cryptorchid testes as Pick's adenomas. Because of their appearance these should be distinguished from the actual Sertoli cell tumors which generally are larger and sometimes there are areas that mimic Call-Exner bodies

4.37.5 Leydig Cell Hyperplasia

- Is seen in testicles with marked tubular atrophy, such as in the Klinefelter syndrome, but it is also possible to see Leydig cell nodules that must be distinguished from the Leydig cell tumors. The interstitial growth without expansive pattern favors hyperplasia.
- Nodules of eosinophilic cells appearing to be Leydig cells are found in the patients with adrenogenital syndrome and Nelson's syndrome are usually bilateral and of a large size with cellular pleomorphism and pigmentation.

4.37.6 Hyperplasia of the Rete Testis

(Synonym: adenomatous hyperplasia)

- The normal rete testis epithelium is flat, but in some cases with estrogen effect (therapy or hepatic dysfunction, other) can acquire a columnar appearance and rarely a micropapillary growth of bland cells can be observed. In some cases there are intracytoplasmic hyaline eosinophilic globules that should not be mistaken as yolk sac tumor.
- Smooth muscle hyperplasia of the rete testis and other testicular adnexa is a rare idiopathic tumor-like condition observed in men

46–80 years old forming an intrascrotal palpable mass from millimeter to several centimeters.

4.37.7 Cribriform Hyperplasia and Atypical Nuclei in the Epididymis

- The normal epididymis, which usually has a simple columnar epithelium, may display a cribriform epithelial pattern focal or rarely extensive, thus suggesting a hyperplastic process.
- Enlarged and atypical nuclei may also occur in the efferent ductuli, ductos epididymis, and vas deferens.

4.37.8 Reactive Mesothelial Hyperplasia

- Is the most important benign mimicker of the testicular tunics, and is seen in reactive situations as hydrocele or hernia. The mesothelial proliferation has an epithelial appearance occasionally with tubular appearance with retraction artifact, and rarely showing spindle cell features.
- In the differential diagnosis with mesothelioma the bland nuclear features, lack stromal invasion and the associated inflammatory/reactive background is useful. WT1 immunoreactivity confirms the mesothelial nature of the lesion.

4.37.9 Vasitis/Epididymitis Nodosa

- Ductular proliferation with a microglandular appearance mild nuclear atipia and perineural growth or benign vascular invasion, generally after vasectomy or trauma that may be clinically mistaken for malignancy.
- The coincidence with microscopic sperm granulomas and inflammatory reaction can help in the correct diagnosis. An epididymal lesion with similar histology may occur.

4.37.10 Proliferative Funiculitis

(Synonyms: inflammatory myofibroblastic tumor, pseudosarcomatous myofibroblastic proliferation, inflammatory pseudotumr)

- The inflammation of the spermatic cord usually is the result of the extension of a vasitis, but the soft tissues of the spermatic cord are the most common site in the male genital tract of the Inflammatory pseudotumor.
- The lesion is ill defined, mixoid and white-grey color with a moderate cellular proliferation with a loose collagen fibers and irregular inflammatory cells infiltration, exceptionally including mast cells.
- In some cases a prominent spindle cell proliferation mimics a sarcoma (pseudosarcomatous myofobroblastic proliferation) but the finding of no atypical mitosis, variable mitotic index, the capillary pattern and the presence of inflammatory cells is against the diagnosis of sarcoma. Immunohistochemistry may be helpful in differential diagnosis. Inflammatory pseudotumor may be seen also in epididymis or rete testis.

4.37.11 Embryonic Remnants

- Rare embryonic remnants such as the presence of seminiferous tubules within the tunica albuginea; Leydig cells in rete testis, albuginea, spermatic cord, or within sclerotic tubules; prostate gland in the epididymis and muscular rete testis hypertrophy can mimics a neoplasia.

Suggested Reading

Akhtar M, AlDayel F, Siegrist K, et al. Neutrophil-rich Ki-1-positive anaplastic large cell lymphoma presenting as a testicular mass. Mod Pathol. 1996; 9:812–5.

Alvarado-Cabrero I, Hernández-Toriz N, Paner GP. Clinicopathologic analysis of choriocarcinoma as a pure or predominant component of germ cell tumor of the testis. Am J Surg Pathol. 2014;38(1):111–8. doi:10.1097/PAS.0b013e3182a2926e.

Ameur A, al Bouzidi A, Aqira A, Benomar S, Draoui D. Granulomatous orchitis. A case report and review of the literature. Prog Urol. 1998;8:410–2.

Augusto D, Leteurtre E, De La Taille A, et al. Calretinin: a valuable marker of normal and neoplastic Leydig cells of the testis. Appl Immunohistochem Mol Morphol. 2002;10:159–62.

Azua-Romeo J, Alvarez-Alegret R, Serrano P, et al. Primary anaplastic large cell lymphoma of the testis. Int Urol Nephrol. 2004;36:393–6.

Bach AM, Hann LE, Hadar O, Shi W, Yoo HH, Giess CS, Sheinfeld J, Thaler H. Testicular microlithiasis: what is its association with testicular cancer? Radiology. 2001;220:70–5.

Bailey D, Marks A, Stratis M, et al. Immunohistochemical staining of germ cell tumors and intratubular malignant germ cells of the testis using antibody to placental alkaline phosphatase and a monoclonal anti-seminoma antibody. Mod Pathol. 1991;4:167–71.

Ballereau C, Leroy X, Morschhauser F, et al. Testicular natural killer T-cell lymphoma. Int J Urol. 2005;12: 223–4.

Balogh K, Travis WD. Benign vascular invasion in vasitis nodosa. Am J Clin Pathol. 1985;83:426–30.

Bergh A, Cajander S. Immunohistochemical localization of inhibin-alpha in the testes of normal men and in men with testicular disorders. Int J Androl. 1990;13:463–9.

Berney DM, Shamash J, Pieroni K, et al. Loss of CD30 expression in metastatic embryonal carcinoma: the effects of chemotherapy? Histopathology. 2001;39:382–5.

Bode PK, Barghorn A, Fritzsche FR, et al. MAGEC2 is a sensitive and novel marker for seminoma: a tissue microarray analysis of 325 testicular germ cell tumors. Mod Pathol. 2011;24:829–35.

Brauers A, Striepecke E, Mersdorf A, Sohn M, Fuzesi L. Inflammatory pseudotumor of the epididymis. Eur Urol. 1997;32:253–5.

Burke AP, Mostofi FK. Placental alkaline phosphatase immunohistochemistry of intratubular malignant germ cells and associated testicular germ cell tumors. Hum Pathol. 1988a;19:663–70.

Burke AP, Mostofi FK. Intratubular malignant germ cells in testicular biopsies: clinical course and identification by staining for placental alkaline phosphatase. Mod Pathol. 1988b;1:475–9.

Caillaud JM, Bellet D, Carlu C, et al. Immunohistochemistry of germ cell tumors of the testis. Study of beta HCG and AFP. Prog Clin Biol Res. 1985;203:139–40.

Cao D, Humphrey PA, Allan RW. SALL4 is a novel sensitive and specific marker for metastatic germ cell tumors, with particular utility in detection of metastatic yolk sac tumors. Cancer. 2009a;115:2640–51.

Cao D, Li J, Guo CC, Allan RW, et al. SALL4 is a novel diagnostic marker for testicular germ cell tumors. Am J Surg Pathol. 2009b;33:1065–77.

Cao D, Allan RW, Cheng L, et al. RNA-binding protein LIN28 is a marker for testicular germ cell tumors. Hum Pathol. 2011;42:710–8.

Casella R, Nudell D, Cozzolino D, Wang H, Lipshultz LI. Primary testicular amyloidosis mimicking tumor in a cryptorchid testis. Urology. 2002;59:445.

Chan JK, Tsang WY, Lau WH, et al. Aggressive T/natural killer cell lymphoma presenting as testicular tumor. Cancer. 1996;77:1198–205.

Cheng L, Zhang S, MacLennan GT, Poulos CK, Sung MT, Beck SD, Foster RS. Interphase fluorescence in situ hybridization analysis of chromosome 12p abnormalities is useful for distinguishing epidermoid cysts of the testis from pure mature teratoma. Clin Cancer Res. 2006;12:5668–72.

Cheng L, Sung MT, Cossu-Rocca P, et al. OCT4: biological functions and clinical applications as a marker of germ cell neoplasia. J Pathol. 2007;211:1–9.

Cheville JC, Rao S, Iczkowski KA, et al. Cytokeratin expression in seminoma of the human testis. Am J Clin Pathol. 2000;113:583–8.

Chu P, Wu E, Weiss LM. Cytokeratin 7 and cytokeratin 20 expression in epithelial neoplasms: a survey of 435 cases. Mod Pathol. 2000;13:962–72.

Claahsen-van der Grinten HL, Otten BJ, Takahashi S, et al. Testicular adrenal rest tumors in adult males with congenital adrenal hyperplasia: evaluation of pituitary-gonadal function before and after successful testis-sparing surgery in eight patients. J Clin Endocrinol Metab. 2007;92:612–5.

Cools M, van Aerde K, Kersemaekers AM, et al. Morphological and immunohistochemical differences between gonadal maturation delay and early germ cell neoplasia in patients with undervirilization syndromes. J Clin Endocrinol Metab. 2005;90:5295–303.

Cui W, Kong NR, Ma Y, et al. Differential expression of the novel oncogene, SALL4, in lymphoma, plasma cell myeloma, and acute lymphoblastic leukemia. Mod Pathol. 2006;19:1585–92.

Dahl EV, Bahn RC. Aberrant adrenal cortical tissue near the testis in human infants. Am J Pathol. 1962;40:587–98.

de Jong J, Stoop H, Dohle GR, et al. Diagnostic value of OCT3/4 for pre-invasive and invasive testicular germ cell tumours. J Pathol. 2005;206:242–9.

de Jong J, Stoop H, Gillis AJ, et al. Differential expression of SOX17 and SOX2 in germ cells and stem cells has biological and clinical implications. J Pathol. 2008;215:21–30.

Dekker I, Rozeboom T, Delemarre J, et al. Placental-like alkaline phosphatase and DNA flow cytometry in spermatocytic seminoma. Cancer. 1992;69:993–6.

Demirtas E, Krishnamurthy S, Tulandi T. Elevated serum beta-human chorionic gonadotropin in nonpregnant conditions. Obstet Gynecol Surv. 2007;62:675–9.

Dieckmann KP, Henke RP, Zimmer-Krolzig G. Malacoplakia of the epididymis. Report of a case and review of the literature. Urol Int. 1995;55:222–5.

Dotan ZA, Laufer M, Heldenberg E, Langevitz P, Fridman E, Duvdevani M, Ramon J. Isolated testicular polyarteritis nodosa mimicking testicular neoplasm-long-term follow-up. Urology. 2003;62:352.

Dunner PS, Lipsit ER, Nochomovitz LE. Epididymal sperm granuloma simulating a testicular neoplasm. J Clin Ultrasound. 1982;10(7):353–5.

Eble JN, Sauter G, Epstein JI, Sesterhenn IA, editors. Pathology & genetics. Tumors of the urinary system and male genital organs, WHO classification of tumors. Lyon: IARC Press; 2004. p. 218–9.

Eglen DE, Ulbright TM. The differential diagnosis of yolk sac tumor and seminoma. Usefulness of cytokeratin, alpha-fetoprotein, and alpha-1-antitrypsin immunoperoxidase reactions. Am J Clin Pathol. 1987;88:328–32.

Fernandopulle SM, Hwang JS, Kuick CH, Lui J, Tan PH, Siow WY, Wong M. Rosai-Dorfman disease of the testis: an unusual entity that mimics testicular malignancy. J Clin Pathol. 2006;59(3):325–7.

Ferreiro JA. Ber-H2 expression in testicular germ cell tumors. Hum Pathol. 1994;25(5):522–4.

Ferry JA, Harris NL, Young RH, et al. Malignant lymphoma of the testis, epididymis, and spermatic cord. A clinicopathologic study of 69 cases with immunophenotypic analysis. Am J Surg Pathol. 1994;18:376–90.

Ferry JA, Ulbright TM, Young RH. Anaplastic large cell lymphoma presenting in the testis. J Urol Pathol. 1997;5:139–47.

Fridman E, Skarda J, Ofek-Moravsky E, Cordoba M. Complex multilocular cystic lesion of rete testis, accompanied by smooth muscle hyperplasia, mimicking intratesticular Leydig cell neoplasm. Virchows Arch. 2005;447(4):768–71.

Garat JM, Algaba F, Parra L, Gomez L. Meconium vaginalitis. Br J Urol. 1991;68:430–1.

Gopalan A, Dhall D, Olgac S, et al. Testicular mixed germ cell tumors: a morphological and immunohistochemical study using stem cell markers, OCT3/4, SOX2 and GDF3, with emphasis on morphologically difficult-to-classify areas. Mod Pathol. 2009; 22:1066–74.

Gouw AS, Elema JD, Bink-Boelkens MT, de Jongh HJ, ten Kate LP. The spectrum of splenogonadal fusion. Case report and review of 82 reported cases. Eur J Pediatr. 1985;144:316–23.

Hartwick RW, Ro JY, Srigley JR, Ordonez NG, Ayala AG. Adenomatous hyperplasia of the rete testis. A clinicopathologic study of nine cases. Am J Surg Pathol. 1991;15:350–7.

Hasselblom S, Ridell B, Wedel H, et al. Testicular lymphoma–a retrospective, population-based, clinical and immunohistochemical study. Acta Oncol. 2004;43:758–65.

Henley JD, Young RH, Ulbright TM. Malignant Sertoli cell tumors of the testis – a study of 13 examples of a neoplasm frequently misinterpreted as seminoma. Am J Surg Pathol. 2002;26:541–50.

Hirschowitz L, Rode J, Guillebaud J, Bounds W, Moss E. Vasitis nodosa and associated clinical findings. J Clin Pathol. 1988;41(4):419–23.

Hittmair A, Rogatsch H, Hobisch A, et al. CD30 expression in seminoma. Hum Pathol. 1996;27:1166–71.

Hoang MP, Amirkhan RH. Inhibin alpha distinguishes hemangioblastoma from clear cell renal cell carcinoma. Am J Surg Pathol. 2003;27:1152–6.

Hurd DS, Olsen T. Cutaneous sarcoidosis presenting as a testicular mass. Cutis. 2000;66:435–8.

Hustin J, Collette J, Franchimont P. Immunohistochemical demonstration of placental alkaline-phosphatase in various states of testicular development and in germ-cell tumors. Int J Androl. 1987;10:29–35.

Hyland J, Lasota J, Jasinski M, et al. Molecular pathological analysis of testicular diffuse large cell lymphomas. Hum Pathol. 1998;29:1231–9.

Iczkowski KA, Bostwick DG, Roche PC, et al. Inhibin A is a sensitive and specific marker for testicular sex cord stromal tumors. Mod Pathol. 1998;11:774–9.

Iczkowski KA, Butler SL, Shanks JH, et al. Trials of new germ cell immunohistochemical stains in 93 extragonadal and metastatic germ cell tumors. Hum Pathol. 2008;39:275–81.

Idrees M, Saxena R, Cheng L, et al. Podoplanin, a novel marker for seminoma: a comparison study evaluating immunohistochemical expression of podoplanin and OCT3/4. Ann Diagn Pathol. 2010;14:331–6.

Izquierdo MA, Van der Valk P, Van Ark-Otte J, et al. Differential expression of the c-kit proto-oncogene in germ cell tumours. J Pathol. 1995;177:253–8.

Jacobsen GK, Jacobsen M. Alpha-fetoprotein (AFP) and human chorionic gonadotropin (HCG) in testicular germ cell tumours. A prospective immunohistochemical study. Acta Pathol Microbiol Immunol Scand A. 1983;91:165–76.

Jacobsen GK, Norgaard-Pedersen B. Placental alkaline phosphatase in testicular germ cell tumours and in carcinoma-in-situ of the testis. An immunohistochemical study. Acta Pathol Microbiol Immunol Scand A. 1984;92:323–9.

Jones TD, Ulbright TM, Eble JN, et al. OCT4 staining in testicular tumors: a sensitive and specific marker for seminoma and embryonal carcinoma. Am J Surg Pathol. 2004a;28:935–40.

Jones TD, Ulbright TM, Eble JN, et al. OCT4: a sensitive and specific biomarker for intratubular germ cell neoplasia of the testis. Clin Cancer Res. 2004b;10(24):8544–7.

Kao CS, Idrees MT, Young RH, et al. Solid pattern yolk sac tumor in testicular germ cell tumors: a morphologic and immunohistochemical study of 52 cases. Am J Surg Pathol. 2012;36:360–7.

Katergiannakis V, Lagoudianakis EE, Markogiannakis H, Manouras A. Huge epidermoid cyst of the spermatic cord in an adult patient. Int J Urol. 2006;13:95–7.

Kato Y, Sasagawa I, Kaneko M, et al. Aggrus: a diagnostic marker that distinguishes seminoma from embryonal carcinoma in testicular germ cell tumors. Oncogene. 2004;23:8552–6.

Kim YB, Chang SK, Yang WI, et al. Primary NK/T cell lymphoma of the testis. A case report and review of the literature. Acta Haematol. 2003;109:95–100.

Kommoss F, Oliva E, Bittinger F, et al. Inhibin-alpha CD99, HEA125, PLAP, and chromogranin immunoreactivity in testicular neoplasms and the androgen insensitivity syndrome. Hum Pathol. 2000;31:1055–61.
Kraggerud SM, Berner A, Bryne M, et al. Spermatocytic seminoma as compared to classical seminoma: an immunohistochemical and DNA flow cytometric study. APMIS. 1999;107:297–302.
Kryvenko ON, Epstein JI. Testicular hemangioma: a series of 8 cases. Am J Surg Pathol. 2013;37(6):860–6.
Lagmay J, Termuhlen A, Fung B, et al. Primary testicular presentation of ALK-1-negative anaplastic large cell lymphoma in a pediatric patient. J Pediatr Hematol Oncol. 2009;31:330–2.
Lagrange JL, Ramaioli A, Theodore CH, et al. Non-Hodgkin's lymphoma of the testis: a retrospective study of 84 patients treated in the French anticancer centres. Ann Oncol. 2001;12:1313–9.
Lau SK, Weiss LM, Chu PG. D2-40 immunohistochemistry in the differential diagnosis of seminoma and embryonal carcinoma: a comparative immunohistochemical study with KIT (CD117) and CD30. Mod Pathol. 2007;20:320–5.
Lee LY, Tzeng J, Grosman M, Unger PD. Prostate gland-like epithelium in the epididymis: a case report and review of the literature. Arch Pathol Lab Med. 2004;128:60–2.
Leroy X, Augusto D, Leteurtre E, et al. CD30 and CD117 (c-kit) used in combination are useful for distinguishing embryonal carcinoma from seminoma. J Histochem Cytochem. 2002;50:283–5.
Li M, Fogarty J, Whitney KD, Stone P. Repeated testicular infarction in a patient with sickle cell disease: a possible mechanism for testicular failure. Urology. 2003;62:551.
Loftus BM, Gilmartin LG, O'Brien MJ, et al. Intratubular germ cell neoplasia of the testis: identification by placental alkaline phosphatase immunostaining and argyrophilic nucleolar organizer region quantification. Hum Pathol. 1990;21:941–8.
Looijenga LH. Human testicular (non)seminomatous germ cell tumours: the clinical implications of recent pathobiological insights. J Pathol. 2009;218:146–62.
Looijenga LH, Stoop H, de Leeuw HP, et al. POU5F1 (OCT3/4) identifies cells with pluripotent potential in human germ cell tumors. Cancer Res. 2003;63:2244–50.
Lugli A, Forster Y, Haas P, et al. Calretinin expression in human normal and neoplastic tissues: a tissue microarray analysis on 5233 tissue samples. Hum Pathol. 2003;34:994–1000.
Manivel JC, Jessurun J, Wick MR, et al. Placental alkaline phosphatase immunoreactivity in testicular germ cell tumors. Am J Surg Pathol. 1987;11:21–9.
McCluggage WG, Shanks JH, Whiteside C, et al. Immunohistochemical study of testicular sex cord-stromal tumors, including staining with anti-inhibin antibody. Am J Surg Pathol. 1998a;22:615–9.
McCluggage WG, Ashe P, McBride H, et al. Localization of the cellular expression of inhibin in trophoblastic tissue. Histopathology. 1998b;32:252–6.
McClure J. Malakoplakia of the testis and its relationship to granulomatous orchitis. J Clin Pathol. 1980;33:670–8.
Miettinen M, Wang Z, McCue PA, et al. SALL4 expression in germ cell and non germ-cell tumors: a systematic immunohistochemical study of 3215 cases. Am J Surg Pathol. 2014;38:410–20.
Mikuz G. Clinical pathology of urologic tumors. Boca Raton: Informa Health Care; 2006.
Niehans GA, Manivel JC, Copland GT, et al. Immunohistochemistry of germ cell and trophoblastic neoplasms. Cancer. 1988;62:1113–23.
Nistal M, Regadera J, Paniagua R. Cystic dysplasia of the testis. Light and electron microscopic study of three cases. Arch Pathol Lab Med. 1984;108:579–83.
Nistal M, Paniagua R, Leon L, Regadera J. Ectopic seminiferous tubules in the tunica albuginea of normal and dysgenetic testes. Appl Pathol. 1985;3:123–8.
Nistal M, Iniguez L, Paniagua R. Histological classification of spermatic cord cysts in relation to their histogenesis. Eur Urol. 1987;13:327–30.
Nistal M, Castillo MC, Regadera J, Garcia-Cabezas MA. Adenomatous hyperplasia of the rete testis. A review and report of new cases. Histol Histopathol. 2003;18(3):741–52.
Nonaka D. Differential expression of SOX2 and SOX17 in testicular germ cell tumors. Am J Clin Pathol. 2009;131:731–6.
Ota S, Hishinuma M, Yamauchi N, et al. Oncofetal protein glypican-3 in testicular germ-cell tumor. Virchows Arch. 2006;449:308–14.
Pallesen G, Hamilton-Dutoit SJ. Ki-1 (CD30) antigen is regularly expressed in tumor cells of embryonal carcinoma. Am J Pathol. 1988;133:446–50.
Parveen T, Fleischmann J, Petrelli M. Benign fibrous tumor of the tunica vaginalis testis. Report of a case with light, electron microscopic, and immunocytochemical study, and review of the literature. Arch Pathol Lab Med. 1992;116:277–80.
Perez-Ordonez B, Srigley JR. Mesothelial lesions of the paratesticular region. Semin Diagn Pathol. 2000;17:294–306.
Ponti G, et al. The impact of histopathologic diagnosis on the proper management of testis neoplasms. Nat Clin Pract Oncol. 2008;5:619–22.
Rajpert-De Meyts E, Skakkebaek NE. Expression of the c-kit protein product in carcinoma-in-situ and invasive testicular germ cell tumours. Int J Androl. 1994;17:85–92.
Rajpert-De Meyts E, Jorgensen N, Brondum-Nielsen K, et al. Developmental arrest of germ cells in the pathogenesis of germ cell neoplasia. APMIS. 1998;106:198–204.
Ramalingam P, Malpica A, Silva EG, et al. The use of cytokeratin 7 in differentiating yolk sac tumors from endometrioid and clear cell carcinomas of the ovary. Mod Pathol. 2003;16:207A.
Renshaw AA, Granter SR. A comparison of A103 and inhibin reactivity in adrenal cortical tumors: distinction from hepatocellular carcinoma and renal tumors. Mod Pathol. 1998;11:1160–4.

Rorth M, Rajpert-De Meyts E, Andersson L, et al. Carcinoma in situ in the testis. Scand J Urol Nephrol Suppl. 2000;205:166–86.

Santagata S, Ligon KL, Hornick JL. Embryonic stem cell transcription factor signatures in the diagnosis of primary and metastatic germ cell tumors. Am J Surg Pathol. 2007;31:836–45.

Skakkebaek NE, Berthelsen JG, Giwercman A, et al. Carcinoma-in-situ of the testis: possible origin from gonocytes and precursor of all types of germ cell tumours except spermatocytoma. Int J Androl. 1987;10:19–28.

Stoop H, Honecker F, van de Geijn GJ, et al. Stem cell factor as a novel diagnostic marker for early malignant germ cells. J Pathol. 2008;216:43–54.

Strohmeyer T, Reese D, Press M, et al. Expression of the c-kit proto-oncogene and its ligand stem cell factor (SCF) in normal and malignant human testicular tissue. J Urol. 1995;153:511–5.

Sung MT, Jones TD, Beck SD, et al. OCT4 is superior to CD30 in the diagnosis of metastatic embryonal carcinomas after chemotherapy. Hum Pathol. 2006;37:662–7.

Thompson JE, van der Walt JD. Nodular fibrous proliferation (fibrous pseudotumour) of the tunica vaginalis testis. A light, electron microscopic and immunocytochemical study of a case and review of the literature. Histopathology. 1986;10:741–8.

Tolhurst SR, Lotan T, Rapp DE, Lyon MB, Orvieto MA, Gerber GS, Sokoloff MH. Well-differentiated papillary mesothelioma occurring in the tunica vaginalis of the testis with contralateral atypical mesothelial hyperplasia. Urol Oncol. 2006;24:36–9.

Tyagi G, Munn CS, Kiser LC, Wetzner SM, Tarabulcy E. Malignant mesothelioma of tunica vaginalis testis. Urology. 1989;34:102–4.

Ulbright TM. Germ cell tumors of the gonads; a selective review emphasizing problems in differential diagnosis, newly appreciated, and controversial issues. Mod Pathol. 2005;18 Suppl 2:S61–79.

Ulbright TM. The most common, clinically significant misdiagnoses in testicular tumor pathology, and how to avoid them. Adv Anat Pathol. 2008;15:18–27.

Ulbright TM, Gersell DJ. Rete testis hyperplasia with hyaline globule formation. A lesion simulating yolk sac tumor. Am J Surg Pathol. 1991;15:66–74.

Ulbright TM, Tickoo SK, Daniel M, Berney DM, et al. Best practices recommendations in the application of immunohistochemistry in testicular tumors – report from the international society of urologic pathology consensus conference. Am J Surg Pathol. 2014;38:e50–9.

Ushiku T, Uozaki H, Shinozaki A, et al. Glypican 3-expressing gastric carcinoma: distinct subgroup unifying hepatoid, clear-cell, and alpha-fetoprotein-producing gastric carcinomas. Cancer Sci. 2009;100:626–32.

Wiesenthal JD, Ettler H, Razvi H. Testicular epidermoid cyst: a case report and review of the clinicopathologic features. Can J Urol. 2004;11:2133–5.

Wittekind C, Wichmann T, Von Kleist S. Immunohistological localization of AFP and HCG in uniformly classified testis tumors. Anticancer Res. 1983;3:327–30.

Woodward PJ, Mostofi FK, Talerman A, et al. Germ cell tumours. In: Eble JN, Sauter G, Epstein JI, Sesterhenn IA, editors. Pathology and genetics of tumours of the urinary system and male genital organs. Lyon: IARC Press; 2004. p. 221–49.

Yu H, Pinkus GS, Hornick JL. Diffuse membranous immunoreactivity for podoplanin (D2-40) distinguishes primary and metastatic seminomas from other germ cell tumors and metastatic neoplasms. Am J Clin Pathol. 2007;128:767–75.

Zhang M, Kao CS, Ulbright TM, Epstein JI. Testicular fibrothecoma: a morphologic and immunohistochemical study of 16 cases. Am J Surg Pathol. 2013; 37(8):1208–14.

Zynger DL, Dimov ND, Luan C, et al. Glypican 3: a novel marker in testicular germ cell tumors. Am J Surg Pathol. 2006;30:1570–5.

Zynger DL, Gupta A, Luan C, et al. Expression of glypican 3 in hepatoblastoma: an immunohistochemical study of 65 cases. Hum Pathol. 2008;39:224–30.

Zynger DL, McCallum JC, Luan C, et al. Glypican 3 has a higher sensitivity than alpha-fetoprotein for testicular and ovarian yolk sac tumour: immunohistochemical investigation with analysis of histological growth patterns. Histopathology. 2010;56:750–7.

Penis and Scrotum

5

Contents

5.1 **Basic Anatomy and Histology** 374
5.1.1 Penis 374
5.1.2 Scrotum 374

5.2 **Carcinoma of the Penis** 374
5.2.1 Overview 374
5.2.2 Preneoplastic and Other Intraepithelial Lesions 376
5.2.3 Squamous Cell Carcinoma, Usual Type 387
5.2.4 Variants of Squamous Cell Carcinoma 393
5.2.5 Other Carcinomas 409

5.3 **Benign Tumors and Tumor-Like Conditions** 411
5.3.1 Benign Tumors of Epithelial Origin 411
5.3.2 Benign Human Papillomavirus-Associated Lesions 411
5.3.3 Myointimoma 413
5.3.4 Other Benign Tumors 416

5.4 **Malignant Soft Tissue Tumors** 416
5.4.1 Kaposi Sarcoma 417
5.4.2 Leiomyosarcoma 418
5.4.3 Epithelioid Sarcoma 419
5.4.4 Other Soft Tissue Sarcomas 419

5.5 **Other Rare Tumors** 420
5.5.1 Primary Malignant Melanoma of the Penis 420
5.5.2 Clear Cell Sarcoma (Malignant Melanoma of Soft Parts) 420
5.5.3 Lymphoma 420

5.6 **Secondary Tumors** 421

5.7 **Carcinoma of the Scrotum** 422
5.7.1 Overview 422
5.7.2 Preneoplastic Lesions 423
5.7.3 Squamous Cell Carcinoma 423

5.8 **Other Carcinomas** 423
5.8.1 Basal Cell Carcinoma 423
5.8.2 Merkel Cell Carcinoma 423
5.8.3 Extramammary Paget Disease 423

5.9 **Benign Tumors and Tumor-Like Conditions** 427
5.9.1 Scrotal Calcinosis 427
5.9.2 Sclerosing Lipogranuloma of the Scrotum 429
5.9.3 Angiokeratoma 429
5.9.4 Fat Necrosis 430
5.9.5 Verruciform Xanthoma 430
5.9.6 Spindle Cell Nodule (Inflammatory Myofibroblastic Tumor) 432
5.9.7 Epidermal Cyst 432
5.9.8 Other Benign Lesions 432

5.10 **Soft Tissue Tumors** 433

5.11 **Other Rare Tumors** 433

5.12 **Secondary Tumors** 433

Suggested Reading 435

A. Lopez-Beltran et al., *Rare Tumors and Tumor-like Conditions in Urological Pathology*,
DOI 10.1007/978-3-319-10253-5_5, © Springer International Publishing Switzerland 2015

5.1 Basic Anatomy and Histology

5.1.1 Penis

- Penile anatomical regions are glans, foreskin, and shaft. Glans is distal, formed by corpus spongiosum covered by squamous mucosa. Distal urethra opens up into meatus, a ventrally located slit-like orifice in glans.
- Glans corona separates glans from coronal sulcus. Coronal sulcus is cul-de-sac between glans and foreskin. Frenulum connects foreskin to ventral portion of glans corona. Foreskin covers glans and presents mucosal (inner) and cutaneous (outer) surface.
- Penile root anchors penis to perineal membrane and pubic arc. Penile shaft is composed mainly by ventral column of corpus spongiosum and two dorsal columns of corpora cavernosa.
- Glans, coronal sulcus, and inner foreskin are covered by nonkeratinized squamous epithelium overlying loose lamina propria.
- Penile erectile tissues comprising two corpora cavernosa and corpus spengiosum surrounding penile urethra form body of penile shaft.
- Irregular vascular spaces with intermingling elastic connective tissue form penile erectile tissues. Vascular spaces of corpus spongiosum are more widely spaced and irregular when compared with corpus cavernosum.
- Corpus spongiosum is also covered by tunica albuginea. Tunica albuginea composed of dense connective tissue encompasses both corpus cavernosus and separates them from corpus spongiosum.
- Outer foreskin and shaft are covered by skin. Bundles of dartos muscle extend underneath dermis throughout shaft and foreskin.

5.1.2 Scrotum

- Contains the testes and the lower parts of the spermatic cords. Consists of skin, the dartos muscle, and external spermatic, cremasteric, and internal spermatic fasciae. The internal fascia is loosely attached to the parietal layer of the tunica vaginalis.
- The scrotum is divided into right and left halves by a cutaneous raphe which continues ventrally to the inferior penile surface and dorsally along the midline of the perineum to the anus. A median raphe of fibrovascular connective tissue separates the two halves.
- Its blood supply derives from the external and internal pudendal arteries. Additional blood comes from the cremasteric and testicular arteries that traverse the spermatic cords. Lymphatic drainage is to the superficial inguinal nodes.
- The epidermis covers the dermis. The deepest layer of the dermis merges with the smooth muscle bundles of the dartos tunic. There is no subcutaneous adipose tissue layer, but scattered fat cells are usually present. The dermis contains sebaceous and eccrine, apocrine glands, and hair follicles.

5.2 Carcinoma of the Penis

5.2.1 Overview

- Squamous cell carcinoma represents most common malignant tumor of penis. Keratinocytic differentiation is characteristic. Most penile squamous cell carcinomas originate from squamous mucosal surface of distal penis (glans, coronal sulcus, and foreskin). Glans is most common affected site followed by inner foreskin and coronal sulcus. Squamous cell carcinoma of penile shaft is exceedingly rare.
- Major risk factors for penile cancer are phimosis and human papillomavirus (HPV) infection (especially by high-risk HPV). History of genital warts, poor hygiene, and smoking is common. Treatment with ultraviolet A (PUVA) therapy is a recently recognized factor.
- Thirty to forty percent of all squamous cell carcinomas are HPV-related. High-risk HPV predominates, and HPV16 is most common genotype encountered. HPV18 is second most

common genotype. Other reported genotypes include 45, 52, and 74. Low-risk HPV (genotypes 6 and 11) infection is uncommon.

- Most frequent in sixth to seventh decades of life. There is wide range of geographical variation with low incidence in USA and Europe and high incidence in South America, Asia, and Africa.
- Squamous cell carcinoma of the penis represents approximately 0.5 % of all cancers among men in the United States and other developed countries. Only one-half of patients survive beyond 5 years.
- Ulceration may be present but urinary obstruction secondary to urethral tumoral extension is uncommon. About 50 % of penile carcinomas affect multiple anatomic compartments and frequently present as painless tumoral mass.
- Patterns of growth include superficial spreading, vertical growth, verruciform, and multicentric, but mixed forms of growth are common.
- Superficial spread includes intermediate risk cases with horizontal or superficial extension involving one or more anatomical compartments. The in situ component, usually extensive, shows invasion confined to lamina propria.
- Vertical growth is common in deeply infiltrative tumors with frank invasion of corpus spongiosum or corpus cavernosum. Vertical growth tumors show poor outcome and higher rate of nodal involvement.
- Verruciform tumors may reach large sizes but tend to be a localized, low metastatic rate and characteristically exophytic, cauliflower-like tumor mass, usually invading only superficial anatomical levels.
- Multicentric tumors with presence of two or more independent foci of squamous cell carcinoma are also seen. Each foci should be separately evaluated and reported
- Mixed patterns with combinations of any of patterns of growth may be seen.
- There is striking correlation of HPV presence and tumor histologic classification. Basaloid and warty (condylomatous) squamous cell carcinoma are HPV related in most cases.
- HPV incidence is low in squamous cell carcinoma, usual type, sarcomatoid, and papillary squamous cell carcinoma. Verrucous, pseudohyperplastic, and cuniculatum squamous cell carcinoma are typically HPV negative tumors. Lichen sclerosus and other chronic inflammatory conditions are common in these variants of carcinoma.
- Although the diagnosis and classification of penile tumors is straightforward in most cases, a few entities are problematic, especially to pathologists from countries in which penile cancer is rarely encountered.

Pathologic Prognostic Parameters

- Over 50 % of the invasive penile squamous cell carcinoma cases are associated with HPV, using p16 (INK4a) as a surrogate marker of HPV infection. These patients had a statistically significant survival advantage, independent of other prognostic factors. The prognosis in high grade cases lacking p16 (INK4a) is worse.
- Tumor extension follows local invasion of penile levels with extension to adjacent tissues, scrotum, perineum, prostate and metastasis to inguinal superficial and deep nodes. Metastases to pelvic lymph nodes also occur and when present, this is an adverse prognostic marker, with a 3-year overall survival rate of approximately 12 % (Tables 5.1 and 5.2).
- Systemic dissemination (nonregional lymph nodes) presents in up to 30 % of patients in high-risk regions. Liver is most common site of metastatic dissemination followed by lungs, heart, and rarely bone involvement (Tables 5.3 and 5.4).
- Lymphatic or vascular invasion, primary tumor expression of p53, number of metastatic inguinal lymph nodes and lymph node density are predictors of pathologic pelvic lymph node involvement.

Table 5.1 Prognostic factors for squamous carcinoma of the penis

Grade 3
Perineural invasion
Invasion of corpora cavernosa
Tumor depth or thickness greater than 10 mm
Sarcomatoid and basaloid subtypes
Vertical growth pattern

Table 5.2 Prognostic index score to predict regional nodal involvement and mortality

Histologic grade	
Grade 1	1 point
Grade 2	2 point
Grade 3	3 point
Level of infiltration	
Level 1 (lamina propria)	1 point
Level 2 (corpus spongiosum-Dartos)	2 point
Level 3 (corpus cavernosum-preputial skin)	3 point
Perineural invasion	
Absent	0 point
Present	1 point

Modified from Chaux et al.
It is represented by number 2–7. Score 2–3:0 % node+, 6 % dead of disease. Score 4 20 % Node +, 9 % mostality. Score 5 50 % node+, 30 % mortality. Score 6 66 % node +, 30 % mortality. Score 7 79 % node +, 49 % mortality

Table 5.3 TNM staging system for penile carcinoma (2010)

Primary tumor (T)
Tx Primary tumor cannot be assessed
T0 No evidence of primary tumor
Tis Carcinoma in situ
Ta Verrucous carcinoma
T1a Tumor invades subepithelial connective tissue. No lymphovascular invasion. No poorly differentiated (No grade 3–4)
T1b Tumor invades subepithelial connective tissue with lymphovascular invasion or is poorly differentiated
T2 Tumor invades corpus spongiosum or cavernosum
T3 Tumor invades urethra
T4 Tumor invades other adjacent structures (perineum, scrotum, psotate)
Pathologic stage (based upon biopsy or surgical excision) (pN)
pNX Regional lymph node cannot be assessed
pN0 No regional lymph node metastasis
pN1 Metastasis in a single inguinal lymph node
pN2 Metastasis in multiple or bilateral lymph nodes
pN3 Extranodal extension of lymph node metastasis or pelvic lymph nodes unilateral or bilateral
Distant metastasis (M)
M0 No distant metastasis
M1 Distant metastasis (lymph node metastasis outside of the true pelvis in addition to visceral or bone sites)

Table 5.4 Pathologic stages/prognostic groups of penile carcinomas

Group	T	N	M
Stage 0	Tis, Ta	N0	M0
Stage I	T1a	N0	M0
Stage II	T1b, T2, T3	N0	M0
Stage IIIa	T1-3	N1	M0
Stage IIIb	T1-3	N2	M0
Stage IV	T4	Any N	M0
	Any T	N3	M0
	Any T	Any N	M1

5.2.2 Preneoplastic and Other Intraepithelial Lesions

5.2.2.1 Penile Intraepithelial Neoplasia

- Penile intraepithelial neoplasia (PeIN) is considered intraepithelial lesion of invasive squamous cell carcinoma (synonyms: Erythroplasia of Queyrat, Bowen disease, squamous cell carcinoma in situ, squamous intraepithelial lesion (SIL)) (Table 5.5).
- PeIN may present as uni- or multifocal, flat to slightly elevated hyperkeratotic, sharp, or ill-defined borders or even papillary lesions. Clinically seen as moist, white, erythematous, dark brown or black macules, papules, or plaques.
- Real incidence is unknown, but most are associated with invasive squamous cell carcinoma, differentiated PeIN (65 %) and undifferentiated PeIN (35 %). Most cases present in fifth and sixth decades.

Table 5.5 Types of penile intraepithelial neoplasia (PeIN)

Differentiated
Undifferentiated
Warty
Warty-Basaloid
Basaloid
Other
Mixed differentiated-undifferentiated

- Differentiated or simplex PeIN is unrelated to HPV. Lichen sclerosus may be implicated in pathogenesis of differentiated PeIN. Frequently affects foreskin.
- Warty, warty/basaloid, and basaloid (undifferentiated) PeIN are HPV-related, with frequent HPV16 genotype. Usually affects glans, perimeatal region. Usually not associated with lichen sclerosus. Patients may have history of condyloma or genital warts (Figs. 5.1, 5.2, 5.3, 5.4, 5.5, 5.6, 5.7, 5.8, 5.9 and 5.10).

Pathology

Differentiated or Simplex PeIN

- Thickened acanthotic epithelium with elongated and anastomosing rete ridges. Subtle abnormal maturation (enlarged keratinocytes with abundant eosinophilic cytoplasm). Parakeratosis is frequent on the surface. Absence of koilocytosis.
- Atypical basal cells with hyperchromatic nuclei. Occasionally, keratin pearl formation (in deep rete ridges). Prominent intercellular bridges (spongiosis and sometimes acantholysis).
- Lichen sclerosus, chronic scarring, or other inflammatory dermatosis usually seen in adjacent epithelium.
- Preferential association with HPV-unrelated variants of invasive squamous cell carcinoma.
- Squamous hyperplasia or lichen simplex chronicus may enter differential diagnosis. Basilar atypia and abnormal maturation are not seen in reactive conditions.

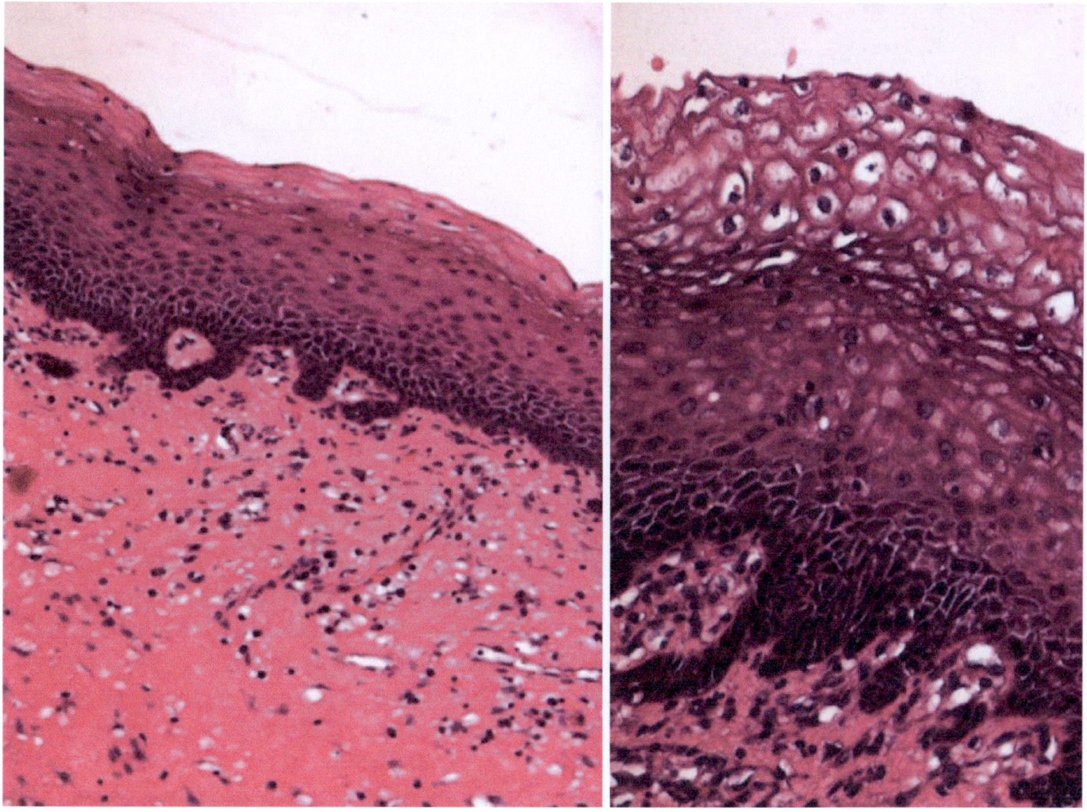

Fig. 5.1 Differentiated-PeIN. Low (*left*) and high (*right*) power view with koilocytosis

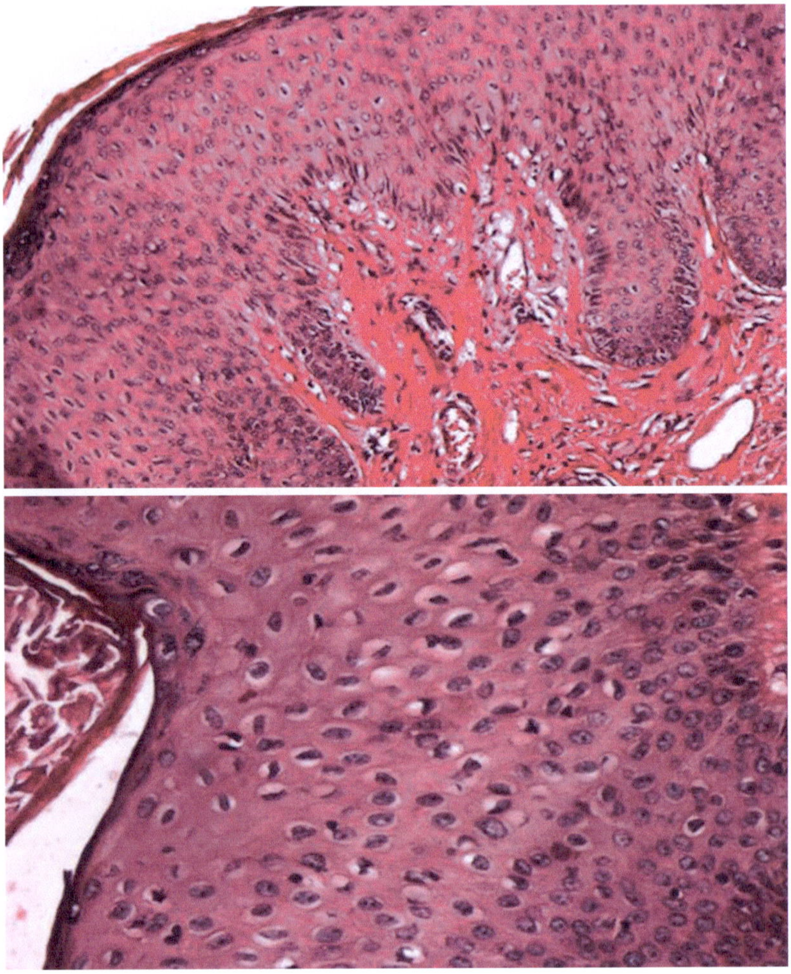

Fig. 5.2 High grade-PeIN (*upper*) with koilocytosis (*lower*)

Basaloid PeIN

- Epithelium replaced by monotonous population of small immature cells with high nuclear/cytoplasmic ratio. Mitotic figures are numerous.

Warty PeIN

- Epithelium replaced by pleomorphic cells with koilocytic changes including multinucleation, nuclei with irregular contours, perinuclear halo, and dyskeratosis. Undulating or spiky surface with atypical parakeratosis. Frequent mitoses.

Mixed PeIN (Warty/Basaloid)

- Combined features of basaloid and warty types of PeIN. Warty/basaloid PeIN is usually seen adjacent to HPV-related variants of invasive squamous cell carcinoma (basaloid and warty)
- Lower part of epithelium is replaced by small, basaloid cells, with high nuclear/cytoplasmic ratio. Upper portion shows features of warty PeIN.
- Differential diagnosis includes condyloma acuminatum. Koilocytosis is restricted to upper epithelium, there is absence of nuclear pleomorphism, and mitoses are scant and confined to lower epithelium. Bowenoid papulosis may be indistinguishable from warty/basaloid PeIN on histology alone. Clinical correlation is essential.

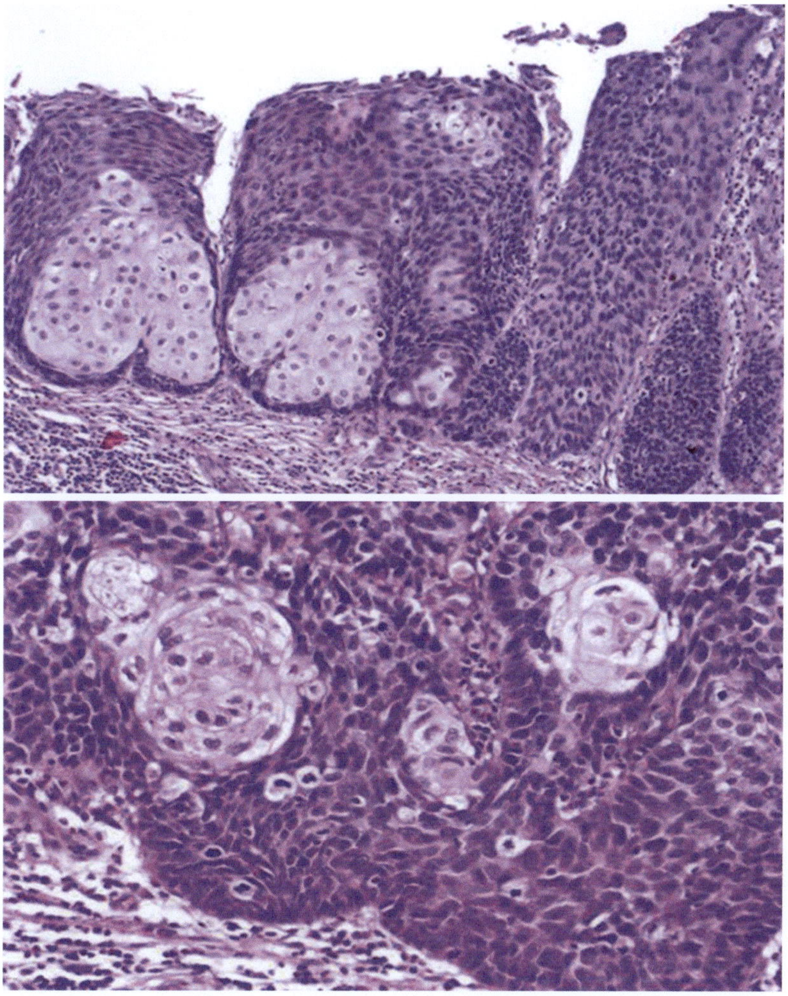

Fig. 5.3 Mixed-basaloid-PeIN. Low (*upper*) and high (*lower*) power view

5.2.2.2 Bowenoid Papulosis

- HPV-related multifocal papular condition typically seen in anogenital region in young adults. May be pruritic, painful or asymptomatic. Usually transmitted via sexual contact. Related to high-risk HPV, especially HPV 16. Other HPV types have also been implicated.
- Lesions are often small, brown, or red-colored and exhibit histologic spectrum of changes from dysplasia to in situ carcinoma. Usually affect skin of shaft and surface may be verruciform. May also affect epithelium of glans, coronal sulcus or foreskin. Spontaneous regression has been reported, but minority of lesions evolves to invasive squamous cell carcinoma.

Pathology

- Proliferation of atypical basaloid cells that may be scattered throughout epidermis, often with preserved maturation. Koilocytic-like changes are also seen.
- Atypia ranges from scattered atypical cells of low-grade dysplasia to full thickness atypia of the squamous epithelium. Most lesions are indistinguishable from squamous cell carcinoma in situ. Variable increased pigmentation of basal layer.
- Differential diagnosis with squamous cell carcinoma in situ requires clinical correlation.

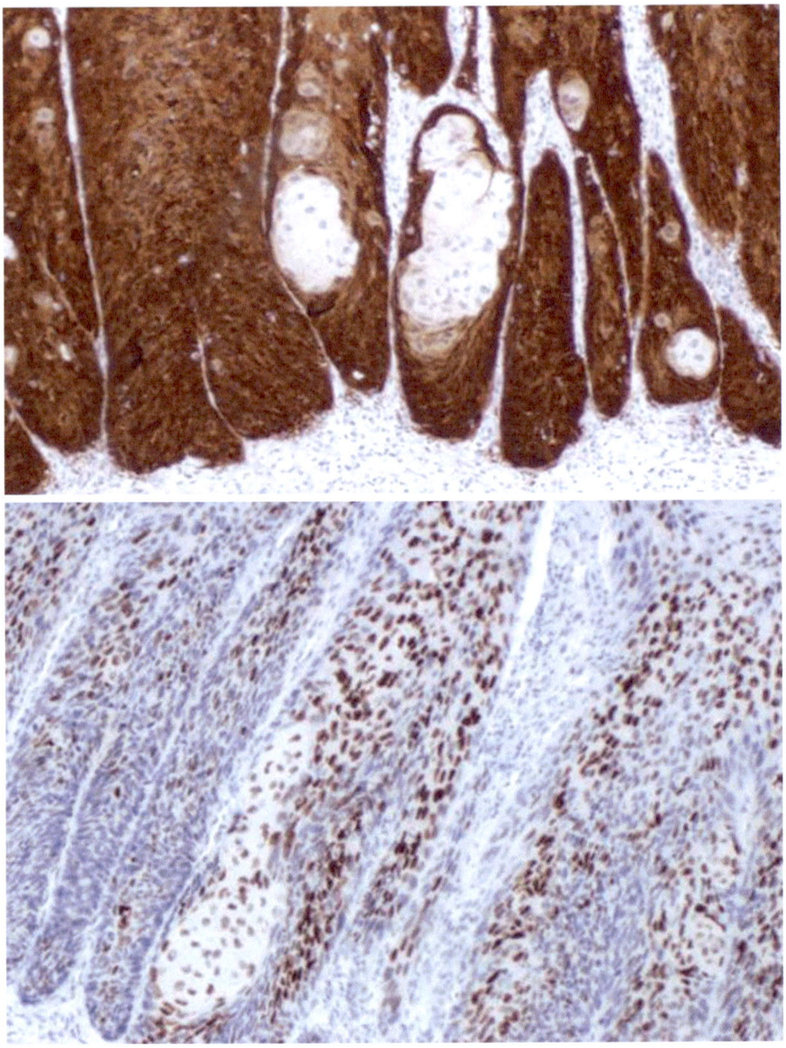

Fig. 5.4 Mixed-basaloid-PeIN. p16 (*upper*) and p53 (*lower*)

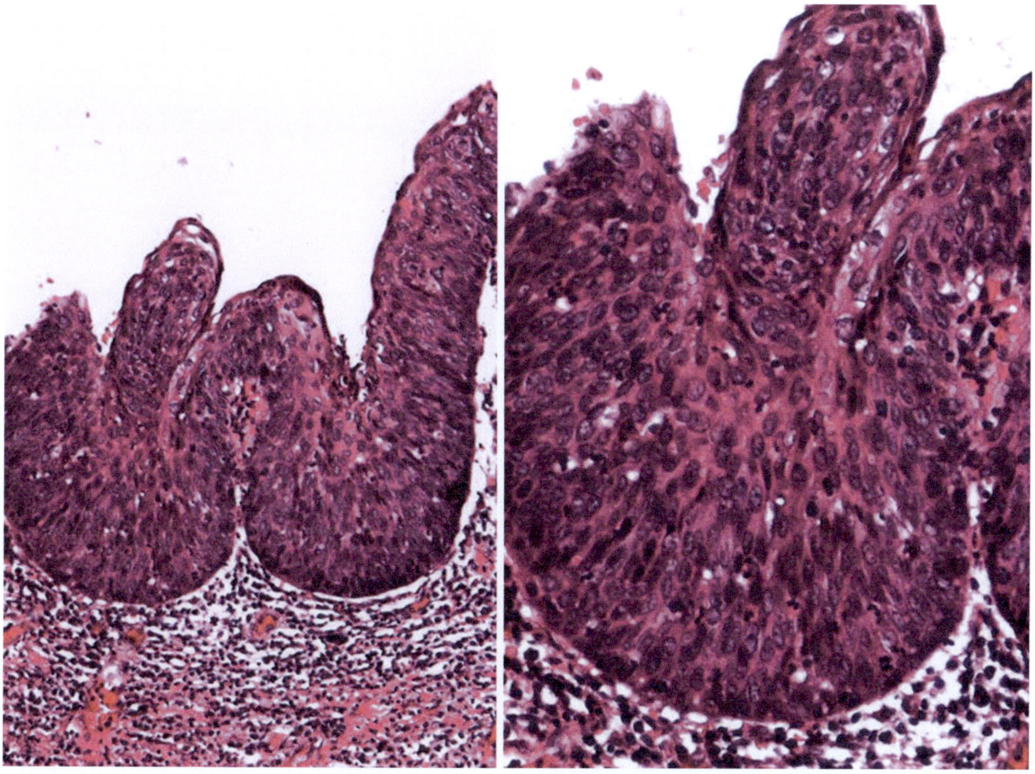

Fig. 5.5 High grade basaloid-PeIN with papillary configuration seen a low (*left*) and high (*right*) power

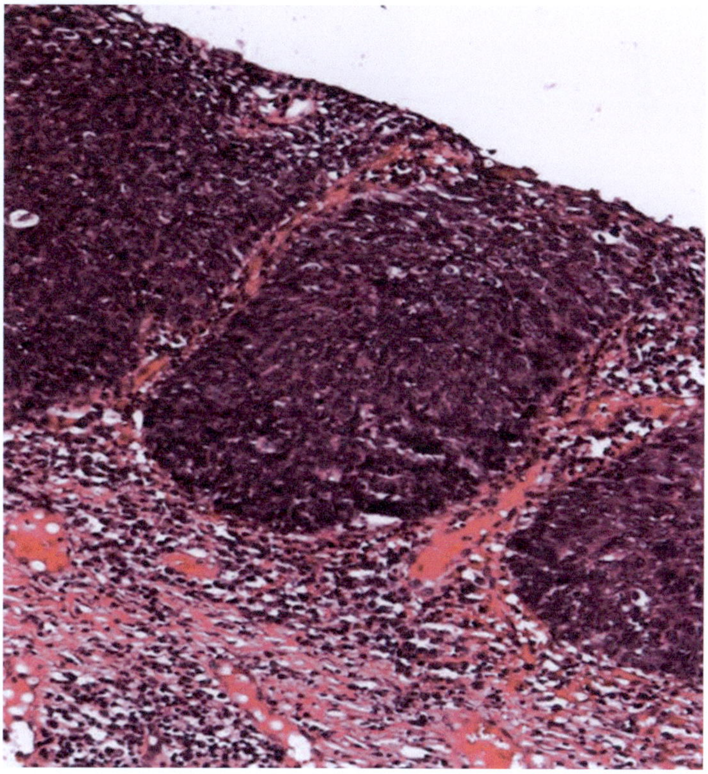

Fig. 5.6 Basaloid-PeIN

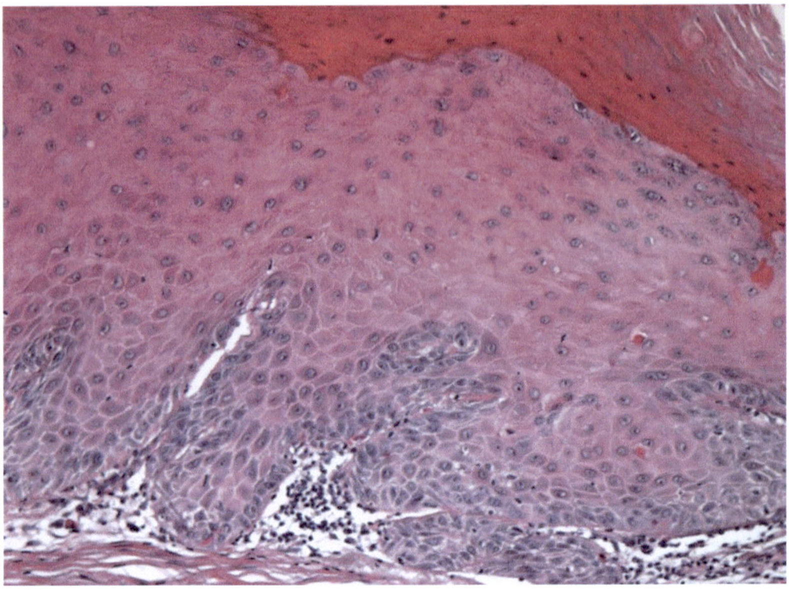

Fig. 5.7 Verrucous-PeIN. The lesion was adjacent to a verrucous carcinoma

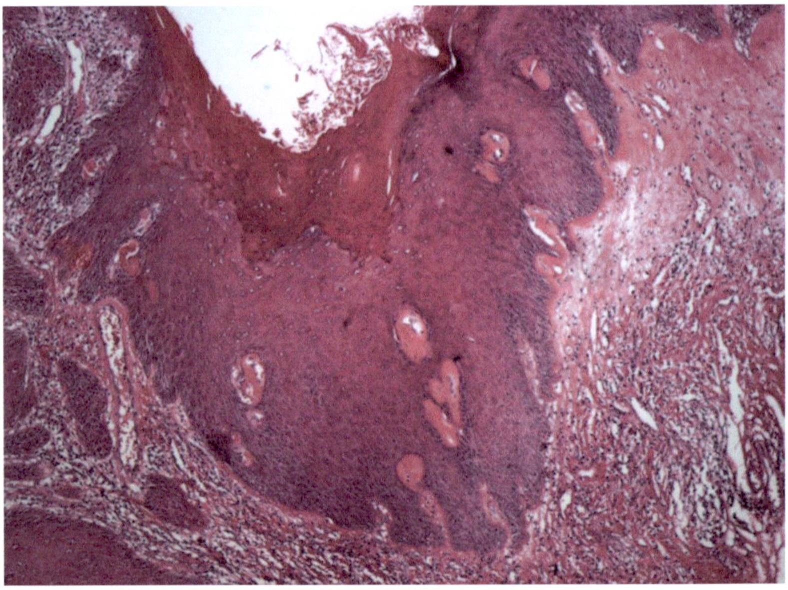

Fig. 5.8 This verrucous lesion was adjacent to a papillary carcinoma (*left*). Lichen sclerosus is also present (*upper-right*)

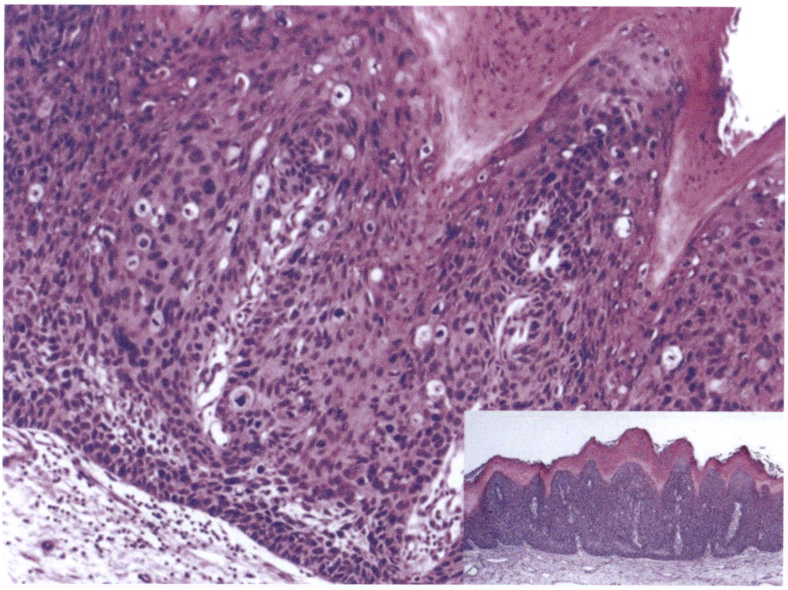

Fig. 5.9 Warthy-PeIN. Lesion at low power (Inset)

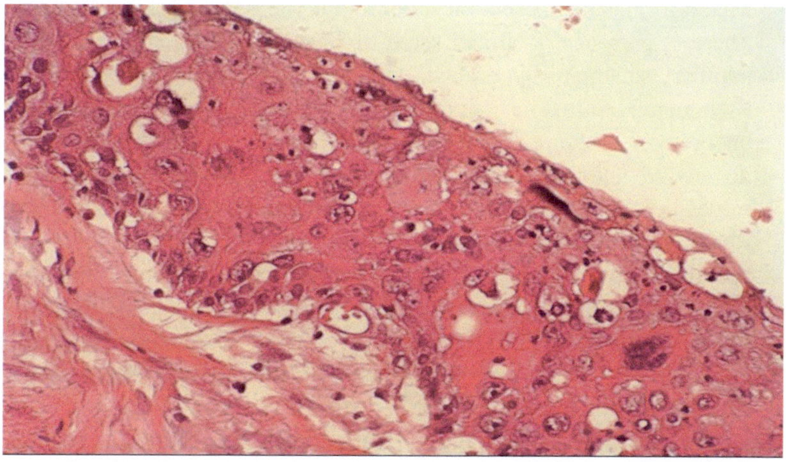

Fig. 5.10 High grade PeIN (Bowen-disease, carcinoma in situ)

5.2.2.3 Squamous Hyperplasia

- Most common epithelial change associated with penile cancer. Almost all keratinizing squamous cell carcinoma have associated squamous hyperplasia. There is thickening of mucosal squamous epithelium without cytologic atypia. It seems to be a reactive condition rather than specific entity. May be associated with reactive inflammatory conditions.
- Clinically, it may be difficult to distinguish from PeIN. Micaceous balanitis and penile horn are clinically florid forms of squamous hyperplàsia with prominent hyperkeratosis. Usually found in continuity or slightly distant from in situ or invasive carcinoma. Maybe precursor lesion of HPV-unrelated squamous cell carcinoma.
- The differential diagnosis of squamous hyperplasia from differentiated PeIN or from extremely low-grade invasive neoplasms (e.g., pseudohyperplastic and verrucous carcinomas) may be particularly difficult.

Pathology

- Whitish areas with irregular borders with acanthosis with orthokeratotic and minimal to absent parakeratosis with normal epithelial maturation. Chronic inflammation may be present. There is absence of cytologic atypia, koilocytosis, and intraepithelial keratin pearls. Frequently associated with differentiated PeIN and with lichen sclerosus in some cases. Usually found in association with usual, papillary, and verrucous squamous cell carcinoma (HPV-unrelated variants). Rarely present adjacent to condylomatous (warty) or basaloid squamous cell carcinoma.

Histological Subtypes

- Flat is the most common subtype. There is non-atypical acanthosis, hyperkeratosis with orthokeratosis, and linear interface between basal layer and stroma.
- Mixed form is the second most common type. There is presence of mixed areas of flat and papillary squamous hyperplasia.
- Pseudoepitheliomatous hyperplasia is an uncommon pattern. There is acanthosis, downward elongated proliferation of rete ridges that appear detached from epithelium. Regular epithelial nests with peripheral palisading and stromal reaction are not prominent. Some cases are associated to papillary squamous hyperplasia.
- Papillary, represents minority of cases with serrated appearance on low-power view and jagged interface with underlying stroma. There is non-atypical acanthosis with short hyperkeratotic papillae.
- Verrucous pattern presents adjacent to verrucous carcinoma with marked acanthosis with no atypia, hyperkeratosis with hypergranulosis, and slight papillomatosis.
- Differential diagnosis of squamous hyperplasia includes differentiated PeIN that shows aberrant keratinization with cytologic basal atypia.
- Warty/basaloid PeIN with cytologic atypia with loss of squamous maturation and monotonous population of small cells with scant cytoplasm throughout epithelium in basaloid PeIN. Detection of HPV in high proportion of cases and immunohistochemical overexpression of p16 is the rule.
- Pseudohyperplastic squamous cell carcinoma simulating pseudoepitheliomatous hyperplasia in which there is prominent stromal reaction and mass forming clinically.
- Verruciform xanthoma, an exophytic lesion with acanthosis, hyperkeratosis, and "xanthoma" cells (foamy histocytes) in lamina propria.
- Warty, papillary, and verrucous carcinomas show evidence of destructive stromal invasion. Diagnosis may be difficult in small biopsies (Figs. 5.11, 5.12, 5.13 and 5.14).

5.2.2.4 Lichen Sclerosus et Atrophicus (Balanitis Xerotica Obliterans)

- Affect inner aspect of foreskin, glans, and perimeatal region, and may be focally hyperkeratotic. About 9 % of patients will develop penile squamous cell carcinoma, usual type.
- Well-established lesions appear as white-gray, atrophic, and geographic with frequent erosion or ulceration. Early lesions appear as pink macules that become papules. It is a chronic process of unknown pathogenesis that tends to be broad and multifocal, and affect epithelium and superficial dermis/lamina propria.

Pathology

- Typical case shows interface vacuolar or lichenoid dermatitis with thickened papillary dermis/lamina propria with band-like hyalinization (sclerosis). Scattered melanophages may be sen in superficial dermis and occasionally there is prominent edema of papillary dermis/lamina propria. Dermal-epidermal clefting or blisters may form secondary to marked basal cell vacuolar alteration.
- In well-established lesions, a band-like lymphoid infiltrate underneath band of sclerosis. Early lesions show more superficial lymphoid infiltrate underneath epithelium without

well-formed sclerotic band, but late lesions are sclerotic with minimal inflammation.

- Rare cases of chronic lichen sclerosus may be associated with atypical foci in epithelium raising concern of epithelial dysplasia.
- Lichen Planus enters differential diagnosis, shows a wedge-shaped hypergranulosis and band-like lymphoid infiltrate obscuring dermal-epidermal junction. Hyalinized band in superficial dermis/lamina propria is absent (Fig. 5.14).

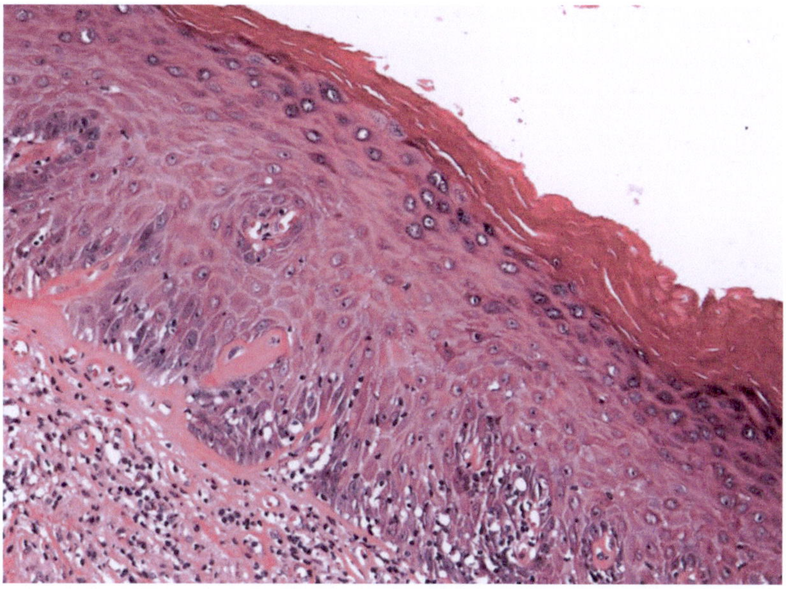

Fig. 5.11 Squamous hyperplasia

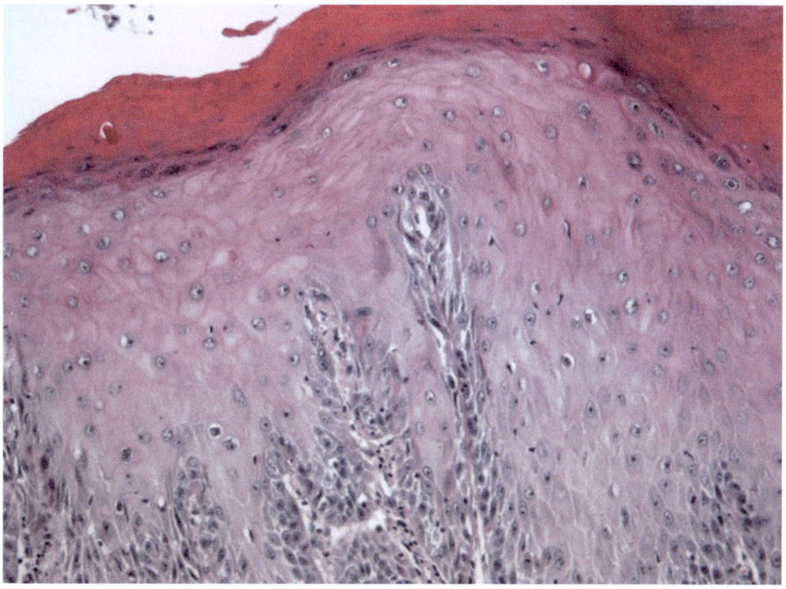

Fig. 5.12 Verrucous Squamous hyperplasia adjacent to verrucous carcinoma

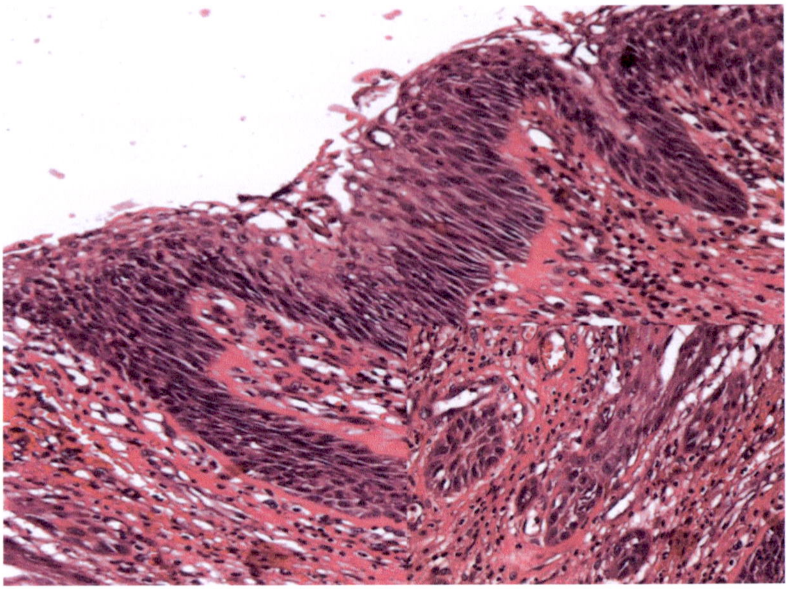

Fig. 5.13 Pseudo-epitheliomatous hyperplasia with infiltrating nests (*inset*)

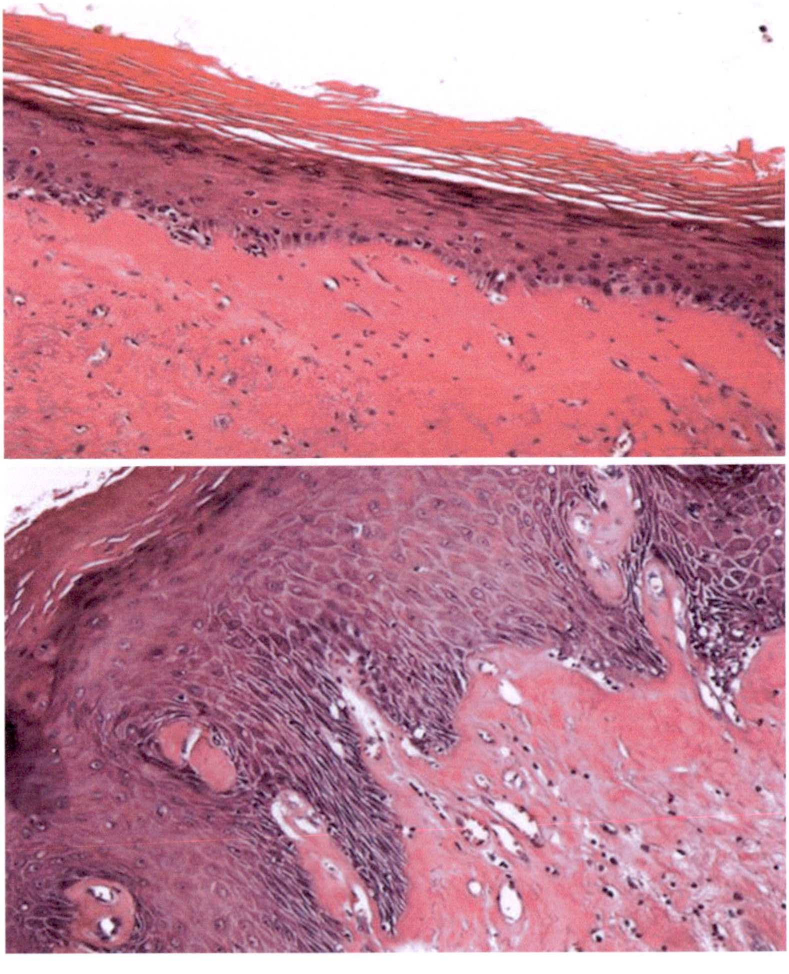

Fig. 5.14 Lichen sclerosus et atroficus (balanitis xerotica obliterans). Microscopic features (*upper and lower view*)

5.2.3 Squamous Cell Carcinoma, Usual Type

- Also known as epidermoid carcinoma, is and invasive carcinoma with keratinization and or intercellular bridges. Most common histologic subtype of penile squamous cell carcinoma (60 % of cases). HPV DNA is present in 25 % of cases.
- Presents as solid mass most frequently affecting glans, with ulceration, pain, or bleeding. Superficial spreading is predominant pattern of growth. Size ranges 2–5 cm. Tumors exclusive of foreskin are rare (Table 5.6)

Pathology

- Tumor nests of well to moderately differentiated squamous cell carcinoma with neoplastic cells with ample, eosinophilic, frequently keratinized cytoplasm and distinctive cellular borders.
- Histologic grade heterogeneity is the rule and pure grade 1 or 3 tumors are very rare. Level of keratinization is the key for histologic grading. Only highest grade is considered for tumor grading. In some cases there are focal areas of spindle, trabecular, solid, or clear cells.
- Differentiated PeIN, squamous hyperplasia or lichen sclerosus commonly found in adjacent areas. Associated basaloid and warty PeIN is rare.

Table 5.6 Histologic types of squamous cell carcinoma of the penis

Squamous cell carcinoma, usual type
Variants of squamous cell carcinoma
Warty (condylomatous)
Basaloid
Verrucous
Pseudohyperplastic
Papillary
Sarcomatoid
Pseudoglandular (acantholytic)
Carcinoma cuniculatum
Adenosquamous
Mixed (hybrid)
Other

- Associated stromal reaction includes lymphocytes and plasma cells, and occasionally desmoplastic reaction. Vascular and perineural invasion is seen in about 30 % of cases, and extension to distal urethra in one-half of cases. Extension to multiple compartments is also common.
- Pathologic prognostic factors include histologic grade, the level of infiltration (pathologic stage), vascular, lymphatic, and perineural invasion. Inguinal nodal metastases seen in about 30 % of patients. Some patients may experience tumor recurrences after definitive therapy.
- Lesions entering differential diagnosis include pseudoepitheliomatous hyperplasia because of pseudoinfiltrative pattern of growth, but epithelial nests are orderly disposed, there is peripheral palisading and no stromal reaction and no or only mild cytologic atypia.
- Pseudohyperplastic Carcinoma is extremely well differentiated, frequently multicentric, with inconspicuous peripheral palisading and prominent stromal reaction. Urothelial carcinoma of distal urethra is also an important differential; there is usually previous history of urothelial carcinoma, urothelial carcinoma in situ seen in adjacent areas. Immunohistochemistry with CK20, GATA3 and uroplakin-3 positive urothelial carcinoma and negative or only focal in squamous cell carcinoma may help in selected cases.
- In mixed squamous cell carcinoma there are foci of usual squamous cell carcinoma intermingled with other subtypes. Verrucous carcinoma is the commonest (Figs. 5.15, 5.16, 5.17, 5.18, 5.19, 5.20, 5.21, 5.22, 5.23, 5.24 and 5.25)
- Metastatic squamous cell carcinoma to penis may occur. Most are from genitourinary origin. Prominent squamous differentiation may be seen in urothelial and less frequently in prostate cancer. Tumor nests located mainly in vascular spaces of penile erectile tissues but squamous mucosa covering glans, coronal sulcus, or inner foreskin is usually unaffected. Clinical correlation may be necessary.

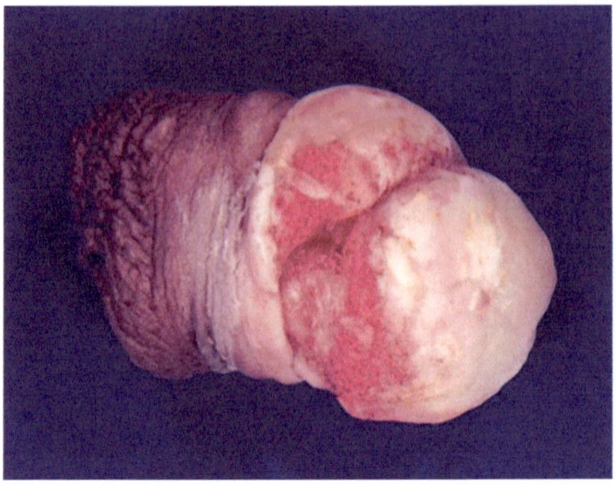

Fig. 5.15 Ulcerated squamous cell carcinoma with adjacent leukoplakia

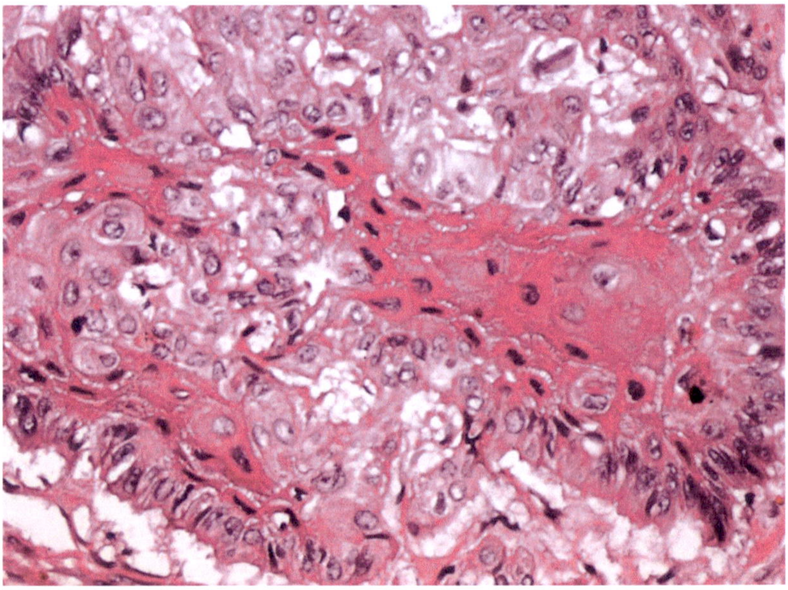

Fig. 5.16 Squamous cell carcinoma with intercellular bridges

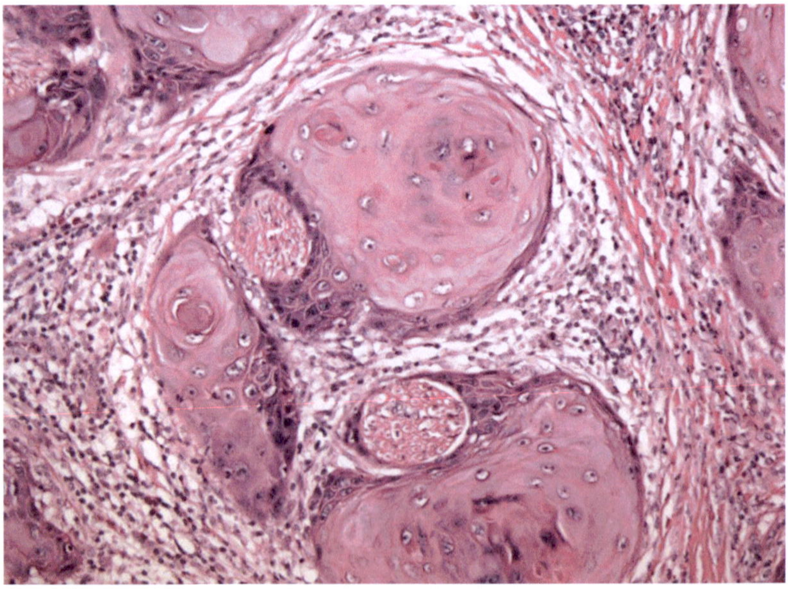

Fig. 5.17 Squamous cell carcinoma with perineural invasion

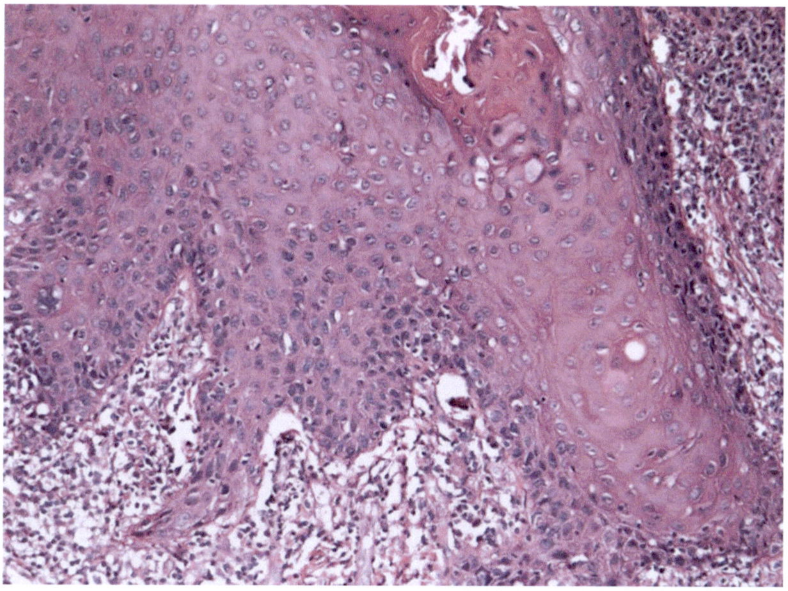

Fig. 5.18 Lack of maturation in squamous cell carcinoma

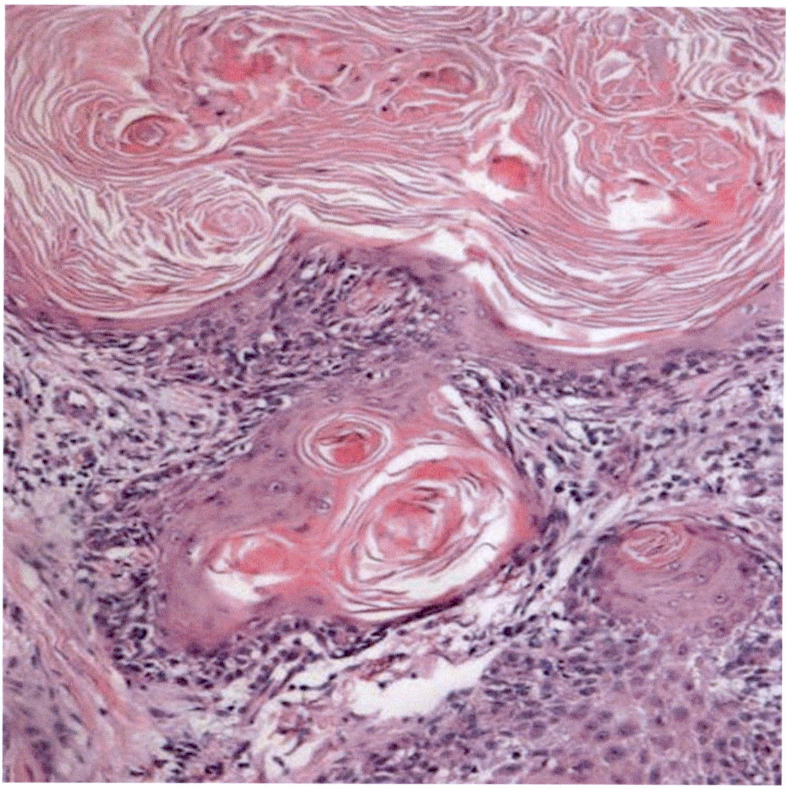

Fig. 5.19 Well differentiated-grade 1 squamous cell carcinoma

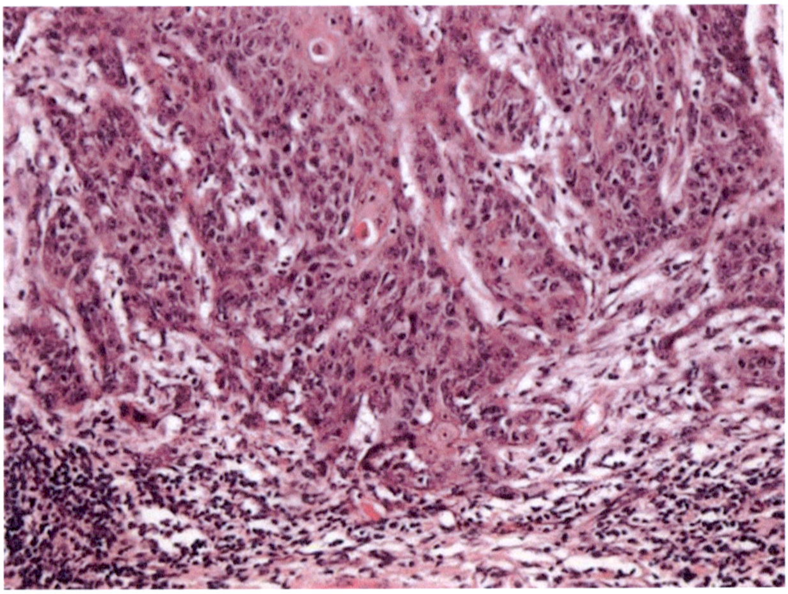

Fig. 5.20 Moderately differentiated-grade 2 squamous cell carcinoma

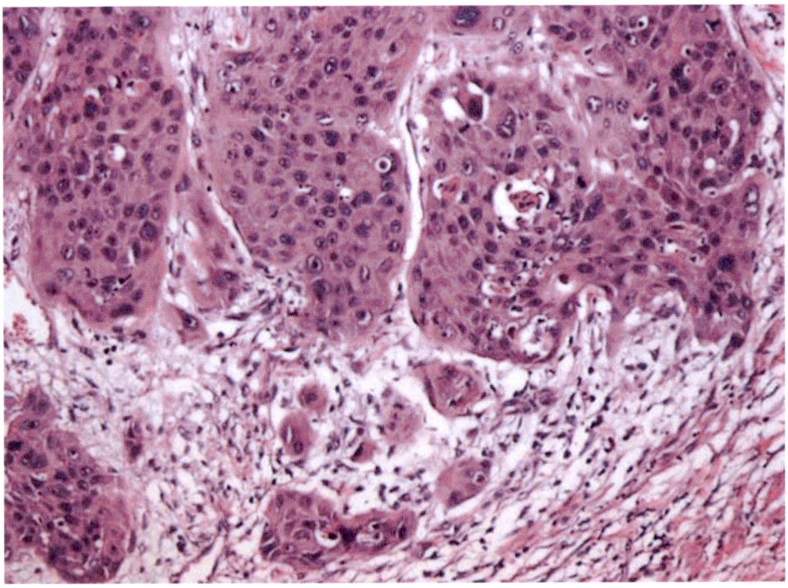

Fig. 5.21 Poorly differentiated grade 3 squamous cell carcinoma

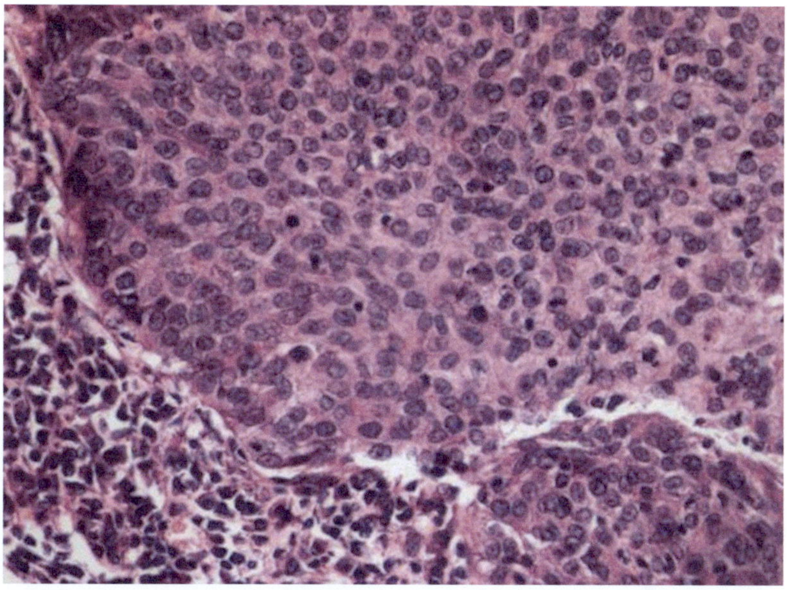

Fig. 5.22 Undifferentiated squamous cell carcinoma showing high mitotic ratio, and lack of keratin

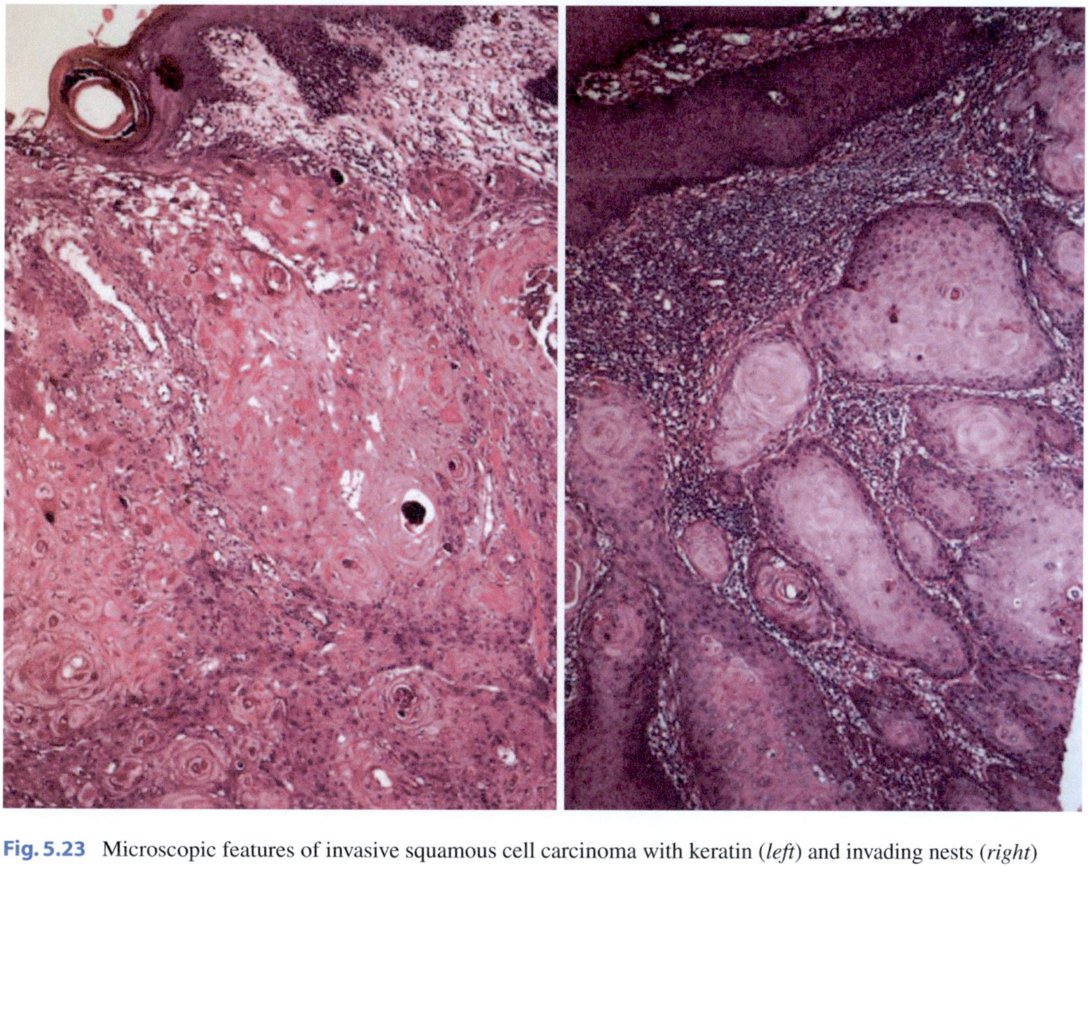

Fig. 5.23 Microscopic features of invasive squamous cell carcinoma with keratin (*left*) and invading nests (*right*)

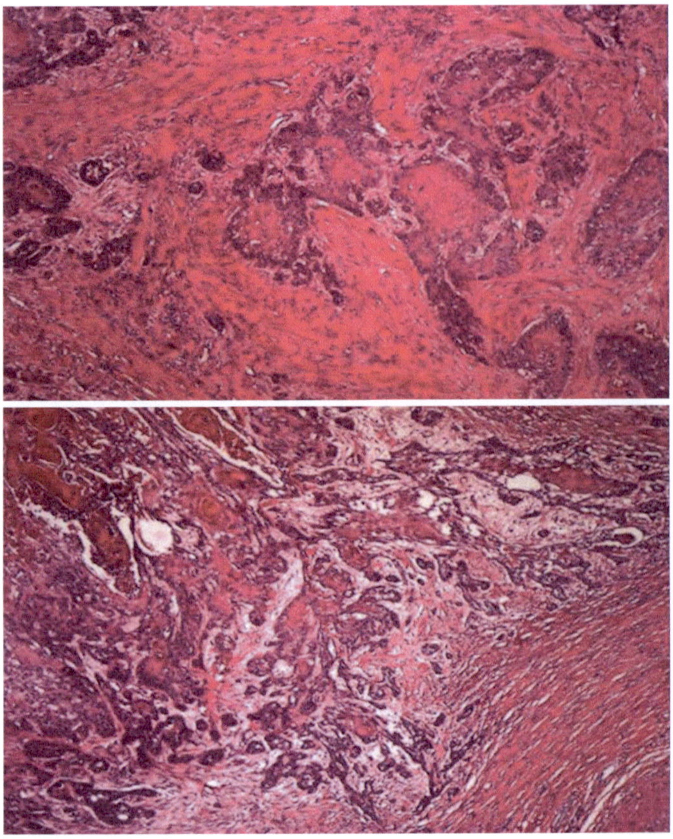

Fig. 5.24 Microscopic features of squamous cell carcinoma showing infiltrating neoplastic cords (*upper*) and associated stromal reaction (*lower*)

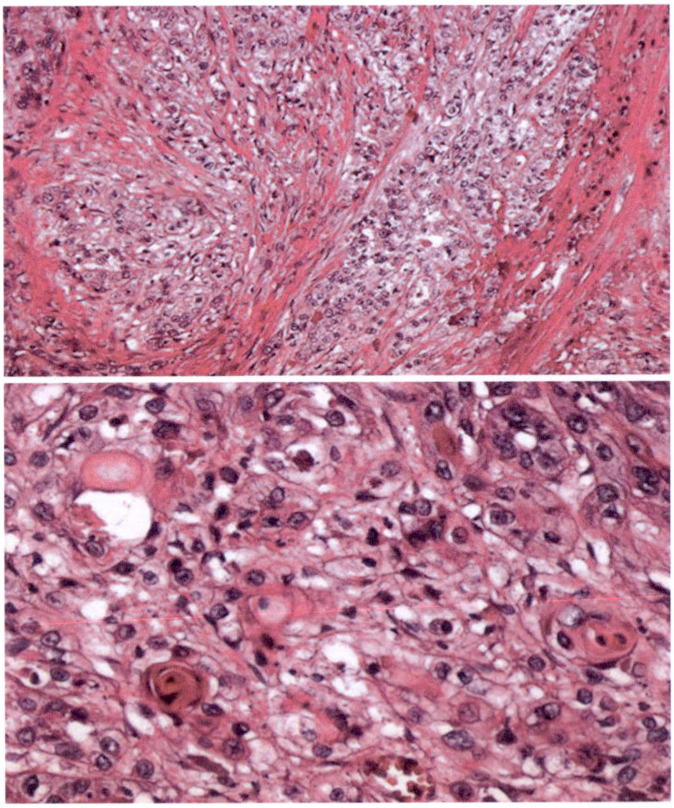

Fig. 5.25 Clear cell change in squamous cell carcinoma. Low (*upper*) and high (*lower*) power view

5.2.4 Variants of Squamous Cell Carcinoma (Figs. 5.26, 5.27, 5.28, 5.29, 5.30, 5.31, 5.32, 5.33, 5.34, 5.35, 5.36, 5.37, 5.38, 5.39, 5.40, 5.41, 5.42, 5.43, 5.44, 5.45, 5.46, 5.47 and 5.48)

5.2.4.1 Pseudohyperplastic Carcinoma

- Rare nonverruciform low-grade squamous cell carcinoma preferentially affecting foreskin in elderly patients (eighth decade) strongly associated with lichen sclerosus et atrophicus. Most unrelated to HPV infection. It is often multicentric. Other concurrent tumor pattern may be verrucous carcinoma. Minority of cases may recur showing higher grade areas.

Pathology

- Nonverruciform tumors usually affecting foreskin that may be hyperkeratotic flat or slightly elevated, often multicentric, on a background of lichen sclerosus. Mean size is 2 cm.
- Extremely well-differentiated tumor that May be confined to subepithelial connective tissue or infiltrate dartos in foreskin. There is downward proliferation of keratinizing nests of squamous cells. Keratin-pearl formation within infiltrating nests. Occasional individual cell keratinization and mild atypia of basal cells. Lack of kolocytosis. Uneven or jagged infiltrative borders. Asymmetrical infiltrative nests surrounded by reactive fibrous stroma with mild inflammation. Adjacent epithelium may show differentiated PeIN.
- Differential diagnosis may include pseudoepitheliomatous hyperplasia. Infiltration of dartos or corpus spongiosum is not seen in hyperplasia. Downward proliferation is more organized with elongated rete ridges. Keratin pearl formation is less frequent and inflammation is more prominent.

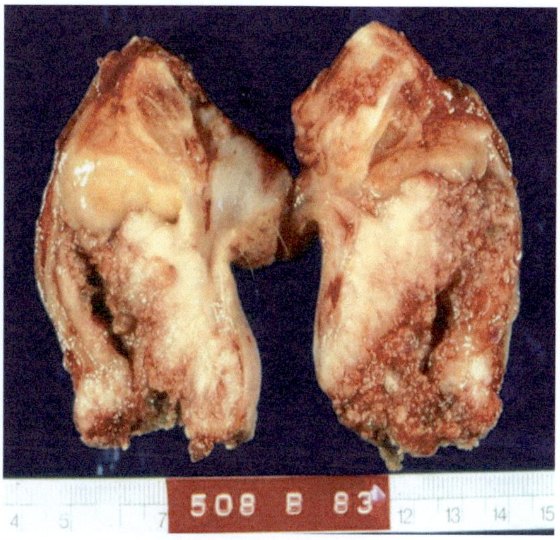

Fig. 5.26 Gross appearance of Warthy squamous cell carcinoma

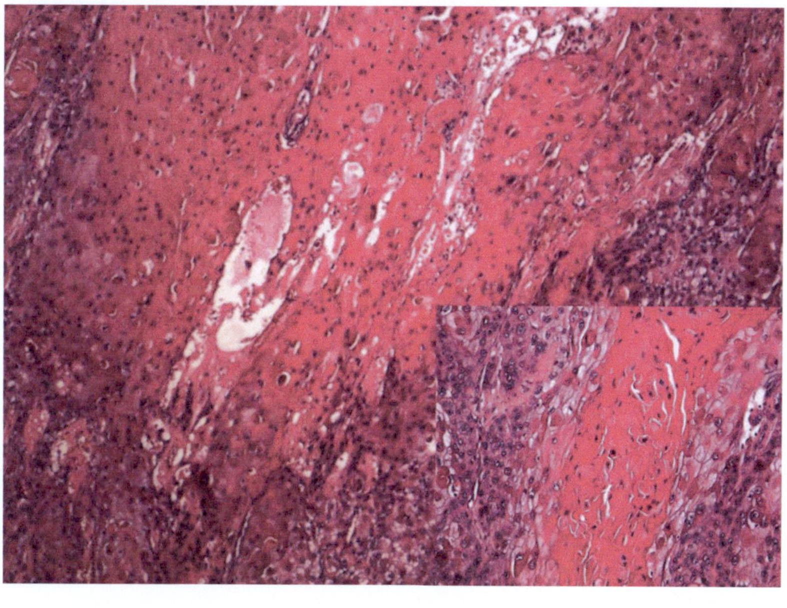

Fig. 5.27 Exophytic appearance of Warthy squamous cell carcinoma. High power view in *inset*

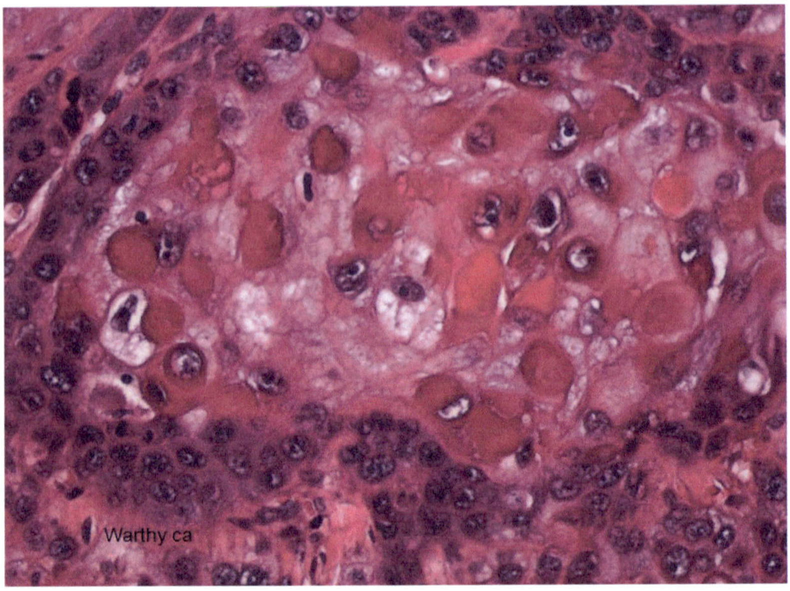

Fig. 5.28 Warthy squamous cell carcinoma with atypical parakeratosis and rhabdoid-like features

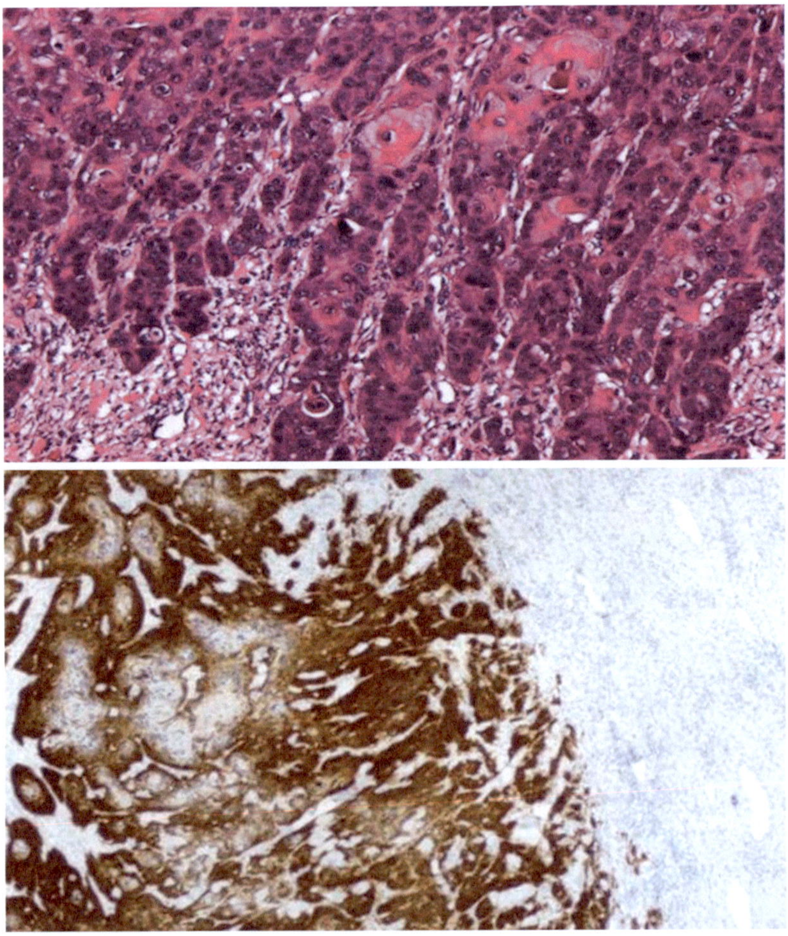

Fig. 5.29 Infiltrative aspect (*upper*) of Warty squamous cell carcinoma and p16 expression (*lower*)

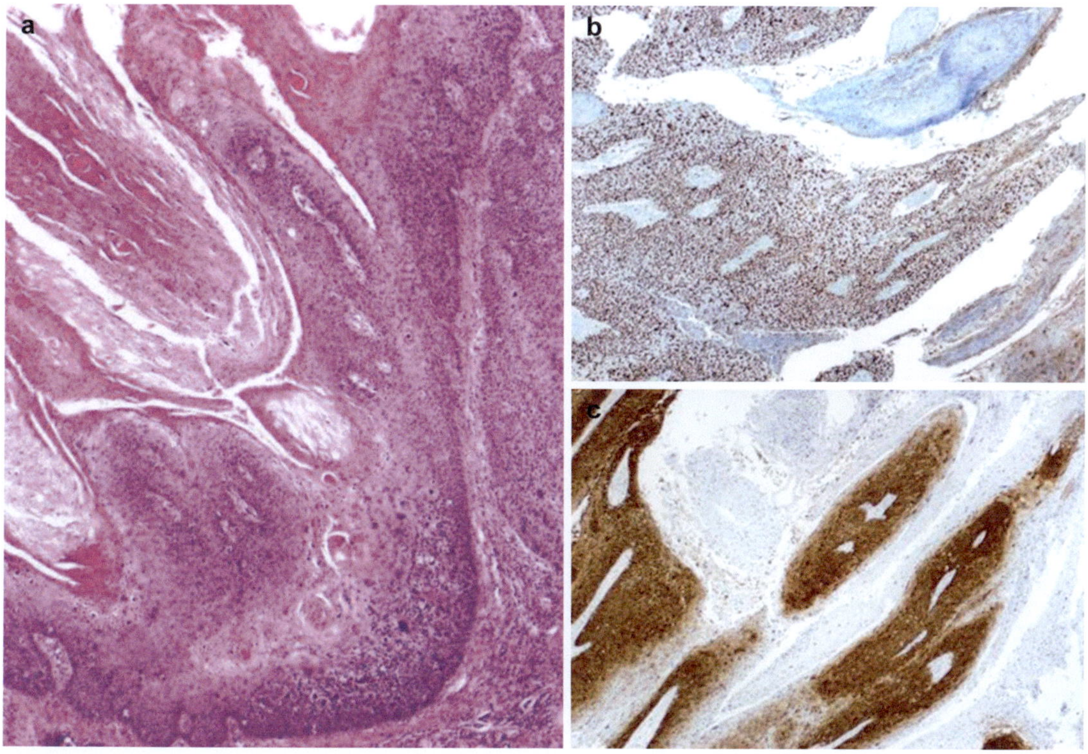

Fig. 5.30 Warthy squamous cell carcinoma (**a**) with ki67 proliferation (**b**) and p16 (**c**) expression

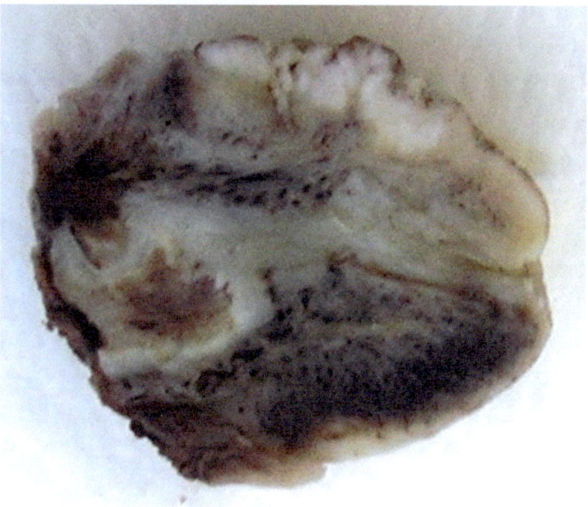

Fig. 5.31 Verrucous squamous cell carcinoma. Gross features

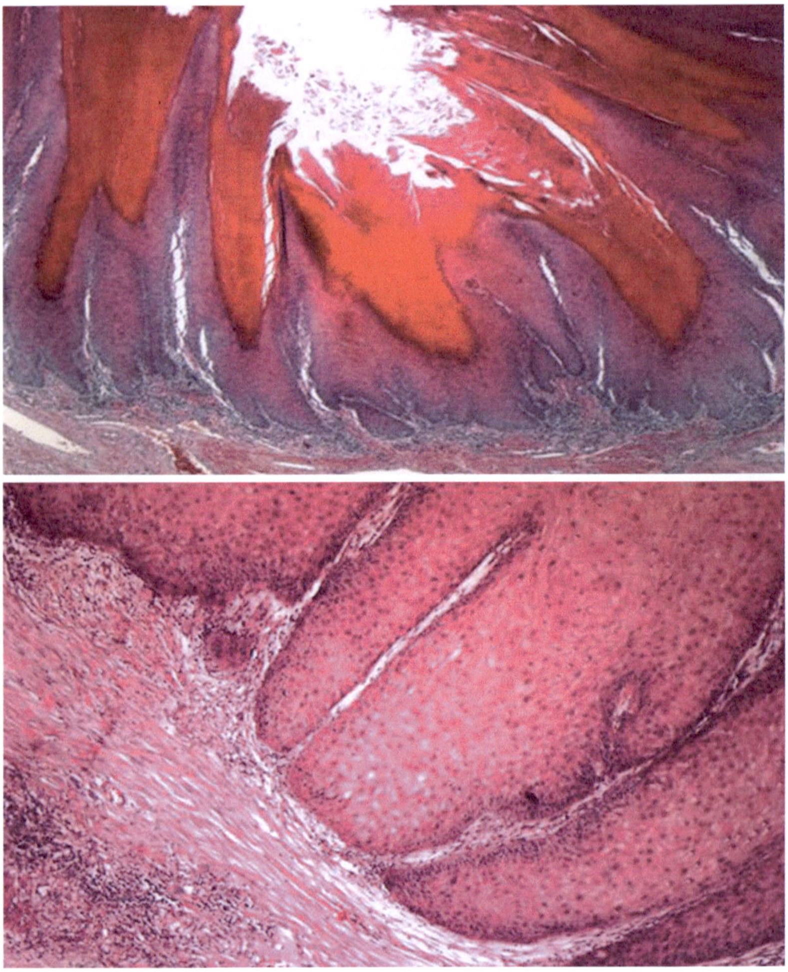

Fig. 5.32 Verrucous squamous cell carcinoma microscopic features (*upper*) and deep aspect of the lesion (*lower*)

5.2.4.2 Warty (Condylomatous) Carcinoma

- Slow-growing verruciform tumor usually affecting glans, but also, coronal sulcus, and/or foreskin. It is related to HPV infection (most frequent HPV16). Shares some gross and microscopic characteristics with condyloma but has definitive malignant potential. May represent up to 10 % of penis carcinomas and is more frequent in patients in their 50s.
- It is placed as an intermediate aggressiveness between that of low risk verrucous or papillary carcinomas and high risk squamous cell carcinoma, usual type. It may present with inguinal nodal metastasis. Level of invasion and higher histologic grade are important prognostic factors.

Pathology

- Rare verruciform, cauliflower-like tumor, with exo- to endophytic growth and papillomatous surface on cut sections. Usually affects at least two anatomical compartments (glans, coronal sulcus, and foreskin). Variable deep borders, pushing and/or jagged, usually penetrate into corpora spongiosum and or cavernosa.
- Long and undulating papillae with prominent central fibrovascular core and arborescent papillae. Frequent atypical parakeratosis containing large nuclei. Mixture of basaloid (lower epithelial layers) and koilocytotic cells (upper epithelial layers) gives classic light and dark low-power pattern.
- Cells with enlarged nuclei with irregular contours, binucleation or multinucleation, clear

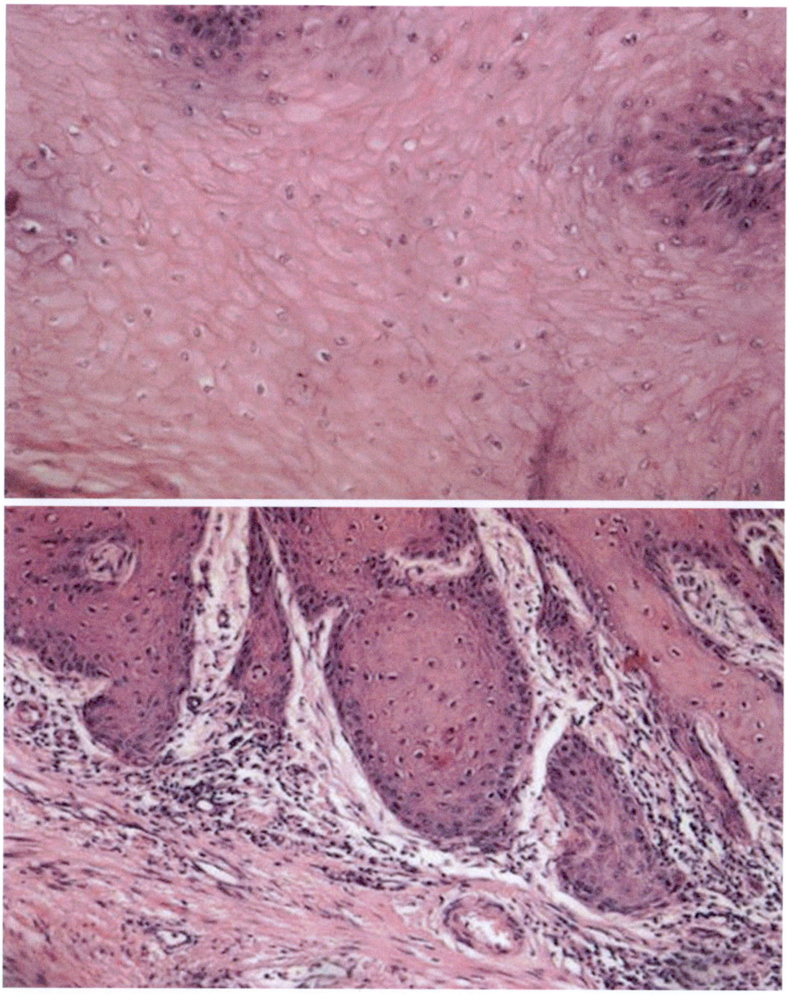

Fig. 5.33 Verrucous squamous cell carcinoma with focal koilocytic-like change

perinuclear halo, and dyskeratosis are prominent. Koilocytosis is present throughout tumor and not restricted to surface. Clear cell changes may be prominent and diffuse. Cellular anaplasia is usually marked. There are numerous mitotic figures (including atypical ones). Microabscesses may be prominent.

- Adjacent epithelium shows PeIN of warty/basaloid-type with p16 positive and diffuse by immunohistochemistry, in majority of cases. Mixed warty/basaloid carcinoma is important to recognize since basaloid component has worse prognosis.
- Differential diagnosis of warty carcinoma includes giant condyloma, an extremely well-differentiated lesion with bulbous base and koilocytosis confined to surface showing no anaplasia or stromal invasion. Mild nuclear atypia may be seen focally.
- Verrucous carcinoma also enters differential diagnosis. It is an extremely well-differentiated lesion with bulbous base that lacks of koilocytosis
- Clear cell carcinoma is rare an aggressive tumor with exophytic but not papillomatous pattern of growth. Affects inner portion of foreskin and seems to be of sweat gland origin. Tumor clear cells are CEA positive, and have intracytoplasmic PAS-D positive material
- Papillary carcinoma, a well-differentiated tumor with jagged infiltrative base and lack of koilocytosis
- Metastatic carcinomas with clear cells are usually not connected to overlying epithelium and lack papillomatous surface or true koilocytosis.

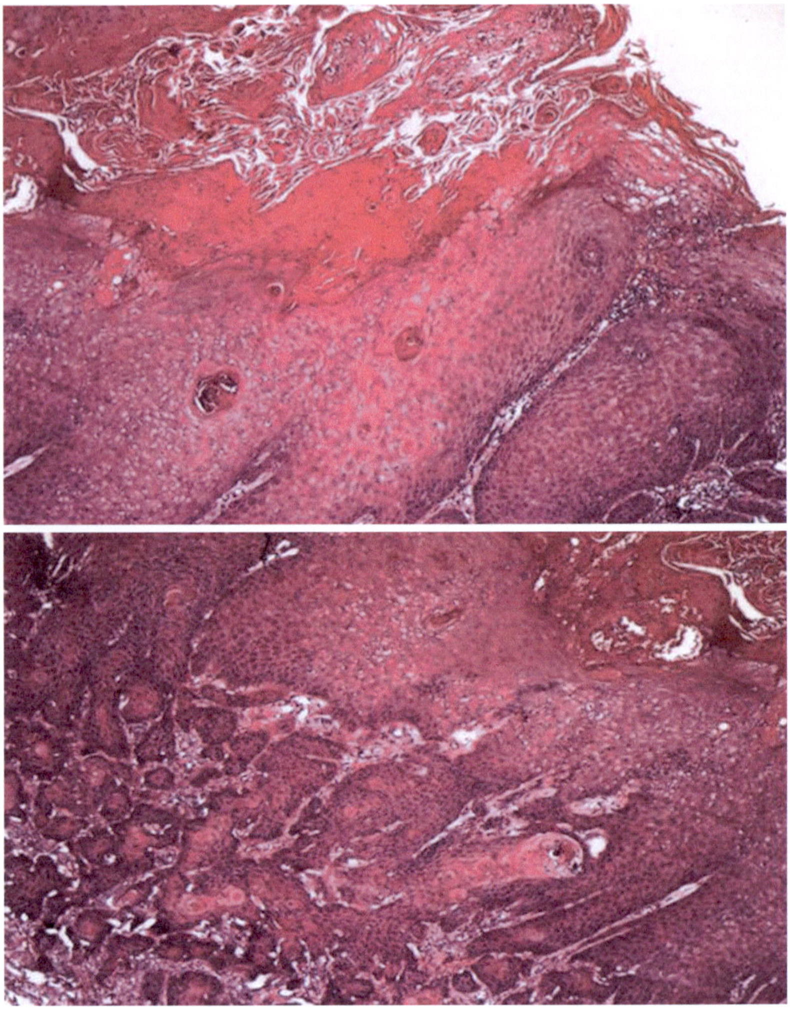

Fig. 5.34 Warthy squamous cell carcinoma simulating verrucous squamous cell carcinoma. Surface (*upper*) and infiltrative aspect (*lower*)

5.2.4.3 Verrucous Carcinoma

- Rare, extremely well-differentiated verruciform squamous cell carcinoma with bulbous deep borders. It represents about 4 % of all penile carcinoma. Koilocytic-like changes may be focally present but no true koilocytosis is present. Some cases are associated with lichen sclerosus et atrophicus and is likely HPV-unrelated carcinoma.
- White-gray 1–3 cm exophytic neoplasm with patients in their sixties. Some are multicentric tumors most frequently located in glans, coronal sulcus, and/or foreskin. Spiky surface and well-demarcated tumor base is characteristic. Tumors are usually confined to lamina propria.
- Pure verrucous carcinomas have excellent prognosis, may recur, but almost never metastasize.

Pathology

- Thick acanthotic papillae with slender fibrovascular core, orthokeratosis with variable presence of granular layer and occasional parakeratosis. Absent koilocytosis and pushing deep borders are common features.
- Abundant keratin-filled craters are common in verrucous carcinoma. Sarcomatoid transformation is a rare occurrence. Irregular jagged borders or foci of necrosis are not features of pure verrucous carcinoma.

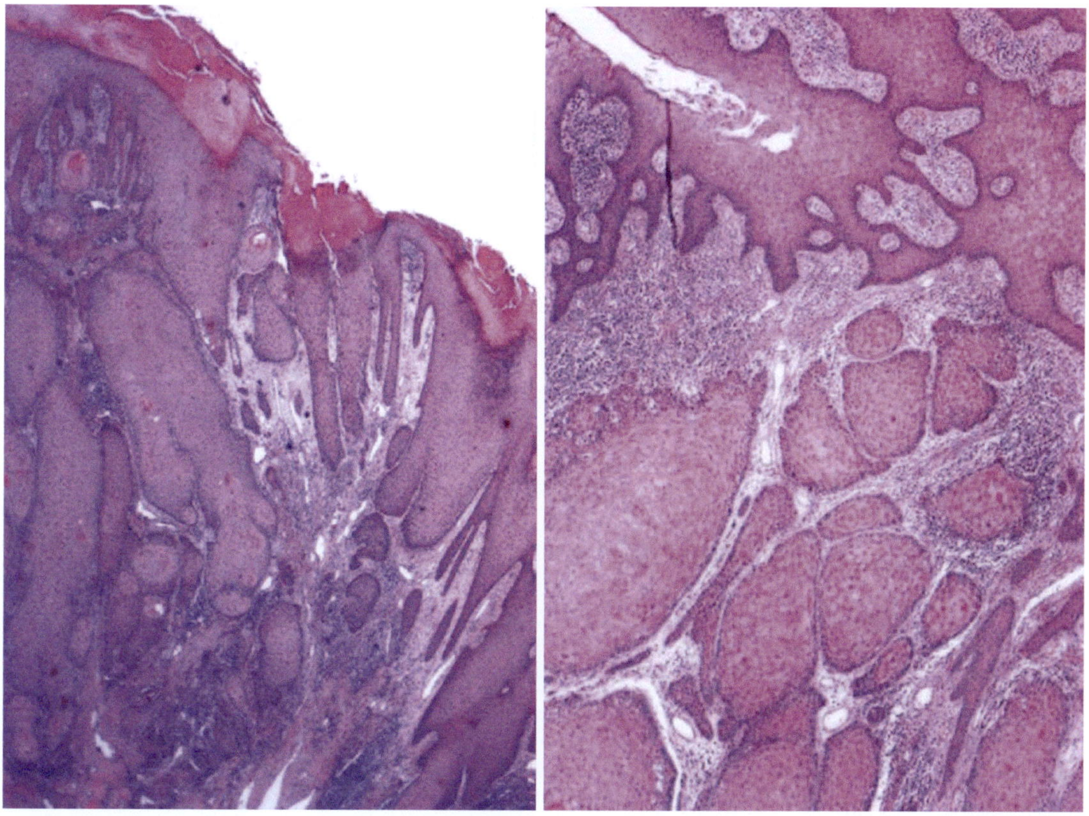

Fig. 5.35 Peudohyperplastic squamous cell carcinoma. Microscopic features (*left*) and infiltrating nests (*right*)

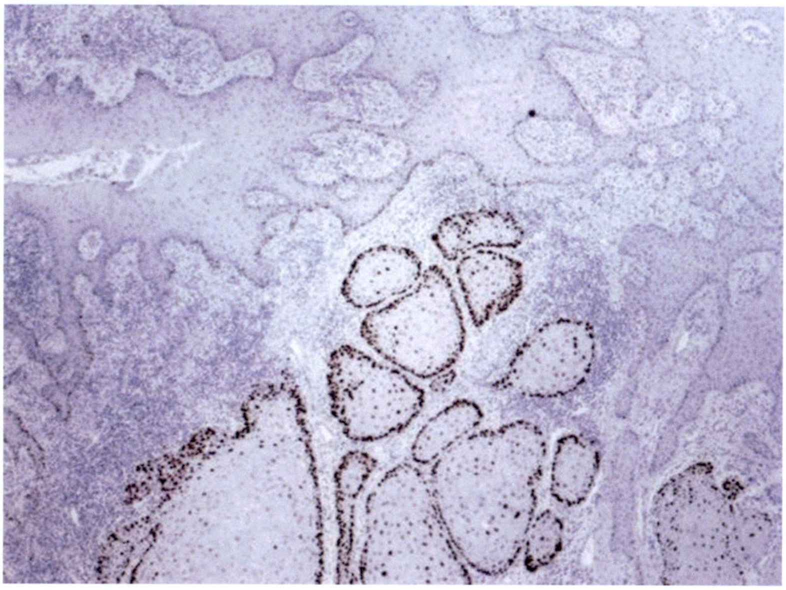

Fig. 5.36 p53 expression in peudohyperplastic squamous cell carcinoma

- Adjacent epithelium often shows verrucous type squamous hyperplasia and/or differentiated penile intraepithelial neoplasia.

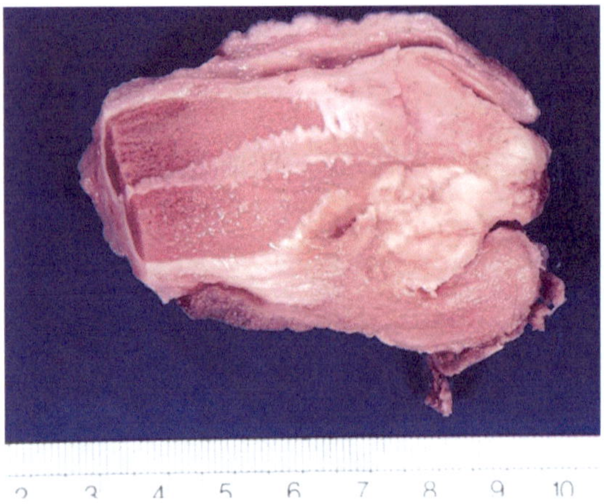

Fig. 5.37 Mixed-Basaloid squamous cell carcinoma. Gross features

- Differential diagnosis includes giant condyloma having more rounded arborescent papillae and true koilocytosis on surface.
- Papillary carcinoma shows well to moderately differentiate infiltrative neoplasm.
- Warty carcinoma shows higher histological grade, prominent koilocytosis and frequent infiltrative borders
- Carcinoma cuniculatum present the characteristic burrowing pattern, focal higher grade areas or jagged invading borders
- Mixed (hybrid) verrucous carcinoma shows admixed foci of squamous cell carcinoma, usual type with focal infiltrative, jagged borders, and focal higher grade areas. About 25 % of cases are associated with lymph node metastasis.

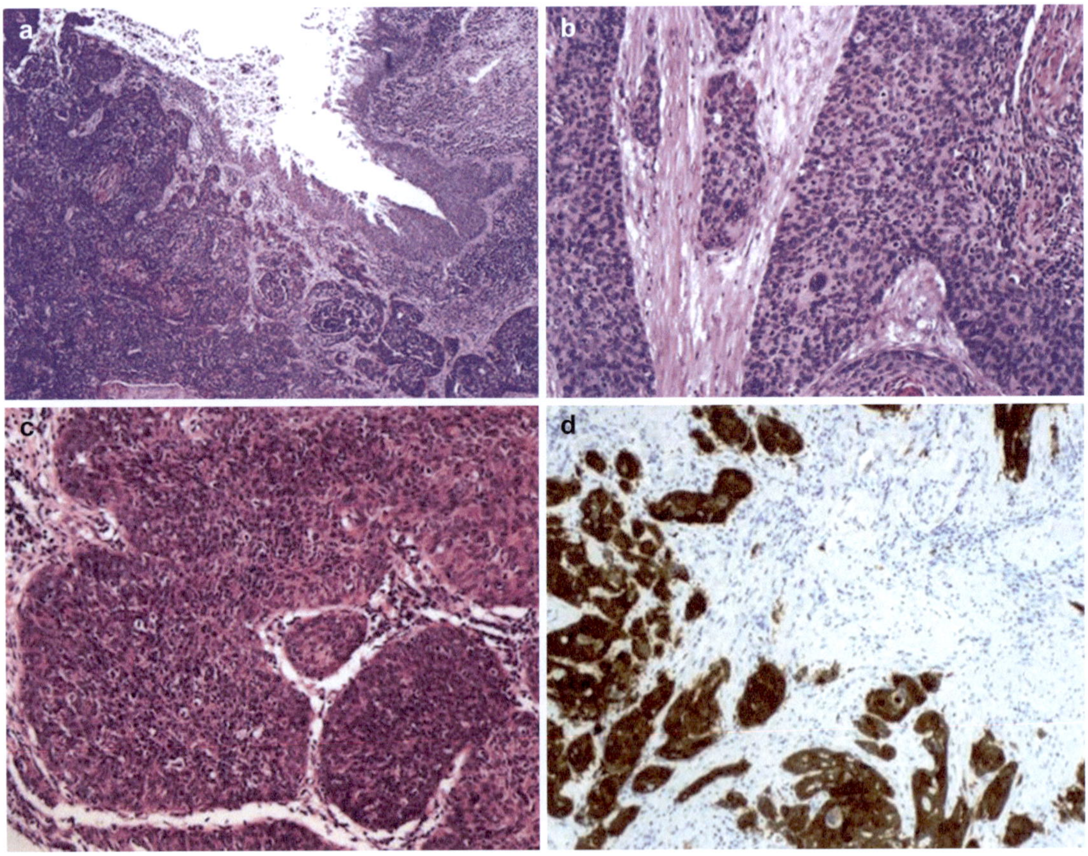

Fig. 5.38 Basaloid squamous cell carcinoma. Surface (**a**) infiltrative aspects (**b**, **c**), and p16 expression (**d**)

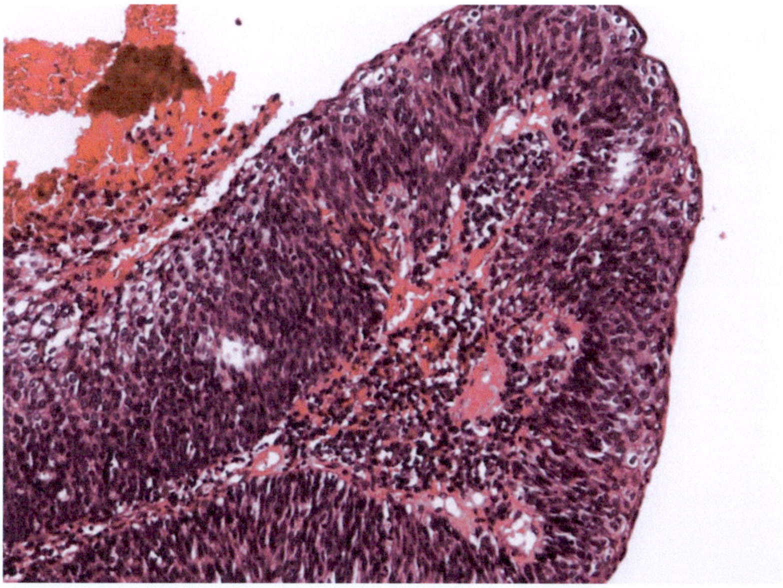

Fig. 5.39 Basaloid squamous cell carcinoma. Papillary architecture

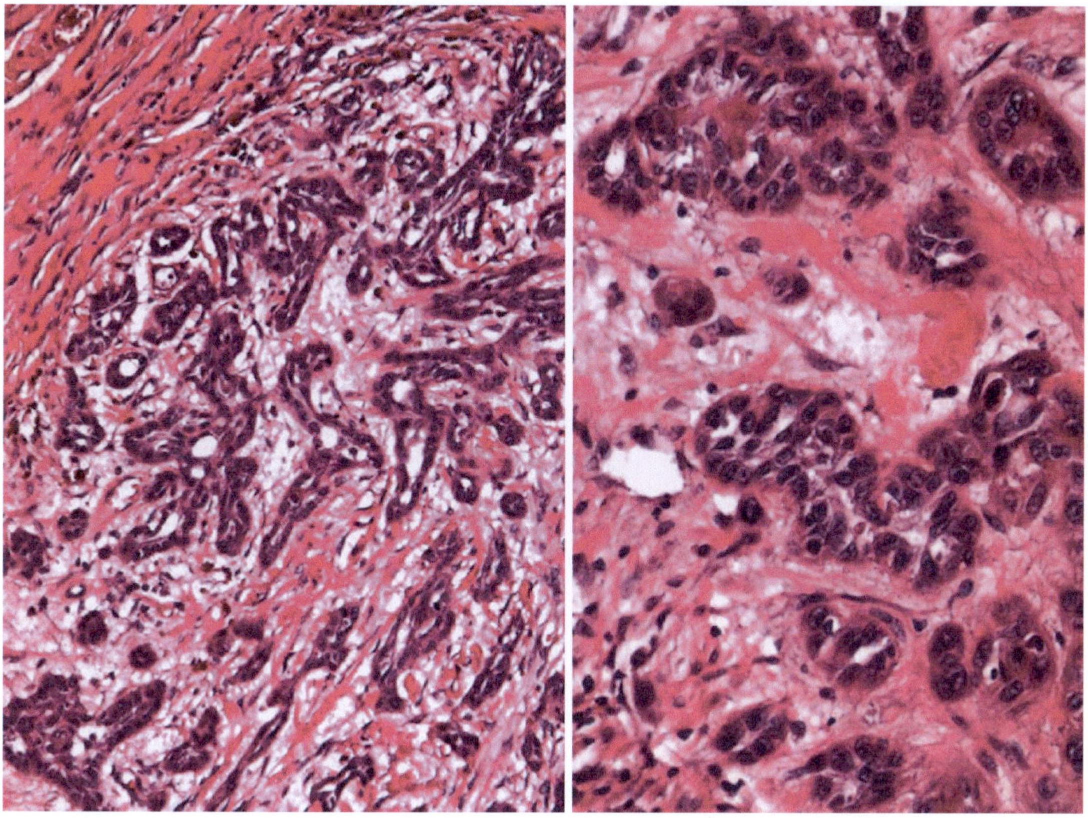

Fig. 5.40 Acantholytic/pseudoglandular squamous cell carcinoma. Low (*left*) and high (*right*) power

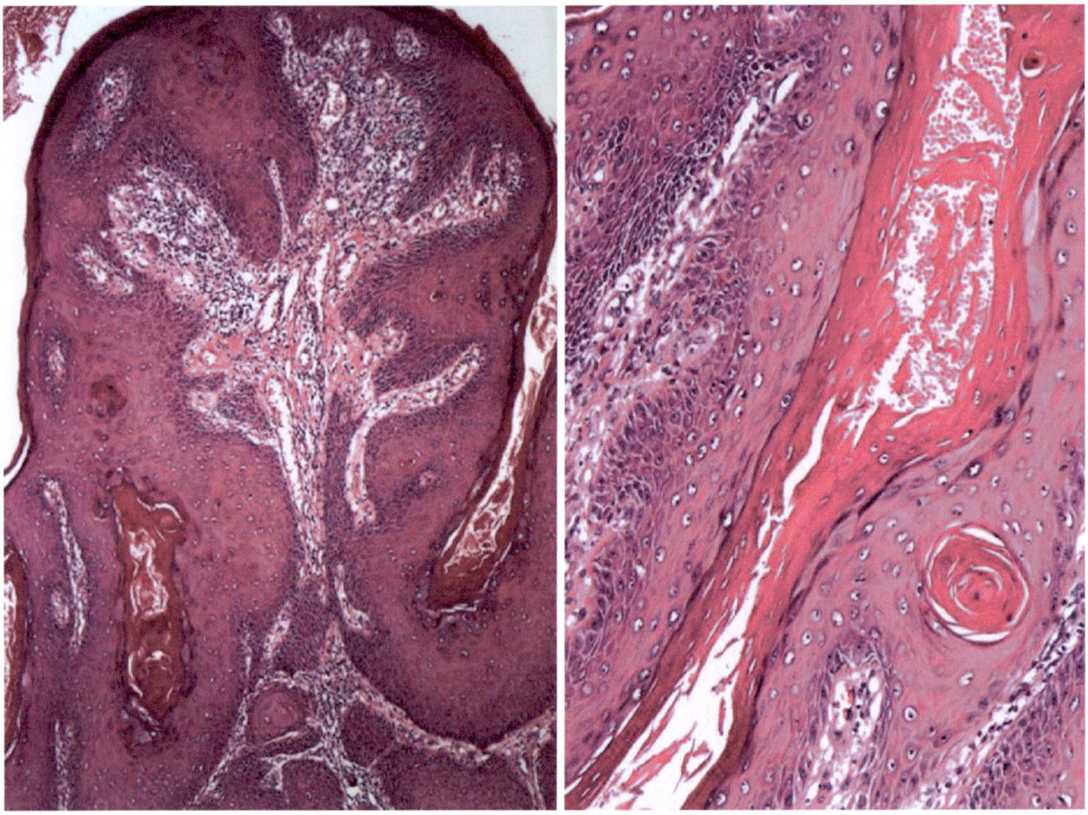

Fig. 5.41 Papillary squamous cell carcinoma at low (*left*) and high (*right*) power

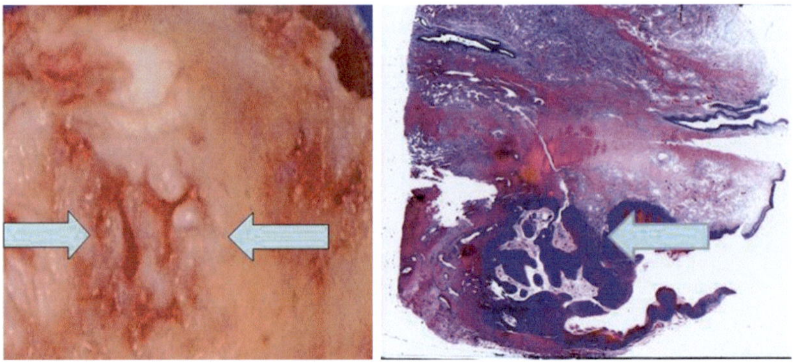

Fig. 5.42 Gross aspects of carcinoma Cuniculatum (*left* and *right*). Arrows point out gross (*left*) and microscopic view (*right*)

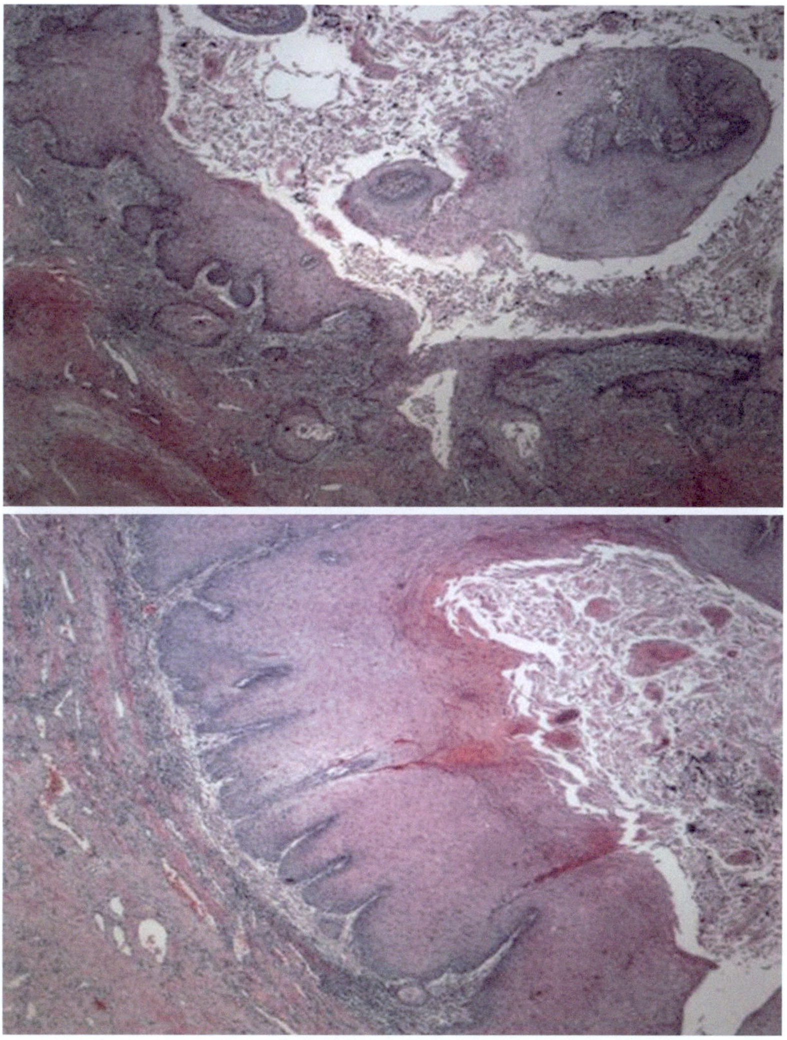

Fig. 5.43 Carcinoma Cuniculatum. Microscopic features (*upper* and *lower*)

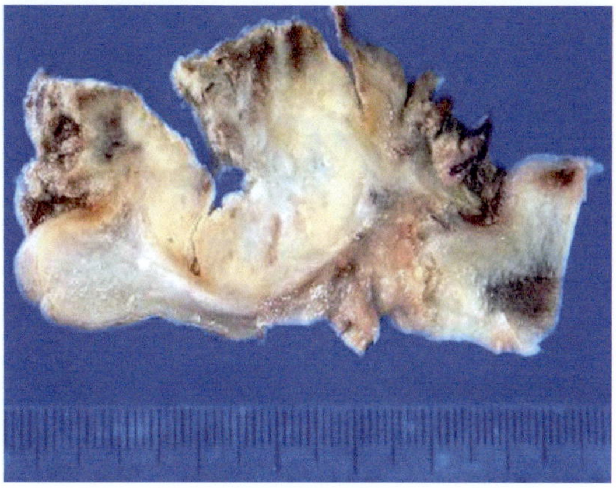

Fig. 5.44 Sarcomatoid squamous cell carcinoma. Gross features

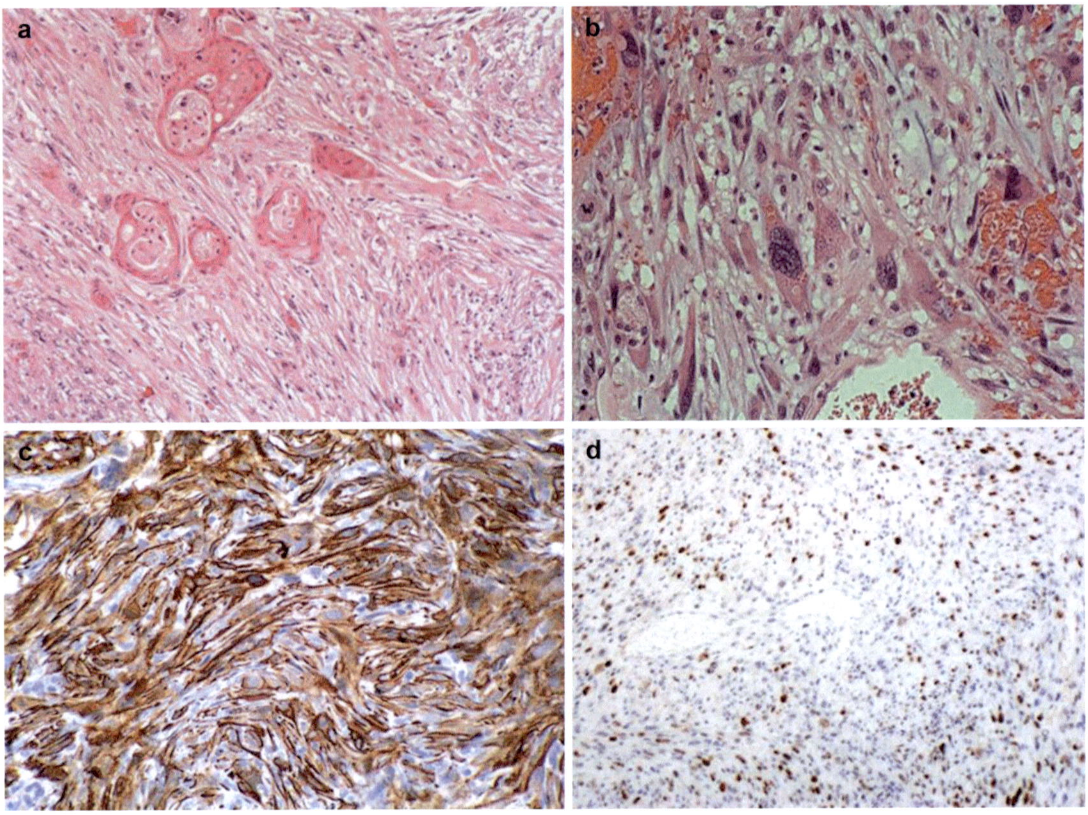

Fig. 5.45 Sarcomatoid squamous cell carcinoma. Microscopic features (**a**, **b**). Immunohistochemical expression of CKAE1/AE3 (**c**) and p63 (**d**)

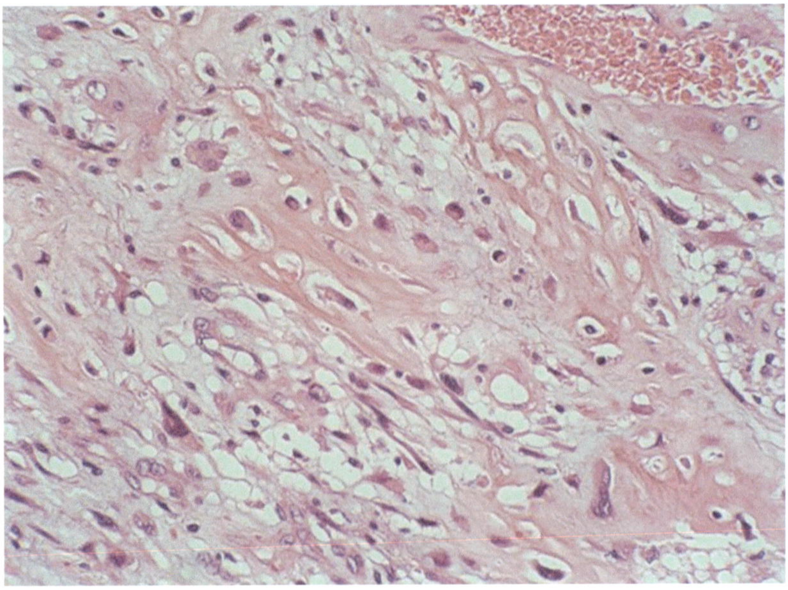

Fig. 5.46 Sarcomatoid squamous cell carcinoma with osteosarcomatous heterologous elements

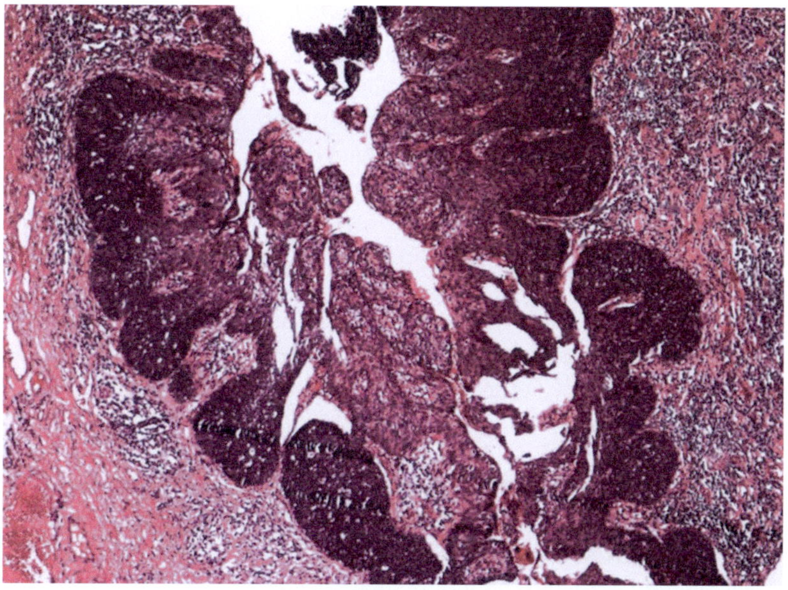

Fig. 5.47 Mixed-Basaloid squamous cell carcinoma

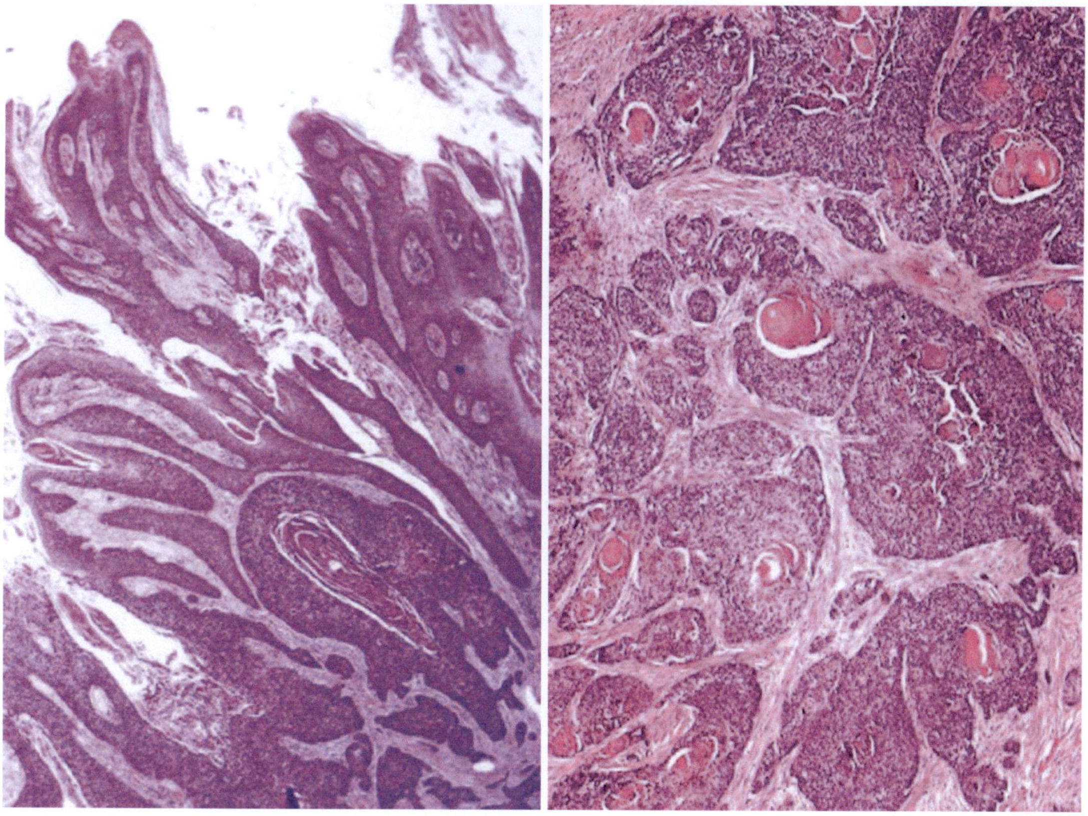

Fig. 5.48 Mixed Warty-Basaloid squamous cell carcinoma

5.2.4.4 Basaloid Carcinoma

- Rare and aggressive variant of nonkeratinizing squamous cell carcinoma composed of small to intermediate-sized basaloid cells, frequently associated HPV (HPV16 genotype in most cases). It represents about 15 % of all penile carcinomas.
- Patients in their fifties present with large, ulcerated, nonexophytic mass. Many patients have positive inguinal nodes at diagnosis and local recurrence after definitive therapy seen in 30 % of cases. Cancer-specific mortality in these patients is high.

Pathology

- Basaloid tumors are unifocal, usually affect glans, and may extend to coronal sulcus and foreskin. Exclusive foreskin location is uncommon. Basaloid carcinoma shows deeply invasive solid tumor with vertical growth pattern. Grossly is tan-gray to yellow in color. Invasion of corpus cavernosum at diagnosis is common.
- Tumoral nests with variable intervening stroma are frequently surrounded by retraction artifact; peripheral palisading is inconspicuous to absent. Focal and abrupt central keratinization may be seen, as well as comedo type necrosis, in some nests.
- Neoplastic cells are small to medium-sized and round to oval blue cells with high nuclear:cytoplasmic ratio and mild to moderate nuclear pleomorphism. Numerous mitoses and prominent apoptosis with "starry sky" pattern are common.
- Rarely, an adenoid cystic-like morphology secondary to extensive acantholysis may predominate. Perineural invasion and extension to distal urethra is common.
- Clear cell changes and spindle cell features may be focally seen in rare cases. Basaloid type of PeIN is frequent in adjacent areas.
- Differential diagnosis may include warty/basaloid (mixed) carcinoma variant composed of admixture of warty and basaloid carcinomas. Frequently warty and basaloid areas are intimately admixed but may be separated.
- Urothelial carcinoma of distal urethra also enters differential diagnosis. Patients have previous or concurrent history of urinary tract urothelial carcinoma. Urothelial features are usually recognizable as well as associated urothelial carcinoma in situ. Squamous and/or glandular differentiation is frequent. Immunohistochemistry for uroplakin-3, thrombomodulin, or GATA3 may support urothelial origin.
- Cutaneous basal cell carcinoma may present in penile shaft. It shows typical peripheral palisade and myxoid stroma, but less pleomorphism than basaloid carcinoma of penis.
- Small cell undifferentiated (neuroendocrine) carcinoma is extremely rare. It may be difficult to differentiate from basaloid carcinoma on morphology alone. Clinical correlation and immunohistochemical stains for neuroendocrine markers chromogranin, synaptophysin, or CD57 may be necessary in most cases.

5.2.4.5 Sarcomatoid Carcinoma

- Also known as spindle cell carcinoma, carcinosarcoma, or metaplastic carcinoma, it represents an undifferentiated carcinoma arising from squamous epithelium predominantly composed of malignant spindle cells with pleomorphic nuclei and mitoses. Some examples may be HPV-related.
- Most originate from glans, often extending to coronal sulcus and foreskin. Frequently, presents as large, deeply invasive, polypoid, and ulcerated tumor that extensively invades the corpora spongiosum and cavernosa.
- It is rare and aggressive, and represents about 4 % of penile carcinomas. Patients are in their sixties with frequent lymph node metastasis.

Pathology

- The cut surface shows solid white/gray/yellow to hemorrhagic. Predominantly composed of patternless atypical spindle cells or those in interlacing fascicles. May resemble fibrosarcoma or leiomyosarcoma or pleomorphic malignant fibrohistiocytoma.
- Myxoid changes and pseudovascular pattern mimicking angiosarcoma may be seen. Mitotic figures are numerous and necrosis may be prominent in some cases. Bone and cartilaginous heterologous differentiation may be observed.

Table 5.7 Immunohistochemistry in spindle cell lesions of the penis

Antibody	Sarcomatoid ca	Leiomyosarcoma	Angiosarcoma	Spindle cell melanoma
Actin sm	–/+	+	+	+
Calponin	–	+	–	–
Pan-CK	+/–	–/+ focal	–	–
HMWCK	+	–	–	–
P63	+	–	–	–
Vimentin	+	+	+	+
S100	–	–	–	+
FLI1	–	–	+	–
CD34	–	–	+	–
CD31	–	–	+	–

- Frequent lymphovascular and perineural invasion. Squamous cell carcinoma in situ and clear-cut squamous invasive component may be present, at least focally.
- Spindle cells are positive for p63, vimentin, and cytokeratins. Cytokeratin expression (especially AE1/AE3 and CAM5.2) by spindle cells may be only focally present. AE1/AE3 and high molecular weight cytokeratin (34βE12) tend to be more diffusely expressed by spindle cells. Smooth muscle actin is usually negative but focal positive staining may be seen in rare cases. Desmin and S100 are both negative.
- Differential diagnosis includes soft tissue tumors located deep within corpora spongiosum or cavernosa with no connection to surface epithelium unless ulcerated samples; squamous differentiation is absent. Immunohistochemistry may be necessary. Most are negative for cytokeratins and p63, and positive for markers depending on histogenesis. Leiomyosarcoma is positive for SMA, desmin, calponin and angiosarcoma is positive for CD31, FLI-1, and CD34 (Table 5.7).
- Spindle cell melanoma may enter differential diagnosis. Recognition of associated melanoma in situ is helpful. Immunohistochemistry is usually necessary. S100 positive (may be the only positive melanocytic marker), Melan-A usually negative, and cytokeratins and p63 are negative.

5.2.4.6 Carcinoma Cuniculatum

- Rare variant of verrucous (low grade) squamous cell carcinoma characterized by deep burrowing growth pattern mimicking rabbit burrows (cuniculi) seen in patients in their seventies. Likely not HPV-related tumor. Similar to epithelioma cuniculatum seen in other organs. Usually affects glans and extends to coronal sulcus and foreskin. No reported metastases.

Pathology

- Histologically represents hybrid (mixed) verrucous carcinoma with unique growth pattern. Deep and narrow complex tumor invaginations connect to surface through sinus tracts
- Deeply endophytic tumoral invaginations mimicking rabbit burrows (cuniculi). Neoplastic invaginations invade through lamina propria and corpus spongiosum to involve tunica albuginea and corpora cavernosa. Most frequently, there are large, papillomatous lesions with cobblestone or spiky appearance.
- Deeply invasive keratin-filled pseudocysts or crypts are common findings. Interanastomosing channels and pseudocystic structures are lined by well-differentiated squamous cell carcinoma. Bulk of lesion may have features of verrucous carcinoma with acanthotic papillae and thin fibrovascular cores, piling up of keratin among papillae, bulbous deep borders, and lack of koilocytosis.
- In some cases, minor component showing features of squamous cell carcinoma, usual type.

Also focal higher grade areas with infiltrative borders may be seen.
- Differential diagnosis includes verrucous carcinoma, warty carcinoma, papillary carcinoma, or condyloma acuminatum/giant condyloma, all lacking classic burrowing pattern.

5.2.4.7 Mixed (Hybrid) Carcinoma

- Penile mixed tumors, harboring more than one histologic subtype and grade, constitute a frequent finding in routine pathology.
- Typically, there is coexistence of two or more histologic subtypes, and represents about 30 % of all penile carcinomas. Most patients are in their 50s and glans is most frequently affected site. Foreskin location is rare.
- Prognosis related to relative proportion of different components and the presence of higher histologic grade. Tumor recurrences may occur but inguinal nodal involvement is rarely seen and cancer-specific mortality rate is low.

Pathology

- Most frequent patterns include mixture of HPV-related histologic subtypes. Mixtures of usual squamous cell carcinoma with other HPV-related and unrelated variants are also common. Histologic grade distribution is variable and depends on subtypes present. Gross appearance is variable and multicentricity is not uncommon. Vascular invasion, perineural invasion, and extension to distal urethra may be seen in about 30 % of cases. Mixtures of differentiated, basaloid, and/or warty PeIN may be identified in adjacent mucosa. One-half of cases are associated with typical condylomata.
- Warty/basaloid carcinoma is the most frequently observed mixed squamous cell carcinoma, and clinically it behaves as basaloid squamous cell carcinoma. Warty pattern may be superficial and basaloid histology is present in invasive carcinoma. Warty and basaloid areas may occasionally be randomly intermingled. Occasionally, papillae may be composed of both clear warty and small basaloid cells. HPV and p16 positivity is present in most cases.
- Usual type squamous cell carcinoma admixed with verrucous carcinoma (hybrid verrucous carcinoma) represents approximately 25 % of all mixed carcinomas. Biological behavior is dictated by highest histologic grade. Even small foci of high-grade tumor impart metastatic potential. Verrucous carcinoma is always low grade. Usual type squamous cell carcinoma may be well, moderately well, or poorly differentiated. Pure verrucous may locally recur as hybrid verrucous carcinoma.
- Squamous cell carcinoma with mixed sarcomatoid features are observed in one-half of sarcomatoid carcinomas. In some cases, typical areas of verrucous, papillary, and basaloid may be present. Regardless of presence of other histologic subtypes, all of these tumors are considered and reported as sarcomatoid carcinoma.
- Other mixed patterns including usual type-warty squamous cell carcinoma are rare. Mixtures of basaloid with usual squamous cell carcinoma are also uncommon. Papillary squamous cell carcinoma admixed with usual type squamous cell carcinoma may be seen occasionally. Other mixtures may occur since virtually any combination is possible.
- Differential diagnosis is important because of different prognostic significance. Tumors should be adequately sampled in order to identify minor clinically relevant mixed areas. Also, pathologist should follow strict criteria in histologic subtyping. Special attention should be paid in separating hybrid verrucous carcinoma from pure verrucous carcinoma.
- Sarcomatoid carcinoma is clinically aggressive regardless of presence and extension of other morphological components. Biological behavior of mixed squamous cell carcinoma with basaloid features seems to be similar to pure Basaloid carcinoma.

5.2.4.8 Papillary Carcinoma

- Represents 15 % of all penile squamous cell carcinoma and about 40 % of all verruciform tumors. The pattern of growth is exophytic, and the histology is of low-grade malignant epithelial tumor. Diagnosis need to exclude other verruciform tumors. Associated lichen sclerosus is common. A minority of cases show evidence of HPV infection.

- Patients range 43–85 years in age. Recurrence rate of about 10 % of cases, most probably due to insufficient surgery. Inguinal metastases are found in about 10 % of patients, but cancer-specific mortality rate is very low, similar to other verruciform tumors. Most tumors invade up to corpus spongiosum or dartos at diagnosis. Invasion of deep corpus cavernosum is unusual

Pathology

- Tumors (4–6 cm) present exophytic verruciform, cauliflower-like pattern of growth. Glans is most frequently affected with extension to multiple anatomical compartments in one-half of cases. Foreskin exclusively affected is rare. There is poorly defined tumor-stroma interface.
- There is papillomatous pattern of growth with mild to moderate acanthosis, hyperkeratosis with parakeratosis. Papillae are architecturally complex and can be short or elongated. Central fibrovascular cores may be noted and tips of papillae may be blunt or spiky. Areas of intraepithelial keratin pearls are not uncommon. Most tumors are well- to moderately well differentiated squamous cell carcinoma. High-grade areas are unusual and focal. No koilocytotic atypia is present.
- Microabscesses, acantholysis, and clear cell changes may be focally observed in some cases. Tumoral base is irregular and jagged with destructive stromal invasion and invasive nests at tumoral front are surrounded by reactive stroma. Extension to distal urethra is uncommon and vascular and perineural invasion may be observed in small subset of cases.
- Differentiated PeIN, lichen sclerosus and or squamous hyperplasia frequently seen in adjacent areas.
- Differential diagnosis includes warty carcinoma showing more pleomorphic neoplastic cells, koilocytotic atypia, jagged and irregular tumoral base, and high-risk HPV detected and p16 positive immunohistochemistry in most cases.
- Verrucous carcinoma present less pleomorphic neoplastic cells, broad tumoral base with pushing borders, fibrovascular cores absent or very inconspicuous, absent koilocytic changes, and invasion up to lamina propria or superficial corpus spongiosum. HPV negative.
- Carcinoma cuniculatum shows presence of cysts and sinus-like tracts connecting tumoral surface with deeper invaded areas. It is HPV negative.
- Mixed usual-verrucous carcinoma (hybrid verrucous carcinoma) with well-differentiated areas intermingled with more pleomorphic foci of neoplastic cells and irregular tumoral base due to presence of usual type squamous cell carcinoma.
- Giant condyloma shows condylomatous papillae, koilocytic changes, and absence of pleomorphic or clearly malignant cells. A broad tumoral base with pushing borders is present. It is HPV positive.

5.2.5 Other Carcinomas

5.2.5.1 Paget Disease

- Primary extramammary Paget disease exclusively affecting penis is rare.
- Secondary extramammary Paget disease tends to affect glans and especially perimeatal region. May also affect perianal area extending to perineum and scrotum. Secondary extramammary Paget disease is related to the underlying carcinoma and is usually poor. Secondary extramammary Paget disease may represent extension from urethral, bladder, or anal/rectal carcinoma (Fig. 5.49).

Pathology

- Focal with a few mm in size or multicentric. Microscopic examination identifies intraepithelial proliferation of large round atypical cells (Paget cells). Mitoses may be numerous. Nuclei are large and vesicular with prominent nucleoli.
- Primary extramammary Paget disease is positive for CEA, low molecular weight cytokeratins (especially CK7 and CAM5.2) EMA/MUC1, and GCDFP-15. It is negative for CK20 and melanocytic markers such as S100, Melan-A, tyrosinase, and HMB45 (Table 5.8).

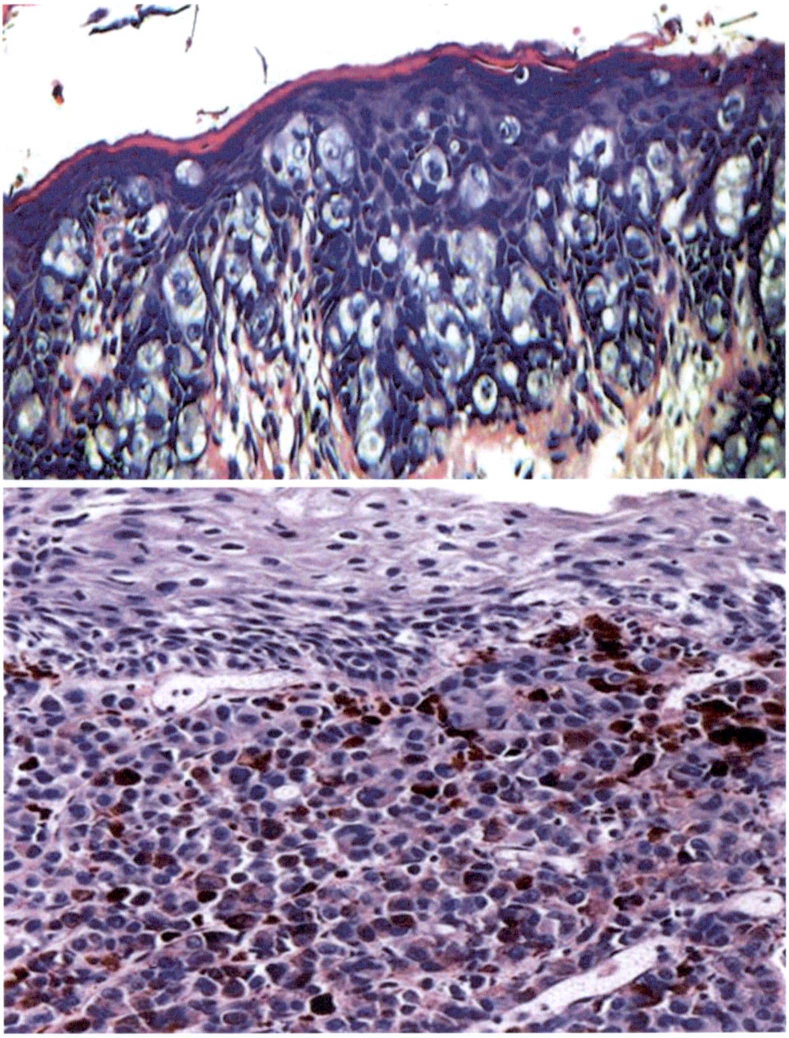

Fig. 5.49 Paget disease (*upper*) and melanoma (*lower*) of penis

Table 5.8 Immunohistochemistry of extramamary Paget disease

Antibody	Primary	Secondary-urothelial carcinoma	Secondary-anal/rectal carcinoma	Squamous cell carcinoma in situ	Melanoma in situ
CEA	+	−	+	−	−
CK7	+	+	−	−	−
GCDEFP-15	+	−	−	−	−
CK20	−	+	+	−	−
S100	−	−	−	−	+
Melan A	−	−	−	−	+
Uroplakin 3	−	+	−	−	−
CDX2	−	−	+	−	−

- Main differential diagnosis includes melanoma in situ, squamous cell carcinoma in situ with pagetoid pattern, clear cell papulosis, pagetoid dyskeratosis pagetoid reticulosis and benign mucinous metaplasia of penis (see also pages 424–426 scrotum)

5.2.5.2 Merkel Cell Carcinoma

- Rare in the penis, presents small round blue cells with scarce cytoplasm, no glandular formations and characteristic dot-like pattern with cytokeratin AE1/AE3 and CK20. Positive expression of neuroendocrine markers chromogranin and synaptophysin is the rule. Some cases may coexpress CK7, focally.

5.2.5.3 Penile Tumors with Glandular Features: Adenosquamous and Mucoepidermoid Carcinomas

- Very rare forms of penile cancer.
- The presence of a biphasic population of neoplastic cells, one with glandular and the other with squamous carcinoma characterizes adenosquamous carcinoma. The clinical features are similar to those of usual squamous cell carcinoma.
- Squamous component usually predominates. PeIN is usually present adjacent to the invasive carcinoma. CEA is present in glandular component and 34ßE12 has been reported in both components.
- Adenosquamous carcinoma with solid areas punctuated by mucinous cells and mucin containing glands are also referred to as mucoepidermoid carcinoma.
- Penile tumors with glandular features may be confused with the more common pseudoglandular (adenoid, acantholytic) variant of squamous cell carcinomas, their main mimicker.

5.2.5.4 Clear Cell Carcinoma

- HPV-related tumors composed of periodic acid-Schiff positive clear cells are aggressive tumors with a high incidence of inguinal nodal metastases.

5.3 Benign Tumors and Tumor-Like Conditions

5.3.1 Benign Tumors of Epithelial Origin

- Rare examples of squamous cell papilloma with clinical and pathologic features similar to those seen in the skin have been described (Fig. 5.50; Table 5.9).

5.3.2 Benign Human Papillomavirus-Associated Lesions

- Evidence of HPV infection found in most cases. Low-risk genotypes (6, 11) predominate. Incidence of HPV6 is higher than HPV11. Other genotypes identified include 76, 18, 30–32, 42–44, and 51–55.

5.3.2.1 Condyloma Acuminatum

- Very common in sexually active young males and ranges from few mm to several cm.
- Papillary cauliflower-like exophytic tumor with arborescent papillae, prominent fibrovascular cores, and variable parakeratosis and orthokeratosis. Conspicuous surface koilocytosis. Typical koilocytes exhibit perinuclear vacuolization, wrinkled and hyperchromatic nuclei with frequent binucleation. Sharply defined broad pushing base.
- Glans is most frequently affected site, following foreskin, meatus urethralis, and penile shaft (Figs. 5.51 and 5.52).

5.3.2.2 Giant Condyloma (Buschke-Löwenstein Tumor)

- It is very unusual and patients tend to be older than those with condyloma acuminatum. Tumors shows evident endophytic pattern of growth measuring 4–10 cm. Giant condyloma may harbor focal squamous cell carcinoma.

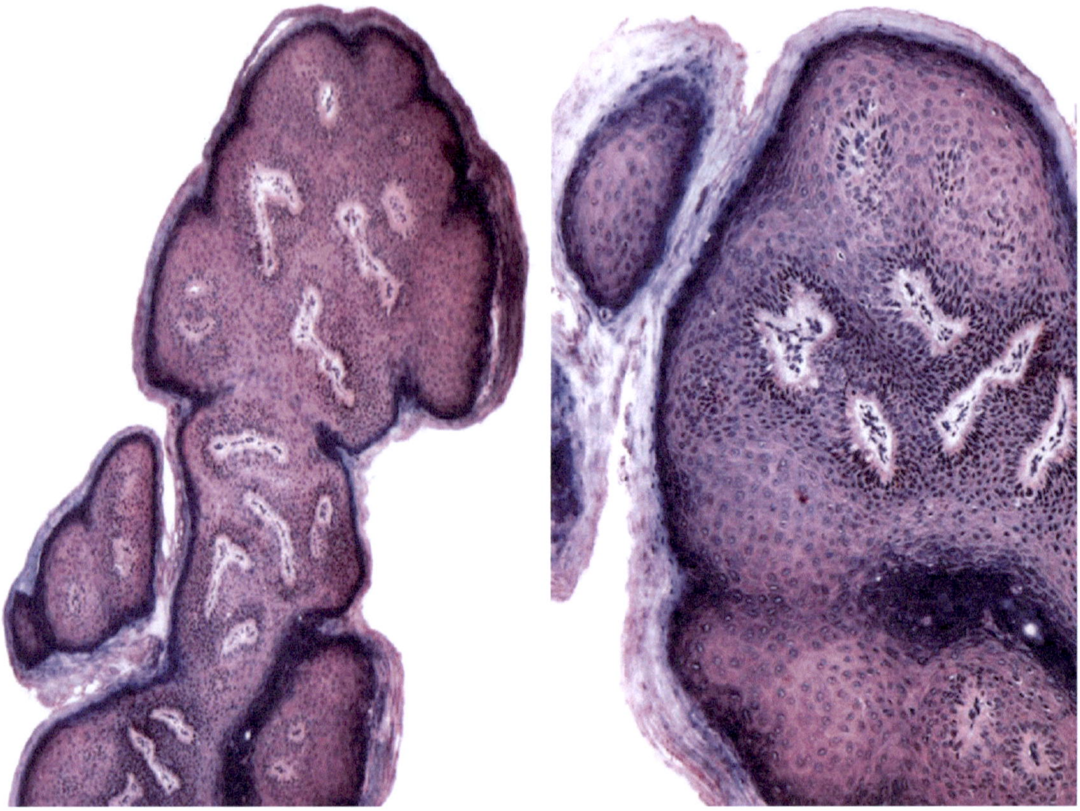

Fig. 5.50 Low (*left*) and high (*right*) power of squamous cell papilloma

Table 5.9 Nonepithelial neoplasms

Melanocytic
Nevi
Malignant melanoma
Mesenchymal
Benign
Angiokeratoma
Hemangioma
Leiomyoma
Other
Malignant
Kaposi Sarcoma
Angiosarcoma
Rhabdomyosarcoma
Leiomyosarcoma
Epithelioid sarcoma
Other
Malignant lymphomas
Other rare primary tumors

- Usual type squamous cell carcinoma is most commonly associated subtype. Most commonly affects foreskin and coronal sulcus (Figs. 5.53 and 5.54)

5.3.2.3 Differential Diagnosis of Condylomatous Lesions

- Given the morphologic features shared by all verruciform tumors (ie, verrucous, warty, papillary, and cuniculatum carcinomas, along with giant condylomas), it is challenging at times to distinguish one from another.
- Warty carcinoma is the most frequent consideration since it is high-risk HPV positive with immunohistochemical p16 overexpression. Other considerations include verrucous carcinoma or papillary carcinoma. Both are not associated with HPV infection and tend to be

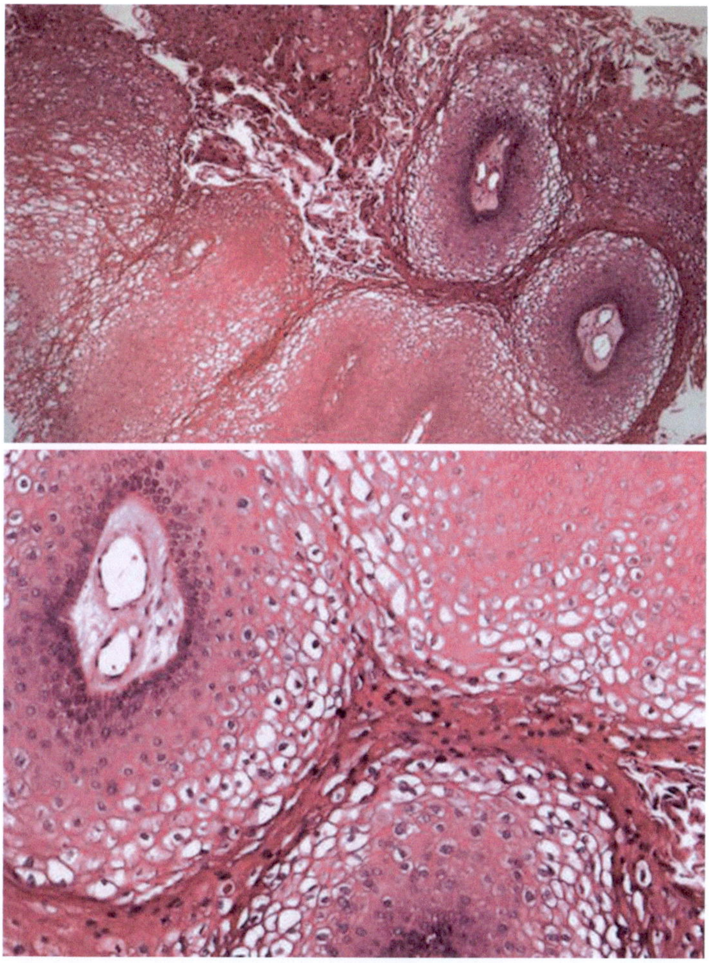

Fig. 5.51 Condyloma acuminatum. Low (*upper*) and high (*lower*) power view showing koilocytosis

negative for p16. Papillomatosis of glans corona (pearly penile papules) characterized by small fibroepithelial papillomas, also enters differential diagnosis.

5.3.3 Myointimoma

- Myointimal rare benign proliferation occurring exclusively in corpus spongiosum of glans penis characterized by small palpable nodular lesion seen most frequently in children with some examples reported in variable aged adults. No recurrences reported after treatment. Some cases may spontaneously regress.

Pathology

- Single nodule less than 2 cm with occasional presentation as multinodular growth.
- There is an intravascular growth extension within preexisting vascular network of corpus spongiosum. Proliferating cells have a spindled myofibroblastic appearance with eosinophilic cytoplasm and associated fibrous and myxoid stroma. They expand the vascular spaces with atrophy of the vessel walls and loss of the lumen. There is no significant nuclear atypia. A surrounding collarette of residual, desmin positive, smooth muscle is generally present at periphery.
- There is immunohistochemical expression of smooth muscle actin, muscle-specific actin

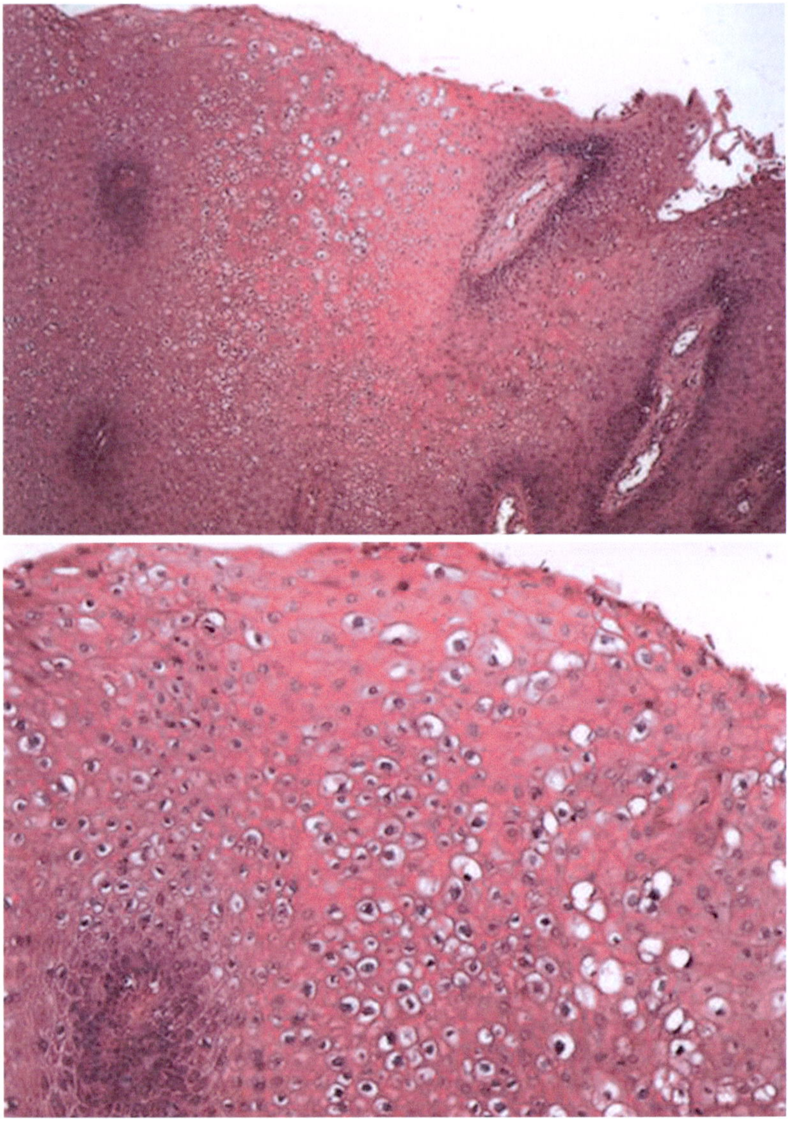

Fig. 5.52 Condyloma acuminatum. Low (*upper*) and high (*lower*) power view showing koilocytosis

(HHF35), and calponin. CD31 and CD34 highlight residual endothelial cells at periphery

- Differential diagnosis includes intravascular fasciitis showing myofibroblastic proliferation and intralesional inflammatory cells including occasional osteoclast-like giant cells.
- Nerve sheath tumors. Rare cases of neurofibroma, schwannoma, or nerve sheath myxoma may have multinodular growth pattern and diffuse nuclear reactivity for S100.
- Myoid nodules in myofibroma are similar in morphology to myointimoma cells. Myofibroma often have classic biphasic appearance.
- Leiomyoma has intersecting fascicular architecture with more eosinophilic cells that express desmin.
- Epithelioid hemangioendothelioma is morphologically similar also with myxoid stroma. Usually more epithelioid but may be spindled. Rare in children. Very uncommon in penis. Epithelioid hemangioma is seen in penis. However, there is less morphologic overlap with myointimoma. Immunoreactivity for CD31 and CD34 in epithelioid population is characteristic (Fig. 5.55).

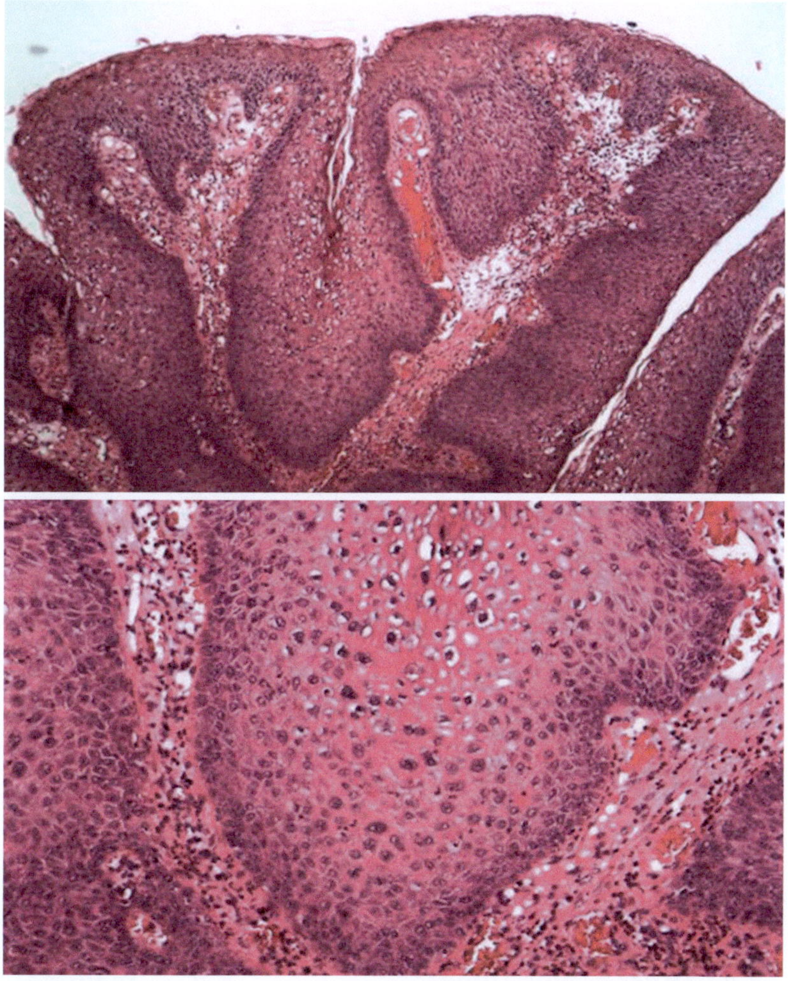

Fig. 5.53 Giant Condyloma. Exophytic (*upper*) and endophytic (*lower*) components with evident nuclear atypia

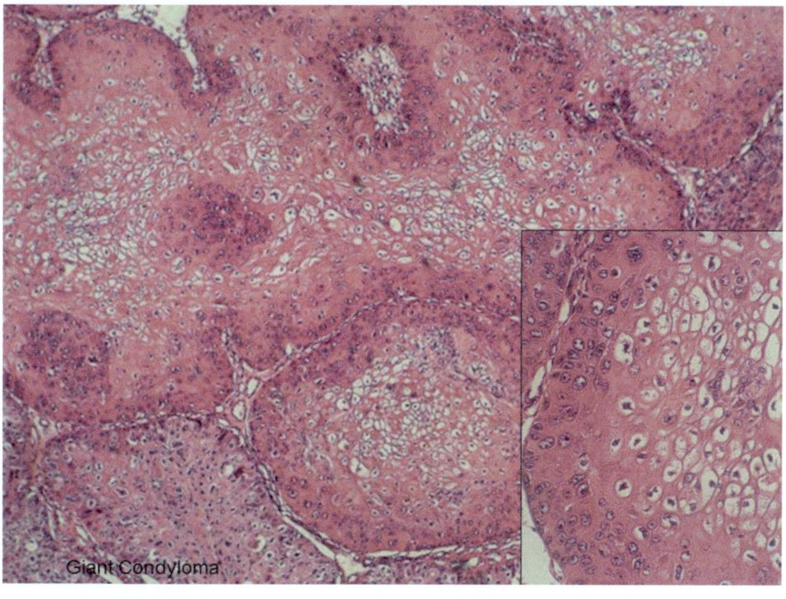

Fig. 5.54 Giant Condyloma with evident nuclear atypia and prominent koilocytosis (*inset*)

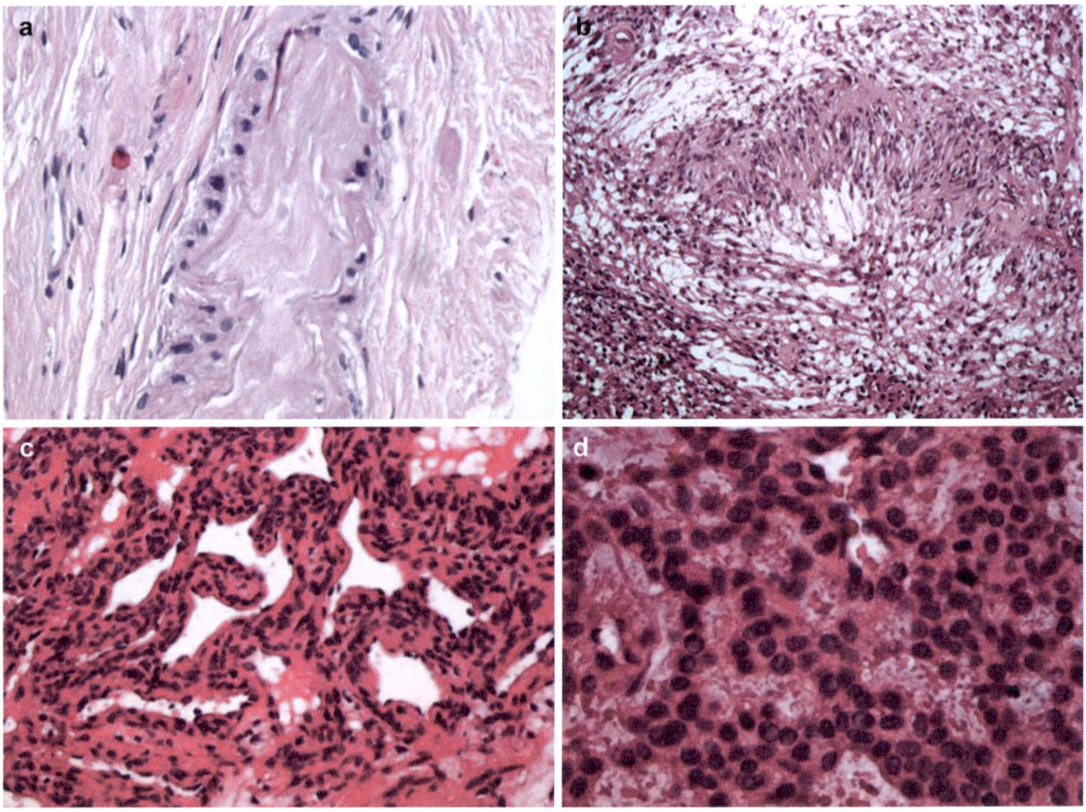

Fig. 5.55 Myointimoma (a). Schwannoma (b). Glomus tumor (c, d)

5.3.4 Other Benign Tumors

- Among the benign soft tissue tumors of the glans penis, tumors of vascular origin, including capillary or cavernous hemangioma, epithelioid hemangioma, and lymphangioma, are the most common, followed by neurofibroma, schwannoma, leiomyoma, glomus tumor, fibrous histiocytoma, and granular cell tumor (Fig. 5.55; Table 5.9).
- Epithelioid hemangioma can be exuberant and often confused with epithelioid hemangioendothelioma and epithelioid angiosarcoma. Benign soft tissue tumors are more common located on the distal part, and malignant lesions are more common on the proximal penis.

5.4 Malignant Soft Tissue Tumors

- Less than 5 % of all penile malignancies are sarcomas. Sarcoma arises in men of all ages, with a peak occurrence in late fifties or sixties; exceptions include rhabdomyosarcoma most common in children and epithelioid sarcoma in young adults. Sarcoma is most frequently located on the shaft. Sarcomas of myogenic, neurogenic, and fibrous origin are rarities in penis.
- Histologic features of these lesions are similar to those of their counterparts arising at other locations.
- Vascular sarcomas, including Kaposi sarcoma, epithelioid hemangioendothelioma,

and angiosarcoma, are the most common type of penile sarcoma (Table 5.5).

5.4.1 Kaposi Sarcoma

- Virus-associated vascular tumor related to Human herpesvirus-8. Proliferating cell in Kaposi sarcoma appears to be lymphatic in origin.
- Four main groups of Kaposi sarcoma are recognized: Classic, endemic/African, AIDS-associated, and iatrogenic/transplantation-associated Kaposi sarcoma.
- Penile Kaposi sarcoma usually affects HIV positive patients or patients affected by other forms of immunosuppression. AIDS-related Kaposi sarcoma and endemic forms affect younger patients. Classic Kaposi sarcoma and transplant-related Kaposi sarcoma tend to affect older patients. Classic and endemic forms of Kaposi sarcoma affecting penis are extremely rare.

Pathology

- Most common location is the glans. But may also affect coronal sulcus, foreskin, and skin of shaft. Frequently multifocal, forms ill-defined erythematous macules to violaceous plaques and nodules (Figs. 5.56 and 5.57).

Patch Stage

- Proliferation of slit-like and or angulated vessels separating collagen bundles within dermis with promontory sign, that is adnexal structures and preexisting vessels protruding within newly formed vessels. Extravasated red blood cells, siderophages and dermal infiltrate of lymphoid cells and plasma cells

Plaque Stage

- Vascular proliferation diffusely involves dermis and may extend to subcutis. Relatively bland spindle cell component appears at this stage. PAS-D positive hyaline globules may be seen intra- and extracellularly.

Nodular Stage

- Spindle cell proliferation becomes confluent to form well-defined nodules. Fascicles of spindle cells intersect one another and are intimately admixed/separated by slit-like spaces containing erythrocytes. Spindle cells are devoid of significant pleomorphism. At periphery of nodules, dilated blood vessels, inflammatory cells, and siderophages are often seen.

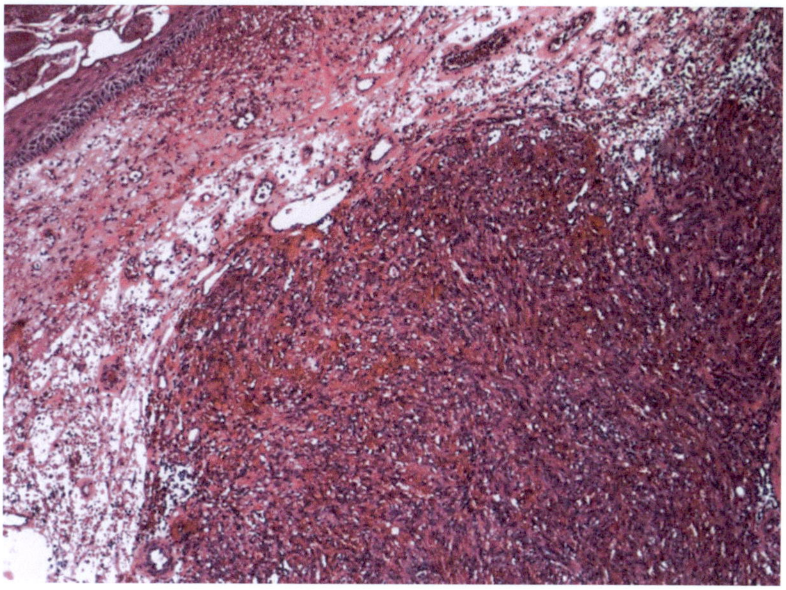

Fig. 5.56 Kaposi's sarcoma of penis

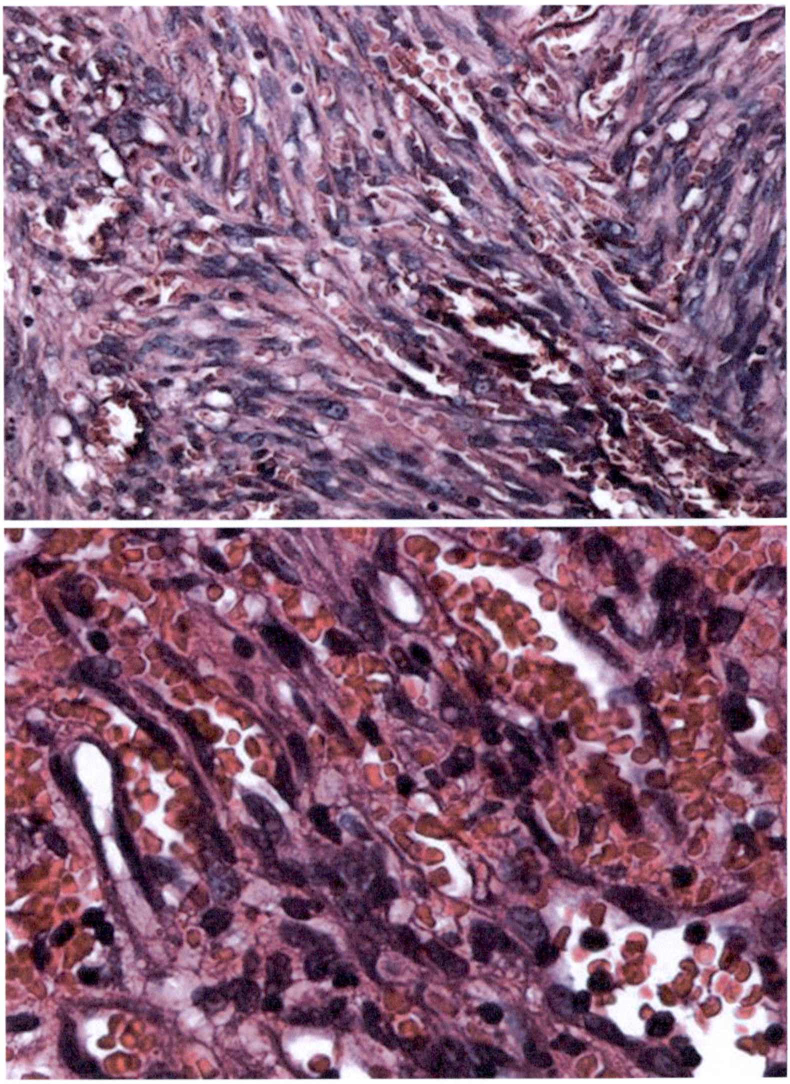

Fig. 5.57 Microscopic appearance of Kaposi's sarcoma of penis at low (*upper*) and high (*lower*) power view

- Differential diagnosis includes angioma or angiosarcoma that usually is more pleomorphic.

5.4.2 Leiomyosarcoma

- Very rare in the penis and involves the prepuce, distal shaft, circumcision scar line, or base of the penis. It usually occurs in the fifth to seventh decades of life. Superficial leiomyosarcoma usually forms subcutaneous nodules, and is thought to arise from the smooth muscle of the glans, frenulum, or the dermis of the shaft. Deep leiomyosarcoma is yet less common, arising from the smooth muscle of the corpora cavernosa and tending to invade the urethra and to produce early metastases.
- Tumor depth and size (<5 cm vs. >5 cm) are currently the best predictors of outcome for primary leiomyosarcoma (Fig. 5.58).

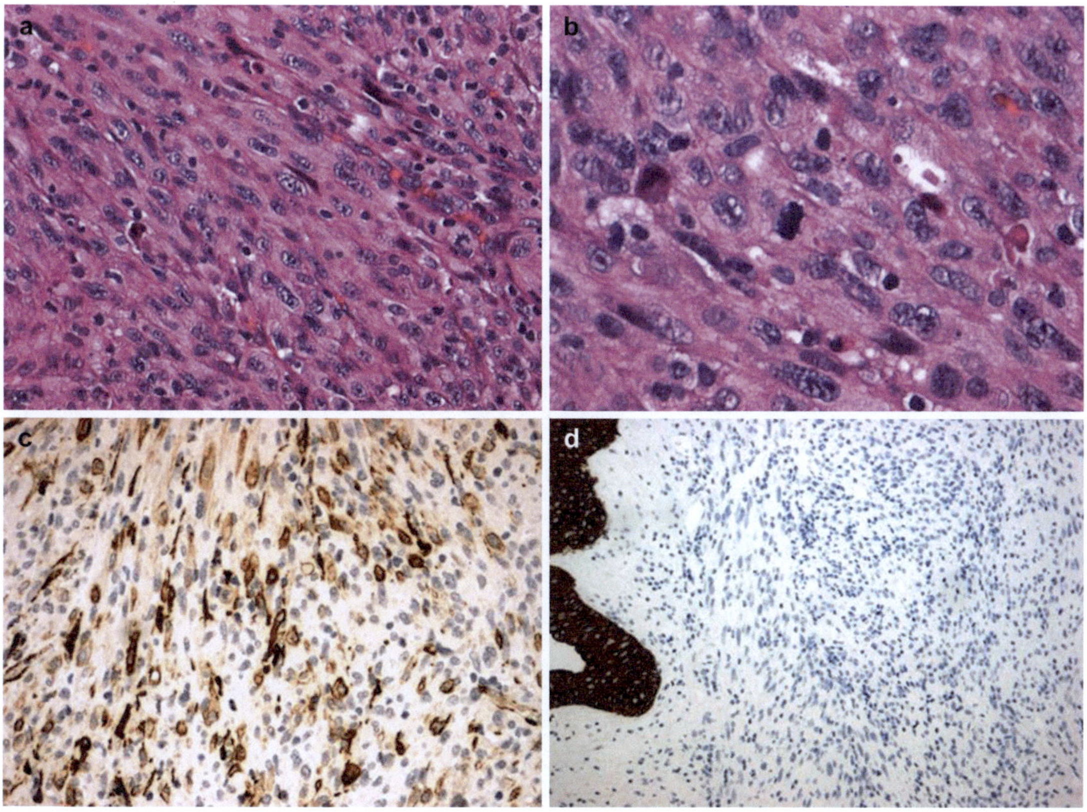

Fig. 5.58 Leiomyosarcoma seen at low A and high power B with brisk mitotic figures. Smooth muscle actin expression C and negative expression of CK AE1/AE3 D

5.4.3 Epithelioid Sarcoma

- Patients range in age from 23 to 43 years. The sarcoma presented as single or multiple, firm, slow-growing, painless subcutaneous nodules. Epithelioid sarcoma is a slow-growing but aggressive tumor in the penis, as elsewhere in the body.
- The masses may produce surface ulceration, resulting in erectile pain or dysuria. Therefore, epithelioid sarcoma may mimic Peyronie disease, urethral stricture, or ulcerating carcinoma. Regardless of therapy, up to 80 % recur locally. Lung metastases may occur (Fig. 5.59).

5.4.4 Other Soft Tissue Sarcomas

- Hemangiopericytoma, malignant schwannoma, and extraskeletal osteosarcoma with malignant fibrous histiocytoma-like component may arise in the penis.

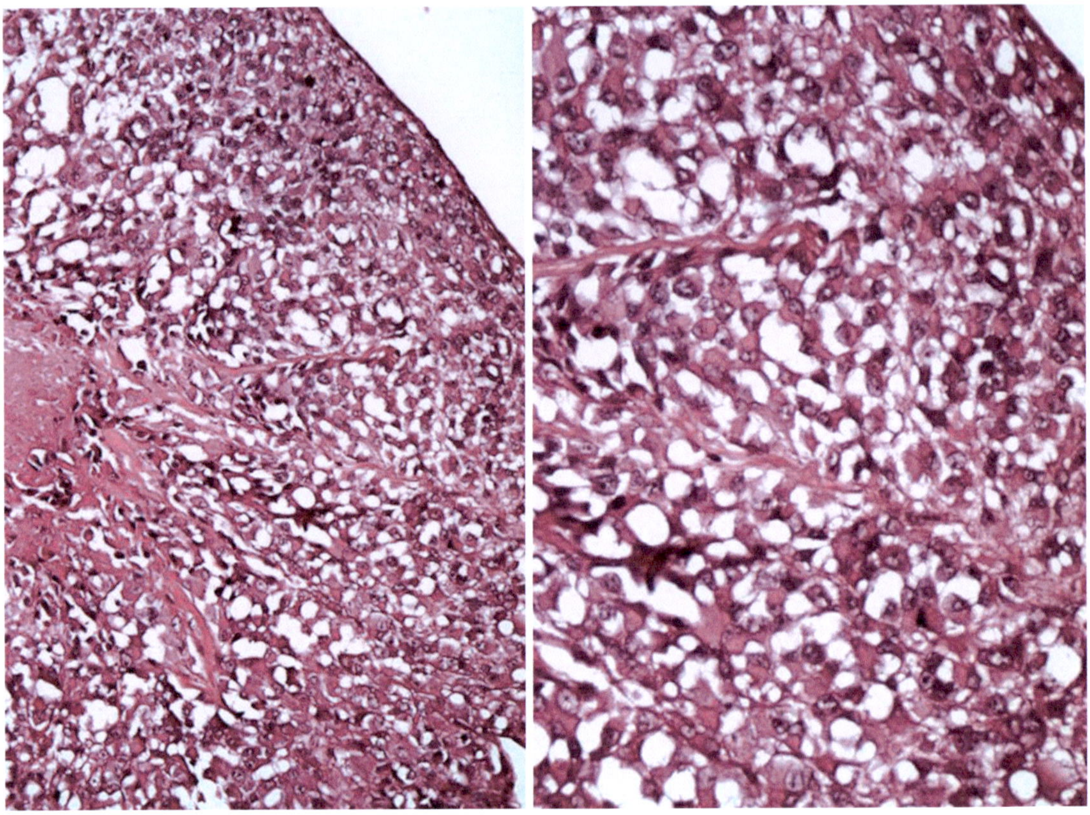

Fig. 5.59 Low (*left*) and high power (*right*) view of an epithelioid sarcoma of penis

5.5 Other Rare Tumors

5.5.1 Primary Malignant Melanoma of the Penis

- Including melanoma in situ, malignant melanoma of the penis accounts for less than 1 % of all penile cancers. Most occur in white men in their fifth and sixth decades of life and is rare in men of African ancestry.
- Patients present with a black, brown, or blue variegated papule or ulcerated plaque. In the majority of cases it arises on the glans.
- The histologic findings are identical to those in other mucosal or cutaneous sites. Histologic variants of penile malignant melanoma include nodular, superficial spreading and acral lentiginous types, similar to other anatomic locations.
- The prognosis is similar to skin melanoma and depends on the depth of invasion and the stage. Penile melanoma with a thickness of 0.75 mm or less has an excellent prognosis, whereas a depth of invasion of 1.5 mm or more carries a poor prognosis because of the high frequency of metastases.

5.5.2 Clear Cell Sarcoma (Malignant Melanoma of Soft Parts)

- This uncommon neoplasm occurs most frequently in the aponeuroses or tendons of the extremities with rare cases reported in the penis.

5.5.3 Lymphoma

- Primary lymphoma of the penis is extremely rare. Patients present with painless swelling or ulceration of the shaft or glans, and may simulate

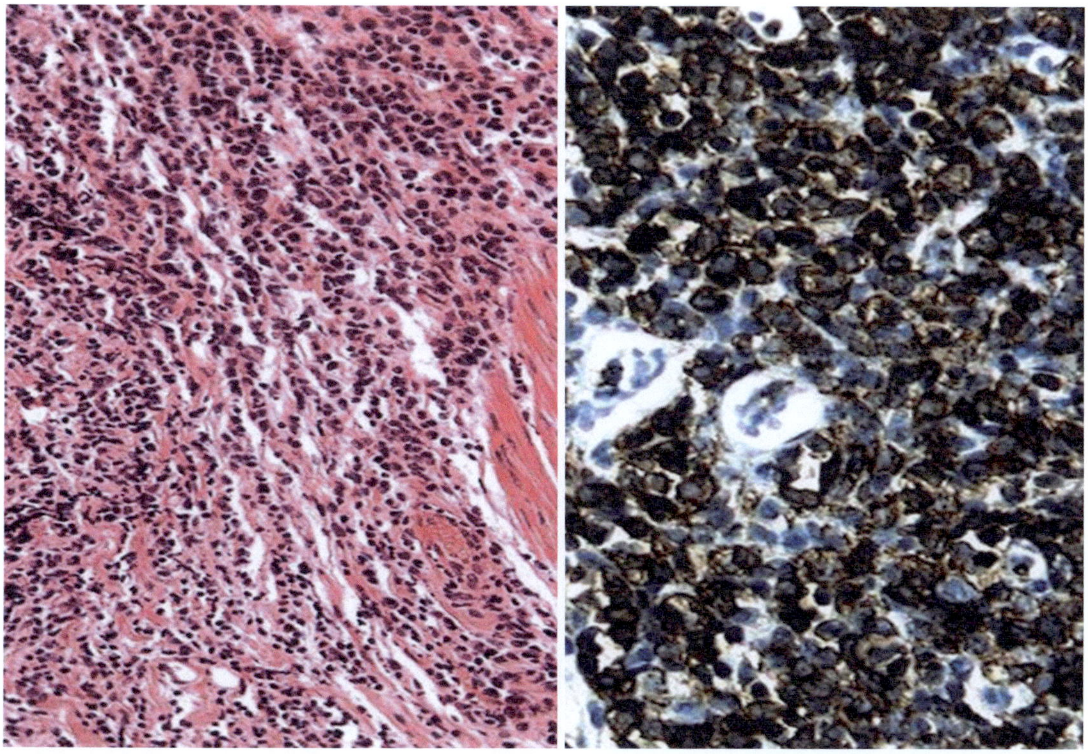

Fig. 5.60 Lymphoma of penis seen on H&E (*left*). CD45 Immunorreactivity of the proliferating cells (*right*)

Peyronie disease, occasionally. Primary lymphoma appears to have a good prognosis after definitive therapy.

- Most are high-grade diffuse large B cell lymphoma, but other subtypes, including T cell lymphomas, MALT lymphoma, and Hodgkin disease, have been reported (Fig. 5.60).

5.6 Secondary Tumors

- Genitourinary tumors are most common metastatic tumors to penis, although only a minority of genitourinary tumors metastasizes to penis. Prostatic adenocarcinomas and bladder urothelial carcinoma account for most primaries. Renal cell carcinoma and seminoma are extremely rare (Fig. 5.61).
- Penile metastasis as initial manifestation is rare since most cases are detected concurrently with the primary. Common symptoms include urinary retention, dysuria, or priapism due to massive erectile tissue involvement.
- Colonic adenocarcinomas are most common among gastrointestinal tumors. Pancreatic, gastric, and esophageal primaries are rarities. Malignant lymphomas may also secondarily affect penis. Rare primary sites include melanoma, lung, or thyroid gland, among others. Examples of synovial sarcoma, chondrosarcoma, and angiosarcoma have been rarely reported.
- Most secondary tumors portend a poor prognosis related to advanced pathologic stage.

Pathology

- Vascular spaces of penile erectile tissues are occupied by malignant cells with corpora cavernosa most frequently involved. Histologic picture is consistent with morphology of primary tumor. Corpus spongiosum, glans or skin of shaft, and foreskin are rarely involved.
- Primary squamous cell carcinoma enters differential diagnosis, in situ changes in surface epithelium are commonly present and of value in suggesting primary.
- Urothelial carcinoma of urethra, papillary, solid infiltrating, or carcinoma in situ may

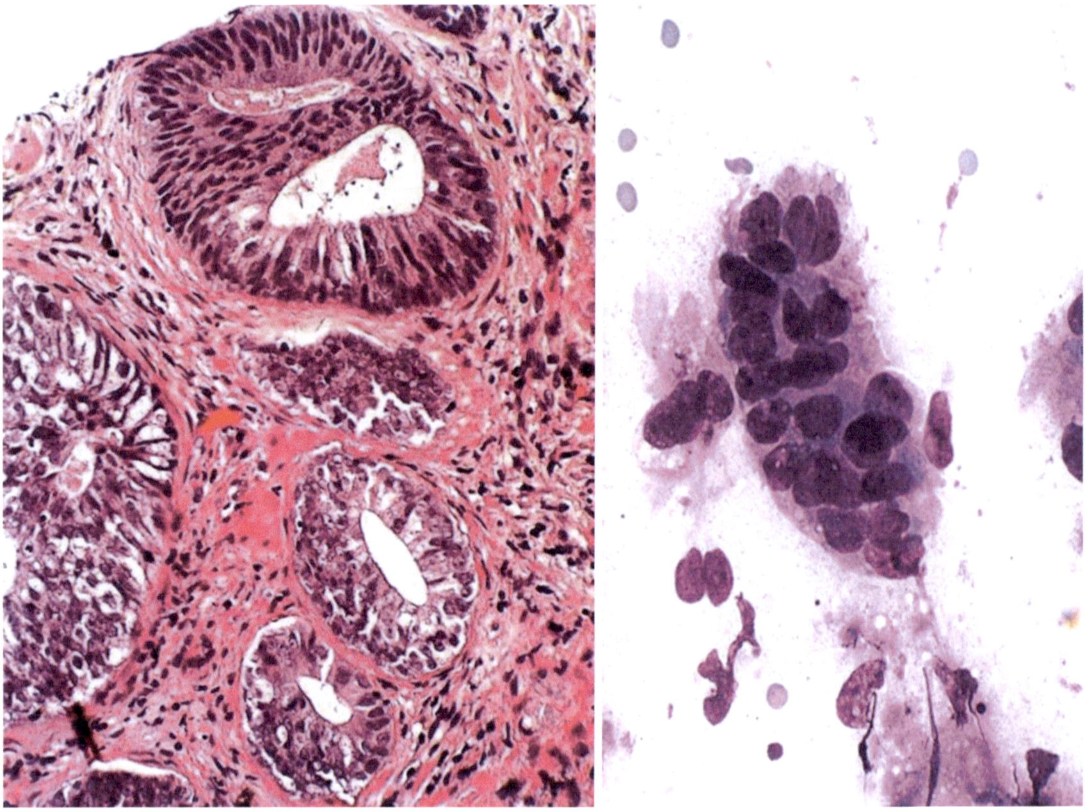

Fig. 5.61 Prostate cancer metastatic to penis as seen on H&E (*left*) and cytologic appearance following fine needle aspiration cytology (*right*)

secondary involve surface or deep penile tissues. Immunohistochemistry for uroplakin-3, thrombomodulin, or GATA3 is usually helpful.

- Primary penile sarcoma is often considered in differential diagnosis as mucosa/skin is usually uninvolved. There is predilection for deep erectile tissues and parenchyma with histology and immunohistochemistry typical of primary sarcoma.

5.7 Carcinoma of the Scrotum

- Benign and malignant tumors of the scrotum are rare; most arise from the skin and adnexal structures or penile soft tissues. Squamous cell carcinoma is the most common scrotal cancer but skin type basal cell carcinoma and Merkel cell carcinoma may also arise in the scrotum.

5.7.1 Overview

- The incidence of squamous cell carcinoma of the scrotum has dramatically decreased over the years and, now, these tumors are extraordinarily infrequent.
- Incidence rate of less than 2 per 1,000,000 person-years, most frequently being squamous cell carcinoma (27 %), basal cell carcinoma (19 %) and Bowen disease (15 %). Overall 5-year relative survival was 82 %, being 77 and 95 % for patients with squamous and basal cell carcinoma, respectively.
- This tumor was the first cancer to be directly linked to exposure to occupational carcinogens; for example, it was a common occurrence among chimney workers. In recent years, PUVA treatments have been shown to be associated with male genital malignancies. The risk to penis and scrotum for development of squamous cell carcinoma is ten times

greater than for other parts of the body, at similar level of exposure.
- Another risk factor is HPV infection since HPV16 genotype has been found in some cases.

5.7.2 Preneoplastic Lesions

- Bowenoid papulosis may occur in the scrotum, typically as multifocal papules in young adults. As mentioned before, is a HPV-related condition. Intraepithelial lesions exhibit spectrum of changes from dysplasia to in situ carcinoma (Bowen disease). Morphological features are similar to HPV-related PeIN (see also page 380 penis).

5.7.3 Squamous Cell Carcinoma

- Squamous cell carcinoma is usually a solitary, slow-growing nodular lesion, affecting men in their 50s that most commonly is ulcerated at presentation. Advanced lesions show invasion of the testis or penis. About one-half of the patients have palpable ipsilateral inguinal lymphadenopathy at presentation.
- Clinical history of condyloma or multiple skin cancers is seen in some cases.
- The significance of histologic grade remains controversial because of limited experience due to rarity of the tumor. The most commonly used staging system is Lowe's modification of the system proposed by Ray and Whitmore (Table 5.10).

Pathology

- The tumor is usually well to moderately differentiated, keratinizing, and identical to conventional cutaneous squamous cell carcinoma. Rare and more common histologic variants of squamous cell carcinoma seen in penis (including basaloide or warthy) may also be seen occasionally in scrotum as primary carcinomas (Fig. 5.62).
- About half of cases show p16 positivity and suprabasal Ki67 expression.
- The epidermis adjacent to the ulcerated neoplasm may show dysplastic changes and is frequently acanthotic with hyperkeratosis.

Table 5.10 Staging system for scrotal squamous carcinoma

Stage	Description
A1	Disease localized to the scrotum
A2	Locally extensive tumor invading adjacent structures such as testis, spermatic cord, penis, pubic bone, and perineum
B	Metastatic disease involving inguinal lymph nodes only
C	Metastatic disease involving pelvic lymph nodes without evidence of distant spread
D	Metastasis beyond the pelvis lymph nodes, to involve distant organs

Squamous cell carcinoma in situ (Bowen disease) may be seen in some cases. The tumor may be heavily pigmented (Fig. 5.63).
- Differential diagnosis may include malignant tumors such as basal cell carcinoma, adnexal tumors, malignant melanoma, Paget disease with invasive component, and sarcoma.

5.8 Other Carcinomas

5.8.1 Basal Cell Carcinoma

- Basal cell carcinoma, similar to its nongenital cutaneous counterpart, is a rare scrotal tumor. As a difference with more common cutaneous form, some may metastasize.
- Rarely may coexist with squamous cell carcinoma.

5.8.2 Merkel Cell Carcinoma

- Also very rare, it is characterized by solid sheets of small round blue cells with scarce cytoplasm and the characteristic dot-like pattern with CK20 and cytokeratin AE1/AE3. Positive expression of neuroendocrine markers, such as chromogranin and synaptophysin is the rule (Fig. 5.64).

5.8.3 Extramammary Paget Disease

- Extramammary Paget disease is an adenocarcinoma involving epidermis and extending

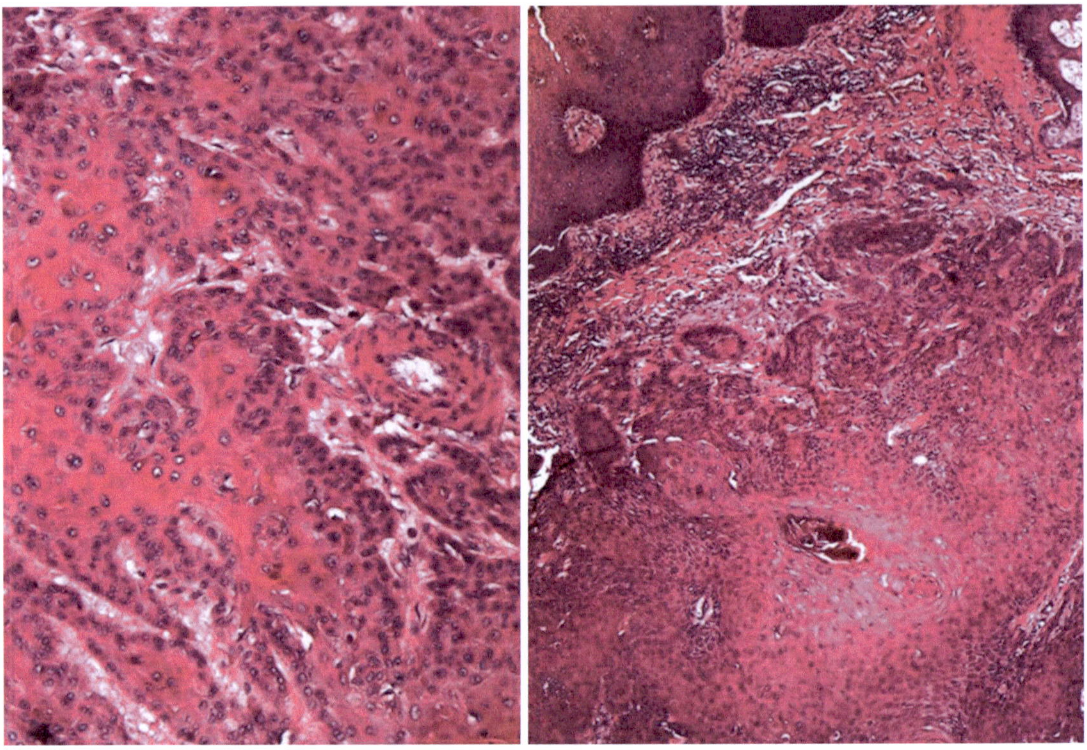

Fig. 5.62 Well differentiated squamous cell carcinoma of the scrotum showing keratin formation (*left*) and stromal infiltration (*right*)

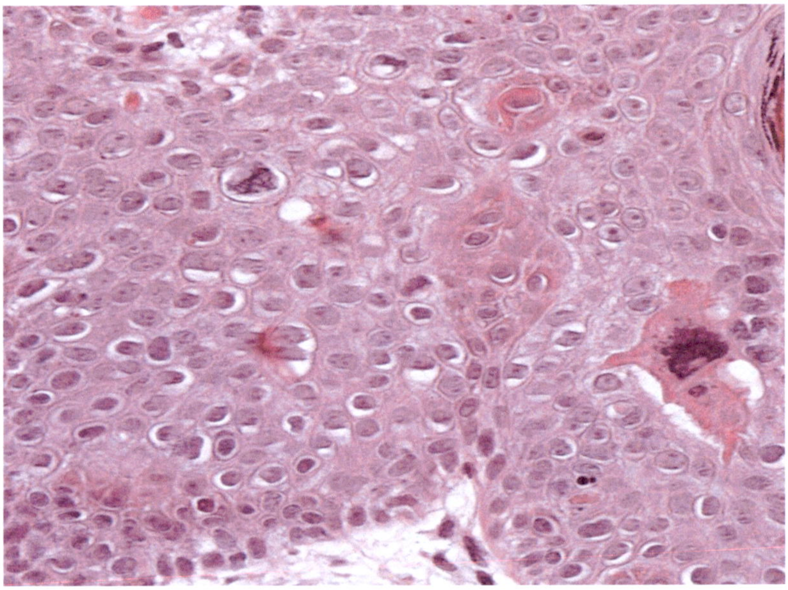

Fig. 5.63 Bowen disease (carcinoma in situ) of the scrotum

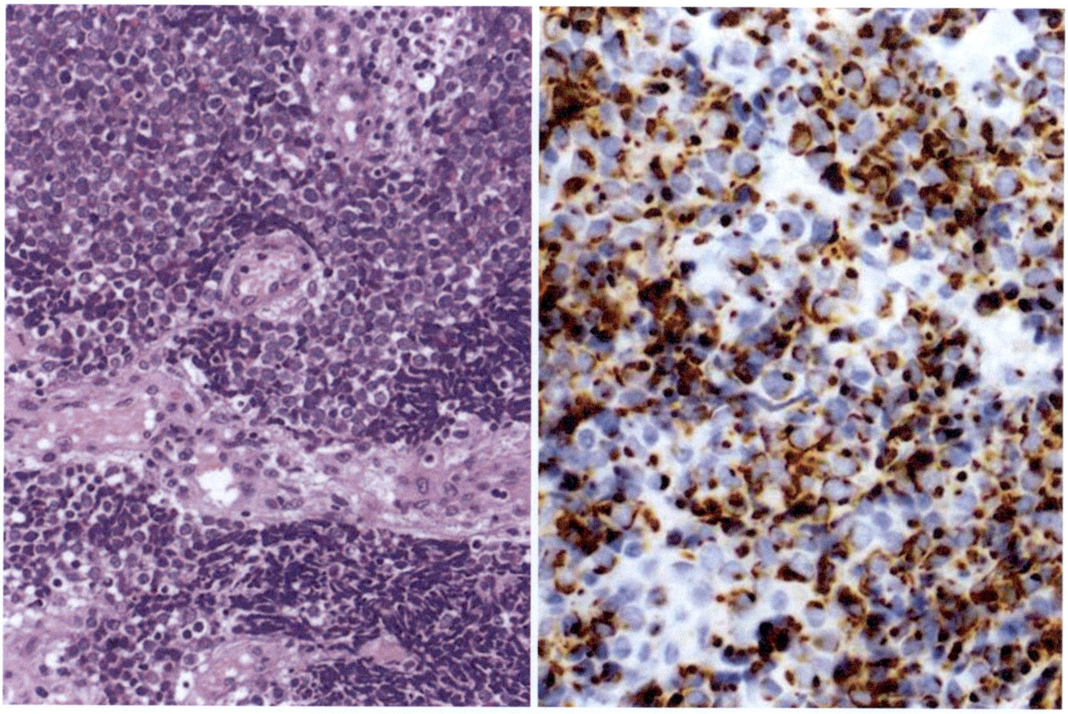

Fig. 5.64 Merkel-cell carcinoma of the scrotum seen on H&E (*left*) showing dot-like CK20 expression (*right*)

to epithelium of apocrine glands follicles (adenocarcinoma in situ). Rarely, primary extramammary Paget disease is associated with underlying sweat gland adenocarcinoma. Cases limited to epidermis are postulated to originate from intraepidermal portion of sweat glands or from intraepidermal stem cells.

- Classified as primary (cutaneous origin) and secondary (extracutaneous origin). Most cases arise in their sixties or seventies. Secondary extramammary Paget disease may represent extension from urethral, bladder, or anal/rectal carcinoma.
- Scrotum and perineum with extension to adjacent areas are most frequent sites in primary lesions. Primary extramammary Paget disease confined to epidermis and epithelium of adnexal structures (in situ carcinoma) has good prognosis.
- Secondary extramammary Paget disease tends to affect perianal area extending to perineum and scrotum. Secondary extramammary Paget disease is related to the underlying carcinoma and is usually poor.

Pathology

- Range from lesions with a few mm in size to lesions that broadly involve entire anogenital area. Microscopic examination identifies intraepithelial proliferation of large round atypical cells (Paget cells). Epithelium varied from hyperplastic to atrophic and may be eroded or ulcerated. Cytoplasm of neoplastic cells is abundant and pale or vacuolated and mucicarmine positive. Intercellular bridges are not appreciated, but melanin pigment may be present within cytoplasm of Paget cells. Mitoses may be numerous. Nuclei are large and vesicular with prominent nucleoli.
- As lesions evolve, Paget cells are more numerous, arranged as single cells or aggregates. Flattened compressed basal keratinocytes lying between neoplastic cells and underlying dermis are observed. Neoplastic cells often extend to epithelium of adnexal structures and may form true intraepidermal glandular lumina. Early lesions show only scattered single Paget cells in epidermis. Dermal involvement by tumoral cells may occur (Fig. 5.65).

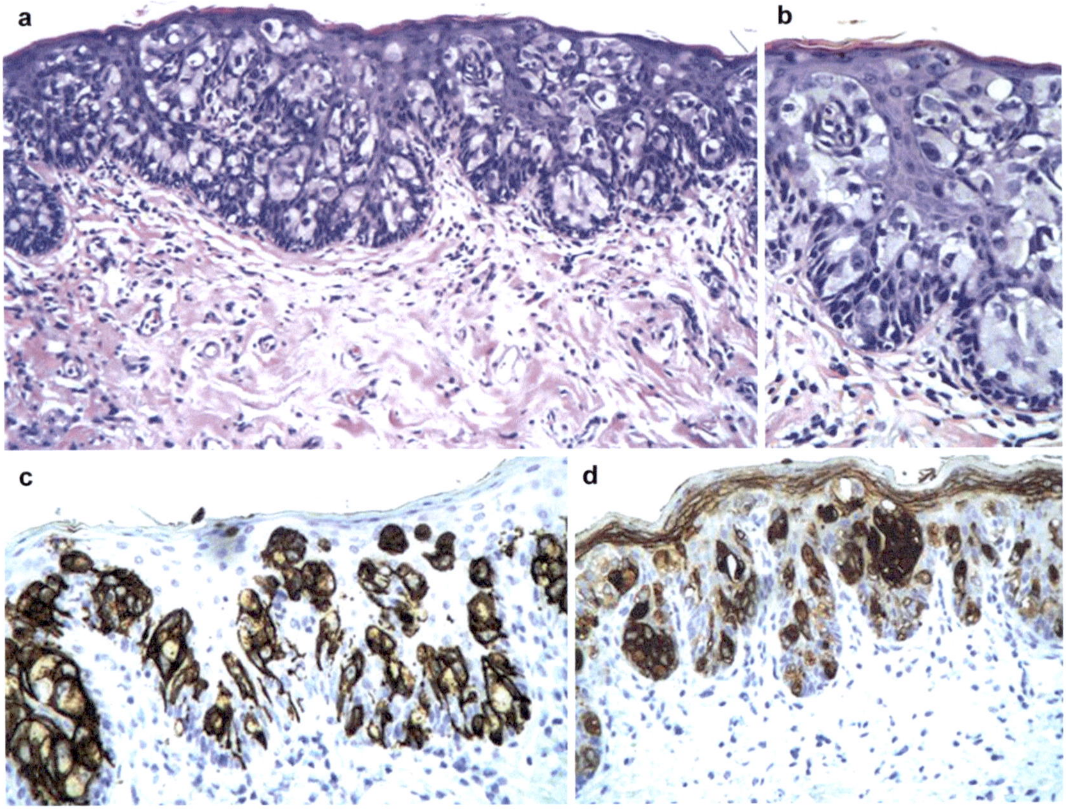

Fig. 5.65 Paget disease of the scrotum seen at low (**a**) and high (**b**) power, and immunohistochemical expression of CK 7 (**c**) and CEA (**d**)

- Morphologic patterns of growth may include glandular, and acantholysis-like as the most common.
- Primary extramammary Paget disease is positive for CEA, low molecular weight cytokeratins (especially CK7 and CAM5.2) EMA/MUC1, and GCDFp-15. Primary Extramammary Paget disease is negative for CK20 and melanocytic markers such as S100, Melan-A, tyrosinase, and HMB45.
- Secondary extramammary Paget disease is related to associate carcinoma. When associated with urothelial carcinoma usually expresses both CK7 and CK20. Also expresses uroplakin-3 and is negative for CEA and high molecular weight cytokeratin. If secondary to anal/rectal carcinomas expresses CK20 and CEA. CDX2 expression would be another indicator of associated anal/rectal malignancy but CK7 usually negative and GCDFP-15 negative.
- Main differential diagnosis includes melanoma in situ with cells present in all levels of epidermis, including basal layer. No flattened basal cells are seen between melanoma cells and dermis. Immunohistochemical expression of melanocytic markers, such as 5,100, Melan-A, and HMB45 is helpful.
- Squamous cell carcinoma in situ with pagetoid pattern is positive for high molecular weight cytokeratin (34ßE12) and p63. Negative for mucicarmine. Negative for CEA, GCDFP-15, CK7, and CK20.
- Clear cell papulosis seen in young children also enters differential diagnosis. Clear cells with pagetoid features in lower part of epidermis; predominantly milk line location. Cytokeratin AE1/AE3 and CEA positive.
- In pagetoid dyskeratosis, lesional cells are keratinocytes showing early keratinization

- Pagetoid reticulosis is a rare variant of cutaneous T cell lymphoma with epidermal infiltration by medium to large sized T cells with abundant pale cytoplasm. T cells are CD45 (LCA) and CD3 positive. T cell gene rearrangement can be demonstrated
- Benign mucinous metaplasia of penis seen in prepuce or glans of elderly patients showing benign mucin containing cells in squamous epithelium.

5.9 Benign Tumors and Tumor-Like Conditions

- Benign tumors of the scrotum are rare and most arise from the skin and adnexal structures with some examples of soft tissue tumors.
- A hamartoma with muscular hyperplasia or angioleiomyomatous features rarely occurs in the scrotum and may simulate malignancy (Fig. 5.66).
- A fibrous pseudotumor is also rarely seen in the scrotum (Figs. 5.67, 5.68 and 5.69).
- Hemangioma, leiomyoma, lymphangioma, neurofibroma, and angiokeratoma are common benign scrotal neoplasms. Examples of fibrous histiocytoma, lipoblastoma, ganglioneuroma, aggressive angiomyxoma, angiomyofibroblastoma, and granular cell tumor have also been reported.

5.9.1 Scrotal Calcinosis

- Also known as idiopathic calcinosis of the scrotum is a benign uncommon condition characterized by the presence of single or multiple calcified nodules in the scrotal skin. The lesion seems to develop from dystrophic calcification of cyst contents.

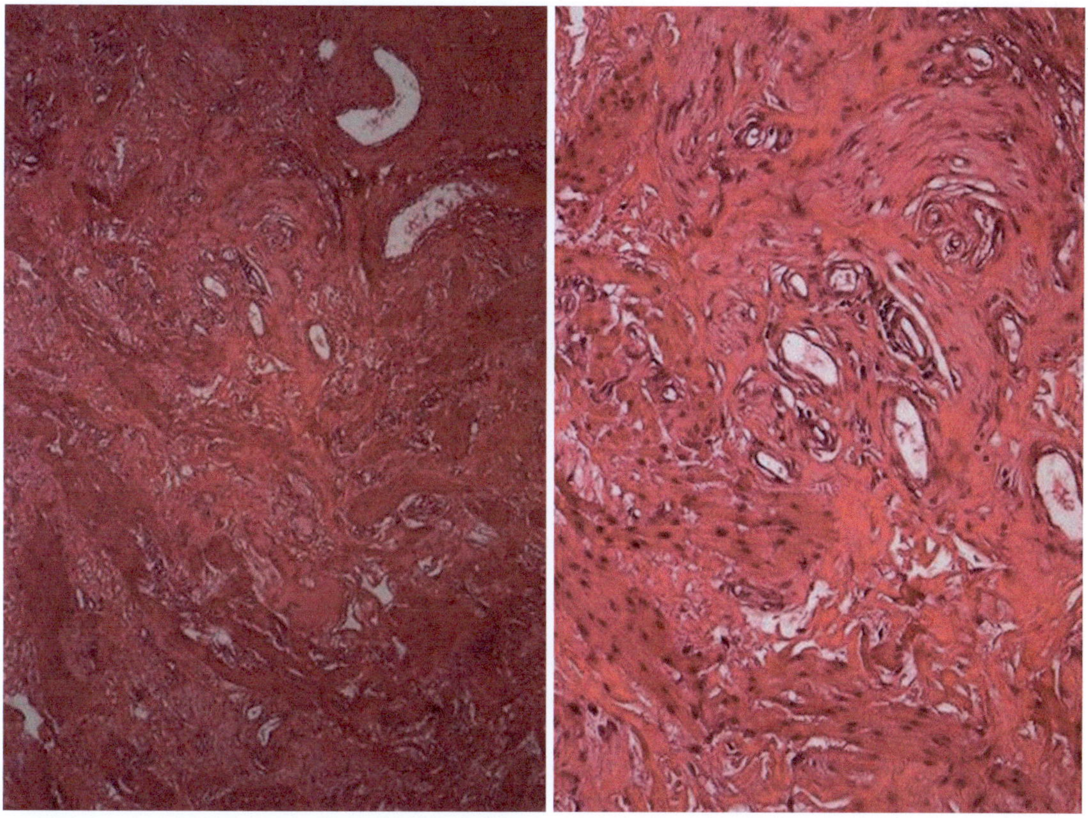

Fig. 5.66 Angyioleyomiomatous hammartoma of the scrotum. Low (*left*) and high (*right*) power view

Fig. 5.67 Gross features of fibrous pseudotumor of the scrotum

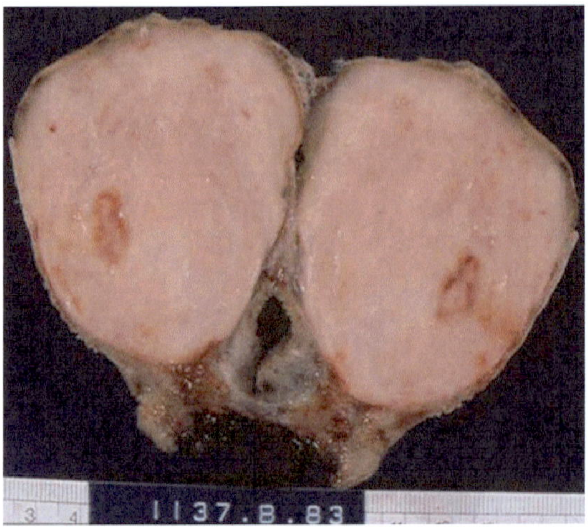

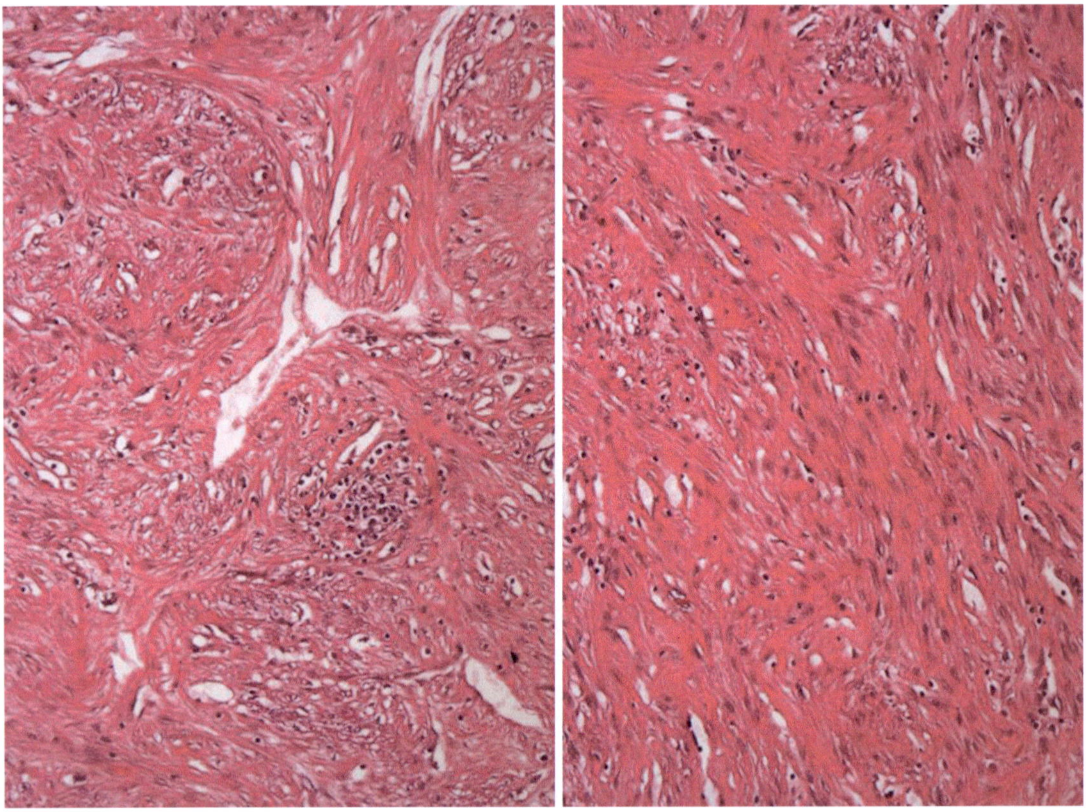

Fig. 5.68 Microscopic features of fibrous pseudotumor of the scrotum showing mild chronic inflammation (*left*) and fibroblastic cellular proliferation (*right*)

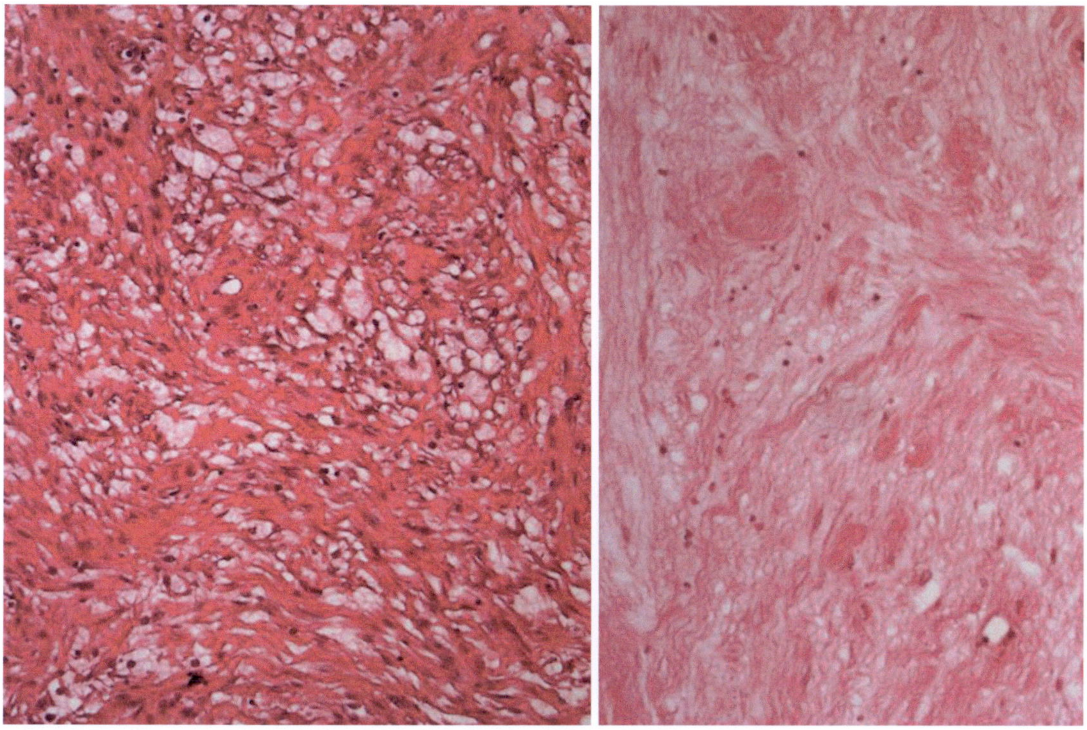

Fig. 5.69 Microscopic features of fibrous pseudotumor of the scrotum showing early myxoid change (*left*) and hypocellular (*right*) areas

Pathology

- Granular deposition of basophilic calcified material with a histiocytic/giant cell granulomatous reaction associated with deposits. Histologic remnants of preexisting epidermoid cyst or adnexal cystic tumors may be identified (Fig. 5.70).

5.9.2 Sclerosing Lipogranuloma of the Scrotum

- Also known as paraffinoma, it is a foreign body histiocytic/xanthogranulomatous and sclerotic reaction to oil-based substances. Most cases are secondary to injection of paraffin or silicone; or may be related to trauma. It seems to be a T cell mediated immune reaction seen in patients under 40 years of age, and may affect penis and/or scrotum. Biopsy is necessary to exclude true neoplastic process.

Pathology

- Firm yellow to gray pieces of tissue with solid or cystic appearance with numerous lipid vacuoles of variable size embedded in sclerotic stroma. Infiltrate of foamy histiocytes admixed with multinucleate giant cells is the rule together with some lymphoid cells typically CD3 positive. Multinucleate giant cells and histiocytes express CD68 (Fig. 5.71).
- Differential diagnosis of liposarcoma, metastatic carcinoma with signed or clear cells features, adenomatoid tumor, or lymphangioma are rare considerations.

5.9.3 Angiokeratoma

- Angiokeratoma of Fordyce is the most common form of angiokeratoma affecting the scrotal skin. It is a distinctive vascular lesion of the scrotum, regarded as a variant distinct

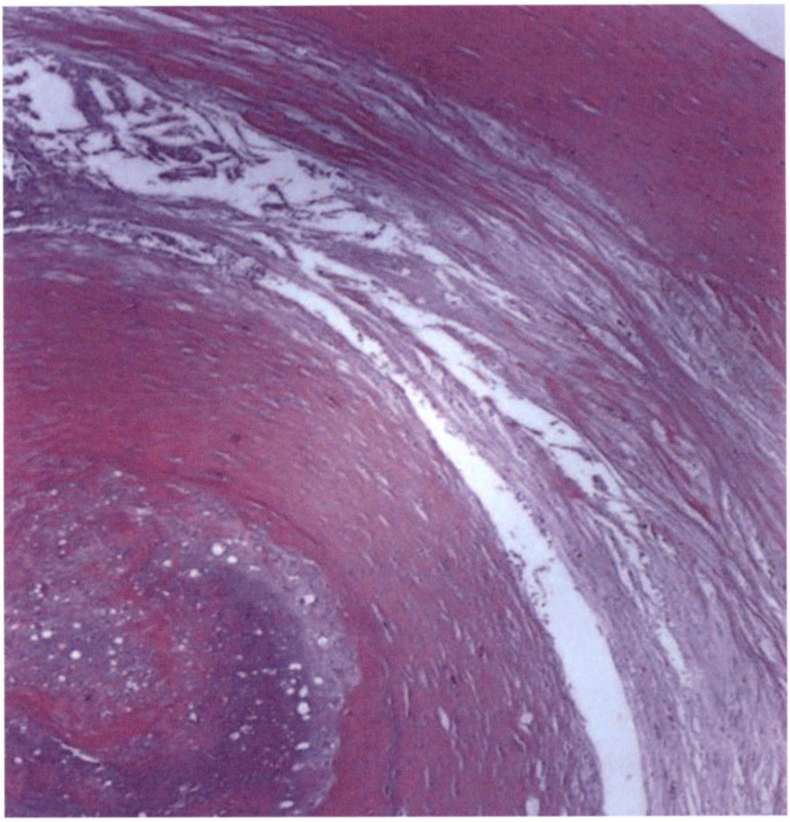

Fig. 5.70 Scrotal idiopathic calcinosis

from systemic angiokeratoma corporis diffusum. Angiokeratomas are multiple, 1–4 mm in size, soft, and affect middle-aged to elderly patients.

Pathology

- Histologic appearance of angiokeratomas includes marked dilatation of the papillary dermal vasculature with acanthosis and elongation of rete ridges forming a collarette circumferentially engulfing vascular lacunae. Thrombi may be present.
- There is moderate to marked hyperkeratosis and parakeratosis, dermal fibrosis, chronic inflammation, atrophy of the dartos muscle, and degeneration of the elastic tissue (Fig. 5.72).

5.9.4 Fat Necrosis

- Fat necrosis of the scrotum usually occurs in obese children and adolescents.

Pathology

- Firm ill-defined, gray-yellow nodules in the lower portion the scrotal wall. May be bilateral. It has been suggested that the lesion develops when scrotal fat crystallizes following exposure to very low temperature.

5.9.5 Verruciform Xanthoma

- Warty lesion characterized by acanthosis, hyperkeratosis, parakeratosis, and long rete ridges. The dermis between the rete ridges is frequently occupied by a neutrophilic and a variable, often prominent xanthomatous infiltrate.
- This lesion is usually solitary and may occur in scrotal, penile, and vulvar areas). Most likely is HPV-unrelated lesion.
- The xanthoma cells are positive, sometimes focally for CD68, MAC387, Factor XIIIa and cytokeratin, and negative for S100 (Fig. 5.73).

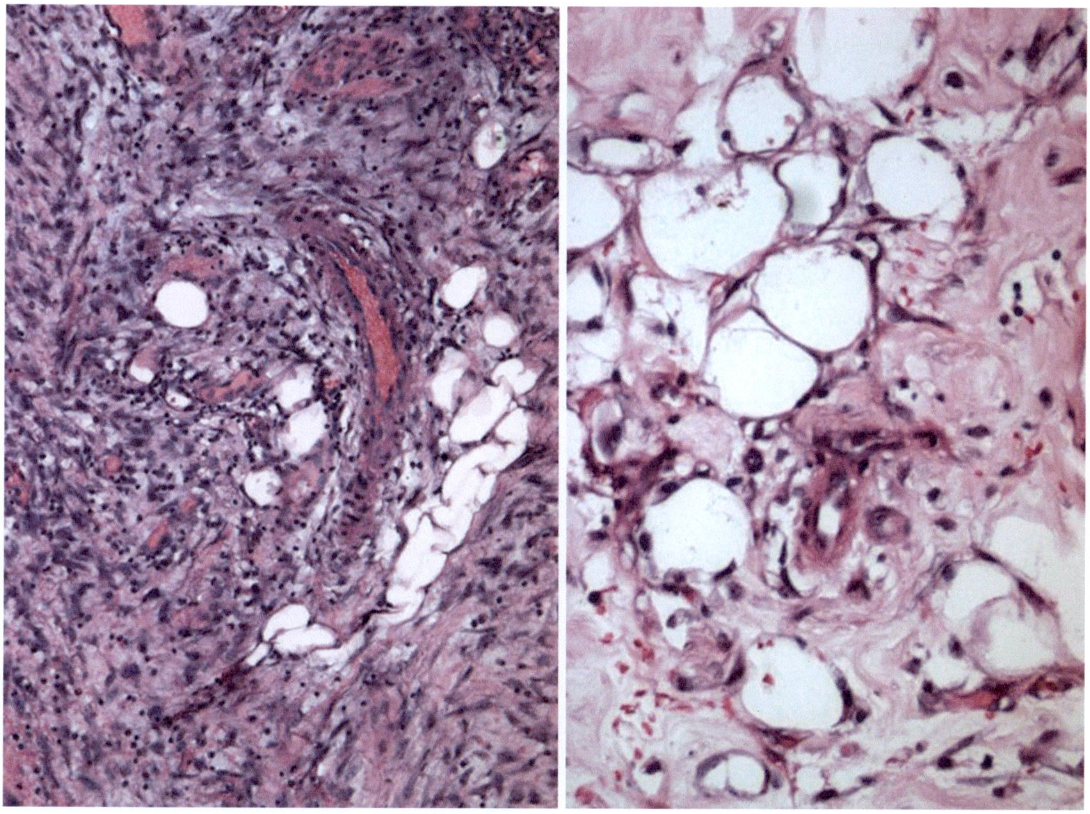

Fig. 5.71 Microscopic appearance of sclerosing lipogranuloma of the scrotum. Low (*left*) and high power (*right*) view

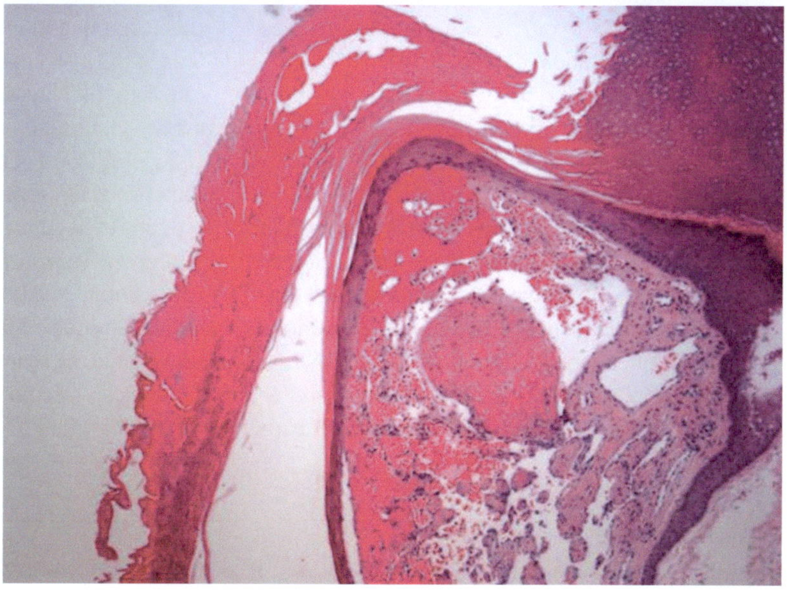

Fig. 5.72 Microscopic appearance of angiokeratoma of the scrotum

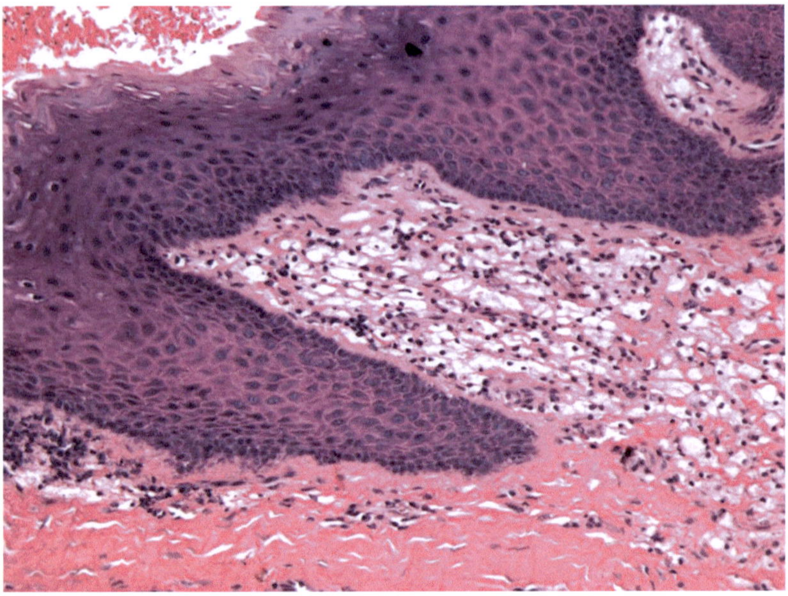

Fig. 5.73 Verruciform xanthoma with subepithelial accumulation of xanthoma cells

5.9.6 Spindle Cell Nodule (Inflammatory Myofibroblastic Tumor)

- Scrotal myofibroblastic proliferation following trauma, with similar histology to nodular fasciitis. May mimic sarcoma. Clinicopathologic evaluation is mandatory in these cases to avoid misinterpretation. (See also page 151 bladder) (Fig. 5.74).

5.9.7 Epidermal Cyst

- Epidermal cyst (keratinous cyst) is common in the scrotum; it contains gray-white cheesy material resulting from exfoliation of the keratinizing, granular layer containing squamous epithelium covering internal surface of cys.
- Occasionally, there is an associated granulomatous reaction mainly associated with rupture (Fig. 5.75).

5.9.8 Other Benign Lesions

Hidradenitis Suppurativa

- It is an inflammatory process of apocrine and eccrine glands that are obstructed by follicular hyperkeratosis that extrudes keratin and eccrine and apocrine products and commensal bacteria into dermis then initiating the acute necrotizing and granulomatous reaction. Some cases may be seen by surgical pathologists as a tumor-like condition in scrotum.

Fournier Gangrene

- Idiopathic form of necrotizing fasciitis of the subcutaneous tissue and skeletal muscle of the genitals and perineum, particularly that of the scrotum. Rarely, it forms a tumor-like lesion entering in differential diagnosis of primary or secondary scrotal tumors. Squamous cell carcinoma may develop in the scar of Fournier gangrene.
- Diabetes, alcoholism, immunosuppression, recent surgical intervention, trauma, and morbid obesity are predisposing factors,

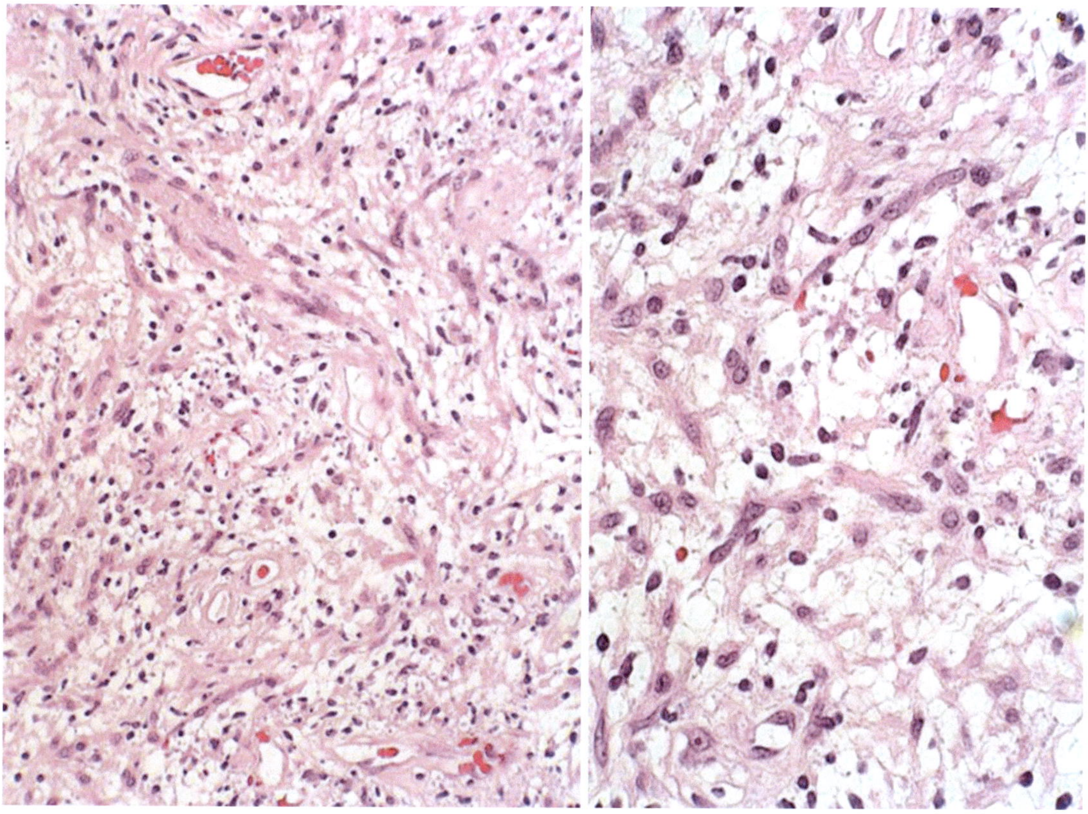

Fig. 5.74 Low (*left*) and high (*right*) power view of nodular fasciitis (myofibroblastic proliferation) seen in the scrotum

5.10 Soft Tissue Tumors

- Sarcoma of the scrotum is extremely rare. The most common type is leiomyosarcoma, which arises from dartos muscle. The age at presentation ranges from 35 to 89 years. Scrotal leiomyosarcoma appears to behave similarly to subcutaneous leiomyosarcoma. Lymph node metastases are rare, but late visceral metastases or recurrence may occur.
- Rare cases of liposarcoma, malignant fibrous histiocytoma, rhabdomyosarcoma, epithelioid sarcoma, and synovial sarcoma arising from the scrotal wall have also been reported in children or young adults (Fig. 5.76). A case of gastrointestinal stromal tumor (GIST) extending through the right inguinal canal that presented as a scrotal mass has also been reported.
- When dealing with a sarcoma of the scrotum, it is mandatory excluding the extension of sarcoma from the spermatic cord.

5.11 Other Rare Tumors

- Malignant lymphoma and melanoma are extremely rare in the scrotum.

5.12 Secondary Tumors

- Cases of metastatic carcinoma to the scrotum have been also reported. Most are the extension of a groin primary tumor or metastasis extending secondarily to scrotum.

Fig. 5.75 Epidermal-cyst

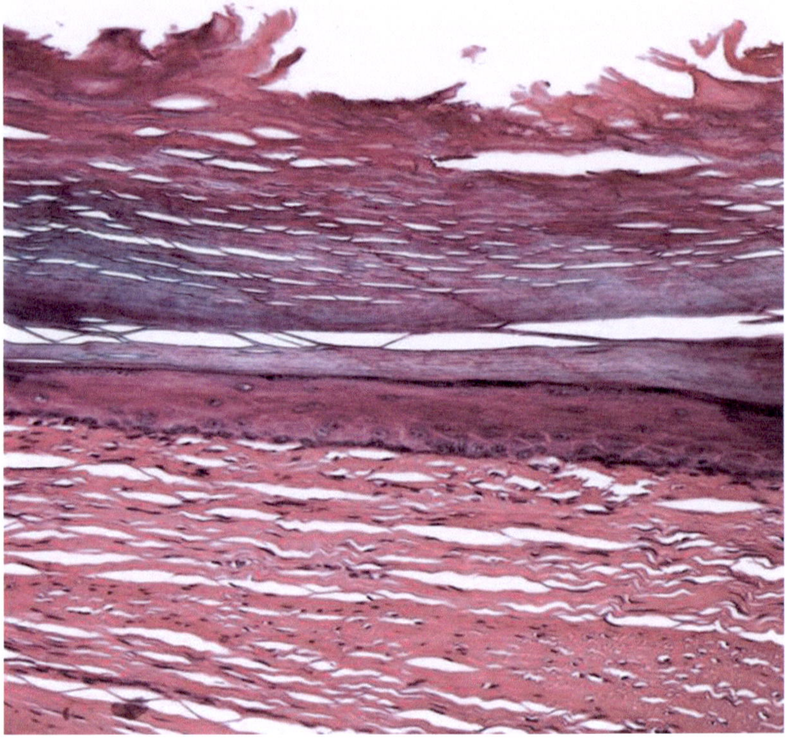

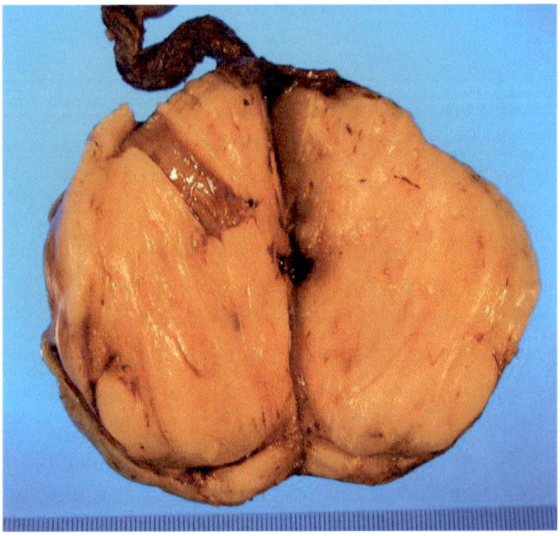

Fig. 5.76 Gross features of rhabdomyosarcoma of the scrotum with testicular involvement

Suggested Reading

Azike JE. A review of the history, epidemiology and treatment of squamous cell carcinoma of the scrotum. Rare Tumors. 2009;1(1):e17. doi:10.4081/rt.2009.e17.

Barreto JE, et al. Carcinoma cuniculatum: a distinctive variant of penile squamous cell carcinoma: report of 7 cases. Am J Surg Pathol. 2007;31(1):71–5.

Bates AW, et al. Secondary tumours of the penis. J R Soc Med. 2002;95(3):162–3.

Berkmen F, Celebioğlu AS. Adult genitourinary sarcomas: a report of seventeen cases and review of the literature. J Exp Clin Cancer Res. 1997;16:45–8.

Bethune G, Campbell J, Rocker A, Bell D, Rendon R, Merrimen J. Clinical and pathologic factors of prognostic significance in penile squamous cell carcinoma in a North American population. Urology. 2012;79(5):1092–7.

Bhargava MK. Paratesticular tumours of mesenchymal origin. Indian J Cancer. 1976;13:108–22.

Brown HM, et al. Uroplakin-3 to distinguish primary vulvar Paget disease from Paget disease secondary to urothelial carcinoma. Hum Pathol. 2002;33(5):545–8.

Buechner SA. Common skin disorders of the penis. BJU Int. 2002;90(5):498–506.

Carroli PA, et al. Kaposi's sarcoma-associated herpesvirus infection of blood éndothelial cells induces lymphatic differentiation. Virology. 2004;328(1):71–8.

Chaux A, Cubilla AL. Diagnostic problems in precancerous lesions and invasive carcinomas of the penis. Semin Diagn Pathol. 2012;29(2):72–82.

Chaux A, et al. Histologic grade in penile squamous cell carcinoma: visual estimation versus digital measurement of proportions of grades, adverse prognosis with any proportion of grade 3 and correlation of a Gleason-like system with nodal metastasis. Am J Surg Pathol. 2009a;33(7):1042–8.

Chaux A, et al. The prognostic index: a useful pathologic guide for prediction of nodal metastases and survival in penile squamous cell carcinoma. Am J Surg Pathol. 2009b;33(7):1049–57.

Chaux A, et al. Comparison of morphologic features and outcome of resected recurrent and nonrecurrent squamous cell carcinoma of the penis: a study of 81 cases. Am J Surg Pathol. 2009c;33(9):1299–306.

Chaux A, et al. Comparison of subtypes of penile squamous cell carcinoma from high and Low incidence geographical regions. Int J Surg Pathol. 2010a;18:268–77.

Chaux A, et al. Metastatic tumors to the penis: a report of 17 cases and review of the literature. Int J Surg Pathol. 2010b;19:597–606.

Chaux A, Velazquez EF, Barreto JE, Ayala E, Cubilla AL. New pathologic entities in penile carcinomas: an update of the 2004 world health organization classification. Semin Diagn Pathol. 2012a;29(2):59–66.

Chaux A, Velazquez EF, Amin A, Soskin A, Pfannl R, Rodríguez IM, Barreto JE, Lezcano C, Ayala G, Netto GJ, Cubilla AL. Distribution and characterization of subtypes of penile intraepithelial neoplasia and their association with invasive carcinomas: a pathological study of 139 lesions in 121 patients. Hum Pathol. 2012b;43(7):1020–7.

Cherian J, et al. Secondary penile tumours revisited. Int Semin Surg Oncol. 2006;3:33.

Clark PE, Spiess PE, Agarwal N, Biagioli MC, Eisenberger MA, Greenberg RE, Herr HW, Inman BA, Kuban DA, Kuzel TM, Lele SM, Michalski J, Pagliaro L, Pal SK, Patterson A, Plimack ER, Pohar KS, Porter MP, Richie JP, Sexton WJ, Shipley WU, Small EJ, Trump DL, Wile G, Wilson TG, Dwyer M, Ho M. Penile cancer. J Natl Compr Canc Netw. 2013;11(5):594–615.

Collin T, Blackburn AV, Milner RH, Gerrand C, Ragbir M. Sarcomas in the groin and inguinal canal – often missed and difficult to manage. Ann R Coll Surg Engl. 2010;92:326–9.

Cubilla AL, et al. Basaloid squamous cell carcinoma: a distinctive human papilloma virus-related penile neoplasm: a report of 20 cases. Am J Surg Pathol. 1998;22(6):755–61.

Cubilla AL, et al. Morphological features of epithelial abnormalities and precancerous lesions of the penis. Scand J Urol Nephrol Suppl. 2000a;205:215–9.

Cubilla AL, et al. Warty (condyiomatous) squamous cell carcinoma of the penis: a report of 11 cases and proposed classification of 'verruciform' penile tumors. Am J Surg Pathol. 2000b;24(4):505–12.

Cubilla AL, et al. Histologic classification of penile carcinoma and its relation to outcome in 61 patients with primary resection. Int J Surg Pathol. 2001;9(2):111–20.

Cubilla AL, et al. Pseudohyperplastic squamous cell carcinoma of the penis associated with lichen sclerosus. An extremely well-differentiated, nonverruciform neoplasm that preferentially affects the foreskin and is frequently misdiagnosed: a report of 10 cases of a distinctive clinicopathologic entity. Am J Surg Pathol. 2004;28(7):895–900.

Cubilla AL, et al. Epithelial lesions associated with invasive penile squamous cell carcinoma: a pathologic study of 288 cases. Int J Surg Pathol. 2005;12(4):351–64.

Cubilla AL, Lloveras B, Alemany L, Alejo M, Vidal A, Kasamatsu E, Clavero O, Alvarado-Cabrero I, Lynch C, Velasco-Alonso J, Ferrera A, Chaux A, Klaustermeier J, Quint W, de Sanjosé S, Muñoz N, Bosch FX. Basaloid squamous cell carcinoma of the penis with papillary features: a clinicopathologic study of 12 cases. Am J Surg Pathol. 2012;36(6):869–75.

Da Cunha Santos G, et al. Penile metastasis of urothelial carcinoma diagnosed by fine-needle aspiration. Cytojournal. 2009;6:10.

De Nisi MC, et al. Usefulness of CDX2 in the diagnosis of extramammary Paget disease associated with malignancies of intestinal type. Br J Dermatol. 2005;153(3):677–9.

Du X, Yin X, Zhou N, Zhang G, Shi H, Cao S. Extramammary Paget's disease mimicking acantholytic squamous cell carcinoma in situ: a case report. J Cutan Pathol. 2010;37(6):683–6.

Edge SB, Byrd DR, Compton CC, Fritz AG, Greene FL, Trotti A. AJCC cancer staging handbook. 7th ed. New York: Springer; 2010.

el Mejjad A, et al. Giant condyloma acuminata –Buschke Lowenstein tumor. Report of 3 cases. Prog Urol. 2003;13(3):513–7.

Froehner M, Lossnitzer A, Manseck A, Koch R, Noack B, Wirth MP. Favorable long-term outcome in adult genitourinary low-grade sarcoma. Urology. 2000;56:373–7.

Froehner M, Schober RR, Koch R, Lossnitzer A, Laniado M, Wirth MP. Adult urologic sarcoma: Experience during 2 decades. Urol Oncol. 2013;31(7):985–9. doi: 10.1016/j.urolonc.2011.10.002.

Froehner M, et al. Adult inguinoscrotal sarcomas: outcome analysis of 21 cases and systematic review of the literature. World J Urol. 2014;32(2):445–51. doi: 10.1007/s00345-013-1124-1.

Fukunaga M, et al. Penile verrucous carcinoma with anaplastic transformation following radiotherapy. A case report with human papillomavirus typing and flow cytometric DNA studies. Am J Surg Pathol. 1994;18(5):501–5.

Guimarães GC, et al. Penile squamous cell carcinoma clinicopathological features, nodal metastasis and outcome in 333 cases. J Urol. 2009;182(2):528–34; discussion 534.

Kato N, et al. Penile hybrid verrucous-squamous carcinoma associated with a superficial inguinal lymph node metastasis. Am J Dermatopathol. 2000;22(4):339–43.

Katona TM, et al. Soft tissue tumors of the penis: a review. Anal Quant Cytol Histol. 2006;28(4):193–206.

Lee JY. Clear cell papulosis: a unique disorder in early childhood characterized by white macules in milk-line distribution. Pediatr Dermatol. 1998;15(4):328–9.

Lee HR, Han TY, Lee JH, Son SJ. Pagetoid dyskeratosis of the scrotum: histologic findings resembling extramammary Paget's disease. Am J Dermatopathol. 2011;33(7):755–7.

Liegl B, et al. Penile clear cell carcinoma: a report of 5 cases of a distinct entity. Am J Surg Pathol. 2004;28(11):1513–7.

Liegl B, et al. Mammary and extramammary Paget's disease: an immunohistochemical study of 83 cases. Histopathology. 2007;50(4):439–47.

Liu H, et al. Expression of p16 and hTERT protein is associated with the presence of high-risk human papillomavirus in Bowenoid papulosis. J Cutan Pathol. 2006;33(8):551–8.

Liu JY, Li YH, Zhang ZL, Yao K, Ye YL, Xie D, Han H, Liu ZW, Qin ZK, Zhou FJ. The risk factors for the presence of pelvic lymph node metastasis in penile squamous cell carcinoma patients with inguinal lymph node dissection. World J Urol. 2013;31:1519–24.

Lont AP, et al. Sarcomatoid squamous cell carcinoma of the penis: a clinical and pathological study of 5 cases. J Urol. 2004;172(3):932–5.

Lowe FC, et al. Kaposi's sarcoma of the penis in patients with acquired immunodeficiency syndrome. J Urol. 1989;142(6):1475–7.

McKenney JK, et al. Penile myointimoma in children and adolescents: a clinicopathologic study of 5 cases supporting a distinct entity. Am J Surg Pathol. 2007;31(10):1622–6.

Micali G, et al. Primary classic Kaposi's sarcoma of the penis, report of a case and review. J Eur Acad Dermatol Venereol. 2003;17(3):320–3.

Nordenvall C, et al. Cancer risk among patients with condylomata acuminata. Int J Cancer. 2006;119(4):888–93.

Oertel YC, et al. Sclerosing lipogranuloma of male genitalia. Review of 23 cases. Arch Pathol Lab Med. 1977;101(6):321–6.

Oh YJ, Lew BL, Sim WY. Acantholytic anaplastic extramammary Paget's disease: a case report and review of the literature. Ann Dermatol. 2011;23 Suppl 2:S226–30.

Ohnishi T, et al. The use of cytokeratins 7 and 20 in the diagnosis of primary and secondary extramammary Paget's disease. Br J Dermatol. 2000;142(2): 243–7.

Salamanca J, et al. Paget's disease of the glans penis secondary to transitional cell carcinoma of the bladder: a report of two cases and review of the literature. J Cutan Pathol. 2004;37(4):371–5.

Sanchez-Ortiz R, et al. Melanoma of the penis, sctotum and male urethra: a 40-year single institution experience. J Urol. 2005;173(6):1958–65.

Seehafer JR, et al. Epithelioma cuniculatum: verrucous carcinoma of the foot. Cutis. 1979;23(3):287–90.

Shah V, et al. Scrotal calcinosis results from calcification of cysts derived from hair follicles: a series of 20 cases evaluating the spectrum of changes resulting in scrotal calcinosis. Am J Dermatopathol. 2007;29(2):172–5.

Shiomi T, Yoshida Y, Shomori K, Yamamoto O, Ito H. Extramammary Paget's disease: evaluation of the histopathological patterns of Paget cell proliferation in the epidermis. J Dermatol. 2011;38(11):1054–7.

Terada T, Kamo M, Sugiura M. Apocrine carcinoma of the scrotum with extramammary Paget's disease. Int J Dermatol. 2013;52(4):504–6.

Turner BM, et al. Penile myointimoma. J Cutan Pathol. 2009;36(7):817–9.

Val-Bernal JF, et al. Benign mucinous metaplasia of the penis. A lesion resembling extramammary Paget's disease. J Cutan Pathol. 2000a;27(2):76–9.

Val-Bernal JF, et al. Pagetoid dyskeratosis of the prepuce. An incidental histologic finding resembling extramammary Paget's disease. J Cutan Pathol. 2000b;27(8):387–91.

Vardar E, et al. Myointimoma of the glans penis. Pathol Int. 2007;57(3):158–61.

Velazquez EF, et al. Lichen sclerosus in 68 patients with squamous cell carcinoma of the penis: frequent atypias and correlation with special carcinoma variants suggests a precancerous role. Am J Surg Pathol. 2003;27(11):1448–53.

Velazquez EF, et al. Epithelial abnormalities and precancerous lesions of anterior urethra in patients with penile carcinoma: a report of 89 cases. Mod Pathol. 2005a;18(7):917–23.

Velazquez EF, et al. Sarcomatoid carcinoma of the penis: a clinicopathologic study of 15 cases. Am J Surg Pathol. 2005b;29(9):1152–8.

Verhoeven RH, Louwman WJ, Koldewijn EL, Demeyere TB, Coebergh JW. Scrotal cancer: incidence, survival and second primary tumours in the Netherlands since 1989. Br J Cancer. 2010;103(9):1462–6.

Wade TR, et al. Bowenoid papulosis of the penis. Cancer. 1978;42(4):1890–903.

Wade TR, et al. Bowenoid papulosis of the genitalia. Arch Dermatol. 1979;115(3):306–8.

Wade TR, et al. The effects of resin of podophyllin on condyloma acuminatum. Am J Dermatopathol. 1984;6(2):109–22.

Wang Z, et al. Penile and scrotal Paget's disease: 130 Chinese patients with long-term follow-up. BJU Int. 2008;102(4):485–8.

Wright JL, Morgan TM, Lin DW. Primary scrotal cancer: disease characteristics and increasing incidence. Urology. 2008;72:1139–43.

MIX
Papier aus verantwortungsvollen Quellen
Paper from responsible sources
FSC® C105338

If you have any concerns about our products,
you can contact us on
ProductSafety@springernature.com

In case Publisher is established outside the EU,
the EU authorized representative is:
Springer Nature Customer Service Center GmbH
Europaplatz 3, 69115 Heidelberg, Germany

Printed by Libri Plureos GmbH
in Hamburg, Germany